Pediatric Pelvic and Proximal Femoral Osteotomies

Reggie C. Hamdy • Neil Saran
Editors

Pediatric Pelvic and Proximal Femoral Osteotomies

A Case-Based Approach

Springer

Editors
Reggie C. Hamdy
Shriners Hospital for Children
Montreal
Québec
Canada

Neil Saran
Shriners Hospital for Children
Montreal
Québec
Canada

ISBN 978-3-030-08603-9 ISBN 978-3-319-78033-7 (eBook)
https://doi.org/10.1007/978-3-319-78033-7

Softcover re-print of the Hardcover 1st edition 2018

Printed on acid-free paper

This Springer imprint is published by the registered company Springer International Publishing AG part of Springer Nature.
The registered company address is: Gewerbestrasse 11, 6330 Cham, Switzerland

We dedicate this book to all the children and adolescents with hip problems hoping that it will help improve their quality of life; to our teachers and mentors for everything they taught us, to our wives, Sylvie and Pascale, for their unconditional love and continuous support and our sons-Sebastien, Nicolas and Charles-who will always inspire and motivate us.

Foreword

Reggie C. Hamdy and Neil Saran have produced a superb and comprehensive textbook of current practice of pediatric hip surgery, focusing on contemporary pelvic and proximal femoral osteotomies. The book contains information essential to all orthopedic trainees and those responsible for care of children and adolescents with these complex and disabling conditions. The editors have assembled a stellar cast of pediatric hip surgeons, each a respected expert, to describe the technique for 37 different or closely related variations of osteotomies about the hip.

The case-based and common format for all chapters creates a consistency of approach that will be appreciated by the reader, as it makes navigation through each chapter simple and convenient. This book has beautiful illustrations, both line drawings and intraoperative photographs, which precisely detail the operative technique for each osteotomy. The Pearls and Pitfalls section in each chapter offers advice and wisdom that may only be gained through extensive experience and will serve to reduce major and common errors in the application of a particular operative technique. The Indications and Contraindications section permits the reader to compare the preoperative imaging with the indications for each clinical scenario and thus be able to contrast and compare between chapters to learn how to select the appropriate osteotomy for a particular clinical problem or presentation. In this respect, this book is unique in that all conceivable operative solutions that involve osteotomies have been included, making it a one-stop reference source for the latest information on the subject.

A skeptic may ask two questions. The first is why so much emphasis on osteotomies when there is a universal solution at skeletal maturity in hip replacement arthroplasty? I believe that the value of osteotomies has been discounted because they are more technically demanding, require adaptation for many variations in deformities, and are not applied in situations where they may be more appropriate because of the lack of familiarity with them by most surgeons. The failure of an arthroplasty in a young person following a precipitous decision for this particular intervention is an all too common phenomenon that is exceedingly difficult to salvage for the long term. Familiarity with osteotomies and their thoughtful application may lead to better results over a lifetime, reserving arthroplasty to an age where it may be expected to last in active individuals.

The second question is why a book when almost all "information" is available online? The answer is that this book provides comprehensive "knowledge" in a systematic manner where the reader is able to compare and contrast clinical presentations with their potential solutions in a structured manner, something that is not readily available online.

In summary, I believe that this book is an essential reference source that should be available, in hard copy or electronically, to all surgeons taking care of children with hip disease or deformity. It is best described as an operative manual embedded in extensive knowledge to guide the surgeon in applying the proper osteotomy for any given clinical application that may benefit from surgical intervention.

Toronto, ON, Canada John H. Wedge

Preface

The hip is a complex joint with several important functions including weight bearing and ambulation. Various congenital, developmental and acquired conditions may affect the anatomy and biomechanics of the hip joint during childhood and adolescence and may have a significant impact on ambulation, overall function and quality of life.

In most of these hip pathologies, the anatomy and biomechanics of the hip joint can be restored to normal or near-normal states by various osteotomies of the proximal femur, acetabulum or both.

In this clinical casebook, commonly performed proximal femoral and pelvic osteotomies in the child and adolescent are described in 39 chapters. We enlisted the help of surgeons from around the world for their expertise in order to have each chapter written by a content expert. All of these chapters are written in a systematic format that will allow the reader to easily navigate between chapters.

The book is divided into three parts. The first part includes two chapters on the clinical and radiological examination of the paediatric and adolescent hip. These chapters outline the general approach and management of any hip problem in the paediatric population and the radiologic evaluation of the adolescent or young adult hip. The second part describes various pelvic osteotomies including redirectional osteotomies (Salter, triple, Ganz), acetabuloplasties (Dega, Pemberton) and salvage procedures (Shelf and Chiari). As a specific osteotomy may be indicated in more than one pathology, the same osteotomy may be discussed in more than one chapter depending on the pathology. The third part describes proximal femoral osteotomies in various conditions (Perthes, slipped capital femoral epiphysis, neuromuscular hips, etc.). The last part includes miscellaneous procedures involving combined pelvic and femoral osteotomies and other surgical procedures such as articulated hip distraction.

We believe that this book will be a valuable reference for all orthopaedic surgeons as well as all personnel (medical and paramedical) involved in the management of children and adolescents with hip disorders requiring surgical intervention. We sincerely hope that this book will ultimately help the care of these children and adolescents and improve their quality of life.

Montreal, Québec, Canada — Reggie C. Hamdy
Montreal, Québec, Canada — Neil Saran

Acknowledgements

We would like to acknowledge the great work of our medical illustration department, Mark Lepik, Guylaine Bedard, Roger Aziz, and Denis Alvez. We would like to thank our administrative assistants Josee Perron, Paula Wall and Adina Sbragia for behind the scenes work without which this book would have taken twice as long to complete. Finally, we would like to acknowledge and thank the Springer Editors, Katherine Kreilkamp and Kristopher Spring for their extraordinary work, patience and help in writing and editing this book.

Contents

Contributors

Franck Accadbled, MD, PhD Pediatric Orthopaedics, Hôpital des Enfants, CHU de Toulouse, Toulouse, France

Fahad S. Alhuzaimi, MD, MBBS Division of Paediatric Orthopaedic Surgery, Department of Paediatric Surgery, Montreal Children's Hospital, McGill University Health Centre, Montréal, QC, Canada

Department of Orthopaedic Surgery, Shriners Hospital for Children Canada, Montreal, QC, Canada

Elizabeth Ashby, MB BChir FRCS (Orth) Department of Orthopaedics, Evelina Children's Hospital, London, UK

Yaroslav Basyuk, MD Orthopaedics, University Hospital, Newark, NJ, USA

Paul E. Beaulé, MD, FRCS(C) Division of Orthopaedic Surgery, University of Ottawa, The Ottawa Hospital, Ottawa, ON, Canada

Étienne L. Belzile, MD, FRCS(C) Department of Orthopaedic Surgery, CHU de Québec-Université Laval, Quebec City, QC, Canada

Thierry E. Benaroch, MD, FRCS(C) Division of Paediatric Orthopaedic Surgery, Department of Paediatric Surgery, Montreal Children's Hospital, McGill University Health Centre, Montréal, QC, Canada

Department of Orthopaedic Surgery, Shriners Hospital for Children-Canada, Montréal, QC, Canada

John G. Birch, MD, FRCS(C) Department of Pediatric Orthopedics, Texas Scottish Rite Hospital for Children, Dallas, TX, USA

Ayşegül Bursalı, MD Private Practice, Istanbul, Turkey

Alexander M. Cherkashin, MD Department of Pediatric Orthopedics, Division of Clinical Implementation and Data Management, Center of Excellence for Limb Lengthening and Reconstruction, Texas Scottish Rite Hospital for Children, Dallas, TX, USA

John C. Clohisy, MD Shriners Hospitals for Children, St. Louis, MO, USA

St. Louis Children's Hospital, St. Louis, MO, USA

Barnes-Jewish Hospital, St. Louis, MO, USA

Department of Orthopaedic Surgery, Washington University School of Medicine, St. Louis, MO, USA

John P. Dormans, MD Division of Orthopaedic Surgery, University of Ottawa, The Ottawa Hospital, Ottawa, ON, Canada

Christopher Dowding, MD, FRCS(C) Division of Orthopaedic Surgery, University of Ottawa, The Ottawa Hospital, Ottawa, ON, Canada

Deborah M. Eastwood, MB ChB Department of Orthopaedic Surgery, Great Ormond Street Hospital for Children, London, UK

Mark Eidelman, MD Pediatric Orthopedics, Ruth Children's Hospital, Technion Faculty of Medicine, Haifa, Israel

Dan S. Epstein, MD McGill University, Montreal, QC, Canada

Shriners Hospital for Children – Canada, Montreal, QC, Canada

David S. Feldman, MD Paley Orthopedic and Spine Institute, St. Mary's Medical Center, West Palm Beach, FL, USA

Panagiotis Peter Glavas, MD Sainte-Justine University Hospital Center, University of Montreal, Montreal, QC, Canada

H. Kerr Graham, MD, FRCS (Ed), FRACS Department of Orthopaedic Surgery (NHMRC CP-CRE), Royal Children's Hospital, Parkville, VIC, Australia

Reggie C. Hamdy, MB, MSc (Ortho), FRCS(C) Division of Orthopaedic Surgery, McGill University Health Centre, Montreal, QC, Canada

The Montreal Children's Hospital, Montreal, QC, Canada

Shriners Hospital for Children – Canada, Montreal, QC, Canada

Lee S. Haruno, BS Division of Orthopedic Surgery, Baylor College of Medicine, Texas Children's Hospital, Houston, TX, USA

Simon P. Kelley, MBChB,PhD,FRCS(C)(Tr and Orth) Department of Surgery, University of Toronto, Toronto, ON, Canada

The Hospital for Sick Children, Toronto, ON, Canada

Young-Jo Kim, MD, PhD Department of Orthopedic Surgery, Boston Children's Hospital, Boston, MA, USA

David J. Kirby, BS Division of Pediatric Orthopaedic Surgery, Department of Orthopaedic Surgery, The Johns Hopkins Hospital, Baltimore, MD, USA

Ken N. Kuo, MD Department of Orthopaedic Surgery, Taipei Medical University, Taipei, Taiwan

Department of Orthopaedic Surgery, National Taiwan University Hospital, Taipei, Taiwan

Jill E. Larson, MD Department of Orthopedic Surgery, Harvard University, Boston Children's Hospital, Boston, MA, USA

Michael Leunig, MD Orthopedic Surgery, University of Rochester Medical Center, Rochester, NY, USA

William G. Mackenzie, MD Orthopedic Department, Nemours/Alfred I. duPont Hospital for Children, Wilmington, DE, USA

M. Chad Mahan, MD Henry Ford Health System, Detroit, MI, USA

Hannes M. Manner, MD Department of Orthopedic Surgery, Schulthess Clinic, Zurich, Switzerland

Benjamin D. Martin, MD Division of Orthopaedic Surgery and Sports Medicine, Children's National Health System, Washington, DC, USA

Travis Matheney, MD, MLA Department of Orthopaedic Surgery, Harvard Medical School, Boston Children's Hospital, Boston, MA, USA

Michael B. Millis, MD Department of Orthopedic Surgery, Boston Children's Hospital, Child and Adult Hip Program, Boston, MA, USA

Nicole I. Montgomery, MD Orthopaedic Oncology, University of Texas MD Anderson Cancer Center, Clinical Care Center, Houston, TX, USA

Kishore Mulpuri, MBBS, MS (Ortho), MHSc (Epi) Orthopaedic Surgery, British Columbia Children's Hospital, Vancouver, BC, Canada

Unni G. Narayanan, MBBS, MSc, FRCS(C) The Hospital for Sick Children, University of Toronto, Toronto, ON, Canada

Eduardo N. Novais, MD Department of Orthopedic Surgery, Boston Children's Hospital, Boston, MA, USA

Ryan M. O'Shea, MD Department of Orthopaedic Surgery, Kaiser Permanente San Diego, San Diego, CA, USA

Matthew E. Oetgen, MD, MBA Division of Orthopaedic Surgery and Sports Medicine, Children's National Health System, Washington, DC, USA

The George Washington University School of Medicine and Health Sciences, Washington, DC, USA

Dror Paley, MD, FRCS(C) Paley Orthopedic and Spine Institute, St. Mary's Medical Center, West Palm Beach, FL, USA

Stefan Parent, MD, PhD Sainte-Justine University Hospital Center, University of Montreal, Montreal, QC, Canada

Thierry Pauyo, MD, FRCSC Department of Orthopaedic Surgery, Shriners Hospital for Children Canada, Montreal, QC, Canada

Department of Paediatric Surgery, The Montreal Children's Hospital, Montreal, QC, Canada

Division of Orthopaedic Surgery, Department of Surgery McGill University, Montreal, QC, Canada

Karl E. Rathjen, MD Department of Pediatric Orthopedics, Texas Scottish Rite Hospital for Children, Dallas, TX, USA

Benjamin F. Ricciardi, MD Orthopedic Surgery, University of Rochester Medical Center, Rochester, NY, USA

Sanjeev Sabharwal, MD, MPH Department of Orthopedics, University of California, San Francisco, CA, USA

Division of Pediatric Orthopedics, University Hospital, Newark, NJ, USA

Jérôme Sales de Gauzy, MD, PhD Pediatric Orthopaedics, Hôpital des Enfants, CHU de Toulouse, Toulouse, France

Mikhail L. Samchukov, MD Department of Pediatric Orthopedics, Center of Excellence for Limb Lengthening and Reconstruction, Texas Scottish Rite Hospital for Children, Dallas, TX, USA

Adolfredo Santana, MD Orthopedic Department, Nemours/Alfred I. duPont Hospital for Children, Wilmington, DE, USA

Neil Saran, MD, MHSc (Clin. Epi.), FRCS(C) Department of Orthopaedic Surgery, Shriners Hospital for Children Canada, Montreal, QC, Canada

Department of Paediatric Surgery, The Montreal Children's Hospital, Montreal, QC, Canada

Division of Orthopaedic Surgery, Department of Surgery McGill University, Montreal, QC, Canada

Emily K. Schaeffer, PhD Orthopaedic Surgery, British Columbia Children's Hospital, Vancouver, BC, Canada

Perry L. Schoenecker, MD Shriners Hospitals for Children, St. Louis, MO, USA

St. Louis Children's Hospital, St. Louis, MO, USA

Barnes-Jewish Hospital, St. Louis, MO, USA

Department of Orthopaedic Surgery, Washington University School of Medicine, St. Louis, MO, USA

Mehmet Serhan Er, MD Orthopedic Department, Nemours/Alfred I. duPont Hospital for Children, Wilmington, DE, USA

Claire E. Shannon, MD Division of Orthopaedics, Department of Orthopaedic Surgery, The Hospital for Sick Children, Toronto, ON, Canada

Benjamin J. Shore, MD, MPH, FRCS(C) Department of Orthopaedic Surgery, Harvard Medical School, Boston Children's Hospital, Boston, MA, USA

Paul D. Sponseller, MD, MBA Division of Pediatric Orthopaedic Surgery, Department of Orthopaedic Surgery, The Johns Hopkins Hospital, Baltimore, MD, USA

Daniel J. Sucato, MD, MS Department of Orthopaedic Surgery, Texas Scottish Rite Hospital, University of Texas at Southwestern Medical School, Dallas, TX, USA

Magdalena Tarchala Department of Orthopaedic Surgery, Shriners Hospital for Children Canada, Montreal, QC, Canada

Department of Paediatric Surgery, The Montreal Children's Hospital, Montreal, QC, Canada

Division of Orthopaedic Surgery, Department of Surgery McGill University, Montreal, QC, Canada

Andrew D. W. Tice, MD Department of Orthopaedic Surgery, Texas Scottish Rite Hospital for Children, Dallas, TX, USA

Vidyadhar V. Upasani, MD Rady Children's Hospital San Diego, University of California San Diego, San Diego, CA, USA

Harold J. P. van Bosse, MD Shriners Hospital for Children, Philadelphia, PA, USA

Ting-Ming Wang, MD, PhD Department of Orthopaedic Surgery, National Taiwan University Hospital, Taipei, Taiwan

Dennis R. Wenger, MD Department of Orthopedic Surgery, Pediatric Orthopedic Training Program, Rady Children's Hospital San Diego, University of California, San Diego, San Diego, CA, USA

Timur Yıldırım, MD Orthopaedic and Traumatology Department, Baltalimani Bone Diseases Training and Research Hospital, Istanbul, Turkey

Ira Zaltz, MD Pediatric Orthopaedic Surgery, Beaumont Hospital, Royal Oak, MI, USA

Stephan T. Zmugg, MD Department of Orthopaedic Surgery, Texas Scottish Rite Hospital, University of Texas at Southwestern Medical School, Dallas, TX, USA

1 Preoperative Planning for Pelvic and/or Proximal Femoral Osteotomies

Reggie C. Hamdy and Dan S. Epstein

Introduction

The hip joint is the largest joint in the human body after the knee joint and the most mobile after the shoulder joint. It is a complex joint that plays a major role in daily activities and has a major impact on the quality of life. In this introductory chapter, some specific aspects of its anatomy and biomechanics that are pertinent to pelvic and proximal femoral osteotomies are discussed.

The hip joint serves several important *functions*. First, it supports the weight of the human body, and second, it permits a wide range of movements that are necessary for ambulation and for carrying out various sports and daily activities (walking, running, sitting, squatting, jumping, etc.).

To fulfill these important functions, the hip joint has to be very *mobile*, very *stable*, and at the same time able to withstand various amounts of stresses across its articulating surfaces. During running and jumping, for instance, the force of the body's movements multiplies the forces on the hip joint to many times the force exerted by the body's weight. Normally, the hip joint can accommodate these extreme forces repeatedly during intense physical activities.

Stability of the Hip Joint

Hyaline cartilage lines both the acetabulum and the head of the femur, providing a smooth surface for the moving bones to glide past each other. Hyaline cartilage also acts as a flexible shock absorber to prevent collision of the bones during movement. The acetabulum is formed by the confluence of the three pelvic bones at the triradiate cartilage: the ilium, pubis, and ischium (Fig. 1.1). The hip joint is a very *stable* joint, due to the depth of the bony acetabular socket, which is slightly less than a hemisphere. The tough fibrocartilaginous labrum, lining the rim of the acetabulum, increases its functional depth and like a suction cup helps maintain the negative pressure in the hip joint (Fig. 1.2). The very strong ligaments surrounding the joint capsule (the iliofemoral ligament anteriorly, ischiofemoral ligament posteriorly, and pubofemoral ligament medially) (Fig. 1.3), combined with the powerful muscles surrounding the joint, ensure the stability of the hip joint and prevent it from dislocating, unless subjected to high energy forces.

R. C. Hamdy (✉)
Division of Orthopaedic Surgery, McGill University Health Centre, Montreal, QC, Canada

The Montreal Children's Hospital, Montreal, QC, Canada

Shriners Hospital for Children – Canada, Montreal, QC, Canada
e-mail: rhamdy@shriners.mcgill.ca

D. S. Epstein
McGill University, Montreal, QC, Canada

Shriners Hospital for Children – Canada, Montreal, QC, Canada

R. C. Hamdy, N. Saran (eds.), *Pediatric Pelvic and Proximal Femoral Osteotomies*, https://doi.org/10.1007/978-3-319-78033-7_1

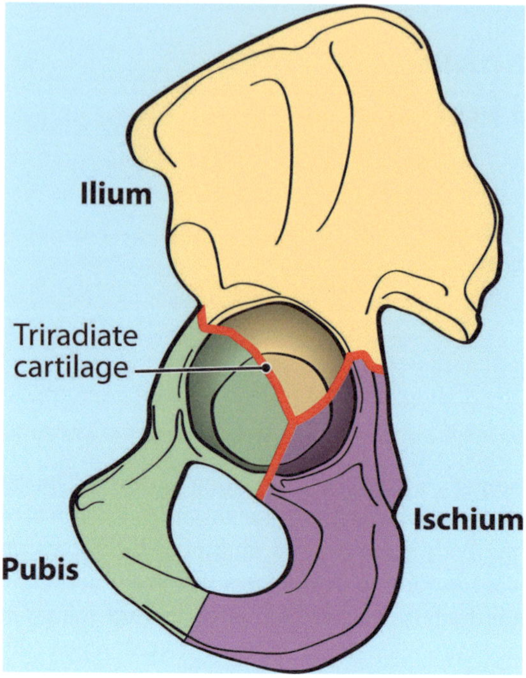

Fig. 1.1 Fusion of the three bones in the pelvis, ilium, ischium, and pubis, forms a cup-shaped socket known as the acetabulum, shown here in lateral view

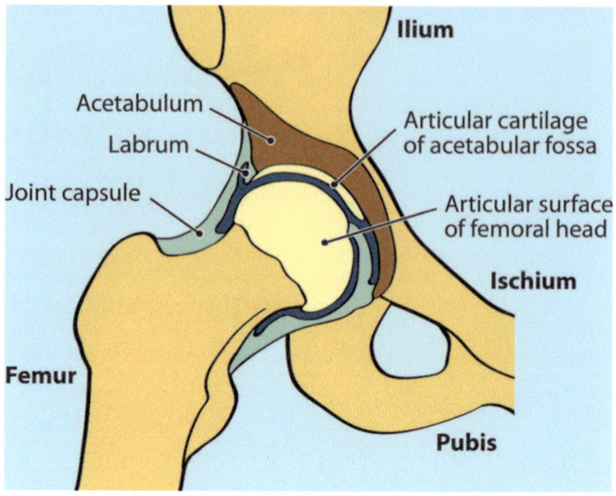

Fig. 1.2 The head of the femur and the acetabulum are in a ball-and-socket configuration. The labrum deepens the socket and allows a negative pressure inside the joint. A thick capsule surrounds the joint

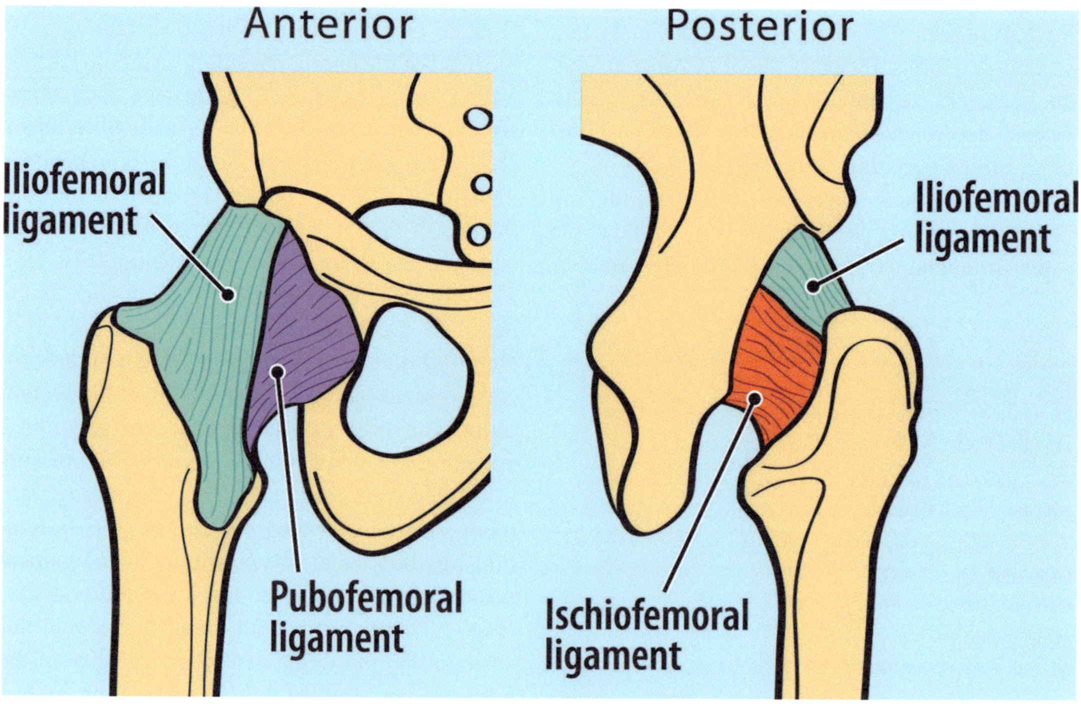

Fig. 1.3 The ligaments surrounding the joint capsule: the iliofemoral anteriorly, ischiofemoral ligament posteriorly, and pubofemoral ligament medially

Mobility of the Hip Joint

Functionally, the hip joint enjoys a very *high range of motion* (*ROM*). Two factors are responsible for this large ROM. First, the ball-and-socket structure of the joint allows the femur to circumduct almost freely through a 360° circle. The second factor that contributes to this large ROM is the shape of the femoral neck. Besides its length, its diameter is smaller than that of the femoral head and that allows this large ROM. A normal hip joint allows about 120° flexion, 20° extension, 60° abduction, 30° adduction, and about 40° of each internal/external rotation. Only the shoulder joint provides as high a level of mobility as the hip joint. Thus any cause leading to a short femoral neck (coxa breva) inevitably leads to a decrease in the hip ROM. In such cases, a femoral neck lengthening procedure may then be indicated (Morsher or Wagner types of proximal femoral osteotomies).

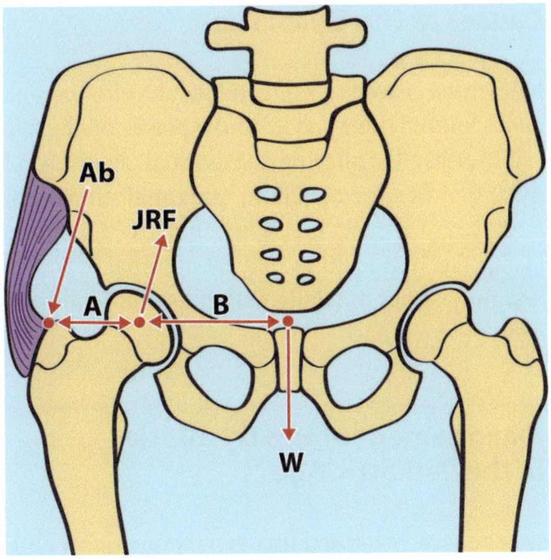

Fig. 1.4 A vector diagram of the joint reaction forces (JRF) generated within the hip joint. *Ab* abductor force, *A* abductor moment arm, *B* moment arm of body weight, *W* body weight

Joint Reaction Forces, Abductor Mechanism, and Role of the Greater Trochanter

The joint reaction forces (JRF) are the forces generated within the hip joint in response to forces acting on the joint and are the result of the need to balance the moment arms of the body weight and abductor tension. This balance is important in order to maintain the pelvis leveled. The JRF equal the combined values of the body weight and the abductor force (Fig. 1.4). During two-leg stance phase, little or no muscular forces are required to maintain equilibrium. However, during walking and running, the JRF are increased several times the body weight. The *greater trochanter* plays a significant role in maintaining the normal biomechanics of the hip joint. The powerful hip abductors (gluteus medius and minimus) are attached to the tip of the greater trochanter, and the abductor muscle length is an important factor in maintaining an adequate abductor force (Fig. 1.5).

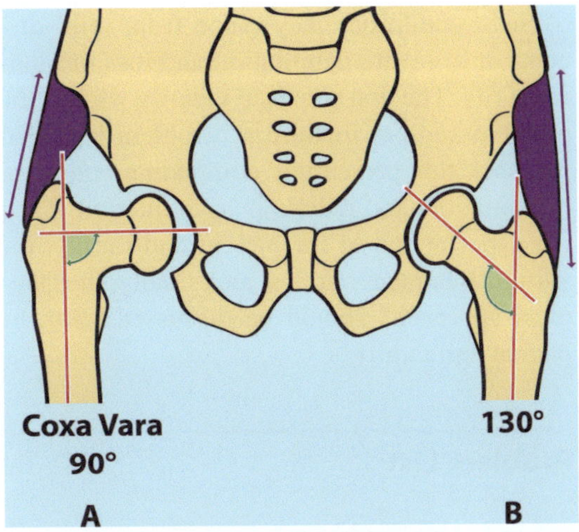

Fig. 1.5 The powerful hip abductors (gluteus medius and minimus) are attached to the tip of the greater trochanter. The abductor muscle length is an important factor in maintaining an adequate abductor force. *A* Coxa vara with decreased neck-shaft angle and decreased abductor muscle length. *B* Normal neck-shaft angle with normal abductor muscle length

Causes of Hip Dysplasia

Numerous causes—congenital, developmental, and acquired—may lead to dysplasia of the hip joint, either by altering the normal anatomy of the hip joint (acetabulum, proximal femur, or both) or by altering the biomechanics of the joint [1, 2]. The implications may be minimal or severe and may affect the daily activities and quality of life of the patient.

Management of Hip Dysplasia in the Pediatric Age

It is generally agreed that hip dysplasia in children should be treated to prevent or delay the onset of degenerative arthritis. The management of various hip pathologies in pediatric patients can be very challenging due to the multitude of causes that can lead to hip dysplasia as well as the complexity of the anatomy and biomechanics of the hip joint. The clinical effects of these conditions may range from mild discomfort to severe debilitation and loss of quality of life. The first step is to identify what is the problem and put forward a "problem list" that includes the presenting complaints, physical examination, and radiological evaluation. Then the expectations of the patient and family, the various treatment options, and, finally, the "surgical approach" should be discussed with the patient and family.

Problem List

What Is the Problem?

The problem is based on the presenting complaint and the findings of the physical examination. It is extremely important to clearly define the reason for the visit. Why did the parents or caregivers bring the child to the clinic? What is their concern? Is there any history of pain? If pain is present, then more details about the pain should be obtained. Is there any limping or stiffness? What is the impact on mobility, daily activities, and quality of life? Is the problem localized to the hip, or is it part of a more generalized systemic problem (such as skeletal dysplasia or metabolic disorder)? Is there any family history of similar problems, previous history of trauma or infection, and similar episodes of pain? In cases of neuromuscular conditions, are there any difficulties with positioning (in wheelchair) or hygiene care (abducting the legs)?

Following a thorough history taking, a complete physical should be performed. The gait of the child is analyzed, specifically, for the presence of a Trendelenburg gait that may point to abductor mechanism pathology (Fig. 1.6). The spine is examined in the standing position. If the pelvis is not horizontal, this may be due to limb length discrepancy (LLD). Wooden blocks under the short leg may be used to determine the amount of LLD. Next, the patient is examined on the bed. The ROM is determined in both the supine and prone position. Assessing rotation in the supine position with the hips flexed 90° relaxes the anterior joint capsule and should eliminate the effects of any hip flexion contractures, thus giving an exaggerated value for hip rotation.

Assessing rotation of the hips is, therefore, more accurate in the prone position, as this is the normal position of the hips during standing and walking. That said, rotational range of motion in the 90° flexed position is useful in cases of suspected femoroacetabular impingement (FAI) as internal rotation is typically decreased on the affected side. The presence of any muscular atrophy and contractures is documented. Pain elicited by any movements—passive or active—should be carefully noted. Anterior and posterior impingement tests should also be performed to detect the presence of any femoroacetabular impingement. A complete neuromuscular examination is a must. In cases of any suspicion of a neuromuscular condition, a neurological consultation and a complete muscular assessment are recommended. A gait laboratory analysis may also be considered.

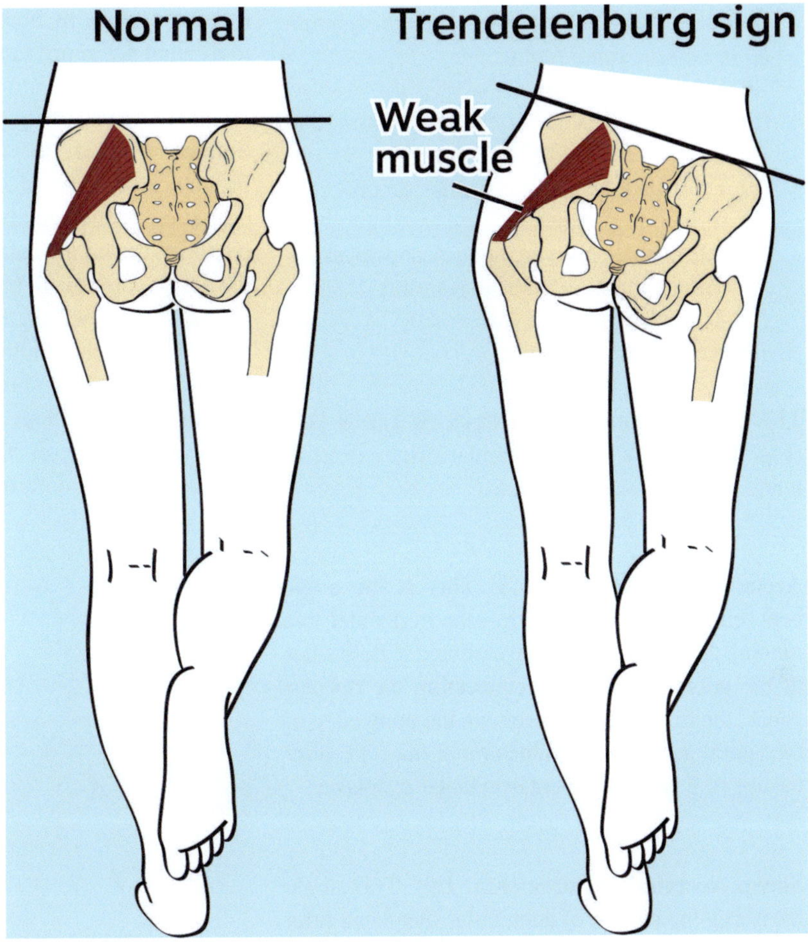

Fig. 1.6 Trendelenburg sign. While standing on one leg, the abductors contract to maintain a leveled pelvis. In case of abductor muscle weakness, the contralateral pelvis "drops"

Where Is the Problem?

This is answered by a careful radiological assessment of the hip joint, as detailed below.

Radiological Assessment of Hip Problems Many modalities can be used for the initial diagnosis and further workup, including ultrasonography in the first 6 months of life, plain radiography, arthrography, computerized tomography with or without three-dimensional (3D) imaging, and magnetic resonance imaging (MRI). Most recently, 3D printing is used in the evaluation and preoperative planning of complex deformities. However, most hip problems could be evaluated on a plain anteroposterior (AP) radiograph, and much can be learned from this simple study. Radiological analysis of the hip joint should include assessment of the acetabulum, the proximal femur, and the relation between the acetabulum and proximal femur.

The most commonly used angles and parameters to assess hip dysplasia include:

1. *To assess acetabular dysplasia*:
   (a) Acetabular index [3]
   (b) Acetabular index of Sharp [4]
   (c) Acetabular depth
   (d) The sourcil
   (e) The teardrop
2. *To assess proximal femoral dysplasia*:
   (a) Neck-shaft angle
   (b) Hilgenreiner epiphyseal angle [5]
   (c) Femoral neck changes: coxa vara and coxa valga
   (d) Changes in the femoral head: coxa breva and coxa magna
   (e) Relation between the greater trochanter and the femoral head

3. *To assess the relationship between the acetabulum and proximal femur*:
   (a) Shenton's line [6]
   (b) Center-edge angle for lateral coverage of the femoral head [7]
   (c) False-profile view for anterior coverage of the femoral head
   (d) AP of the pelvis in neutral and in maximum abduction/internal rotation
   (e) Migration index of Reimers [8]
   (f) Acetabular protrusion

The Hilgenreiner [9] and Perkins Lines [10] (Fig. 1.7) These are the standard lines used in many angular measurements.

Acetabular Index (Fig. 1.8) This is the angle between the Hilgenreiner line—the horizontal line running through the triradiate cartilage of both sides of the pelvis—and a line connecting the deepest part of the triradiate cartilage with the bony edge of the lateral acetabulum. Values more than 20° after the age of 2 years represent acetabular dysplasia.

Sharp Acetabular Index (Fig. 1.9) This angle measures the degree of acetabular dysplasia after the closure of the triradiate cartilage. It is measured on the AP view of the pelvis and represents the angle between the lateral margin of the acetabular roof or lateral sourcil and inferior aspect of the teardrop and the horizontal line between the inferior aspects of both pelvic teardrops. Values more than 42° represent acetabular dysplasia.

Sourcil (Fig. 1.10) The *sourcil* (eyebrow in French) is an area of subchondral osseous condensation in the acetabular roof and represents a response to the articular portion of the ileum to the stress provoked by the compressive forces acting on it. The length of the sourcil is usually about 80% of the width of the femoral head. The lateral extent of the sourcil may appcar—in some cases—different than the lateral edge of the extra-articular ileum. This is important as it may give a false estimate of femoral head coverage.

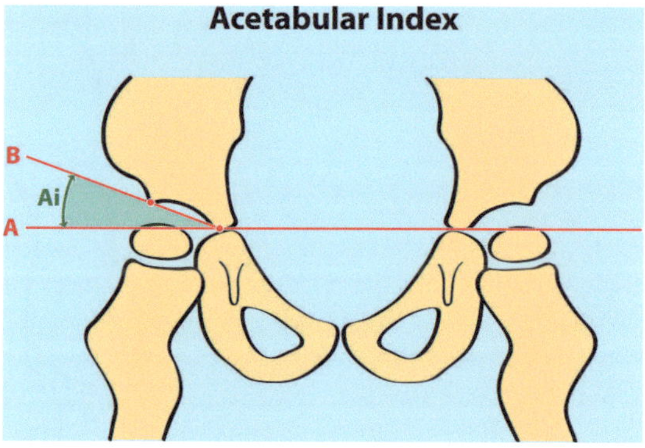

Fig. 1.8 Acetabular index is used to measure acetabular dysplasia in young children prior to the ossification of the triradiate cartilage. It is the angle between the Hilgenreiner line and a line connecting the lateral edge of the acetabulum and the triradiate cartilage. Values more than 20° after the age of 2 years represent acetabular dysplasia

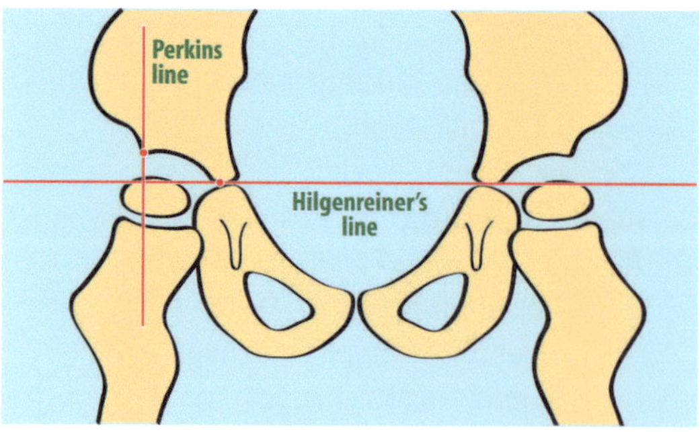

Fig. 1.7 The Hilgenreiner and Perkins lines. The *Hilgenreiner line* is the horizontal line running through the triradiate cartilage of both sides of the pelvis. The *Perkins line* is the vertical line running from the lateral edge of the acetabulum and perpendicular to the Hilgenreiner line

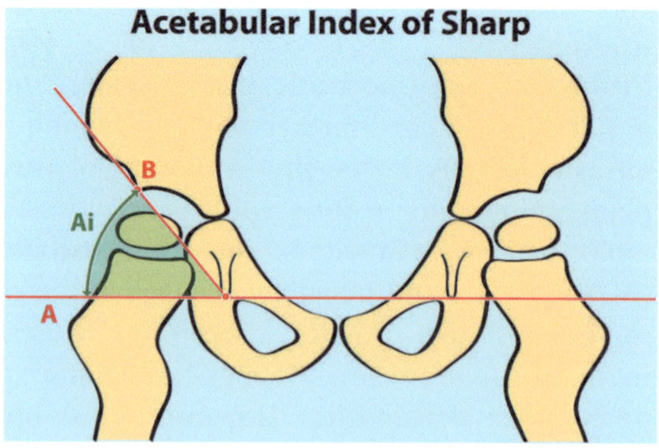

Fig. 1.9 Acetabular index of Sharp is used to measure acetabular dysplasia after ossification of the triradiate cartilage. It is the angle between Hilgenreiner and a line connecting the lateral edge of the acetabulum and the inferior part of the teardrop. Values greater than 42° represent acetabular dysplasia

Tönnis angle is the slope of the sourcil and is normal between 0° and 10°. It measures the inclination or angle of the weight-bearing area of the acetabulum. Tönnis angle is formed between a line joining the medial and lateral ends of the sourcil and a horizontal line. An increase in the slope of the sourcil may be associated with lateral subluxation of the femoral head and represents acetabular dysplasia.

Teardrop (See Fig. 1.10) The acetabular teardrop consists of two vertical lines connected distally. The teardrop is a radiographic condensation of the innominate bone at the inferior end of the acetabulum. A normal teardrop is U-shaped. The medial border of the teardrop is continuous with the ilio-ischial line (named the Kohler line), and the lateral wall is continuous superiorly with the floor of the acetabulum. The width of the teardrop varies with rotation of the pelvis. A wide teardrop is associated with a shallow acetabulum. A very narrow teardrop where the medial and lateral wall touch each other at the floor of the acetabulum or crossover is a sign of a deeper than normal acetabulum causing over coverage of the head called coxa profunda.

The Shenton Line (See Fig. 1.10) The Shenton line is an imaginary line joining the inferior border of the superior pubic ramus to the inferomedial border of the proximal femur. It should be a smooth line. In cases of subluxation, this line is "broken."

Neck-Shaft Angle (Fig. 1.11) The neck-shaft angle represents the angle between the intersection of the femoral neck axis and the long axis of the femoral shaft. The value in adults ranges between 120° and 135°. Values >135° represent

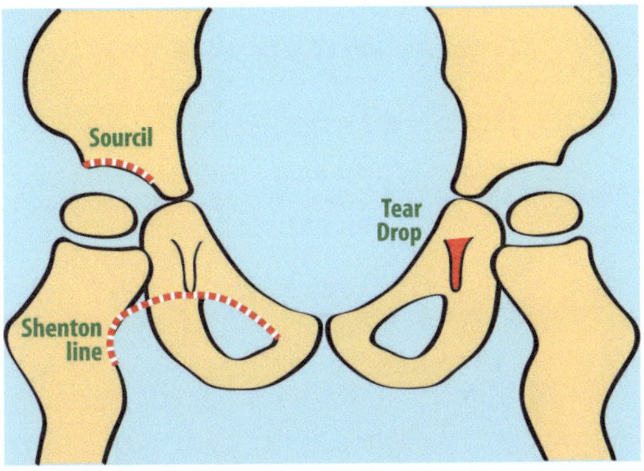

Fig. 1.10 The acetabular teardrop (*marked in red*). The sourcil in the acetabular roof and the Shenton line—the imaginary line joining the inferior border of the superior pubic ramus to the inferomedial border of the proximal femur

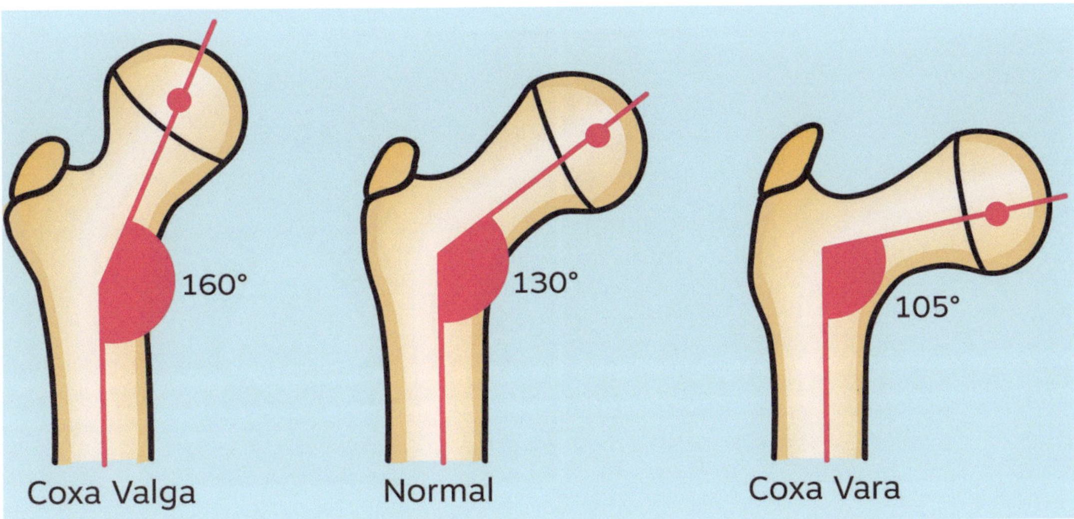

Fig. 1.11 A normal neck-shaft angle ranges between 120° and 135°. Values >135° represent coxa valga. Values of <110–120° represent coxa vara

coxa valga, and values <110–120° represent coxa vara. Internally rotating the hips until the neck is horizontal to the floor shows the true angle, while any external rotation of the femur will increase this value.

Hilgenreiner Epiphyseal Angle (Fig. 1.12) This is an angle used specifically in cases of coxa vara. It is the angle formed between the Hilgenreiner line and a line along the upper femoral physis. Values of more than 60° signify coxa vara.

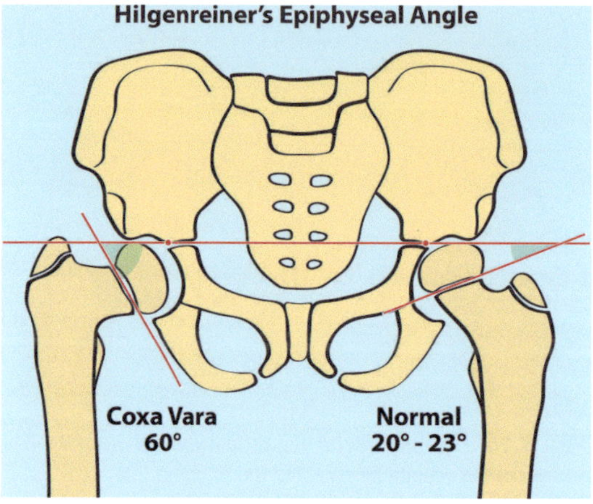

Fig. 1.12 The Hilgenreiner epiphyseal angle is between the Hilgenreiner line and a line along the upper femoral epiphysis. Values >60° signify coxa vara

Shape of the Femoral Head (Fig. 1.13) The femoral head is close to a sphere. Loss of sphericity by flattening (coxa plana) or overgrowth of the epiphysis on to the neck produces a misshapen head that may not be congruous within the acetabulum, and this may lead to degenerative changes in the articular cartilage of both the femoral head and acetabulum. *Coxa magna* (large head) may not be problematic if it is well contained and is congruous in the acetabulum (in certain cases of Perthes disease). However, it may lead to femoroacetabular impingement, labral damage, and degenerative changes. *Coxa breva* (short neck) decreases the abductor resting length and lever arm, increases joint reaction forces, and causes abductor fatigue and Trendelenburg gait.

Articulo-trochanteric Height (Fig. 1.14) The tip of the trochanter lies at the level of the center of the femoral head. In coxa vara, it is superior to the center of the head and in coxa valga; it is inferior to the center of the head (Fig.1.14A). This relation is minimally affected by any rotation of the hips. The articulo-trochanteric height is another measurement used to describe the height of the greater trochanter. It is a line drawn between the tip of the greater trochanter and the superior aspect of the femoral head (Fig.1.14B).

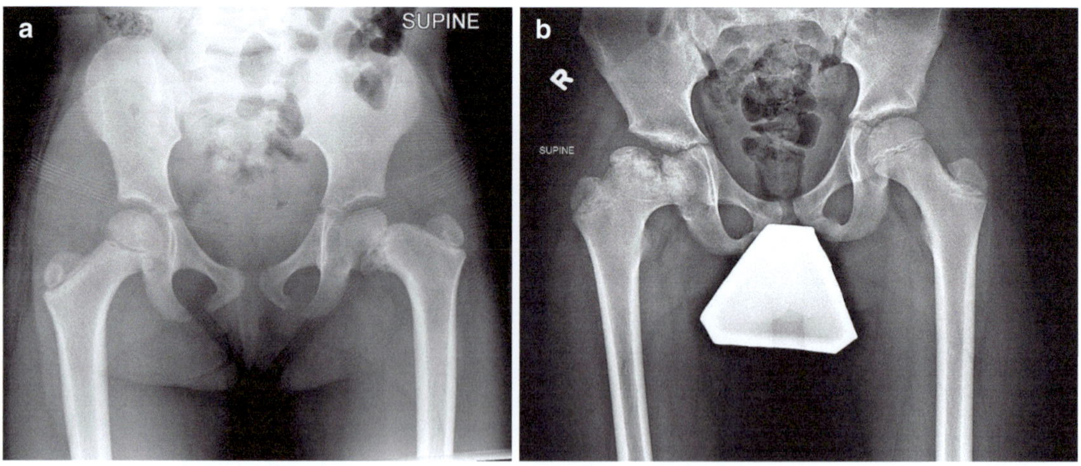

Fig. 1.13 (**a**) The left hip demonstrates coxa breva with varus and high-riding greater trochanter. (**b**) The right hip demonstrates coxa magna coxa breva and coxa irregularis

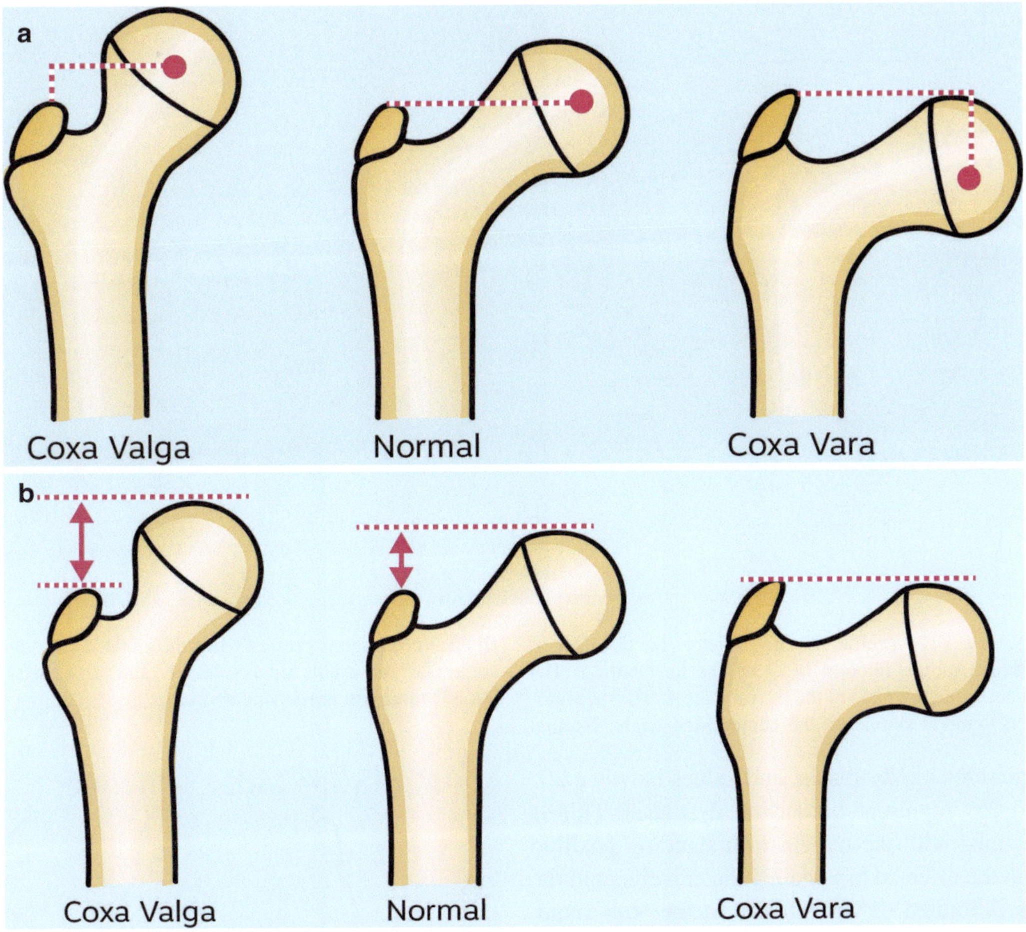

Fig. 1.14 The tip of the trochanter lies at the level of the Centre of the femoral head. In coxa vara, it is superior to the centre of the head and in coxa valga; it is inferior to the center of the head (**a**). This relation is minimally affected by any rotation of the hips. The articulo-trochanteric height is another measurement used to describe the height of the greater trochanter. It is a line drawn between the tip of the greater trochanter and the superorior aspect of the femoral head. The articulo-trochanteric height measurement is used to describe the distance between the tip of greater trochanter and the superior aspect of the femoral head (**b**)

Center-Edge Angle (Wiberg Angle) (Fig. 1.15) This represents the angle between the line connecting the center of the femoral head with the outer bony edge of the acetabulum and the line parallel to the midline of the body drawn from the center of the femoral head. A center-edge angle of more than 25° is normal, and less than 20° represents hip dysplasia. Values of 20–25° are considered borderline dysplasia [11].

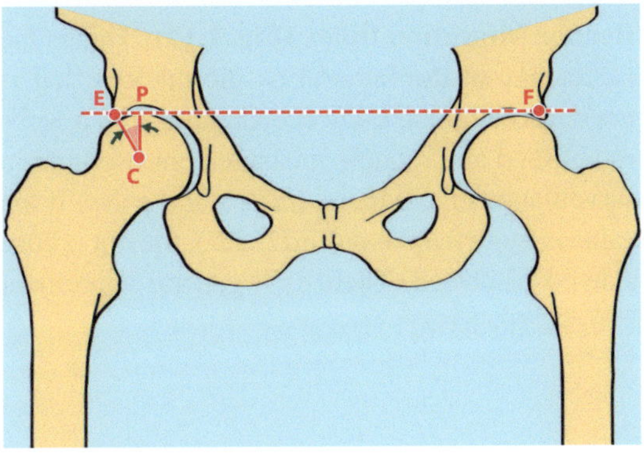

Fig. 1.15 Center-edge angle. The angle between the lateral edge of the acetabulum, the center of the femoral head, and a vertical line. A center-edge angle of more than 25° is normal, and <20° represents hip dysplasia. Values of 20–25° are considered borderline dysplasia

False-Profile View (Fig. 1.16) This view evaluates the anterior coverage of the femoral head by the acetabulum. Normal anterior coverage is present when the angle is >25°. An angle <20°

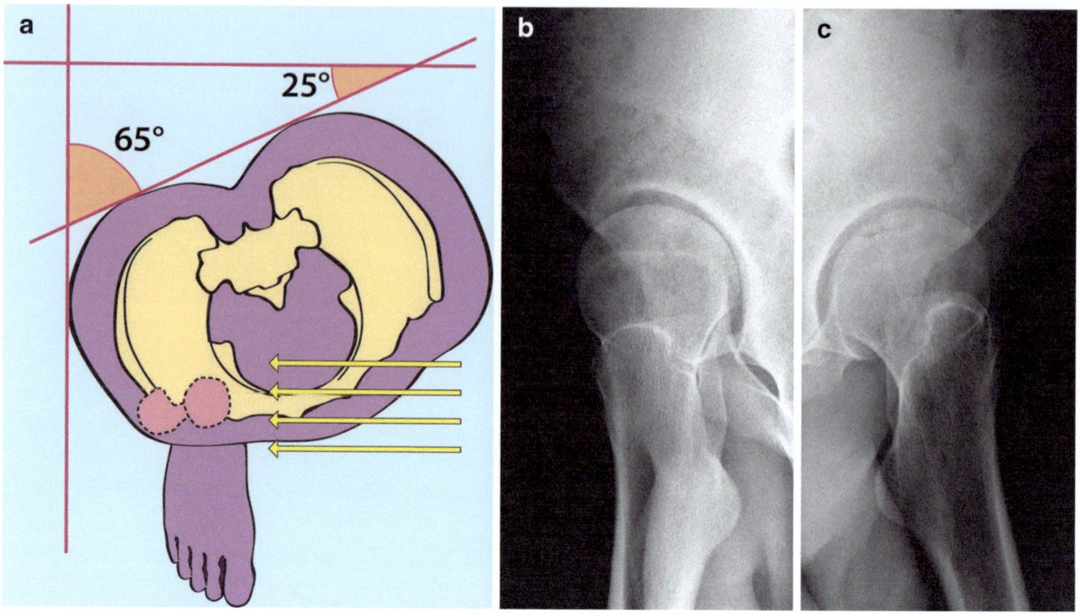

Fig. 1.16 False-profile view helps determine the anterior coverage of the femoral head by the acetabulum. The patient is standing 25° to the lateral view *A*. The measurement is made similar to the center-edge angle. Normal anterior coverage is present when the angle is >25° *B*. An angle <20° represents hip dysplasia *C*, and values between 20–25° represent *borderline dysplasia*

represents hip dysplasia, and values between 20° and 25° represent borderline dysplasia. This is obtained with the patient in a standing position with the affected hip against the cassette, and the pelvis rotated 65° in relation to the wall stand. The foot on the same side as the affected hip should be positioned so that it is parallel to the cassette. The central beam is then centered on the femoral head, with a tube-to-film distance of approximately 102 cm.

Reimer Migration Index (Fig. 1.17) This is the percentage of the femoral ossific nucleus that is not covered by the bony acetabulum. It is a well-established and reliable measurement used in hip surveillance in children with cerebral palsy. If the value is more than one-third (33%), the hip is considered displaced. There is a general agreement

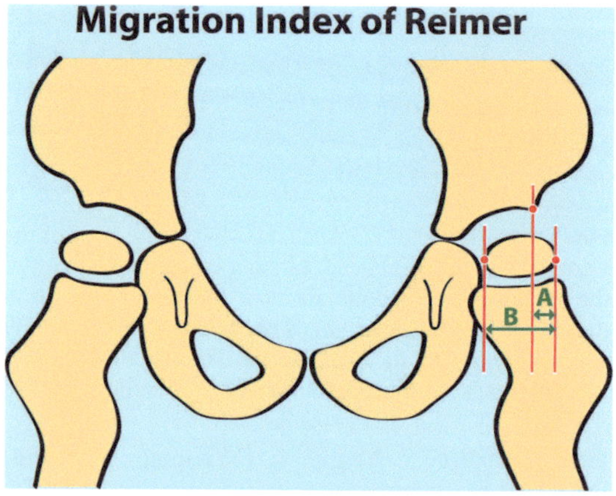

Fig. 1.17 Migration index of Reimer. Three lines are drawn—the Perkins line and two parallel lines: one on the most medial margin of the femoral head and another on the most lateral margin of the femoral head. *A* and *B* distances are measured and divided and converted to a percentage (*A*/*B**100). Above 33% is considered displaced, and above 40% usually requires surgery

that displacement of 40% or more requires a femoral osteotomy and soft tissue releases and a pelvic osteotomy if there is an associated acetabular dysplasia (which is almost always present).

What Are the Expectations of the Patient and Family?

After having clearly identified the cause and nature of the problem, the expectations of the patient and family are then discussed. The expectations may include relief of pain, increase in ROM, ability to partake in sports, correction of gait abnormalities, and improvement in function and ambulation in cases of neuromuscular conditions. Several questions then arise: Can these expectations be met? Are they unrealistic?

How Can These Expectations Be Met?

The various available options are discussed. Is there a role for conservative treatment? Should it be tried first? If surgical intervention is indicated, then a *surgical strategy* is put forward.

Surgical Strategy

The goals of the surgical intervention should be clearly explained and how these goals are in line with the expectations of the patient and family. Sometimes, the goals of the surgery may not fully address the expectations of the patient and family. In some cases, the goal of surgery is to restore normal anatomy and biomechanics of the hip. On the other hand, in other cases, that may be very difficult or even impossible to achieve. However, in most cases, the function of the hip joint and quality of life may be improved without necessarily restoring normal anatomy and biomechanics.

The details of these various surgical interventions, complications, expected outcomes, and long-term implications are reviewed and are discussed in detail in the various chapters of this book.

References

1. Bowen JR, Kotzias-Neto A. Developmental dysplasia of the hip. Towson, MD: Data Trace Publishing Company; 2006.
2. Wedge JH, Wasylenko MJ. The natural history of congenital disease of the hip. J Bone Joint Surg Br. 1979;61-B(3):334–8.
3. Kleinberg S, Lieberman HS. The acetabular index in infants in relation to congenital dislocation of the hip. Arch Surg. 1936;32(6):1049–54.
4. Sharp IK. Acetabular dysplasia. J Bone Joint Surg Br. 1961;43-B(2):268–72.
5. Weinstein JN. Congenital coxa vara. A retrospective review. J Pediatr Orthop. 1984;4(1):70–7.
6. Shenton E. Diseases in bone. London: MacMillan; 1911.
7. Wiberg G. Studies on dysplastic acetabula and congenital subluxation of the hip joint with special references to the complication of osteoarthritis. Acta Chir Scand. 1939;83:58.
8. Reimers J. The stability of the hip in children. A radiological study of the results of muscle surgery in cerebral palsy. Acta Orthop Scand Suppl. 1980;184:1–100.
9. Hilgenreiner H. Zur Frühdiagnose und Frühbehandlung der angeborenen Hüftgelenksverrenkung. Med Klin. 1925;21:1385–8. 1425–9.
10. Perkins G. Signs by which to diagnose congenital dislocation of the hip. Lancet. 1928;211(5457):648–50.
11. Beltran LS, Rosenberg ZS, Mayo JD, De Tuesta MD, Martin O, Neto LP, Bencardino JT. Imaging evaluation of developmental hip dysplasia in the young adult. AJR Am J Roentgenol. 2013;200(5):1077–88.

Radiologic Evaluation of the Adolescent Hip

2

Thierry Pauyo, Magdalena Tarchala, and Neil Saran

Introduction

Radiologic evaluation of the hip in adolescent patients requires a systematic approach in evaluating the various parameters used to identify and quantify both dysplasia and impingement. In dysplasia, the three-dimensional pathology affecting the acetabulum is evaluated with a two-dimensional image, while in impingement, a static image attempts to capture bony abutment often encountered in dynamic movement or at extremes of range of motion. And yet, plain radiographs manage to provide ample information to make a diagnosis and treatment plan in most cases. The following chapter will discuss and illustrate the radiologic parameters utilized to describe acetabular dysplasia and hip impingement in adolescents and young adults.

T. Pauyo · M. Tarchala · N. Saran (✉)
Department of Orthopaedic Surgery, Shriners Hospital for Children Canada, Montreal, QC, Canada

Department of Paediatric Surgery, The Montreal Children's Hospital, Montreal, QC, Canada

Division of Orthopaedic Surgery, Department of Surgery McGill University, Montreal, QC, Canada
e-mail: neil.saran@mcgill.ca

Principles of Radiographic Imaging

Plain radiographs, computed tomography (CT), and magnetic resonance imaging (MRI) are the main imaging modalities of the hip. Plain radiographs are the initial imaging modality of choice to assess hip pathology in young adults as they are readily available and inexpensive. CT and MRI scans provide additional three-dimensional information that may be required in certain instances. MRI scans also provide valuable information regarding the status of the cartilage and labrum if there is a clinical concern for chondral or labral pathology that may warrant intervention. This chapter will focus primarily on the parameters that can be measured on plain radiographs.

Radiographs

Anterior-Posterior (AP) Pelvis Radiograph

The AP pelvis radiograph is the workhorse of radiologic evaluation of the hip in adolescents and young adults. It provides a considerable amount of information regarding the bony morphology of the pelvis, acetabulum, and proximal femur. It is obtained with the patient lying supine or standing with the lower extremities at 15° of internal rotation. The internal

R. C. Hamdy, N. Saran (eds.), *Pediatric Pelvic and Proximal Femoral Osteotomies*,
https://doi.org/10.1007/978-3-319-78033-7_2

rotation compensates for the native femoral anteversion and enables a true AP view of the femoral head and neck [1]. The x-ray beam should be positioned 1.2 m away from the patient and centered at the midpoint between the upper border of the pubis symphysis and a line connecting both anterior superior iliac spines (Fig. 2.1) [2].

It is extremely important to assess the pelvis x-ray for projection errors as the orientation of the pelvis during image acquisition can affect the interpretation of the radiograph. The tilt of the pelvis can be assessed by evaluating the distance between the coccyx and the superior border of the pubic symphysis. This measures 32.3 mm (8–50 mm) in males and 47.3 mm (15–72 mm) in females with neutral pelvic tilt [3, 4]. While a normal range of pelvic tilt has been established, it is important to appreciate that spinopelvic morphology dictates the amount of pelvic tilt that is particular to a patient's individual anatomy. Therefore, no attempt should be made to normalize the distance between coccyx and symphysis by tilting the beam or the pelvis when acquiring an AP pelvis, whether supine or standing (Fig. 2.2). Pelvic rotation is assessed by ensuring that the midline of the sacrum is centered over the pubic symphysis. In addition, this can be verified by looking for symmetric obturator foramen and acetabular teardrops (Fig. 2.3). It is vital that pelvic rotation is neutral for reliable quantification of the various radiologic parameters, as these are greatly affected by pelvic rotation, pelvic tilt, lack of centering of the x-ray beam over the pubic symphysis, and a non-orthogonal x-ray beam [1]. It is important to note that bone morphology that is captured on the radiographic film can be altered by a myriad of factors, and therefore the films must be scrutinized for appropriate technique. For instance, the projection of the hip joint on the radiograph is affected by the centering or the direction of the x-ray beam, as well as pelvic positioning during image acquisi-

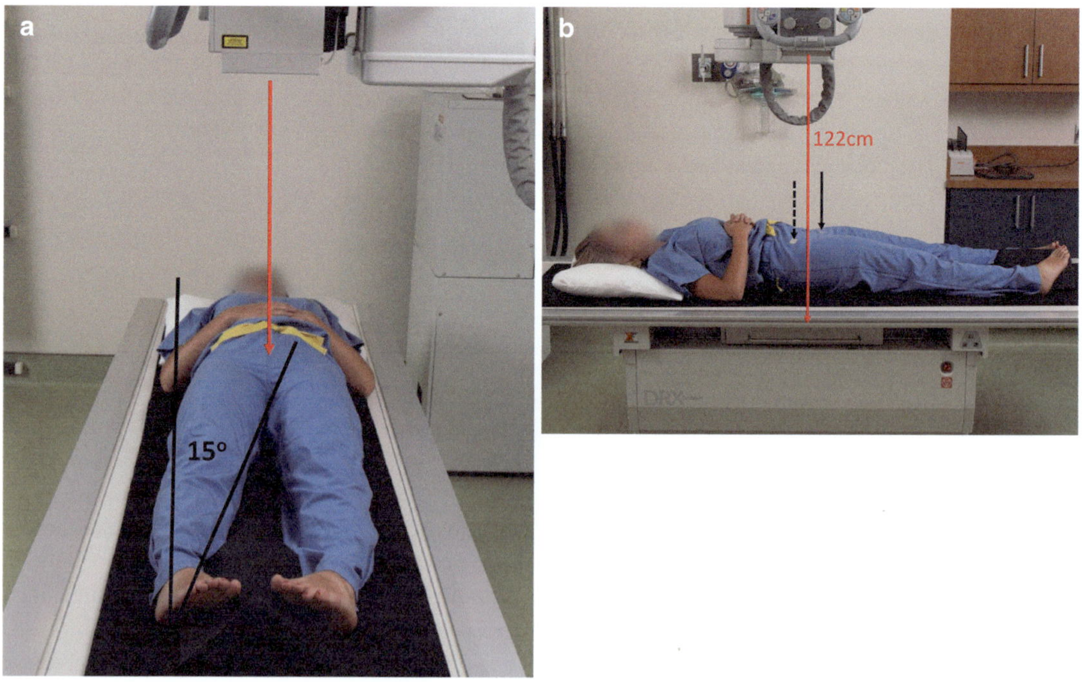

Fig. 2.1 The anterior-posterior (AP) radiograph of the hip is taken with the patient positioned supine and legs rotated inward 15° (**a**). The projector is 122 cm away from the cassette, centered over the pubic symphysis (*solid black arrow*) in the medial-lateral plane and halfway between the pubic symphysis and anterior superior iliac spine (ASIS) (*dashed black arrow*) in the cranial-caudal plane (**b**) (the *red arrow* represents the x-ray beam)

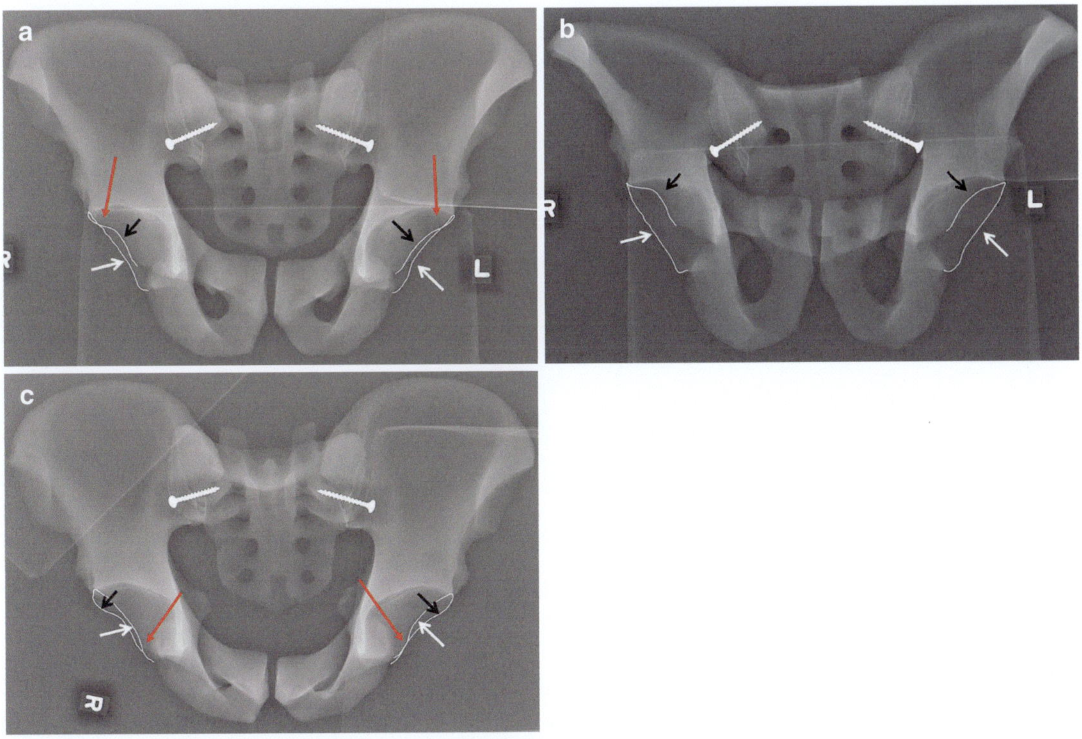

Fig. 2.2 (**a**) Pelvic tilt alters apparent version of the acetabulum by changing the orientation of the acetabulum in space. The sawbones model with wire outlining the acetabulum shows a high crossover sign (*red arrows*) as the anterior wall (*black arrows*) projects lateral to the posterior wall (*white arrows*) at the lateral edge of the acetabulum. Although the coccyx-to-symphysis pubis distance is not "normal" for neutral version, the x-ray will serve as a baseline for what happens as the pelvis is tilted. (**b**) Backward tilt increases apparent acetabular anteversion as the space between the anterior and posterior walls increases and the crossover sign disappears and gives a false impression of acetabular anteversion. (**c**) Forward tilt of the pelvis decreases apparent acetabular version and gives a false impression of acetabular retroversion as seen by the very caudal crossover sign (*red arrows*)

tion [5]. A properly performed AP pelvis radiograph provides valuable information regarding acetabular depth, inclination and version, and femoral head coverage.

Coxa Profunda and Protrusio General acetabular coverage can be assessed with acetabular depth. In an acetabulum with normal depth, the acetabular fossa lies lateral to the ischioischial line (Fig. 2.4a). An acetabulum with overcoverage (pincer impingement) presents with increased depth as seen with coxa profunda and protrusion acetabuli. In coxa profunda, the acetabular fossa lies medial to or touches the ilioischial line (Fig. 2.4b). Protrusio acetabuli is defined as the femoral head lying medial to or touching the ilioischial line (Fig. 2.4c).

Acetabular Index of Depth to Width Acetabular depth can be further quantified with the acetabular index of depth to width (D/W) [6, 7]. The D/W is defined by dividing the depth of the acetabulum by the distance between the inferomedial and superolateral border of the acetabulum (Fig. 2.5). Individuals with hip dysplasia that have a D/W >38% have a positive prognosis regarding the development of osteoarthritis [6].

Angle of Sharp Acetabular dysplasia can be quantified by the angle of Sharp, which measures the inclination of the acetabulum. The angle of Sharp is formed by the angle between a horizontal line joining the inferior border of the teardrops

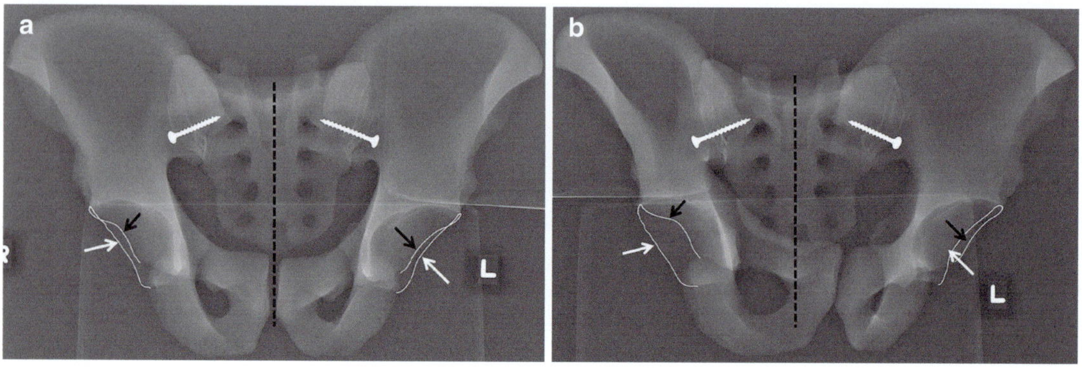

Fig. 2.3 A good AP pelvis radiograph requires neutral rotation of the pelvis (**a**) depicted by alignment of the mid-sacrum with the symphysis pubis. Obturator foramen and iliac wings should also be symmetric unless there is anatomic asymmetry within the pelvis. Acetabular version should similarly be symmetric as depicted by the anterior (*black arrows*) and posterior (*white arrows*) walls. Pelvic rotation (**b**) leads to apparent retroversion on the side toward which the pelvis is rotated and apparent anteversion on the opposite side. In this case, there is slight rotation of the pelvis to the left, and the left hip yields a worsening crossover sign, suggesting acetabular retroversion as the anterior wall is now caudal to the posterior wall. Concurrently, the distance between the anterior and posterior walls of the right hip has increased with the anterior wall now being cranial to the posterior wall, suggesting anteversion

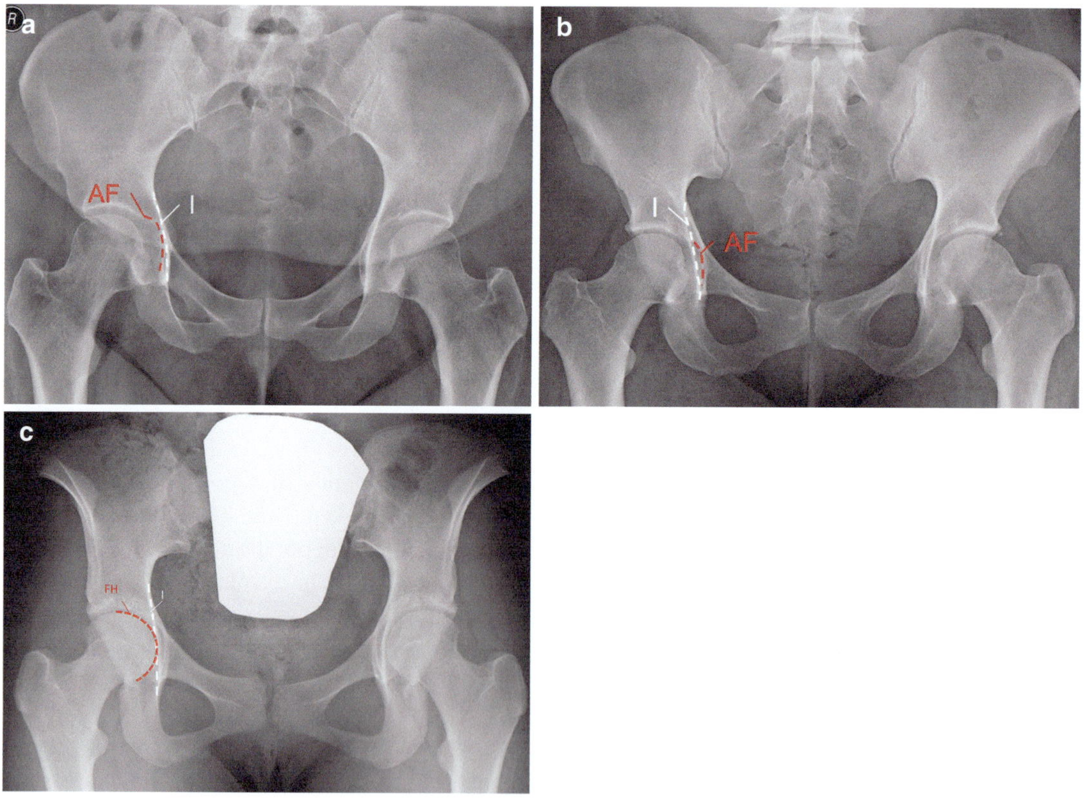

Fig. 2.4 (**a**) The acetabular fossa (AF) normally lies lateral to the ilioischial line (I). (**b**) In coxa profunda, the AF lies medial to or touches the ilioischial line (I). (**c**) In acetabular protrusio, the femoral head (FH) lies medial to or touches the ilioischial (I)

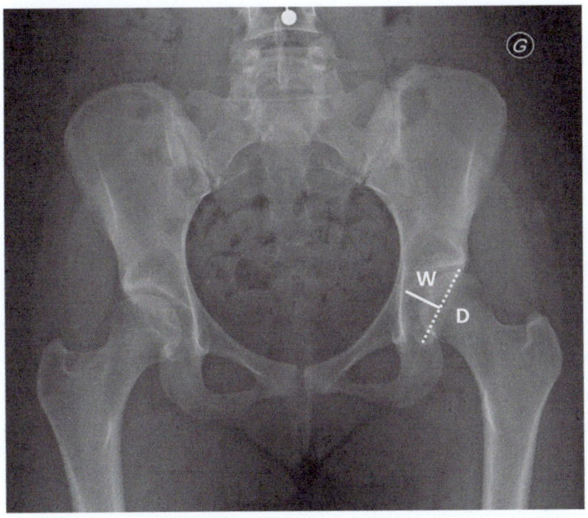

Fig. 2.5 The acetabular index of depth to width quantifies depth or shallowness of the acetabulum and is measured by drawing a line (W, *dashed white line*) from the lateral edge of the sourcil to the inferomedial edge of the acetabulum, which represents acetabular width. The longest possible perpendicular line (D, *solid white line*) is then drawn toward the acetabular roof and represents acetabular depth. The index is calculated as 100% × D/W. A depth <38% is abnormal

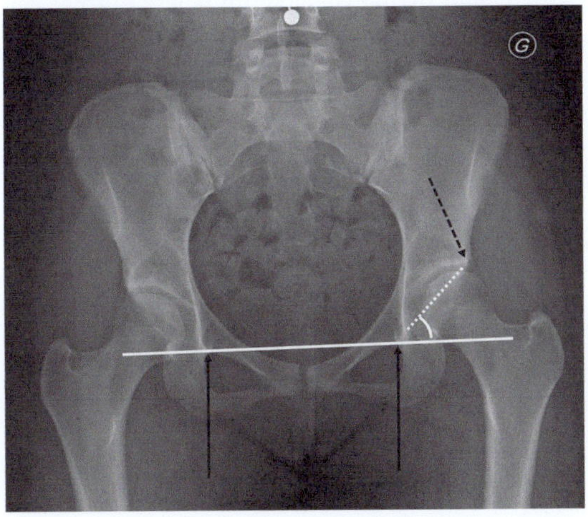

Fig. 2.6 The angle of Sharp is formed by the angle between a horizontal line (*solid white line*) joining the inferior border of the teardrops (*solid black arrows*) and a line (*dashed white line*) from the inferior border of the teardrop to the lateral edge of the sourcil (*dashed black arrow*). The normal value for the angle of Sharp ranges from 33° to 38°

and a line to the lateral sourcil (Fig. 2.6). The normal value for the angle of Sharp ranges from 33–38°. Angles >38° represent acetabular dysplasia [8, 9].

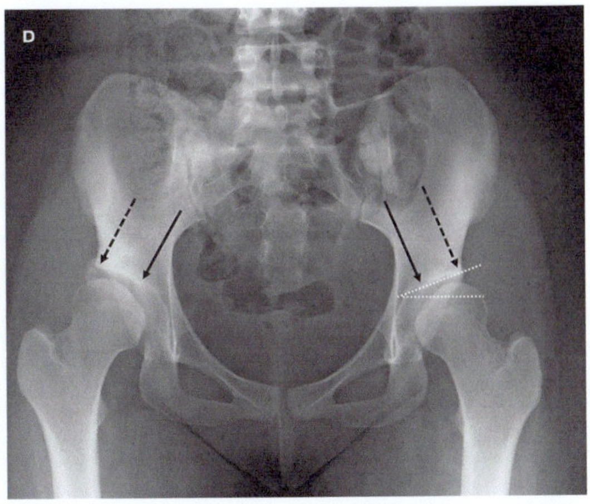

Fig. 2.7 The Tönnis angle is the angle formed from a horizontal line and a line joining the medial (*solid black arrow*) and lateral edge (*dashed black arrow*) of the acetabular sourcil with a normal range from 0° to 10°

Tönnis Angle The Tönnis angle (TA) is another measure that quantifies acetabular inclination on the AP pelvis radiograph. It is defined by the angle formed from a horizontal line and a line joining the medial and lateral edge of the acetabular sourcil (Fig. 2.7). The normal value ranges from 0° to 10° with values from 11° to 14° considered borderline dysplastic. Typically, in cases of overcoverage, the TA will be 0° or negative [10].

Crossover Sign The acetabular orientation is altered in cases of impingement and dysplasia of the hip. In the normal hip, the acetabulum is anteverted with the anterior wall (AW) lying medial to the posterior wall (PW) (Fig. 2.8) [3, 11]. In cases of focal anterior superior overcoverage seen in pincer impingement, the anterior superior AW lies lateral to PW in the proximal aspect of the acetabulum and crosses to the medial side of the PW in the distal acetabulum, effectively forming a figure-of-8 configuration called the "crossover sign" (Fig. 2.9) [1].

Posterior Wall Sign The posterior wall sign is defined by PW lying medial to the center of the femoral head. The PW sign is typically present in acetabular retroversion (see Fig. 2.9).

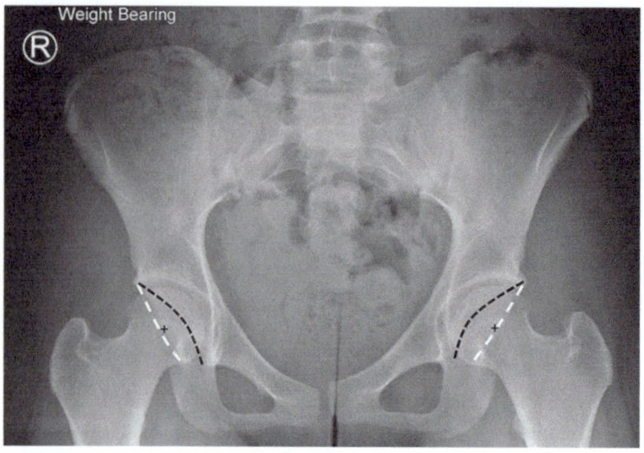

Fig. 2.8 The anterior acetabular wall (*dashed black line*) normally lies medial to the acetabular posterior acetabular wall (*dashed white line*). The posterior wall typically crosses or is just lateral to the center of the femoral head (+)

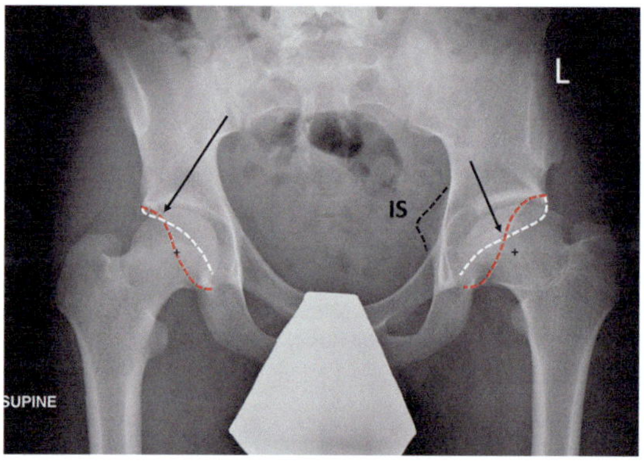

Fig. 2.9 Acetabular retroversion is represented by the crossover sign, the ischial spine sign, and the posterior wall sign. A large crossover sign (*black arrow*) is seen on the left hip represented by the anterior acetabular wall (AW) and posterior wall (PW) crossing over each other such that the AW (*white dashed line*) lies lateral to the proximal aspect of the PW (*red dashed line*). There is also a small crossover seen on the right hip that is located cranially. The ischial spine sign is represented by the ischial spine (IS) (*dashed black line*) protruding past the medial brim and is seen only on the left side. The posterior wall sign is present on the left where the PW passes medial to the center of the femoral head (+), whereas on the right it passes through the center of the femoral head

Ischial Spine Sign The ischial spine sign has also been defined to describe acetabular retroversion present in impingement [12]. It is present when the ischial spine is protruding medial to the pelvic brim (see Fig. 2.9).

Retroversion Index The retroversion index has also been utilized to document the version of the acetabulum. When a crossover sign is present, it is calculated by the ratio of the length of the PW medial to the AW and the total length of the PW [13].

Lateral Center-Edge Angle General coverage of the femoral head, whether under- or overcoverage, can be assessed with the lateral center-edge angle (LCEA). The LCEA is defined as the angle between a vertical line and a line connecting the center of the femoral head and the lateral edge of the acetabulum (Fig. 2.10). The normal value of LCEA in young adults ranges from 25° to 39° [1, 6, 10]. An LCEA smaller than 25° represents acetabular dysplasia and femoral head uncoverage. An LCEA >39° represents overcoverage as seen in pincer impingement.

Extrusion Index The extrusion index (EI) can be measured to evaluate acetabular femoral head coverage. The EI is calculated by measuring the percentage of the diameter of the femoral head that is not covered by the acetabulum where normal values range from 17% to 27% (Fig. 2.11) [14].

Shenton Line Finally, femoral head subluxation seen in dysplasia can be assessed with the Shenton line. This line represents an arc made by the inferior border of the femoral head-neck junction and the superior border of the obturator foramen. A disruption of the Shenton line represents a subluxation of the hip (Fig. 2.12).

Anterior-Posterior (AP) of the Hip

The AP of the hip is obtained with the patient supine or standing with the lower extremity in 15° of internal rotation to account for the native femoral anteversion. The x-ray beam is centered on the femoral head which contrasts with the AP pelvis view. When the x-ray beam is centered on the femoral head, it alters the apparent morphology of the acetabulum by overestimating acetabular anteversion (Fig. 2.13) and produces apparent coxa profunda/protrusio acetabuli; therefore the AP hip view should not be used to assess these

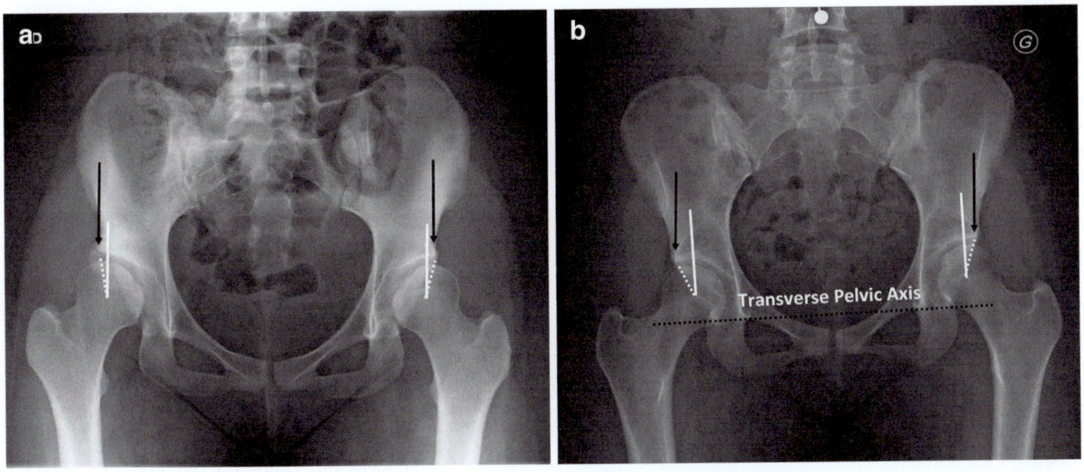

Fig. 2.10 (**a**) The lateral center-edge angle (LCEA) is measured between a vertical line (*solid white lines*) on a weight-bearing film from the center of the femoral head and a line connecting the center of the femoral head and the lateral edge of the sourcil (*dashed white lines*). The normal range is 25–39°. (**b**) On a supine film, the vertical line (*solid white lines*) must be drawn perpendicular to the transverse axis of the pelvis (*dashed black line*) to accommodate for any oblique positioning

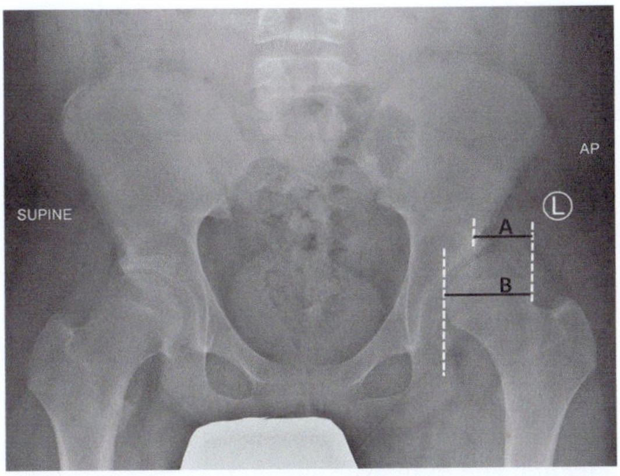

Fig. 2.11 The extrusion index (EI) is calculated by measuring the percentage of the diameter of the femoral head that is not covered by the acetabulum EI = A/B × 100. The left hip is dysplastic with a 65% extrusion index

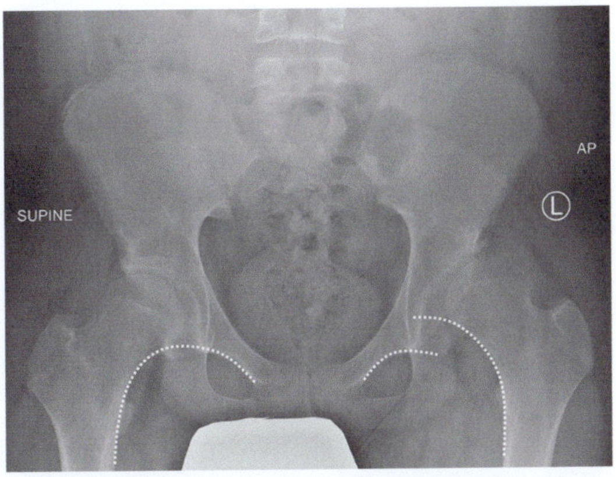

Fig. 2.12 The Shenton line represents an arc made by the inferior border of the femoral head-neck junction and the superior border of the obturator foramen. A normal Shenton line is seen on the right. A disruption of the Shenton line, seen on the left represents subluxation of the hip

parameters [1]. The AP hip view can be used to assess evidence of narrowing or signs of arthritic changes at the lateral, central, and medial sourcil of the acetabulum. The Tönnis grade has been described to characterize the arthritic changes seen in the femoroacetabular joint (Table 2.1) [15, 16]. It can also be used to evaluate the proximal femoral anatomy. When the cam deformity is significant and presents on the superolateral surface of the femoral head-neck junction, a pistol grip deformity can be appreciated.

Lateral Radiographs of the Hip

Typically, lateral radiographs of the hip are obtained to evaluate the anterior superior junction of the femoral head-neck junction for sign of asphericity and cam deformity. The frog-leg lateral view is usually obtained; the axial cross-table view and the modified Dunn view can be used as alternatives.

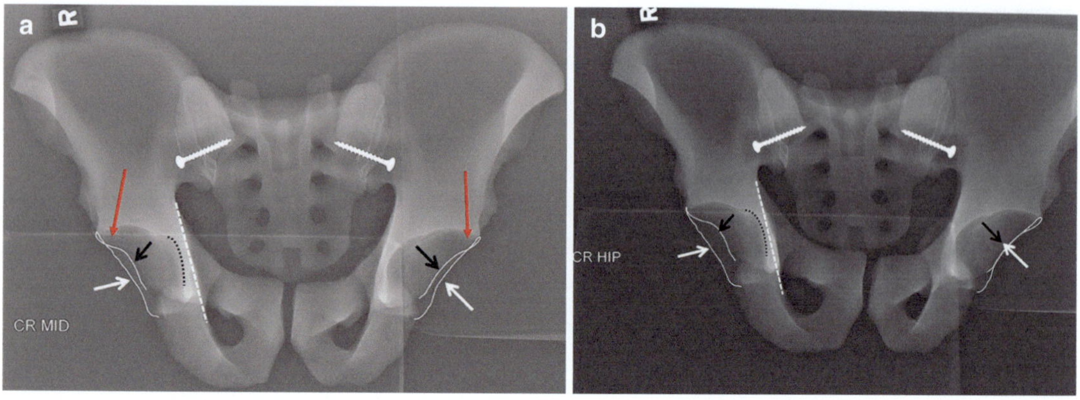

Fig. 2.13 AP pelvis x-ray (**a**) taken with the beam appropriately centered over the symphysis pubis showing mild crossover (*red arrow*) bilaterally. (**b**) An AP pelvis radiograph is taken with the beam centered on the right hip, showing increased apparent anteversion as depicted by the anterior wall (*black arrow*) appearing more cranial and the posterior wall (*white arrow*) appearing more caudal than the image with the beam centered on the pelvis. In addition, centering the beam on the hip increases the appearance of acetabular depth as noted by the decreased space between the ilioischial line (*dashed white line*) and the acetabular fossa (*solid black line*) compared to when the beam is centered on the pelvis

Table 2.1 Tönnis classification for hip joint osteoarthritis

Tönnis grade	Description	Joint space	Femoral head sphericity
0	No sign of osteoarthritis	Normal	Normal
1	Sclerosis and osteophyte formation	Slight narrowing	Normal
2	Small cysts in femoral head or acetabulum	Moderate narrowing (<50%)	Moderate loss of sphericity
3	Large cysts in femoral head or acetabulum and femoral head deformity	Severe narrowing (>50%)	Severe deformity of the femoral head

Axial Cross-Table Lateral The axial cross-table lateral enables evaluation of the anterior and posterior femoral head-neck junction at the 3 o'clock and 9 o'clock position, respectively. It is performed with the patient lying supine with the affected lower extremity in 15° of internal rotation while the contralateral lower extremity is flexed at the hip and elevated. The x-ray beam is centered on the inguinal fold and angled at 45° (Fig. 2.14) [1]. The axial cross-table lateral is useful to evaluate the anterior and posterior contour of the femoral head-neck junction.

Frog-Leg Lateral The frog-leg lateral is obtained with the patient lying supine where both knees and hips are flexed 45° and the lower extremities are externally rotated maximally. The x-ray beam is centered on the hip (Fig. 2.15) [20]. The frog-leg lateral is useful to evaluate the anterior femoral neck at the 1–2 o'clock position, sphericity of the femoral head, and joint congruity. The greater trochanter can often obscure the femoral head-neck junction and limit its evaluation.

Modified Dunn View The modified Dunn view enables an improved evaluation of the superior anterior femoral head-neck junction. It is performed with the patient lying supine with both hips and knees flexed at 45° and the lower leg held in 20° of abduction with neutral rotation. The Dunn view can also be performed with the hip flexed at 70° or at 90° and provides a more inferior and anterior assessment of the femoral head-neck junction at the 1–2 o'clock position as the hip is flexed [17, 18].

The cam deformity can be quantified using the alpha angle (α) and by measuring the anterior offset ratio.

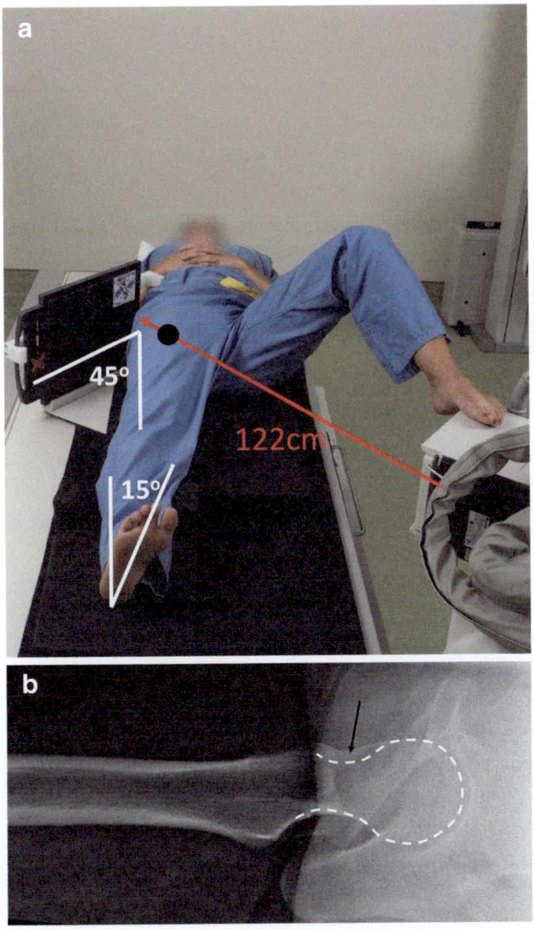

Fig. 2.14 (**a**) The cross-table lateral radiograph of the hip is taken with the patient positioned supine and the limb internally rotated 15°. The projector is positioned 122 cm from the cassette and is angled 45°. The x-ray beam (*red arrow*) points to the center of the femoral head (*black dot*) and is positioned 122 cm from the cassette, which is 45° to the patient and orthogonal to the projector beam. The opposite limb must be positioned out of the way of the x-ray beam. This can be accomplished with a leg holder or, as in this case, with the patient's foot placed on the projector with the hip flexed and abducted. (**b**) The cross-table lateral radiograph is a true lateral of the proximal femur and can reveal abnormalities of the anterior femoral head-neck junction at the 3 o'clock position. In this case, there is loss of normal anterior offset as seen by a cam lesion (*black arrow*) at the head-neck junction

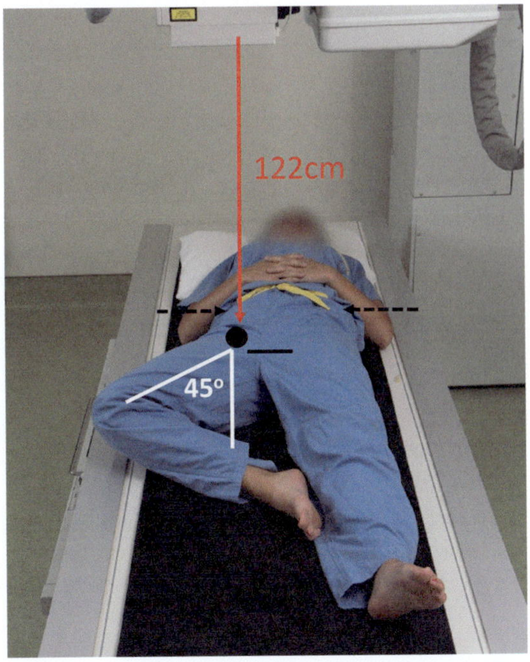

Fig. 2.15 The frog-lateral view of the hip is obtained with the hip flexed 45° and maximally externally rotated. The projector is 122 cm from the cassette and is centered over the hip joint, which is just proximal to the symphysis pubis (*solid black line*) and is approximately halfway between the symphysis pubis and the anterior superior iliac spine in the medial-lateral plane

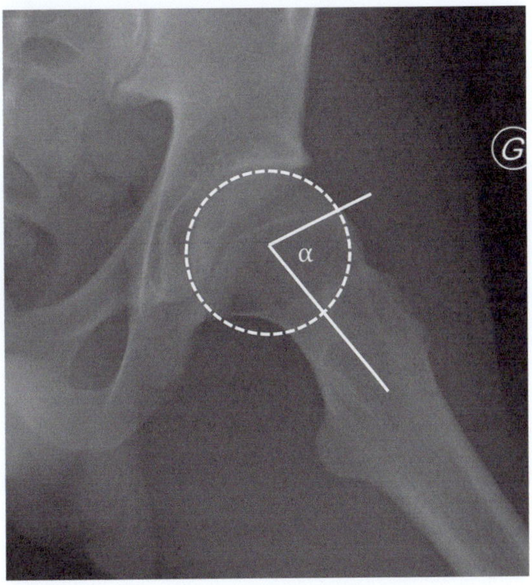

Fig. 2.16 The α angle is formed by the angle between the femoral neck axis and a line joining the center of the femoral head and the point at which the femoral head becomes aspherical. An α angle >50° may represent a cam deformity

Alpha Angle The α angle depicts the point at which the sphericity of the femoral head ends. The α angle is formed by the angle between the femoral neck axis and a line joining the center of the femoral head and the point at which the femoral head becomes aspherical (Fig. 2.16) [19]. A normal α angle measures 42–47°. The true value for an "abnormal" α angle remains controversial. Typically, the larger the value, the more likely it is to be abnormal. Values >65° are definitely abnormal, whereas those between 50° and 65° are borderline abnormal [20]. The anterior offset is another parameter utilized to evaluate the sphericity of the femoral head. The anterior offset is defined by the difference between the radius of the anterior femoral head and the anterior femoral neck where a value of <10 mm is significant for cam impingement [1].

Offset Ratio The offset ratio can further characterize the bone morphology of the femoral head and is calculated as the ratio of the anterior femoral offset and the diameter of the femoral head (Fig. 2.17). A ratio of <0.17 is seen with cam impingement, while an offset >0.21 is considered normal [1].

The False-Profile Radiograph

Anterior acetabular coverage can be evaluated with a false-profile view. The false-profile radiograph is obtained with the patient standing with the pelvis rotated 65° in relation to the plate and the foot parallel to the plate (Fig. 2.18). While the lateral LCEA provides information regarding the lateral coverage of the femoral head, the anterior center-edge angle (ACEA) defines the anterior coverage of the acetabulum. It is formed by the angle between a vertical line and a line joining the center of the femoral head and the anterior acetabular edge (Fig. 2.19). The normal values for the ACEA are 25–39°.

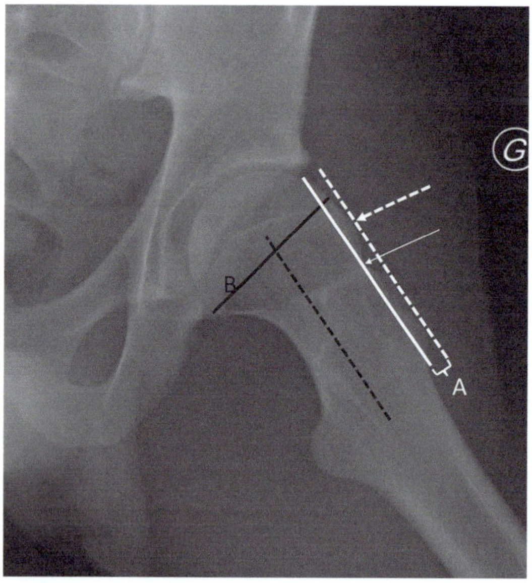

Fig. 2.17 The head-neck offset ratio is calculated as the ratio of the distance between the radius of the anterior femoral head and the anterior femoral neck (A) with the diameter of the femoral head (B, *solid black line*). The anterior offset (A) is measured by drawing a line through the long axis of the femoral neck (*dashed black line*) and the center of the femoral head; a second and third line are drawn parallel to the first line, one through the anterior-most aspect of the femoral neck (*solid white arrow and line*) and the second through the anterior-most aspect of the femoral head (*dashed white arrow and line*). The head-neck offset ratio is calculated by measuring distance A divided by distance B. A cam deformity is suggested when the ratio is <0.17

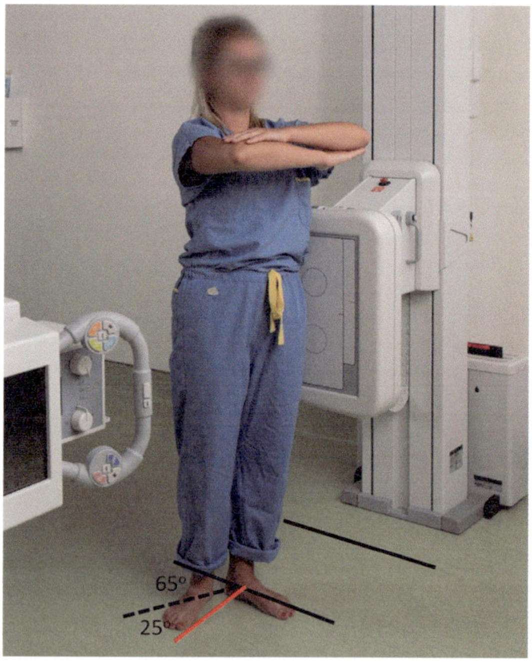

Fig. 2.18 The false-profile view of the hip is performed in the standing position. The pelvis is rotated 65° (*dashed black line*) from the bucky with the foot of the hip being evaluated parallel to the radiographic cassette (*solid black line*). The projector is 122 cm from the cassette and is aimed at the left hip

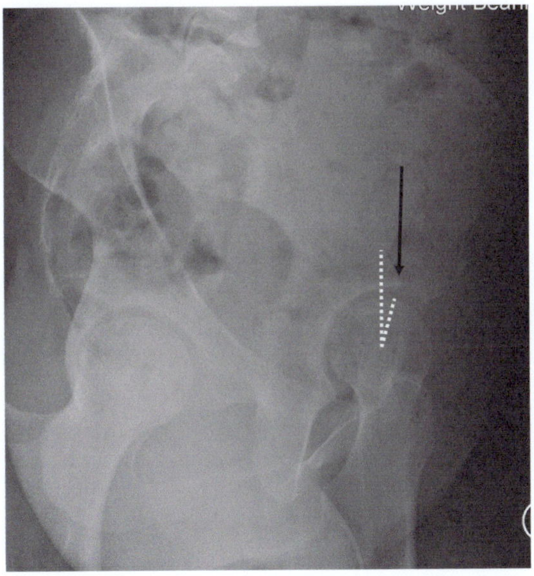

Fig. 2.19 The anterior center-edge angle (ACEA) defines the anterior coverage of the acetabulum and is measured on the false-profile view. The ACEA is formed by the angle between a vertical line and a line joining the center of the femoral head and the anterior acetabular edge. The normal values for the ACEA are 25–39°

The false-profile radiograph can also be used to document subspine impingement which occurs when an enlarged anterior inferior iliac spine (AIIS) impinges on the anterior femoral neck in straight hip flexion [21]. While evident on a false-profile x-ray, this can be mistaken for a crossover sign on an AP pelvis radiograph (Fig. 2.20). The prominent AIIS has been classified into types that express AIIS morphology and protrusion below the acetabular rim (Fig. 2.21) [22].

Computed Tomography (CT)

Some of the diagnostic challenges of evaluating a three-dimensional pathology affecting the acetabulum can be circumvented by using a CT scan. That being said, in most cases, the scans tend to yield more information than we can currently process. CT scans are useful for quantifying the area or volume of the femoral head that is covered by the acetabulum and in determining

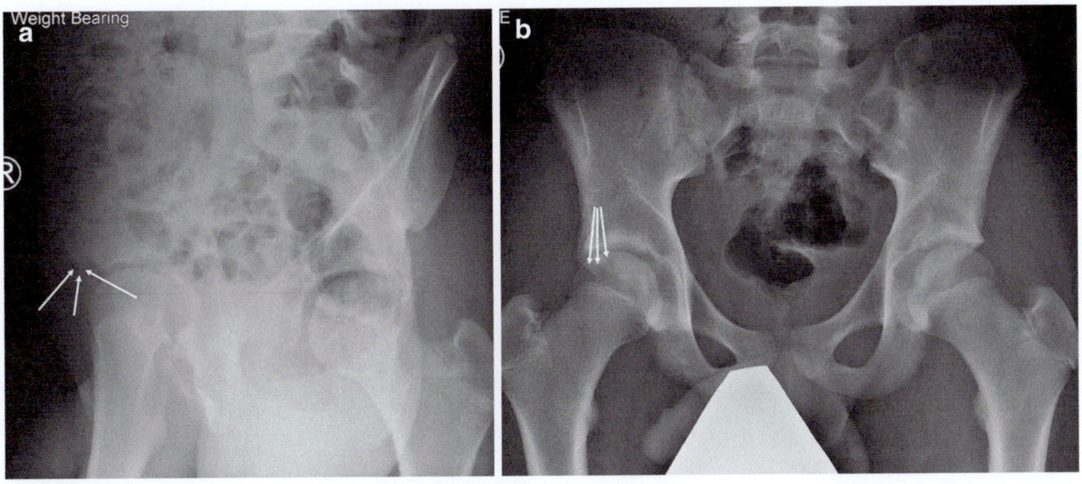

Fig. 2.20 (**a**) A prominent anterior inferior iliac spine (AIIS) (*white arrows*) is seen on the false-profile view. (**b**) AP pelvis in the same patient where the prominent AIIS is seen (*white arrows*). While very clear on the false-profile x-ray, this can easily be mistaken for a crossover sign on the AP pelvis view

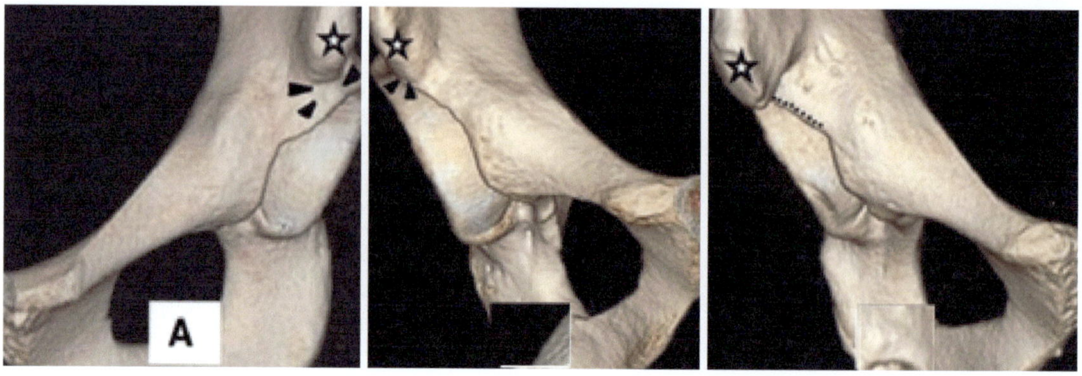

Fig. 2.21 Anterior inferior iliac spine (AIIS) impingement, also known as subspine impingement, is classified by the morphology of the AIIS prominence and its relation to the acetabulum. The three types are as follows: (**a**) There is as smooth ilium wall (*arrowheads*) between the caudal level of the AIIS and the acetabular rim; (**b**) the AIIS sits just at the level of the acetabular rim (*arrowheads*) and appears as a "roof-like" prominence over the hip; (**c**) and the AIIS extends distally to the anterosuperior acetabular rim (*dots*), and it has a downward "spur appearance" (From Hetsroni et al. [22], with permission)

exactly where there is under- and/or overcoverage [23–26]. In addition, CT scans are useful for quantifying acetabular version. Acetabular version can be measured with axial CT or with three-dimensional (3D) CT. In general, 3D CT measurements require reformatting of the CT and special software to allow measurements of acetabular version and inclination [27], whereas acetabular version can be easily calculated using readily available axial and coronal CT slices. This is achieved by selecting an axial plane slice on a coronal scan that correlates with the femoral head equator. The equatorial axial sequence is then used to quantify acetabular version by measuring the angle joining the anterior and posterior bony margins of the acetabulum with a horizontal line joining the posterior margins of both acetabula (Fig. 2.22) [27]. Just as measurements using plain radiographs of various parameters can be altered based on positioning of the patient, the axial CT value of acetabular version is susceptible to error based on pelvic tilt. The average value of acetabular anteversion on CT has been reported as 17° ± 6° [28]. While CT analysis is interesting from an academic point of view, at the current time, it is rarely helpful in the clinical setting other than when acetabular version is not well visualized on the plain radiograph or in revision osteotomy cases where anterior and posterior wall lines can be obscured.

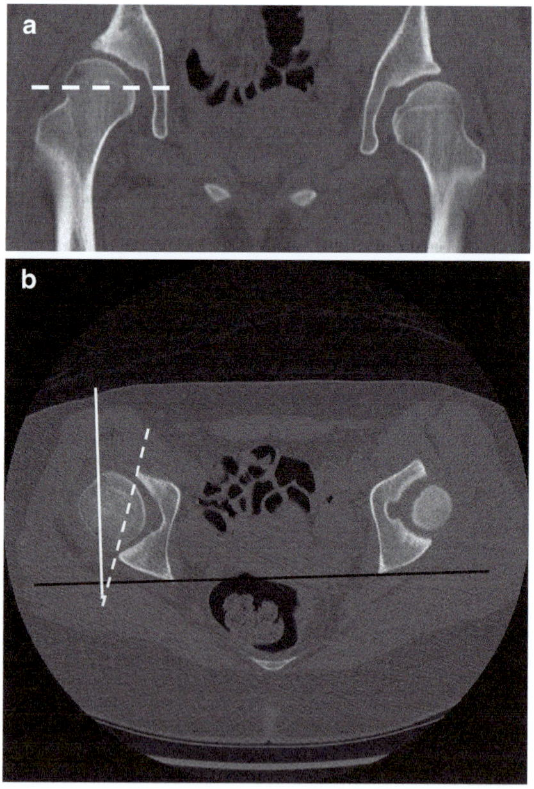

Fig. 2.22 (**a**) Coronal CT is used to find the corresponding axial slice at the level of the femoral head equator. (**b**) The axial CT cut at the equator of the femoral head is used to calculate acetabular version. A reference line (*solid black line*) is drawn on the posterior aspect of both acetabulae. An orthogonal line to the reference line is drawn (*solid white line*). Finally, a line is drawn connecting the anterior and posterior walls of the acetabulum (*dashed white line*). The angle between these two lines quantifies acetabular version

References

1. Tannast M, Siebenrock KA, Anderson SE. Femoroacetabular impingement: radiographic diagnosis--what the radiologist should know. AJR Am J Roentgenol. 2007;188(6):1540–52.
2. Tannast M, Zheng G, Anderegg C, Burckhardt K, Langlotz F, Ganz R, et al. Tilt and rotation correction of acetabular version on pelvic radiographs. Clin Orthop Relat Res. 2005;438:182–90.
3. Siebenrock KA, Schoeniger R, Ganz R. Anterior femoro-acetabular impingement due to acetabular retroversion. Treatment with periacetabular osteotomy. J Bone Joint Surg Am. 2003;85-a(2):278–86.
4. Siebenrock KA, Kalbermatten DF, Ganz R. Effect of pelvic tilt on acetabular retroversion: a study of pelves from cadavers. Clin Orthop Relat Res. 2003;407:241–8.
5. Nho S, Leunig M, Larson CM, Bedi A, Kelly BT, editors. Hip arthroscopy and hip joint preservation surgery, vol. 1. New York: Springer; 2015.
6. Murphy SB, Ganz R, Muller ME. The prognosis in untreated dysplasia of the hip. A study of radiographic factors that predict the outcome. J Bone Joint Surg Am. 1995;77(7):985–9.
7. Heyman CH, Herndon CH. Legg-Perthes disease; a method for the measurement of the roentgenographic result. J Bone Joint Surg Am. 1950;32 a(4):767–78.
8. Ipach I, Rondak IC, Sachsenmaier S, Buck E, Syha R, Mittag F. Radiographic signs for detection of femoroacetabular impingement and hip dysplasia should be carefully used in patients with osteoarthritis of the hip. BMC Musculoskelet Disord. 2014;15:150.
9. Pereira F, Giles A, Wood G, Board TN. Recognition of minor adult hip dysplasia: which anatomical indices are important? Hip Int. 2014;24(2):175–9.
10. Tönnis D, Heinecke A. Acetabular and femoral anteversion: relationship with osteoarthritis of the hip. J Bone Joint Surg Am. 1999;81(12):1747–70.
11. Mast JW, Brunner RL, Zebrack J. Recognizing acetabular version in the radiographic presentation of hip dysplasia. Clin Orthop Relat Res. 2004;418: 48–53.
12. Kalberer F, Sierra RJ, Madan SS, Ganz R, Leunig M. Ischial spine projection into the pelvis: a new sign for acetabular retroversion. Clin Orthop Relat Res. 2008;466(3):677–83.
13. Diaz-Ledezma C, Novack T, Marin-Pena O, Parvizi J. The relevance of the radiological signs of acetabular retroversion among patients with femoroacetabular impingement. Bone Joint J. 2013;95-b(7):893–9.
14. Tannast M, Albers CE, Steppacher SD, Siebenrock KA. Hip pain in the young adult. In: Bentley G, editor. European instructional lectures. Vol 11, 2011. 12th EFORT congress, Copenhagen, Denmark. Berlin: Springer; 2011. p. 141–54.
15. Tönnis D. Congenital dysplasia and dislocation of the hip in children and adults. Berlin: Springer; 1987.
16. Mayo KA, Trumble SJ, Mast JW. Results of periacetabular osteotomy in patients with previous surgery for hip dysplasia. Clin Orthop Relat Res. 1999;363:73–80.
17. Harris MD, Kapron AL, Peters CL, Anderson AE. Correlations between the alpha angle and femoral head asphericity: implications and recommendations for the diagnosis of cam femoroacetabular impingement. Eur J Radiol. 2014;83(5):788–96.
18. Nepple JJ, Martel JM, Kim YJ, Zaltz I, Clohisy JC. Do plain radiographs correlate with CT for imaging of cam-type femoroacetabular impingement? Clin Orthop Relat Res. 2012;470(12):3313–20.
19. Notzli HP, Wyss TF, Stoecklin CH, Schmid MR, Treiber K, Hodler J. The contour of the femoral head-neck junction as a predictor for the risk of anterior impingement. J Bone Joint Surg Br. 2002;84(4):556–60.
20. Clohisy JC, Carlisle JC, Beaule PE, Kim YJ, Trousdale RT, Sierra RJ, et al. A systematic approach to the plain radiographic evaluation of the young adult hip. J Bone Joint Surg Am. 2008;90(Suppl 4):47–66.
21. Bardakos NV. Hip impingement: beyond femoroacetabular. J Hip Preserv Surg. 2015;2(3):206–23.
22. Hetsroni I, Poultsides L, Bedi A, Larson CM, Kelly BT. Anterior inferior iliac spine morphology correlates with hip range of motion: a classification system and dynamic model. Clin Orthop Relat Res. 2013;471(8):2497–503.
23. Larson CM, Moreau-Gaudry A, Kelly BT, Byrd JW, Tonetti J, Lavallee S, et al. Are normal hips being labeled as pathologic? A CT-based method for defining normal acetabular coverage. Clin Orthop Relat Res. 2015;473(4):1247–54.
24. Humbert L, Carlioz H, Baudoin A, Skalli W, Mitton D. 3D evaluation of the acetabular coverage assessed by biplanar X-rays or single anteroposterior X-ray compared with CT-scan. Comput Methods Biomech Biomed Engin. 2008;11(3):257–62.
25. Dandachli W, Kannan V, Richards R, Shah Z, Hall-Craggs M, Witt J. Analysis of cover of the femoral head in normal and dysplastic hips: new CT-based technique. J Bone Joint Surg Br. 2008;90(11):1428–34.
26. Hansen BJ, Harris MD, Anderson LA, Peters CL, Weiss JA, Anderson AE. Correlation between radiographic measures of acetabular morphology with 3D femoral head coverage in patients with acetabular retroversion. Acta Orthop. 2012;83(3):233–9.
27. Dandachli W, Ul Islam S, Tippett R, Hall-Craggs MA, Witt JD. Analysis of acetabular version in the native hip: comparison between 2D axial CT and 3D CT measurements. Skelet Radiol. 2011;40(7):877–83.
28. Reikeras O, Bjerkreim I, Kolbenstvedt A. Anteversion of the acetabulum and femoral neck in normals and in patients with osteoarthritis of the hip. Acta Orthop Scand. 1983;54(1):18–23.

Part I

Pediatric Pelvic Osteotomies

The Salter Innominate Osteotomy

3

Claire E. Shannon and Simon P. Kelley

Introduction

Developmental dysplasia of the hip (DDH), if left untreated in the young child, is known to result in early-onset hip dysfunction. Labral and chondral pathology manifests in the young adult and often results in an accelerated need for joint replacement due to the altered weight-bearing mechanics of the femoral head in a shallow acetabulum. Acetabular reorientation procedures, such as the Salter innominate osteotomy, are performed for DDH in the skeletally immature patient in order to acutely correct anterolateral acetabular deficiency by rotating the acetabular fragment about the symphysis pubis. The Salter innominate osteotomy therefore restores hip stability and may be used in combination with an open reduction and capsulorrhaphy, and/or with femoral osteotomies, as necessary. The improvement of the hip joint mechanics has also been found to induce remodeling of the acetabulum with continued growth of the child, leading to improved clinical outcomes.

C. E. Shannon
Division of Orthopaedics, Department of Orthopaedic Surgery, The Hospital for Sick Children, Toronto, ON, Canada
e-mail: claireshannon@jhmi.edu

S. P. Kelley (✉)
Department of Surgery, University of Toronto, Toronto, ON, Canada

The Hospital for Sick Children, Toronto, ON, Canada
e-mail: simon.kelley@sickkids.ca

Brief Clinical History

A developmentally normal, female child presented at the age of 8 months with concerns of decreased hip range of motion bilaterally. Radiographs revealed bilateral dislocated hips with dysplastic acetabuli. She was treated with adductor tenotomy, closed reduction, and double-leg hip spica casting in the operating room. The spica cast was used for a total of 16 weeks, with two interval cast changes. She achieved successful reduction, and her hips remained located and stable on follow-up. She was monitored regularly with clinical examination and radiographs to assess for the correction of acetabular dysplasia. At the age of 4 years, she was noted to have significant residual acetabular dysplasia (acetabular index >30° bilaterally), and thus staged, bilateral Salter innominate osteotomies were indicated to reorient her acetabulum, improve anterolateral coverage, and restore her radiographic acetabular metrics.

R. C. Hamdy, N. Saran (eds.), *Pediatric Pelvic and Proximal Femoral Osteotomies*,
https://doi.org/10.1007/978-3-319-78033-7_3

Preoperative Imaging (Fig. 3.1)

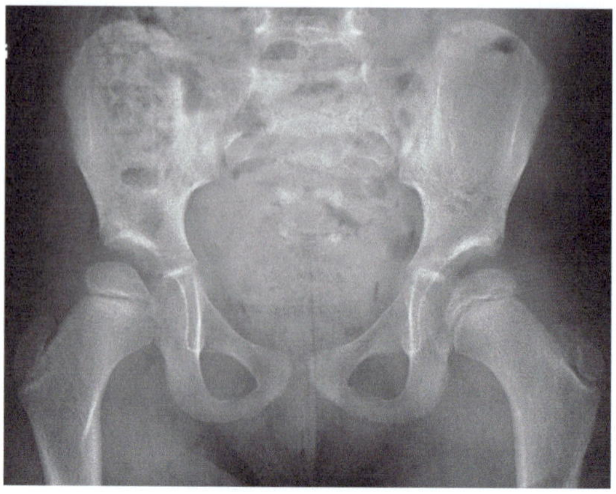

Fig. 3.1 Anteroposterior pelvis radiograph at age 4 years. Bilateral residual acetabular dysplasia after undergoing successful closed reductions at 8 months of age is present. Shenton's line is broken on the right but intact on the left. Bilateral acetabular indices are abnormal and measure 30°. The right and left teardrops are widening

Goals of Treatment

The goals of treatment when performing a Salter innominate osteotomy for acetabular dysplasia are:

- To achieve a concentrically reduced, stable hip
- To normalize the acetabular index
- To minimize early-onset degenerative changes to the hip

Treatment Strategy

The treatment algorithm in developmental hip dysplasia has been well elucidated. Initial presentation in an infant may frequently be managed with nonoperative techniques, such as use of a Pavlik harness or a fixed abduction brace, with highly satisfactory results. In cases of residual dysplasia after treatment or late presentation of dysplasia with or without hip subluxation/dislocation, surgical intervention is often required to correct the acetabular deficiency. Acetabular reorientation procedures such as the Salter innominate osteotomy are recommended for children 18 months of age or older.

As a reorientation procedure, the Salter innominate osteotomy relies on the acetabular segment hinging through the pubic symphysis. This is in contrast to other acetabular reorientation procedures that require multiple osteotomies to create a free acetabular segment or acetabular reshaping procedures that hinge through the triradiate cartilage. The reorientation of the acetabulum aims to improve the anterolateral coverage of the hip in order to restore a stable joint in the functional position required for ambulation. In cases where hip subluxation or dislocation is present, the innominate osteotomy is often combined with an open hip reduction and capsulorrhaphy. In older children who have previously undergone treatment of DDH with or without dislocation/subluxation, a Salter may be performed alone for residual dysplasia. In cases where excessive proximal femoral anteversion (>40°) also exists, a judicious proximal femoral derotation osteotomy may be required in addition. In a dislocated hip, the typical order of surgical elements is as follows: the open reduction of the hip should be performed first, including psoas recession, followed by the femoral osteotomy and then the pelvic osteotomy. The capsulorrhaphy should occur as the last step of the procedure to ensure correct tension of capsulorrhaphy and maintenance of hip reduction.

Surgical Details

Positioning

The patient is positioned supine on a radiolucent operating table with a small gel role under the rib cage of the affected side (Fig. 3.2). Avoid placement of the bump under the buttocks to avoid soft tissue crowding of the incision and approach. The affected side is draped out to include the entire leg, as well as the hip and flank, from the midline anterior and posterior, and up to the inferior most rib proximally.

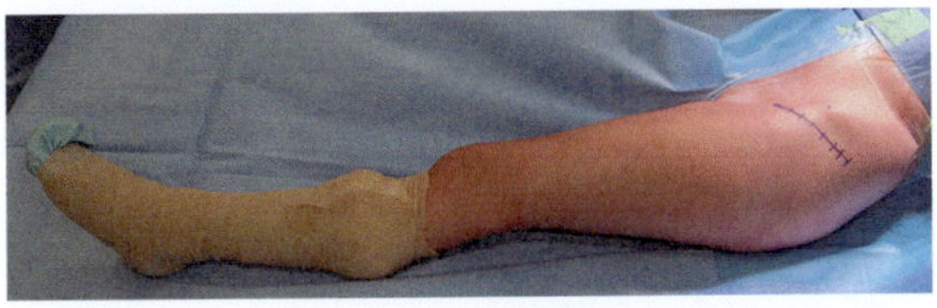

Fig. 3.2 Patient positioning and draping. Note knee remains in surgical field for purposes of orientation

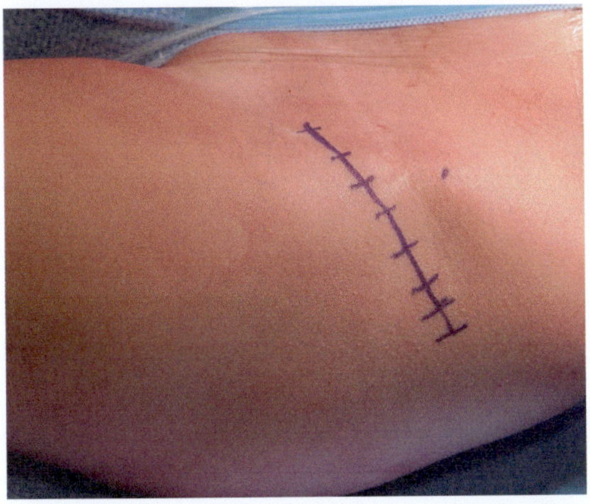

Fig. 3.3 Oblique bikini line incision marked out 2 cm below the iliac crest, in a skin crease. The dot represents the palpable anterior superior iliac spine (ASIS). Two-thirds of the incision should be lateral to the ASIS

Approach

A limited Smith-Peterson approach is used. The oblique portion of the incision is made 2 cm distal to the anterior superior iliac spine (ASIS) overlying the hip joint (Fig. 3.3). An attempt should be made to make this in line with the patient's skin creases for cosmesis, and thus the incision is semi-transverse and will course significantly inferior to the iliac crest. Avoid distal-longitudinal extension of the skin incision, as it does not improve exposure and is cosmetically undesirable.

Exposure

Subcutaneous dissection is carried out in line with the skin incision to expose the iliac apophysis. Identify the interval and expose between sartorius and tensor fascia lata distally. The direct head of

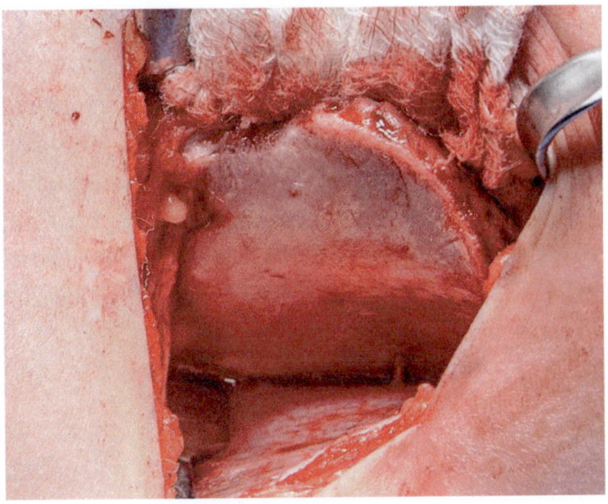

Fig. 3.4 Exposed innominate bone

rectus femoris should be found deep in this interval, attaching to the anterior inferior iliac spine (AIIS). Develop this interval proximally using a broad spade-shaped elevator to expose the ridge between the ASIS and the AIIS. Care is taken to avoid damage to the lateral femoral cutaneous nerve (LFCN) as it pierces the fascia medial to the ASIS within the sartorial compartment.

The external oblique muscle should be carefully dissected from the apophysis just far enough medially to allow the apophysis to be split in its midline. The apophysis is next sharply divided from the midpoint of the iliac crest to the AIIS using a number 10 scalpel blade. Subperiosteal dissection of the inner and outer tables of the ilium is performed with a broad periosteal elevator to expose the sciatic notch (Fig. 3.4). Avoid directing this dissection posteriorly toward the sacroiliac joint, as this is unnecessary for exposure and numerous perforating vessels may be encountered, which may result in excessive bleeding. Sponges should be packed into the subperiosteal spaces on both sides to assist with dissection and hemostasis.

A lengthening of the psoas muscle over the brim is required and should be considered an obligatory part of the surgical procedure. Due to the rotation of the acetabular fragment, the psoas if put under significant tension and left unlengthened can make bony correction difficult and leave a residual hip flexion contracture. The previously elevated periosteum of the inner table may be carefully identified and split at the level of the pelvic brim to facilitate exposure. The intramuscular tendon may be found as it crosses the pelvic brim. The tendon lies deep to the muscle, separating it from the femoral nerve. The psoas should be divided under direct vision, ensuring that only tendon is divided. The rectus tendon may be left intact if an open hip procedure is not being performed.

Salter Innominate Osteotomy

Retractors (Rang, Jantek Engineering, Ontario, Canada) are placed in the sciatic notch from lateral and medial sides. Overlapping the tips of the retractors with the medial placed more superficial will facilitate passage of the Gigli saw. A Gigli saw is pushed from medial to lateral through the sciatic notch with an instrument such as a Kelly clamp. Avoid pulling the saw through to avoid engaging it in the bone before one is ready to perform the osteotomy.

The operating table should be lowered and hands held as wide as allowed by the surgical field. It is of utmost importance that the orientation of the saw in the notch is perpendicular to the ilium rather to the axis of the patient. The Gigli saw is used to make the osteotomy from the midpoint of the sciatic notch to the point just proximal to the AIIS (Fig. 3.5).

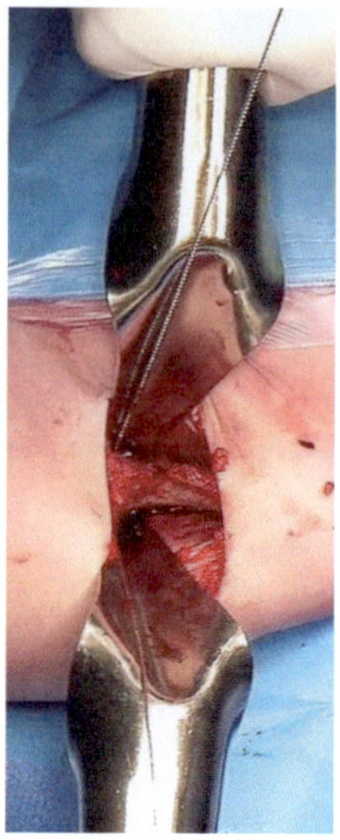

Fig. 3.5 Exposed innominate bone with retractors in sciatic notch and Gigli saw passed in preparation to make the osteotomy. Positioning of the saw perpendicular to the pelvis, rather than to the mechanical axis of the patient, is crucial to obtain the correct orientation of cut and correction

A triangular-shaped bone graft is cut from the ilium with an oscillating saw, whose base is formed between the ASIS and the AIIS and whose apex is at the midpoint of the iliac crest. This produces a 30° tricortical wedge (Fig. 3.6). The osteotomy is wedged open by applying an anterolateral force to the distal segment. This is best affected by placing a towel clamp on the distal fragment and rotating anterolaterally in line with the ilium. Avoid translation in the medial-lateral and anterior-posterior planes, keeping the posterior cortices apposed, with no more than 1–2 mm gap. Never pull up on the proximal ilium, for fear of rotating through the sacroiliac joint, rather than rotating the acetabular fragment about the symphysis pubis. The bone graft is placed in the medial aspect of the osteotomy gap, ensuring medial cortical alignment. Do not place the graft too deeply within the osteotomy to avoid over distraction posteriorly. Two threaded Steinmann pins (2.8–3.2 mm) are used to hold the graft. Position the pins along the medial cor-

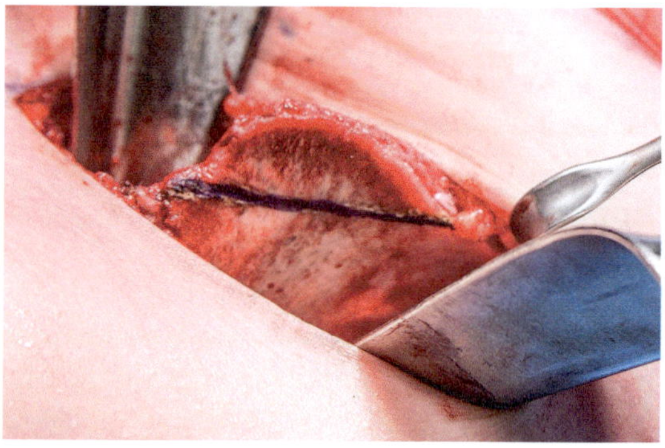

Fig. 3.6 The triangular 30° graft is marked and then cut from the iliac crest using an oscillating saw

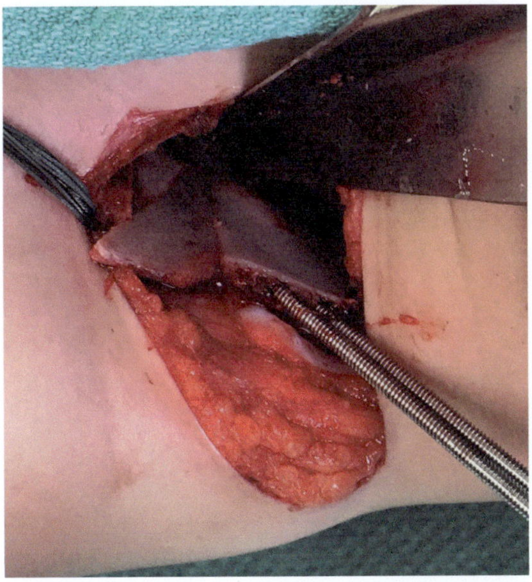

Fig. 3.7 The completed osteotomy with threaded pins transfixing the graft. The excess bone of the graft will be trimmed later in the procedure

tex, passing from superior ilium, through the graft, toward the posteromedial portion of the distal segment, up to the triradiate cartilage. Intraoperative fluoroscopy is used to confirm safe, extra-articular position of the pins (obturator oblique view). Prominent anterior graft may be trimmed and placed into the lateral osteotomy site (Fig. 3.7).

Closure

The iliac apophysis is closed over the ilium, around the Steinmann pins, with interrupted absorbable suture. Pointed towel clips may be used to approximate the apophysis, and care should be taken to appropriately restore the apophysis to avoid growth complications. The pins are cut just above the level of the closed apophysis to avoid prominence but to facilitate future removal if necessary. Subcutaneous fat and skin are closed in standard fashion per surgeon preference.

Postoperative Care

For children under the age of 3, a single-leg spica cast is put on with the patient still under general anesthesia. The affected hip should be positioned for maximal stability in 20–30° of flexion, abduction, and internal rotation. For an isolated Salter innominate osteotomy, 6 weeks of immobilization is recommended. No further bracing is typically required. Older children may be managed with non-weight bearing and recumbent at home, using a wheelchair to mobilize. Weight bearing as tolerated is allowed at 6 weeks postoperatively. Physical therapy is not typically required in children of this age, as they regain a normal range of hip motion within 3–4 months following surgery. The Steinmann pins may be removed at the discretion of the treating surgeon from 12 weeks postoperatively, but this step should not be considered obligatory, as the pins do not interfere with the execution or positioning of hip arthroplasty components in the future. Consequently, the authors leave most Steinmann pins in situ.

Complications

Complications following an isolated Salter innominate osteotomy are rare but may include injury to the sciatic, femoral, or lateral femoral cutaneous nerves; loss of correction; penetration of hip joint with Steinmann pins; and prominence of hardware and wound infection. Meticulous surgical technique will minimize these risks considerably. Avascular necrosis (AVN) and redislocation of the femoral head are the primary complications of concern when performing a pelvic osteotomy in combination with open reduction for the treatment of developmentally dislocated hip. Follow-up of up to skeletal maturity is recommended in order to make assessments of further hip development, or clinically significant AVN, particularly in the setting of a dislocated hip.

Postoperative Imaging (Fig. 3.8)

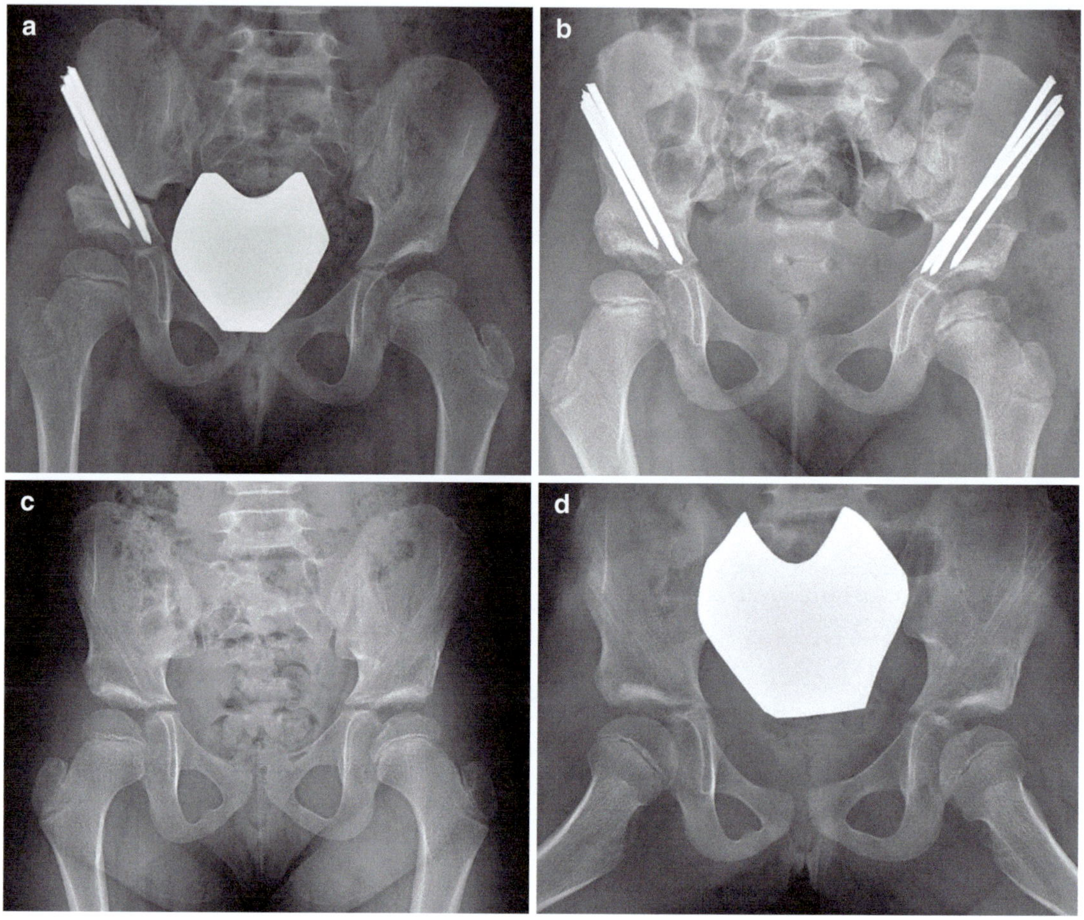

Fig. 3.8 (**a**) Anteroposterior (AP) radiograph shortly after undergoing a right sided Salter innominate osteotomy. Note the improved acetabular index; the asymmetric obliquity of the right obturator foramen, known as the "winking owl" sign; and the slight anterior translation at the posterior aspect of the osteotomy. (**b**) AP radiograph after undergoing left Salter innominate osteotomy 4 months after right side. Bilateral acetabular indices now measure <15°. (**c**) AP and (**d**) frog-leg lateral radiographs taken 2 years after bilateral staged Salter innominate osteotomies and subsequent implant removal. Both femoral heads are well covered with anatomically normal acetabular indices. The left femoral head has continued to remodel from prior avascular necrosis, and the patient remains asymptomatic. Further improvements in acetabular morphology are expected with continuing growth

Pearls and Pitfalls

- Positioning
  - Avoid positioning devices under the pelvis to avoid soft tissue crowding in the surgical field.
  - Maintain a wide surgical field during draping, particularly of the posterior hip.
- Exposure
  - A better cosmetic result is achieved with an oblique skin incision in the patient's skin crease and avoiding a vertical extension.
  - Dissection of the external oblique muscle from the iliac apophysis minimizes bleeding and postoperative pain.
  - Avoid subperiosteal dissection toward the sacroiliac joint as this may result in excessive bleeding and does not contribute to the exposure.
  - Surgical sponges placed in the subperiosteal spaces of the inner and outer tables will assist with hemostasis and exposure.

  - Splitting the periosteum at the pelvic brim enhances exposure of the iliopsoas for recession.
- Osteotomy
  - Ensure the osteotomy is oriented perpendicular to the ilium.
  - Use a pointed towel clip to grasp the distal segment. Use an anterolaterally directed rotation as you hinge the osteotomy open to avoid posterior translation.
  - Place the graft in the medial aspect of the osteotomy with cortical apposition.
  - Avoid lateral Steinmann pin placement to minimize the risk of joint violation.

Indications and Contraindications (Table 3.1)

Table 3.1 The Salter innominate osteotomy: surgical indications and contraindications

Indications
Age >18 months
Developmental dysplasia of the hip
Anterolateral acetabular insufficiency
Concentrically reducible hip
Contraindications
Age <18 months
Posterior acetabular insufficiency
Closed triradiate cartilage
Neuromuscular hip disease

Suggested Reading

Gillingham BL, Sanchez AA, Wenger DR. Pelvic osteotomies for the treatment of hip dysplasia in children and young adults. J Am Acad Orthop Surg. 1999;7:325–37.

Kalamchi A, MacEwen GD. Avascular necrosis following treatment of congenital dislocation of the hip. J Bone Joint Surg Am. 1980;62(6):876–88.

Murphy R, Kim Y. Surgical management of pediatric developmental dysplasia of the hip. J Am Acad Orthop Surg. 2016;24(9):615–24.

Salter RB. Innominate osteotomy in treatment of congenital dislocation of the hip. J Bone Joint Surg Br. 1961;43B:518–39.

Thomas SR, Wedge JH, Salter RB. Outcome at forty-five years after open reduction and innominate osteotomy for late-presenting developmental dislocation of the hip. J Bone Joint Surg Am. 2007;89(11):2341–50.

Wedge JH, Thomas SR, Salter RB. Outcome at forty-five years aftre open reduction and innominate osteotomy for late-presenting developmental dislocation of the hip: surgical technique. J Bone Joint Surg Am. 2008;90(Suppl 2, Part 2):238–53.

Weinstein SL. Natural history of congenital hip dislocation (CDH) and hip dysplasia. Clin Orthop Relat Res. 1987;225:62–76.

Single Anterior Incision Steel Triple Pelvic Osteotomy

4

M. Chad Mahan and Ira Zaltz

Introduction

Untreated acetabular dysplasia is associated with deterioration of labral and chondral structures and the eventual development of osteoarthritis of the hip. The goals of surgical intervention are to relieve pain and to slow the progressive joint deterioration by stabilizing the hip. The triple pelvic osteotomy remains an important treatment for acetabular reorientation in selected skeletally immature patients. This technique allows for dissection of the pelvis enabling osteotomies and acetabular reorientation without violating the periosteum around the triradiate cartilage. This technique includes several modifications of the original described by Le Coeur in 1965. The single-incision technique provides limited soft tissue dissection and improved cosmesis and can be performed in the supine position thereby allowing accurate intraoperative radiographs.

M. Chad Mahan
Henry Ford Health System, Detroit, MI, USA
e-mail: mmahan3@hfhs.org

I. Zaltz (✉)
Pediatric Orthopaedic Surgery, Beaumont Hospital, Royal Oak, MI, USA
e-mail: izaltz@beaumont.edu

Brief Clinical History

This 8-year-old female presented with activity-related hip pain and a history of childhood treatment of congenital hip dislocation. Serial radiographs revealed significant residual acetabular dysplasia with worsening femoral subluxation (Figs. 4.1 and 4.2). Clinical examination demonstrated a Trendelenburg gait and signs of hip irritability. In order to prevent further subluxation, to stabilize the joint while preserving remaining triradiate growth, and to mitigate clinical symptoms, a triple osteotomy was planned. The triple osteotomy described herein enables multiplanar reorientation of the acetabulum and preservation of the remaining triradiate cartilage growth.

Preoperative Imaging

The diagnosis of dysplasia is established based upon plain radiographs. The degree of anterior insufficiency can be estimated using the false profile, and superior acetabular coverage may be assessed intraoperatively using a simulated false profile (60° oblique). Functional radiographs provide an estimate of achievable acetabular coverage and joint congruity. In skeletally immature patients, acetabular version cannot be reliably determined with plain radiographs since the acetabular walls are incompletely ossified. Upper femoral dysplasia and epiphyseal morphology

R. C. Hamdy, N. Saran (eds.), *Pediatric Pelvic and Proximal Femoral Osteotomies*,
https://doi.org/10.1007/978-3-319-78033-7_4

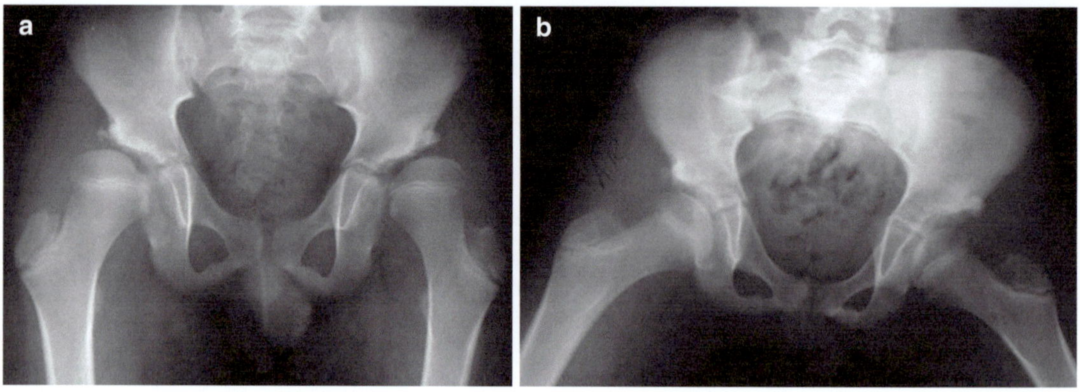

Fig. 4.1 (a) Anteroposterior pelvis and (b) frog lateral radiographs demonstrate open triradiate cartilage in a skeletally immature patient with oblique sourcil (Tonnis angle 18°), lateralization of hip center, and asymmetric sclerosis of the weight-bearing zone

are assessed on both anteroposterior (AP) and frog views. Hip joint congruity and concentricity are established based upon the AP and abduction-internal rotation radiographs and, when necessary, using arthrography.

Additional imaging options include computed tomography, magnetic resonance imaging, and ultrasonography. These modalities may be useful in complex patients such as those who have had multiple surgeries or severe recurrent subluxation.

Goals of Treatment

The goals of treatment are (1) to improve the mechanical environment of the hip joint by reorienting the acetabular weight-bearing zone, improving coverage of the femoral head and stability of the joint, (2) to relieve symptoms, and (3) to improve upon the natural history of the disorder.

Treatment Strategy

The treatment strategy begins with accurate diagnosis through history, physical exam, and imaging studies. In this case, an operative procedure is necessary that allows multiplanar acetabular reorientation to address the complex pattern of acetabular insufficiency. The surgical options are limited by skeletal immaturity, which necessitates preservation of the triradiate cartilage.

Surgical Details

Preoperative Planning

A complete history and physical examination are necessary in the evaluation of children with developmental dysplasia of the hip. In addition to a history of symptoms and prior treatment, the examination should include patient stature, spinal alignment, relative limb length, assessment of joint laxity, and neurological examination. Examination of the hip includes assessment of gait and precise documentation of range of motion. A patient must have at least 20–30° of hip abduction in order to undergo acetabular reorientation. Clinical assessment of hip rotation and femoral version is necessary in order to anticipate the need for a femoral rotational osteotomy.

Patient Positioning

The patient is placed supine on a radiolucent table and placed under general anesthesia. A Foley catheter is inserted to decompress and pro-

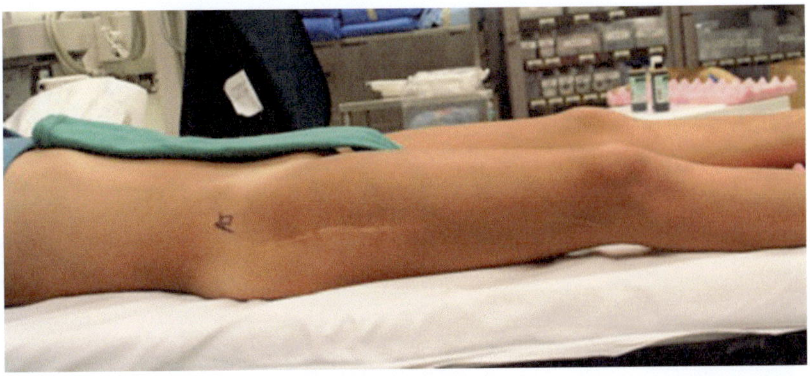

Fig. 4.2 Patient positioned supine on radiolucent table. Note the frontal plane of the pelvis is horizontal and the pelvis is not rotated

tect the bladder during intrapelvic surgery. The patient is carefully positioned to ensure that the frontal plane of the pelvis is horizontal and the pelvis is not rotated (see Fig. 4.2). After positioning a formal AP, pelvis radiograph will establish a baseline for intraoperative comparison after acetabular reorientation. The entire leg, hip, abdomen, and lower chest are included in the surgical field. The surgeon stands on operative side of hip. The assistant and fluoroscope are positioned on the contralateral side. Ensure that the contralateral arm is positioned to facilitate maneuvering of the fluoroscope. The monitor is positioned at the patient's feet.

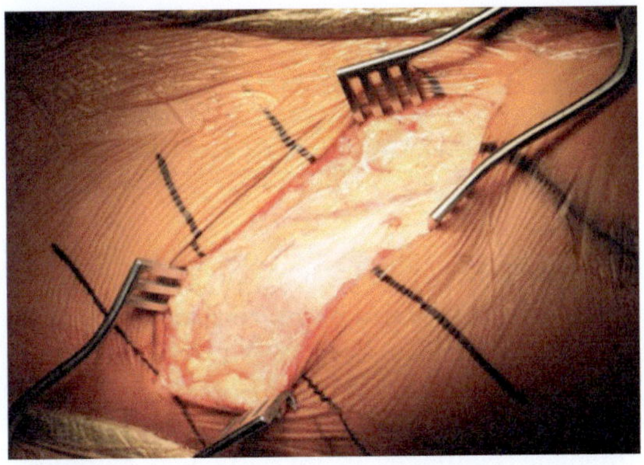

Fig. 4.3 The tensor fascia lata-sartorius interval can be identified distally

Superficial Dissection

There exist many modifications and options for osteotomies. Historically, the procedure has been performed using a two-incision technique where the ischium and/or the pubis are osteotomized through a medial proximal thigh incision or buttock incision depending upon surgeon preference. This chapter describes a single-incision technique that can be performed through an oblique "bikini"-type or a longitudinal Smith-Petersen-type incision. Incision begins just distal to the anterior superior iliac spine. The subcutaneous tissue is divided in line with the skin incision. The fascia of the external oblique muscle is exposed proximally. Distally a subcutaneous flap is elevated to expose the distal tensor fascia lata-sartorius interval (Fig. 4.3). The fascia of the external oblique muscle is incised laterally and the muscle elevated from the iliac apophysis. The tensor-sartorius interval is opened longitudinally with care to preserve the lateral femoral cutaneous nerve. The interval is opened and developed proximally in order to identify the anterior brim of the pelvis. The iliac apophysis is incised along and in line with the iliac crest allowing subperiosteal exposure of the medial and lateral table of the ilium to the sciatic notch. The rectus femoris muscle is identified within the tensor-sartorius interval, and either the tendon is divided or the AIIS apophysis with tendon attached is reflected medially (Fig. 4.4). At this point, the periosteum of the medial ilium is incised enabling medial retraction of the iliacus and psoas muscle and extraperiosteal exposure of the pubis. The iliopectineal membrane is then carefully incised which exposes the retroperitoneum and enables extraperiosteal exposure of the ischium and preservation of the periosteum attached to the

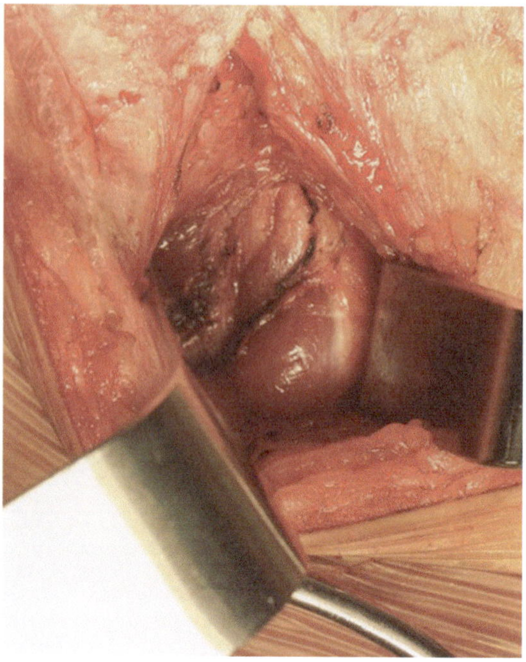

Fig. 4.4 Within the tensor-sartorius interval, the rectus femoris is identified overlying the hip capsule

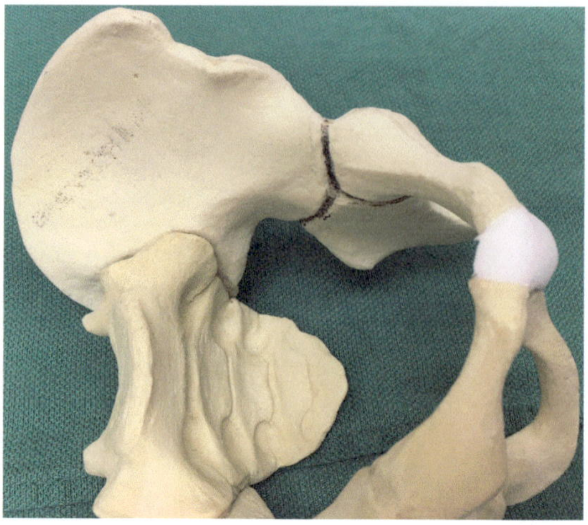

Fig. 4.5 Location of the triradiate cartilage on sawbones model

triradiate cartilage. If intraarticular pathology requires a capsulotomy, the direct and indirect head of the rectus femoris as well as the iliocapsularis muscle need to be released and reflected away from the anterior capsule. Exposure of the acetabular rim may assist the surgeon to identify anterior wall of the acetabulum helping to estimate the degree of acetabular version. The anterior wall in this location is primarily chondral and often difficult to interpret with radiographs. Placing a radiopaque instrument on the anterior wall can help identify its precise location intraoperatively with the assistance of fluoroscopy.

Deep Dissection

Careful dissection around the pubis and medial ischium as well as knowledge of the anatomic location of the triradiate cartilage along the medial ilium, ischium, and pubis is essential so that iatrogenic damage to the triradiate is avoided and growth arrest prevented (Fig. 4.5). The remainder of the pelvis dissection is performed in a supraperiosteal fashion to avoid creating a growth arrest.

Extraperiosteal Dissection of the Distal Ilium The extraperiosteal dissection is performed by incising the iliacus fascia (medial iliac periosteum) from the anterior superior iliac spine to the apex of the sciatic notch. The iliacus muscle must be carefully dissected from the periosteum and then the periosteum carefully elevated from the sciatic notch in order to prevent damage to the superior gluteal artery and sciatic nerve as they exit the greater sciatic notch. The iliacus muscle can now be reflected away from the investing fascia and pubis leaving the periosteum attached to the distal ilium (Fig. 4.6). This can be accomplished through blunt dissection with a small sponge or Kittner. Flexion of the hip and knee relaxes the iliopsoas. Slight adduction can aid in medial retraction of the deep soft tissues. The iliopectineal eminence, now exposed, is the anterior limb of the triradiate cartilage and must not be disturbed.

Exposure of the Anterior Ilium Deep dissection between the psoas tendon and hip capsule can now proceed through either of two similar approaches. The psoas sheath can be dissected from the medial hip capsule exposing the

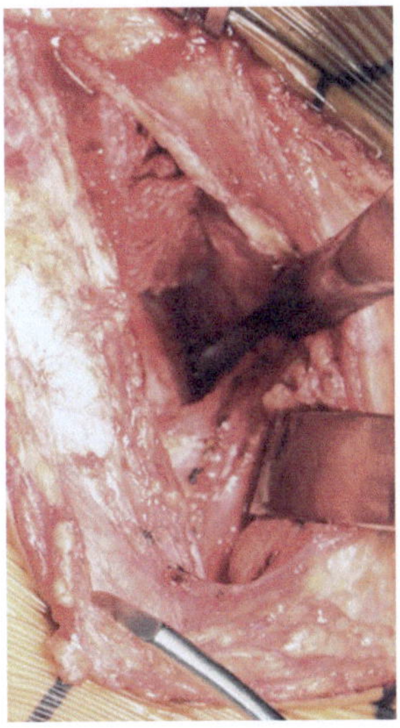

Fig. 4.6 Retractor above is within the sciatic notch, reflecting the iliacus muscle away from the investing fascia and pubis, leaving the periosteum attached to the distal ilium. The second retractor at the bottom of the image is exposing the psoas muscle distally and superifically

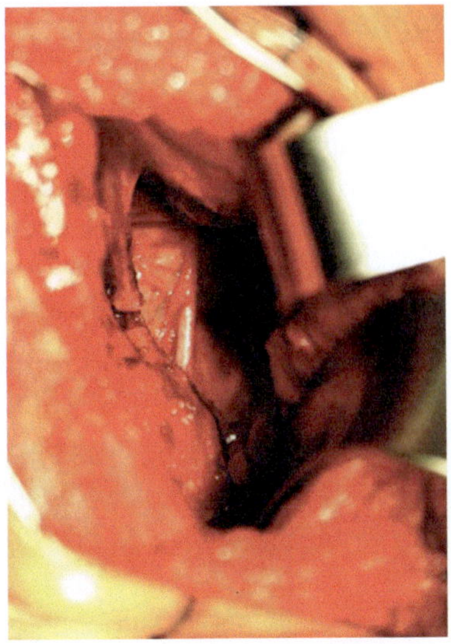

Fig. 4.7 The obturator nerve can be identified within the retroperitoneal fat and will be found coursing distally and laterally toward the superolateral obturator foramen

posteromedial periarticular fat, at which point the anterior ischium is identified by digital palpation. Alternatively, the psoas sheath can be incised longitudinally and the posterior psoas sheath perforated and spread using dissecting scissors in order to access the ischium. Either approach requires the development of planes to access the anterior ischium and pubis that are contiguous; otherwise acetabular mobility may be limited by the restraint of soft tissue attachments.

Extraperiosteal Exposure of the Pubis and Medial Ischial After establishing the anterior ischial plane, the pubis and medial ischial exposures are developed. This exposure necessitates releasing the iliopectineal fascia (medial fascia of the iliacus muscle) from its attachment along the iliopectineal line (medial ilium and posterior pubis). Gentle retraction on the iliacus muscle will expose the iliopectineal fascia and facilitate its release from the iliopectineal line up to the point of the planned pubic osteotomy. Care is taken not to proceed too far medially due to risk of injury to the femoral vessels.

The golden-colored retroperitoneal fat is now visible within the pelvis. The obturator nerve can be identified within the retroperitoneal fat and will be found coursing distally and laterally toward the superolateral obturator foramen (Fig. 4.7). A Deaver or Langenbeck retractor may be used to retract the iliopsoas complex. Ray-Tec sponges are packed along the medial ischium along the course of the planned ischial osteotomy in order to protect the viscera and neurovascular structures from the osteotome that may protrude medially. While osteotomizing the ischium, the ischial periosteum is simultaneously divided using the osteotome.

Finally the pubis is exposed and prepared in an extraperiosteal fashion. A large right-angle dissector can be used to create an opening in the obturator fascia at the junction of the superolateral aspect of the medial pubis and ischium. At this point, the passage of suture through the opening can facilitate passage of the Gigli saw prior to osteotomy. Damage to the pubic component of the triradiate cartilage can occur following exposure of the pubis or posterior column by stripping of the perichondrial ring of LaCroix off of the triradiate cartilage.

Osteotomies

The ischial cut is performed first and is done under radiographic guidance using an angled Ganz-type osteotome. The starting point is identified and confirmed with a 50° cephalad-directed fluoroscopy image (Fig. 4.8). The osteotomy begins medial and distal to the hip capsule at the level of the infracotyloid groove just distal to the acetabulum and is directed into the lesser sciatic foramen just distal to the ischial spine. Using 50° cephalad and 55° oblique fluoroscopic guidance, the ischium is cut in two passes, one medial and another lateral. The medial ischium is cut before the lateral ischium, and the position of the osteotome is confirmed radiographically on both views during the osteotomy (Figs. 4.9 and 4.10). The ischium is wider anterior than posterior, and the osteotome direction must be adjusted to avoid passing into the soft tissue posterolaterally where the sciatic nerve can be injured. Rather than relying on leg position to minimize nerve injury, it is important to monitor the position of the osteotome radiographically to avoid penetrating beyond the cortical margin so as to avoid neurovascular trauma. Finally, rotating or prying the osteotome and observing displacement of the ischium radiographically confirm completion of the osteotomy.

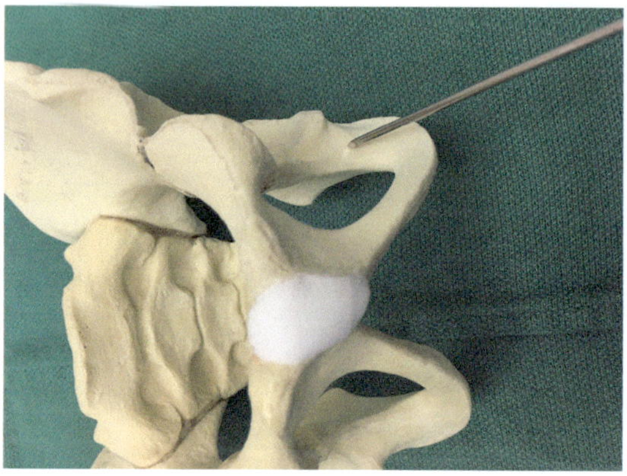

Fig. 4.8 Starting point of ischial cut on sawbones model viewed with 50° cephalad-directed angulation

The pubic osteotomy should be performed second. This osteotomy may be performed using a Gigli saw or osteotome. It is important to protect the obturator nerve no matter the method

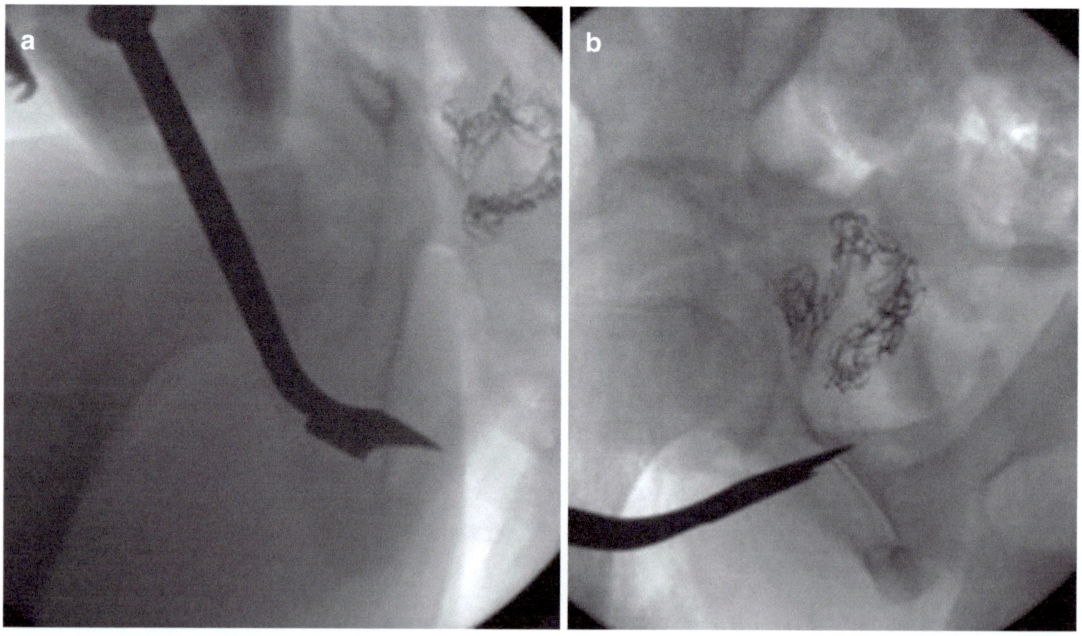

Fig. 4.9 Orthogonal views (**a**, **b**) demonstrating positioning of Ganz osteotome adjacent to infracotyloid groove and directed just distal to the ischial spine at the apex of the lesser sciatic foramen. Note Ray-Tec sponge protecting neurovascular structures

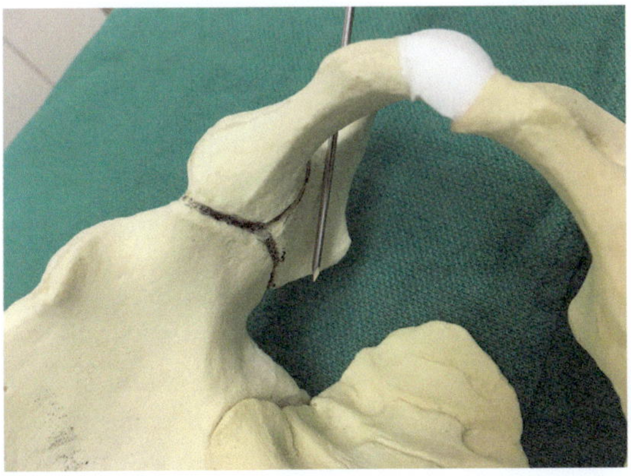

Fig. 4.10 Planned ischial cut viewed from medial aspect of sawbones model at 55° oblique angulation. Note that the osteotomy is directed into the lesser sciatic foramen just distal to ischial spine

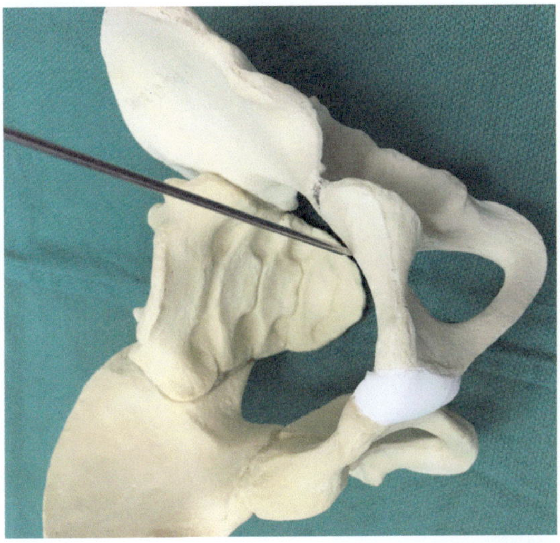

Fig. 4.11 Location of pubic osteotomy on sawbones model

used to osteotomize the pubis. The pubic osteotomy must be located medial to the iliopectineal eminence in order to avoid cutting through and injuring the triradiate cartilage (Fig. 4.11). The suture or tape that was previously passed through the obturator foramen is now used to pass a Gigli saw. A curved Satinsky-type clamp may also assist in the safe passage of the Gigli saw through the obturator foramen (Fig. 4.12). Rang, Crego, or Hohmann retractors can be used to protect surrounding structures around the sciatic notch and

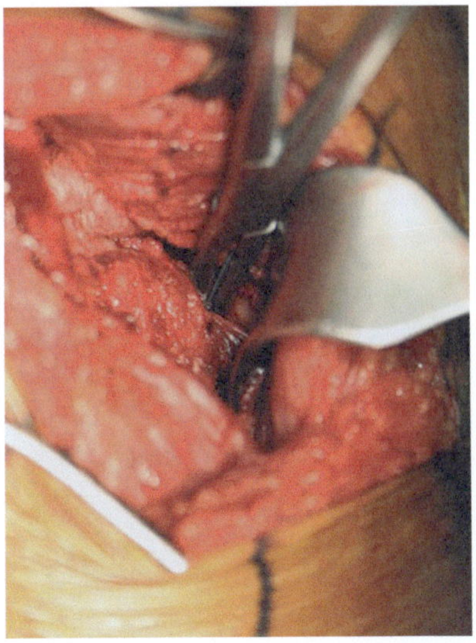

Fig. 4.12 A curved Satinsky clamp is passed from medial to lateral through the obturator foramen assists in safe passage of the Gigli saw

obturator foramen. It is useful to angle the osteotomy approximately 30–45° relative to long axis of the pubis and to incline the osteotomy from slightly medial to lateral to facilitate rotation of the acetabulum. Of note, the periosteum tends to be very thick in this area and needs to be completely divided in order to maximize mobility of the acetabular fragment.

The final cut should be made at the ilium and can be done in one of the two ways. A Gigli saw can be used to make a Salter-like osteotomy, or the ilium can be osteotomized using a saw in a manner similar to the Bernese periacetabular osteotomy. If using a saw, it is important to take care when continuing into the sciatic notch which must be done proximally, whether using either a saw or Gigli saw, making certain to preserve the posterior limb of the triradiate cartilage and to avoid injuring the superior gluteal neurovascular structures (Fig. 4.13). A Kalamchi modification may be used to facilitate "docking" of the ilium. The latter technique is employed if using an abductor-sparing approach. Following the iliac osteotomy, the acetabulum is freely mobile. Two Kirschner wires are used to adjust the position of the acetabulum. One is inserted proximal to the acetabulum and a second medial to the acetabulum, either in the pubis or medial acetabular wall.

Since the bone is immature, it is less dense than adult bone, and great care is used in manipulation. Excessive traction can disrupt the bone and compromise fixation (Fig. 4.14).

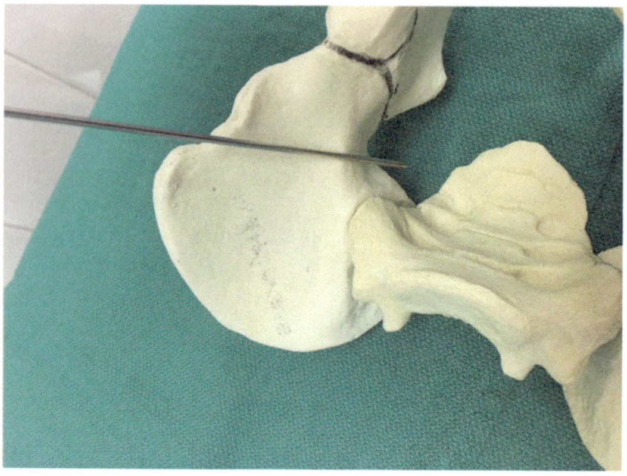

Fig. 4.13 Starting point and trajectory during osteotomy of the ilium on sawbones model. Note the planned trajectory is aimed proximally to avoid damage to the triradiate cartilage

Acetabular Positioning and Fixation

The acetabulum is maneuvered into position to correct the dysplasia based on individual anatomic considerations. Most cases require a combination of acetabular flexion, adduction, and medial rotation. The reoriented acetabulum is now provisionally fixed with Steinmann pins. A formal intraoperative AP pelvis radiograph is obtained which can be compared with the initial baseline radiograph. Again, a marker on the anterior wall of the acetabulum is important to visualize the largely chondral anterior wall in order to approximate acetabular version (Fig. 4.15). Once the appropriate position has been confirmed, fixation is performed with Steinmann pins or screws (see Fig. 4.15). Pin or screw size should be appropriate to ensure adequate stability of the acetabulum. Depending upon the type and shape of the iliac osteotomy, a tricortical iliac graft is used to enhance stability. Allograft or autograft can be

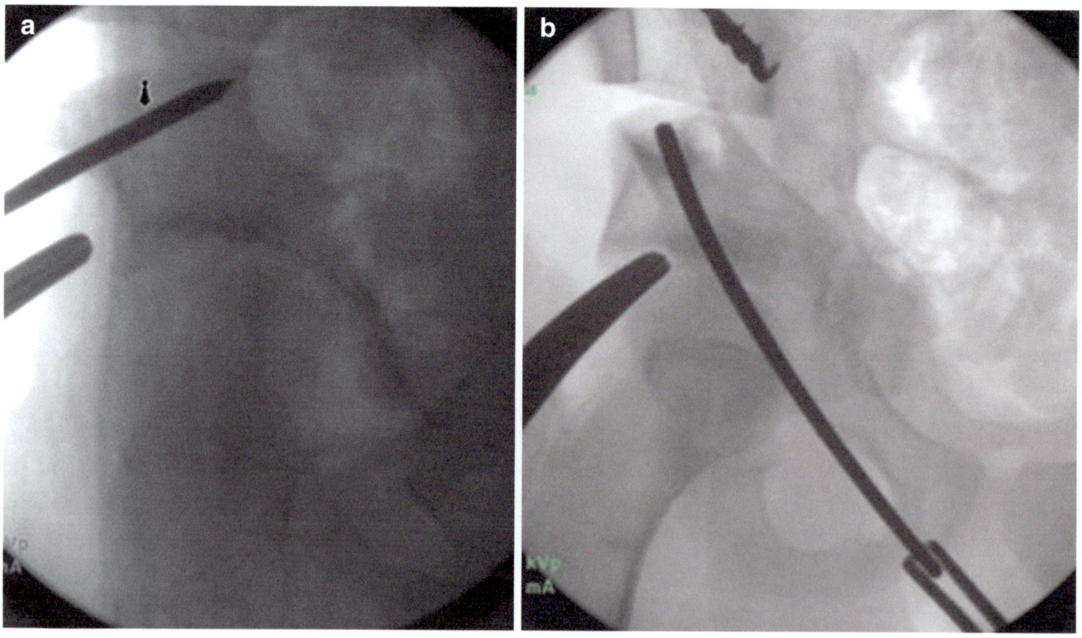

Fig. 4.14 A Kirschner wire is positioned in the supracetabular ilium. Metzenbaum scissors used to mark the anterior acetabular wall on both intraoperative false-profile (**a**) and anteroposterior (**b**) projections

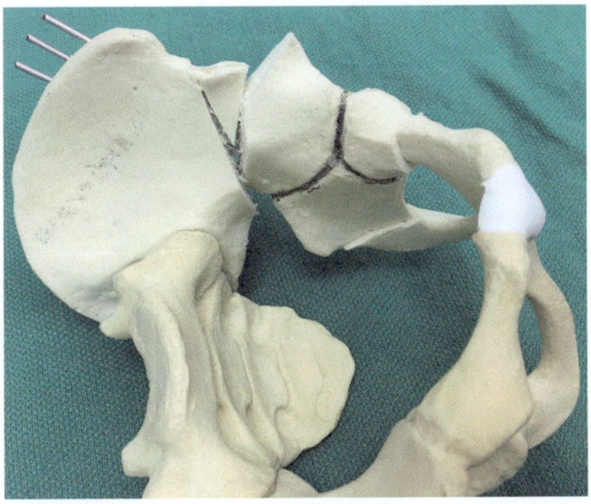

Fig. 4.15 Final fixation option with Steinman pins shown in sawbones model. Notice pins are left proud to allow ease of removal. Also note the autograft carefully harvested and pinned into defect

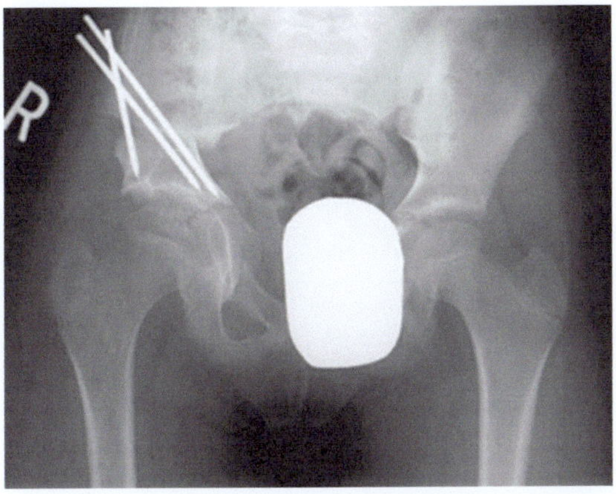

Fig. 4.16 Postoperative views demonstrating final position and fixation of acetabulum. Note that the Steinmann pins are left proud to facilitate removal

used depending on bone size, prior surgery, and need for concomitant limb lengthening. Steinmann pins are cut to appropriate length to facilitate easy removal, and screws are left proud to allow suture fixation of the apophysis as well as ease of removal (Fig. 4.16). If additional intraarticular surgery is needed to address labral pathology or head-neck junction morphology, it can be performed after definitive fixation is secure.

Closure is performed in a layered fashion. Suction drainage is not routinely employed. Spica casting is not routinely necessary.

Patients are admitted to the hospital for analgesia and postoperative antibiotics. Weight bearing is restricted to toe touch, and active hip motion is avoided for the first 6 weeks. Younger patients with poor muscular leg control following surgery are restricted to wheelchair transfers for 2–4 weeks. Once radiographic evidence of union is established, progressive weight bearing is permitted, and muscle strengthening exercises are started under the direction of physical therapy.

Postoperative Imaging

The patient is followed with radiographs taken at 2 weeks and 6 weeks postoperative. Thereafter repeat radiographs are usually performed at 3 and 6 months and then periodically up to the discretion of the physician.

Pearls and Pitfalls

- Acetabular dysplasia can include a combination of anterolateral, lateral, posterior, and global acetabular insufficiency. As such, careful attention must be given to ensuring adequate version of the hip in the final position. Undercoverage can result in instability, and overcoverage can cause femoroacetabular impingement. Since the acetabular rim can be cartilaginous, using a metal marker on fluoroscopy can aid in determining the true version of the redirected acetabulum in the final position. The surgeon must take care to avoid acetabular retroversion.
- This osteotomy is indicated for correction of acetabular dysplasia in skeletally immature individuals in whom osteotomy through the triradiate cartilage may produce a growth arrest that may adversely affect continued acetabular growth and development.

- Simultaneous femoral osteotomies may be necessary in selected cases especially in cases where there is either significant gait dysfunction with either severe intoeing or out-toeing due to femoral malrotation or if the joint is not spherically congruent.
- Failure to fully divide the periosteum, especially that of the pubis, can result in difficulty mobilizing the acetabulum. Therefore, if movement of the acetabulum seems restricted, ensure that the pubic periosteum is completely divided.
- Fixation may be difficult especially in immature bone. Adding an anterior to posterior screw from the acetabulum to the ilium will accentuate stability. If using screws to stabilize the acetabulum, they should be left between 5 and 10 mm proud so that the iliac apophysis can be closed beneath the screw head, theref\genic injury.

Indications and Contraindications (Table 4.1)

Table 4.1 Single anterior incision steel triple pelvic osteotomy: surgical indications and contraindications

Treat either symptomatic individuals or asymptomatic patients with sequentially deteriorating radiographic morphology
Other osteotomies—including single innominate (Salter, Pemberton, or Dega), triple innominate (Steele, Tonnis), and Bernese periacetabular osteotomy—may be considered, depending on the familiarity of the surgeon, age of the patient, and the degree and type of dysplasia
Children with symptomatic acetabular dysplasia, particularly those exhibiting either clinical signs or radiographic signs of hip joint dysfunction, are candidates for surgical reconstruction

Suggested Reading

Kim HT, Wenger D. The morphology of residual acetabular deficiency in childhood hip dysplasia: three-dimensional computed tomographic analysis. J Pediatr Orthop. 1997;17(5):637–47.

Lipton GE, Bowen JR. A new modified technique of triple osteotomy of the innominate bone for acetabular dysplasia. Clin Orthop Relat Res. 2005;434:78–85.

O'Connor PA, Mullhall KJ, Kearns SR, Sheehan E, McCormack D. Triple pelvic osteotomy in Legg-Calve-Perthes disease using a single anterolateral incision. J Pediatr Orthop B. 2003;12(6):387–9.

Steel HH. Triple osteotomy of the innominate bone. J Bone Joint Surg Am. 1973;55(2):343–50.

Tönnis D, Behrens K, Tscharani F. A modified technique of the triple pelvic osteotomy: early results. J Pediatr Orthop. 1981;1(3):241–9.

Pol le Cœur Triple Pelvic Osteotomy

5

Jérôme Sales de Gauzy and Franck Accadbled

Introduction

The Pol le Cœur osteotomy (PLCO) is a triple pelvic osteotomy that combines innominate osteotomy of the ilium and osteotomies of the iliopubic (superior) and ischiopubic (inferior) rami (Fig. 5.1).

The objectives are to improve femoral head coverage and coxofemoral joint stability. It is a reorientation osteotomy. The acetabulum tilts in retroversion, improving the anterior and lateral coverage but reducing posterior femoral head coverage. PLCO maintains hyaline cartilage contact between the femoral head and acetabulum. The main indications are hip dysplasia in childhood and Legg-Calvé-Perthes disease requiring containment.

Brief Clinical History

A 7.5-year-old old boy with Legg-Calvé-Perthes disease

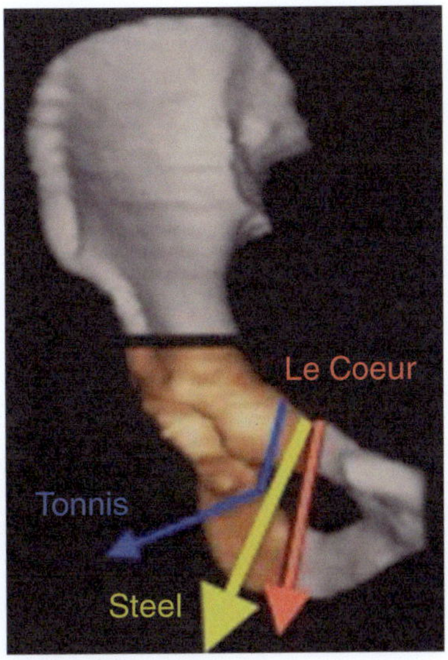

Fig. 5.1 Pol le Cœur osteotomy

J. S. de Gauzy (✉) · F. Accadbled
Pediatric Orthopaedics, Hôpital des Enfants, CHU de Toulouse, Toulouse, France
e-mail: salesdegauzy.j@chu-toulouse.fr; accadbled.f@chu-toulouse.fr

R. C. Hamdy, N. Saran (eds.), *Pediatric Pelvic and Proximal Femoral Osteotomies*,
https://doi.org/10.1007/978-3-319-78033-7_5

Preoperative Imaging

X-ray shows a fragmentation stage, Herring B–C, with medial and lateral subluxation of the femoral head (Fig. 5.2).

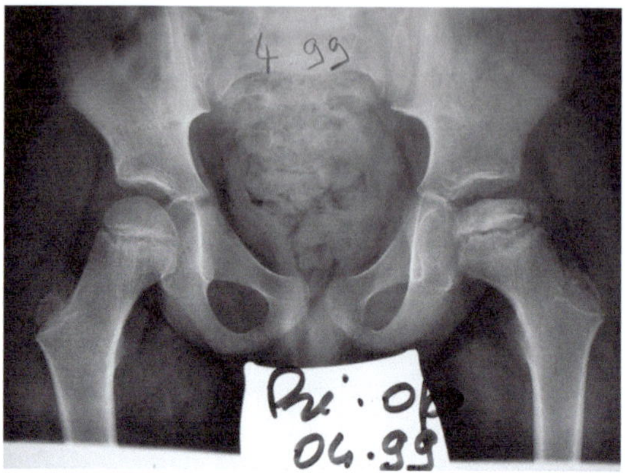

Fig. 5.2 A 7.5-year-old boy with Legg-Calvé-Perthes disease. Preoperative X-ray

Goals of Treatment

The goal of the PLCO is to improve containment of the femoral head to allow for good remodeling during the reossification phase.

Treatment Strategy

Preoperative Arthrography

Preoperative dynamic arthrography is helpful to simulate the effects of the reorientation osteotomy and to verify if the femoral head can be congruently centered into the acetabulum (Fig. 5.3). In case of hinge abduction, the PLCO is not indicated.

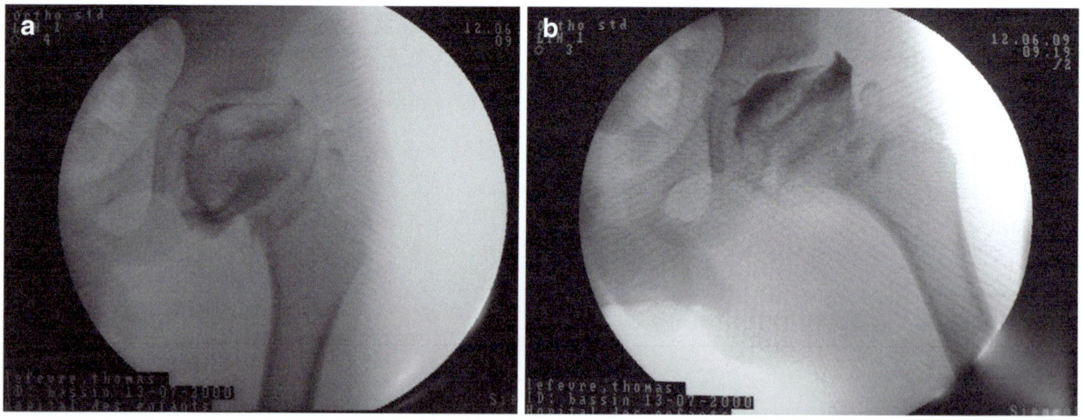

Fig. 5.3 (**a**) Preoperative arthrography. In neutral position, we see flattening and subluxation of the femoral head; (**b**) in abduction, the femoral head is well centered

Surgical Details

Patient Positioning

The surgery is performed under general anesthesia on a radiolucent table. The child is positioned in the three-quarter supine position, and the position is maintained by a sheet rolled behind the child's back. The entire buttock area must be left free to facilitate access for surgical exposure as well as to allow for intraoperative repositioning of the leg as required. The entire leg is draped free (Fig. 5.4).

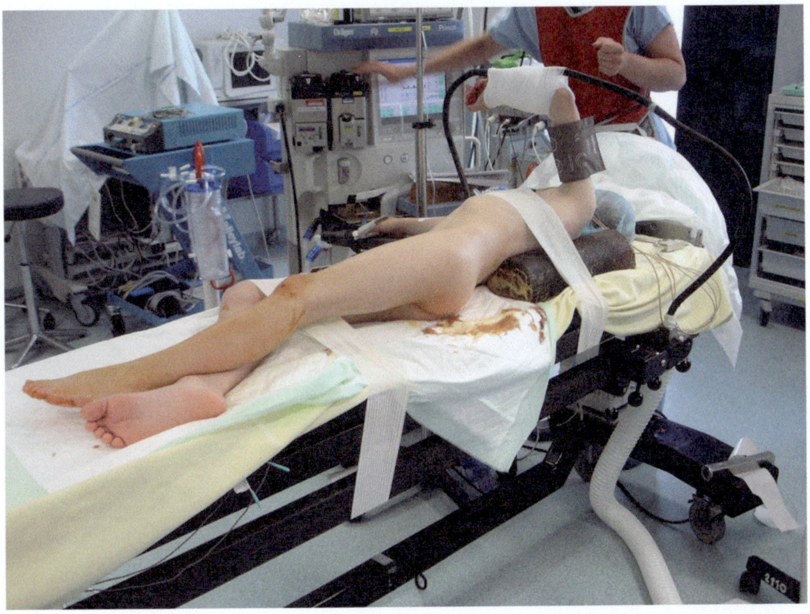

Fig. 5.4 Patient positioning

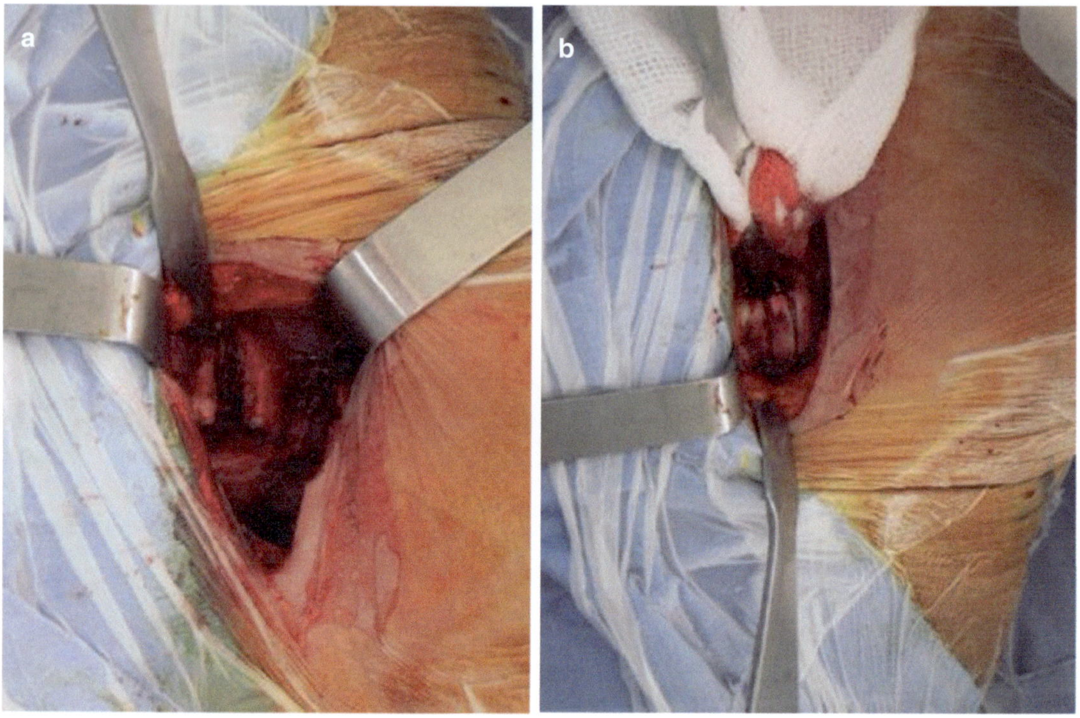

Fig. 5.5 The superior ramus (**a**) and inferior ramus (**b**) osteotomies of a left hemipelvis are seen. A 5mm bone resection is recommended for improved mobilization of the acetabular fragment

Osteotomy of the Iliopubic and Ischiopubic Rami

Approach The procedure begins with the superior and inferior ramus osteotomies. The coxofemoral joint is placed in flexion-abduction and external rotation during the approach.

The incision is vertical in the genitofemoral fold. The adductor muscles are isolated. Adductor longus is detached from the pubic tubercle. Gracilis is detached only if needed to provide adequate exposure. The obturator nerve along the adductor brevis muscle should be preserved. It is not necessary to recess the adductor brevis muscle. The superior ramus is located in the pectineus-adductor longus interval. The inferior ramus is accessed by bluntly dissecting through the adductor magnus which is seen once the adductor longus is reflected.

Osteotomies The inferior ramus is dissected subperiosteally to prevent injury to the cavernous body. The superior ramus can be approached extraperiosteally. Two Hohmann retractors are placed, protecting the soft tissues during the osteotomy. The osteotomies are carried out near the pubis with an osteotome. A 5 mm bone resection using a bone rongeur is recommended to obtain better mobilization (Fig. 5.5). After the osteotomy, deep bleeding may occur, which is normally easily stopped by applying pressure with a hemostatic compress. The adductor muscles are left in place or can be sutured to prevent formation of a dimple. The wound is closed in two layers (subcutaneous and cutaneous) with a suction drain installed.

Innominate Osteotomy

Approach A bikini-type incision is made 1 cm below the anterosuperior iliac spine. It extends from the middle of the iliac crest to the middle of the groin fold.

The tensor-sartorius interval is opened. In this space, the lateral femoral cutaneous nerve should be identified and protected (Fig. 5.6). The tensor fasciae lata and sartorius muscles are separated from bottom to top up to the anterosuperior iliac spine and the anterior perichondrium of the ilium, between the superior and inferior iliac spines. The perichondrium is incised using a scalpel.

Incision of the Iliac Crest The oblique muscles of the abdomen cover the iliac crest. They are detached below the iliac crest and reflected medially and cranially, revealing the cartilaginous iliac crest, which is incised to the bone, using a scalpel. The incision extends from the anterior edge of the anterosuperior iliac spine to the middle third of the iliac crest. It should be linear, taking care to separate the crest into medial and lateral parts equally (Fig. 5.7).

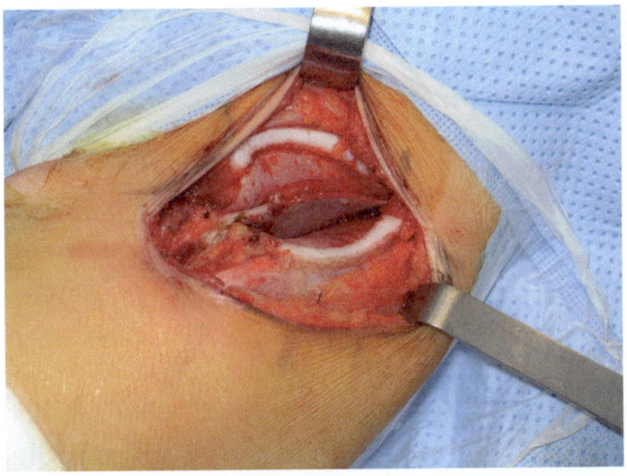

Fig. 5.7 Incision of the iliac crest

Exposure of the Ilium Using a periosteal elevator, the medial and lateral sides of the crest cartilage are detached from the bony iliac crest and left attached to the periosteum. The iliac fossa (the medial iliac fossa) and the gluteal surface can be exposed very easily in a subperiosteal fashion. The dissection extends to the sciatic notch (Fig. 5.8). During the medial dissection, hemostasis of one or two arteries is achieved by coagulation if the arteries are visible or by placing wax if these arteries have been cut.

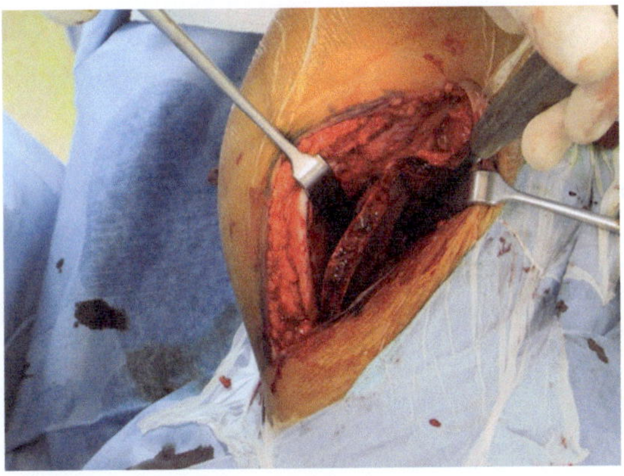

Fig. 5.8 Dissection to the sciatic notch

Psoas Intramuscular Lengthening Psoas lengthening facilitates mobilization of the acetabulum and is performed routinely. It is done extraperiosteally. The psoas-iliac muscle is located in contact with the medial periosteum, facing the iliopubic eminence. The femoral nerve located within the iliac muscle is identified and protected. The approach to the muscle fibers is easy. They are pulled up using a retractor, and then, flexing the hip at least 70°, the tendon of the psoas muscle is revealed. It is sectioned at the tendon-muscle fiber junction.

Positioning of the Gigli Saw The Gigli saw should be positioned in the sciatic notch. It is located just in the vertical direction of the anterosuperior iliac spine. The periosteum is detached both medially and laterally with a curved raspatory. A raspatory with blunt edges (a Chiari-type raspatory) can be useful to enlarge the passage. Two specially designed Rang retractors are positioned in the sciatic notch to improve exposure. To facilitate saw passage, we recommend first passing a suture to which the saw is then attached. The direction should be from inward to outward to prevent damage to the sciatic nerve.

Osteotomy The saw should be new and waxed. Two retractors are positioned in the area to protect the crest cartilage and the skin from the saw. The osteotomy line is perpendicular to the iliac wing. It starts at the sciatic notch and ends just above the anteroinferior iliac spine. The saw action should be regular, wide, rapid, and smooth.

Harvesting the Graft A bicortical graft is harvested using Liston forceps on the anterior and superior part of the ilium. It should be triangular to perfectly match the anterior opening. The base corresponds to the anterior ilium edge.

Mobilization of the Acetabular Block Two sharp bone holders are placed on both sides of the innominate osteotomy line symmetrically positioned as far back as possible. The upper fragment is maintained immobile, whereas the lower fragment is mobilized downward, outward, and forward. Displacement should be assisted with the Salter maneuver, consisting of placing the heel on the contralateral knee. It is very important to check that, at the sciatic notch, the cortices have remained in contact and that there is no posterior displacement of the distal fragment.

Placing the Graft and Fixation The graft is placed at the anterior opening (Fig. 5.9) and then fixed with using two wires (diameter 15–18 depending on the child's age). Smooth wires, which are easier to remove than threaded wires, can be employed, though threaded wires prevent migration. The wires are put in place with a power driver beginning with the wing of the ilium in the graft harvest site. They are directed toward the posterior column. Ideally, the wires transfixate the graft. They should be driven 1–2 cm into the distal pelvic segment. Then the hip must be mobilized to ensure that the wires are not protruding into the hip joint.

Closure

The crest cartilage is carefully closed using cross stitches. We advise removing an additional bone triangle from the iliac wing to facilitate the closure of the crest cartilage. The wires are then bent and cut so as to be flush with the iliac crest (Fig. 5.10). This will facilitate later removal. The oblique muscles are then reinserted. Subcuticular skin closure is generally done using absorbable suture.

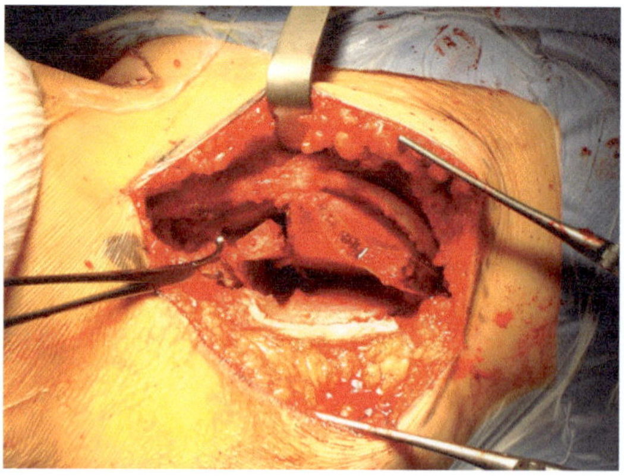

Fig. 5.9 Mobilization of the acetabular block. The acetabulum is mobilized downward, outward, and forward. The graft is placed at the anterior opening

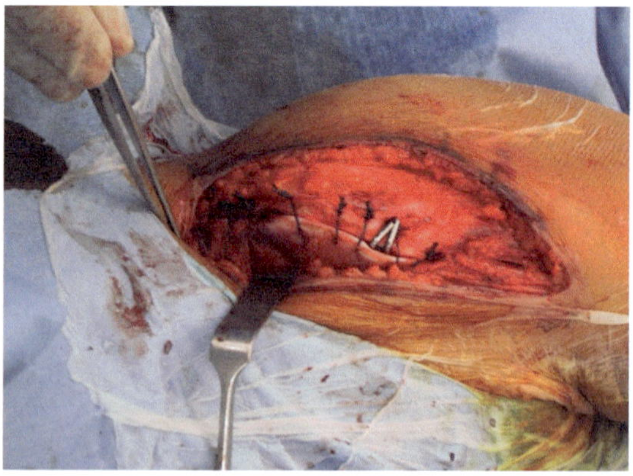

Fig. 5.10 Closure with wires up to the iliac crest

Postoperative Imaging (Fig. 5.11a, b)

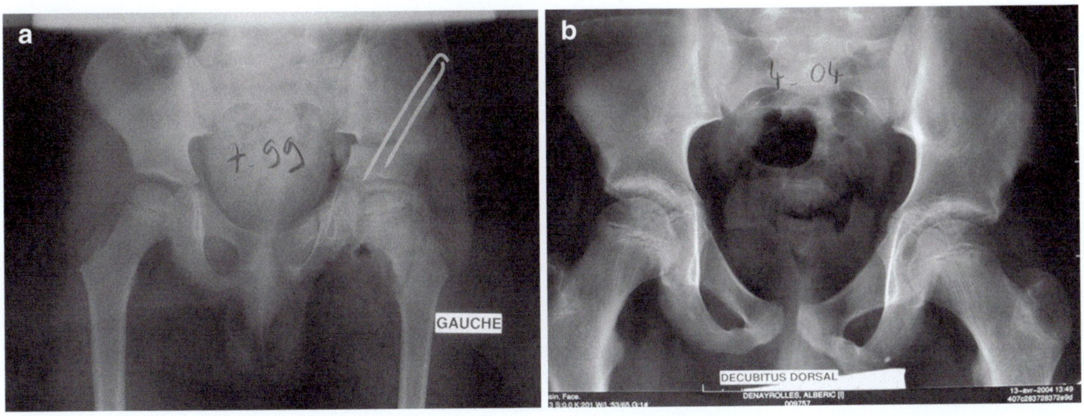

Fig. 5.11 (**a**) postoperative X-ray; (**b**) X-ray at 4-year follow-up

The child is placed supine and an anteroposterior radiograph is taken. It should show ovalization of the obturator foramen, showing the amount of the pelvic tilt and the femoral head coverage with normalization of the center edge angle and the acetabular index as well as improved lateral coverage of the femoral head. One criterion for a good osteotomy is the existence of a posterior hinge between the two iliac fragments with no diastasis or backward displacement of the distal fragment (see Fig. 5.2b, c).

Postoperative Course

A plaster or fiberglass hip spica cast is made with the hip positioned in slight abduction and neutral rotation.

After 45 days, the cast and wires are removed, and clinical and radiological evaluations are performed. Weight bearing is generally authorized 2 weeks after cast removal.

Pearls and Pitfalls

- The PLCO is a redirectional osteotomy. It modifies the orientation of the acetabulum without changing the volume. The acetabulum is redirected forward, downward, and outward. Anterior and lateral femoral head coverage is improved, but posterior coverage is reduced. Therefore, in cases of posterior insufficiency, this osteotomy should be avoided.
- Proper rotation of the acetabulum is the most important part of the procedure. Over-rotation anteriorly will generate anterior impingement. Over-rotation laterally can produce lateral impingement or hinged abduction.
- The femoral head must be fully reducible before considering a PLCO.
- A minimum of 30° abduction is required in considering the PLCO.
- Preoperative arthrogram is useful to simulate the effects of PLCO and to verify joint congruency prior to proceeding.
- Postoperative abduction should reach at least 10°; otherwise, the correction needs to be decreased.

Indications and Contraindications (Table 5.1)

Table 5.1 Pol le Cœur triple pelvic osteotomy: surgical indications and contraindications

Main indication
Hip dysplasia between the ages of 5 and 10 years. Before 5 years old, innominate Salter osteotomy can be sufficient. After 10 years old, Tonnis or Ganz osteotomies are preferable
Legg-Calvé-Perthes disease
Others indications
Sequelae of septic arthritis
Neurological hip, only when insufficiency is anterior and lateral with a normal posterior coverage
Contraindications
Stiff hip
Lack of congruence
Absence of centering in abduction
Posterior acetabular deficiency

Further Reading

Le Cœur P. Correction des défauts d'orientation de l'articulation coxofémorale par ostéotomie de l'isthme iliaque. Rev Chir Orthop. 1965;5:211–2.

Pailhé R, Cavaignac E, Murgier J, Cahuzac JP, de Gauzy JS, Accadbled F. Triple osteotomy of the pelvis for Legg-Calve-Perthes disease: a mean fifteen year follow-up. Int Orthop. 2016;40(1):115–22.

Sales de Gauzy J. Indications de ostéotomies pelviennes chez l'enfant. In: Duparc J, editor. Conférences d'enseignement 1997 (cahiers d'enseignement de la SOFCOT, no. 62). Paris: Expansion Scientifique Publications; 1997. p. 71–90.

Sales de Gauzy J. Pelvic reorientation osteotomies and acetabuloplasties in children. Surgical technique. Orthop Traumatol Surg Res. 2010;96(7):793–9.

Tönnis Triple Pelvic Osteotomy

6

Karl E. Rathjen and Andrew D. W. Tice

Introduction

There are a number of redirectional osteotomies that have been described to treat acetabular dysplasia in patients with an open triradiate cartilage. Classically, these procedures are described by the number of osteotomies made in the ilium and/or the surgeon who described the procedure: single/Salter, double/Sutherland, and triple/Steel, Carlioz, and Tönnis. The most significant alteration in Tönnis's version of the triple innominate osteotomy, described in 1976, is the location of the ischial osteotomy. This osteotomy is proximal to the sacrospinous ligament, which allows greater freedom of movement and, particularly, medialization of the acetabular block (Fig. 6.1). In addition, this technique preserves the ligaments coursing from the sacrum to the ischium. The original description directs the surgeon to perform the operation in a staged fashion; first, the patient is positioned prone to complete the osteotomy of the ischium and then repositioned supine to perform the iliac and pubic osteotomies. Alternatively, the procedure may be performed with the patient in the semi-lateral position, which is described in the technique below.

K. E. Rathjen · A. D. W. Tice (✉)
Department of Orthopaedic Surgery, Texas Scottish Rite Hospital for Children, Dallas, TX, USA
e-mail: karl.rathjen@tsrh.org; tice@ualberta.ca

Brief Clinical History

This 3-year and 7-month-old female was treated for developmental dysplasia of the right hip. The patient's risk factors include female gender, firstborn child, oligohydramnios, and a strong family history. Her mother had also been treated with open hip reduction, complicated by progressive subluxation and avascular necrosis. The patient originally presented at the age of 1 year and 5 months with a right hip dislocation. After 4 weeks of Bryant's traction, the child was taken to the operating room. Closed reduction was unsuccessful, and she underwent open reduction of the hip through an anterior approach with capsulorrhaphy as well as femoral shortening osteotomy and application of a hip spica cast. After four-and-a-half weeks, the cast was removed, satisfactory arthrogram performed, and Petrie cast placed. The Petrie cast was removed after 5 weeks, and the patient had routine clinical and radiographic follow-up. At the age of 3 years and 5 months, the radiographs revealed residual acetabular dysplasia, without improvement, as well as superolateral migration of the femoral head. The abduction internal rotation radiograph showed adequate reduction of the femoral head (Fig. 6.2). Her exam at that time showed a negative Galeazzi test, abduction on the right of 45° compared to 80° on the left, internal rotation of 65°, and external rotation of 40°.

R. C. Hamdy, N. Saran (eds.), *Pediatric Pelvic and Proximal Femoral Osteotomies*,
https://doi.org/10.1007/978-3-319-78033-7_6

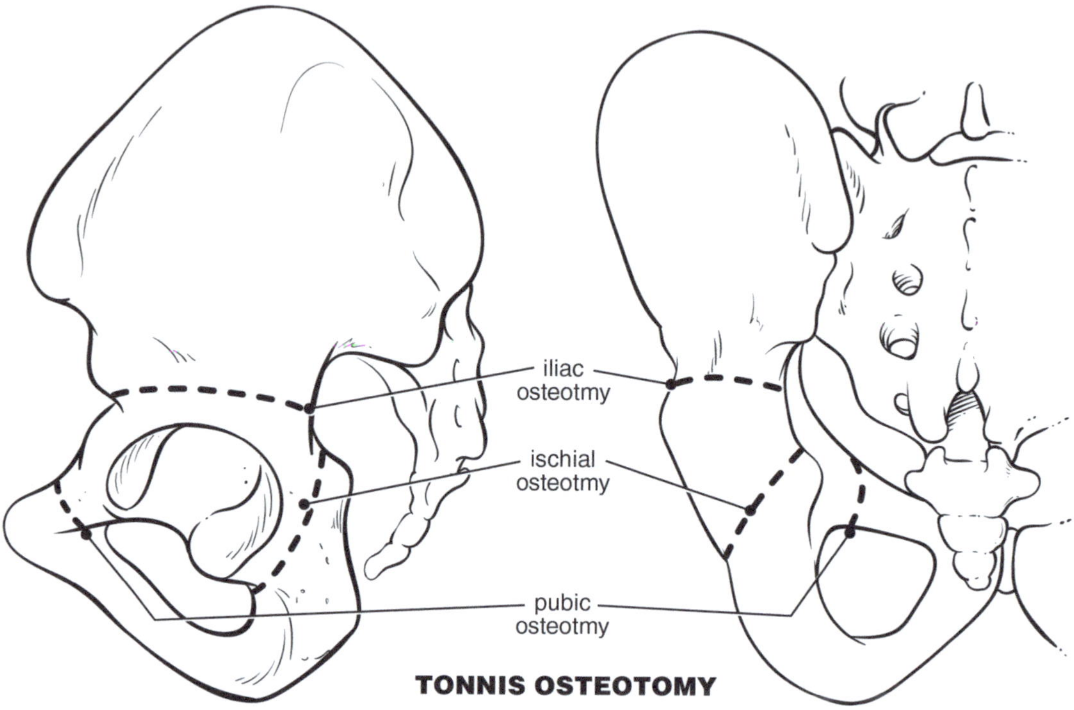

Fig. 6.1 Tönnis osteotomy

Preoperative Imaging (Fig. 6.2)

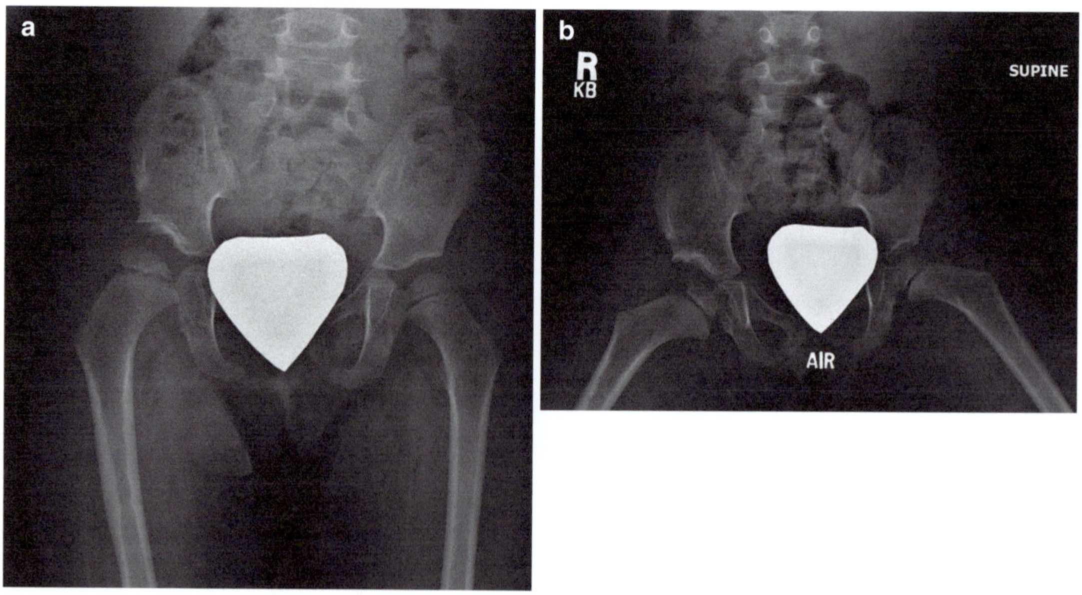

Fig. 6.2 (**a**) Preoperative anteroposterior pelvis radiograph shows the acetabular dysplasia and superolateral migration of the femoral head. (**b**) Preoperative abduction internal rotation view shows reduction of the femoral head

Goals of Treatment

The goals of treatment include redirection of the acetabulum to improve the acetabular index and femoral head coverage, as well as medializing the hip center.

Treatment Strategy

The treatment strategy is to create an acetabular bone block with limited soft tissue restraints to manipulation while maintaining vascularity of the fragment. This involves performing three osteotomies under direct visualization to ensure preservation of all vital neurovascular structures.

Surgical Details

The procedure is performed on a radiolucent table with the patient in the semi-lateral position, with the use of a radiolucent bump under the patient's lumbar spine. The entire lower extremity is prepped and draped free from the costal margin to the toes and medial to the pubic symphysis. The posterior prep extends to the midline (Fig. 6.3). With this preparation, there is no need to reposition during the procedure. The patient is tilted forward after completion of the anterior osteotomies prior to performing the ischial osteotomy, but not repositioned. If indicated, a proximal femoral varus osteotomy is performed first, through a standard lateral approach.

Iliac Osteotomy

The iliac osteotomy is performed through a lateral inguinal, Salter, approach carried posteriorly 6–8 cm along the iliac crest. The incision is made 1–2 cm inferior to the iliac crest to avoid irritation of the scar. Once the skin is incised, the interval between the sartorius and tensor fasciae latae (TFL) is identified in the distal aspect of the incision. The fascia is incised over the TFL and elevated to reduce risk of damaging the lateral femoral cutaneous nerve. This interval is then extended proximally to the iliac crest. The iliac apophysis may be split in its midline or incised laterally and elevated medially in its entirety: we prefer the latter. A transverse incision is made distally through the iliac apophysis to allow the sartorius to mobilize distally and medially. Blunt dissection is carried down both the inner and outer tables of the iliac wing to the sciatic notch. Blunt Hohmann retractors are placed in the notch from both the inner and outer tables. A right-angle hemostat or Rang retractors are used to pass an umbilical tape through the sciatic notch. The umbilical tape is used to pass a Gigli saw through the sciatic notch. The saw is then used to perform the iliac osteotomy, traversing from the sciatic notch to a point mid-

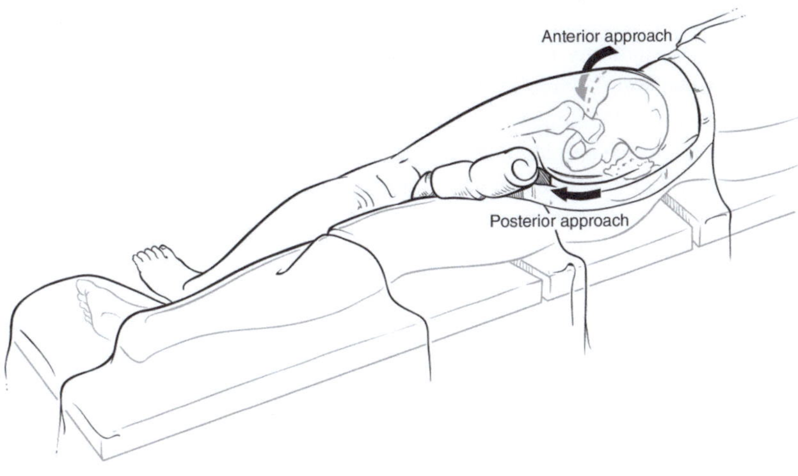

Fig. 6.3 Patient positioning

way between the anterior superior iliac spine and anterior inferior iliac spine.

Superior Pubic Ramus Osteotomy

The superior pubic ramus is then exposed. This can be performed through the same incision by extending the inguinal approach medially. Alternatively, a separate medial incision can be performed. We typically extend the skin incision and then perform a separate fascial incision medial to the femoral vessels. The fascial incision is placed medial to gain access to the superior pubic ramus by elevating some of the insertion of the rectus abdominis. The dissection then proceeds laterally, subperiosteally, in order to elevate the neurovascular bundle and contents of the inguinal canal. This is then used to expose the cranial aspect of the superior pubic ramus. Circumferential subperiosteal exposure of the superior ramus is achieved. Hohmann retractors are placed around the superior pubic ramus, which protect the obturator nerve, and approximately 1 cm of the bone is removed with a Leksell rongeur. Alternatively, this cut may be performed with an osteotome. This osteotomy is typically performed parallel to the acetabulum, in an anterior-superior-lateral to posterior-inferior-medial trajectory, to ensure adequate bony contact for union after the acetabular fragment has been manipulated.

Ischial Osteotomy

The ischial osteotomy is then performed. A longitudinal incision is made in line with the palpable sacrotuberous ligament. In the case that the ligament cannot be palpated, the origin and insertion, lateral sacral tubercles to ischial tuberosity, are used for planning the incision (Fig. 6.4). The gluteus maximus is then bluntly divided to expose the ischium. The sciatic nerve is identified and protected. The sacrotuberous ligament is exposed. Dissection is carried around the medial edge of the sacrotuberous ligament. A Hohmann retractor is placed in this interval into the obturator foramen. The short external rotators are elevated off of the ischium, and a second Hohmann retractor is placed around the lateral aspect of the ischium

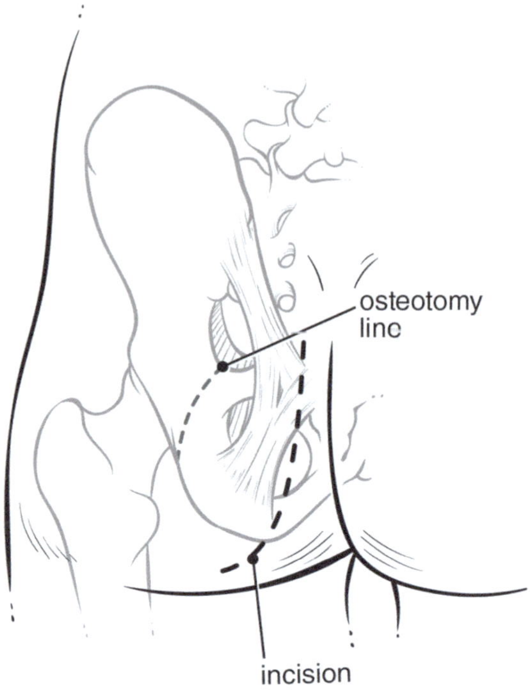

Fig. 6.4 Posterior incision landmarking

into the obturator foramen. The ischial spine is then palpated and sacrospinous ligament identified. Minimizing dissection superiorly, a third Hohmann retractor is then placed superior to the sacrospinous ligament into the sciatic notch. An osteotome is then used to create the osteotomy from above the sacrospinous ligament directed inferolaterally into the obturator foramen. This trajectory is along the two protective Hohmann retractors previously placed (Fig. 6.5). Finger palpation should confirm that the osteotome enters the obturator foramen. Alternatively, a smooth laminar spreader can be used to distract the osteotomy and a Freer elevator used to palpate for completion of the osteotomy. It is important that the periosteum be completely released to allow adequate mobility of the fragment.

Redirection and Stabilization

After completion of all three osteotomies, the acetabular fragment is now free for manipulation. Intraoperative fluoroscopy is used to position the acetabular fragment using two Steinmann pins or a sharp reduction forceps so that the sourcil is

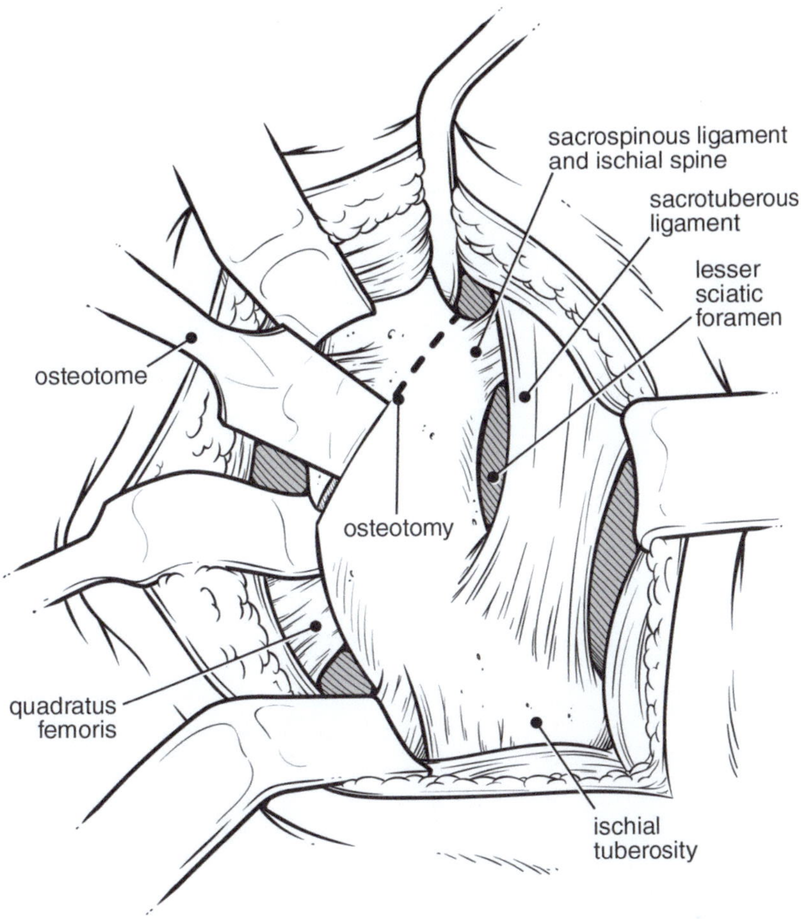

Fig. 6.5 Ischial osteotomy after exposure

horizontal and the hip center is medialized. Version of the acetabulum should also be dialed in to prevent retroversion and impingement. Bone graft is then placed into the iliac osteotomy. If a femoral osteotomy has been performed, we utilize the femoral shaft fragment autograft. Otherwise, we prefer an allograft, having experienced collapse of thin iliac wing autograft. Additionally, iliac wing autograft often produces a permanent radiographically unpleasant deformity in the iliac wing. Two threaded pins are then used for fixation. Layered closure is performed of all wounds, including approximating the iliac apophysis. A one-and-a-half leg hip spica cast is then applied.

Postoperative Imaging (Figs. 6.6, 6.7, 6.8, 6.9, 6.10, and 6.11)

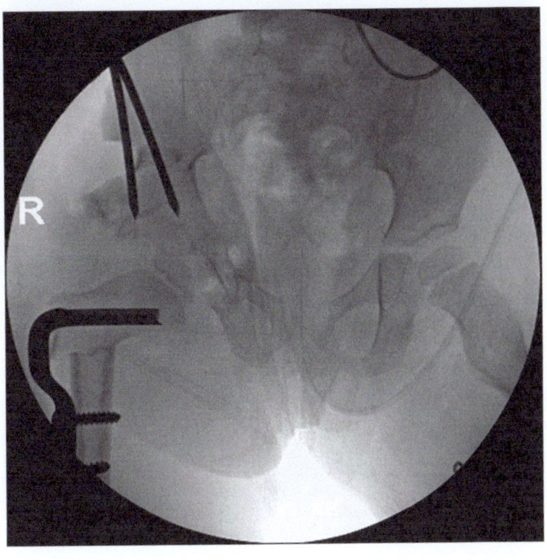

Fig. 6.6 Intraoperative fluoroscopy at conclusion of procedure prior to casting. Note the sloping iliac osteotomy, rotation of the fragment, and medialization of the hip center

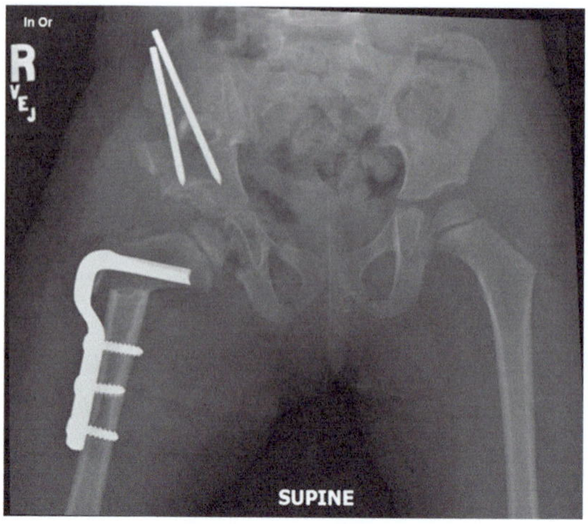

Fig. 6.7 Intraoperative supine anteroposterior radiograph prior to casting

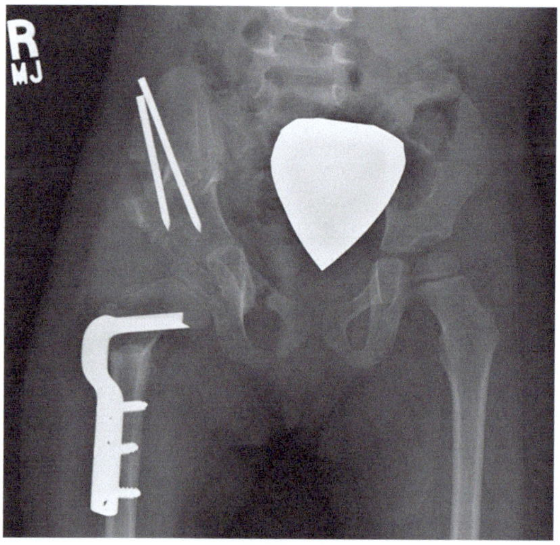

Fig. 6.8 Six-week postoperative anteroposterior pelvis. Maintained reduction and fixation

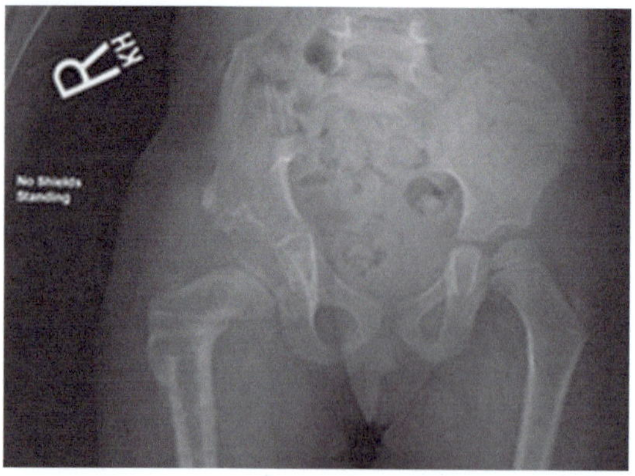

Fig. 6.9 Six-month postoperative standing anteroposterior pelvis. Status post implant removal with healed osteotomy sites

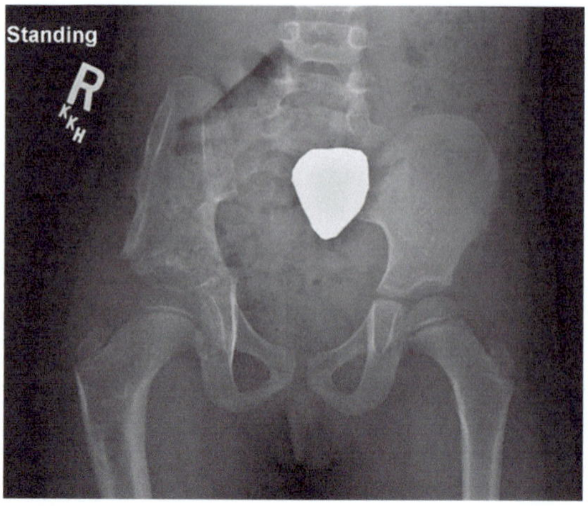

Fig. 6.10 Two-year postoperative standing anteroposterior pelvis

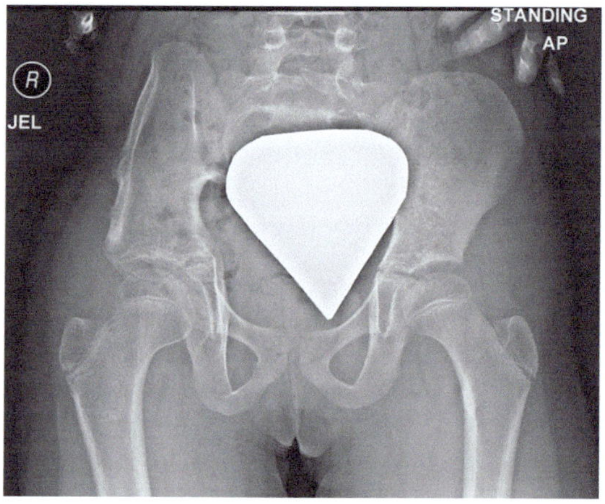

Fig. 6.11 Three-year postoperative (6 years and 5 months) standing anteroposterior pelvis with remodeling of acetabulum

Pearls and Pitfalls

- The ischial osteotomy should be performed in an oblique fashion as described. A more transverse osteotomy reduces surface area for union. This osteotomy should also be checked thoroughly for completeness, using palpation as well as a laminar spreader for visualization.
- The pubic osteotomy should be made as close to the hip joint as possible to allow maximal free motion. Again, this should be performed obliquely, keeping parallel with the acetabulum in order to allow maximal bony surface for union. Attention should be made to insure the

periosteum is released to prevent "tethering"/ allow "free rotation." Occasionally, resection of a small amount of the superior pubis can allow easier positioning of the acetabular fragment.

- In keeping with the other two osteotomies, the iliac osteotomy should be performed, sloping downward toward the sciatic notch to allow maximal free motion and rotation.
- Manipulation of the acetabular fragment can be achieved with a pre-placed Steinmann pin or sharp reduction forceps. In addition to improving the anterior and lateral coverage, attention should be paid to medializing the hip center.
- There is a tendency to create retroversion with redirectional osteotomies. Care should be taken to appropriately position the acetabular fragment such that there is no crossover sign on the fluoroscopic images prior to final stabilization. If a crossover is present, the fragment needs to be either flexed or internally rotated to eliminate anterior over-coverage.

Indications and Contraindications (Table 6.1)

Table 6.1 Tönnis triple pelvic osteotomy: surgical indications and contraindications

Indications
Symptomatic hip dysplasia
Center-edge angle <20°
Acetabular index >40
Spherical femoral head
Contraindications
Tönnis osteoarthritis grade ≥2
Incongruent hip joint
Irreducible hip
Significantly reduced range of motion (<70° arc)

Further Reading

Tönnis D, Legal H, Graf R. Congenital dysplasia and dislocation of the hip in children and adults (Telger TC, translator). Berlin: Springer-Verlag; 1987.

7 Bernese Peri-acetabular Osteotomy

Christopher Dowding and Paul E. Beaulé

Introduction

Hip dysplasia is a common pathology that causes significant morbidity in the young adult population. The abnormal morphology of a dysplastic hip results in nonphysiological loading across the acetabular rim and is associated with labral pathology and the development of osteoarthritis. The goal of corrective surgery in the treatment of hip dysplasia is to improve function by redistributing the load across the hip joint, thereby relieving pain and delaying and possibly preventing end-stage arthritis. In the treatment of adult hip dysplasia, the Bernese peri-acetabular osteotomy (PAO) [1] is the most widely accepted technique for the treatment of hip dysplasia. The PAO provides a method of obtaining a large corrective reorientation of the acetabulum with a single incision and without the need for external immobilization. This is accomplished through a reorientation of the acetabulum which medializes the joint center, improves superolateral inclination, and increases femoral head coverage while keeping the pelvic ring intact. Patient selection is critical to identify patients that stand to benefit the most from this procedure. Factors related to a poor outcome are patient age greater than 35, incongruency of the hip joint, and advanced osteoarthritis. Also, an increased alpha angle can help identify those patients who may benefit from a concomitant arthrotomy or hip arthroscopy to treat a cam deformity of the proximal femur and/or repair the labrum. This procedure can also be used to reorient a retroverted acetabulum in patients with symptoms of anterior impingement and decreased internal rotation.

Brief Clinical History

This 29-year-old female presented with 5 years of worsening right greater than left groin pain. The pain was described as pinching and worsened by long walks. There had been no previous surgical interventions and no history of childhood hip pathology. Physical exam revealed equal leg lengths with a positive flexion/adduction/internal rotation impingement test. She had 110° flexion, 40° external rotation, and 25° internal rotation on that side. Radiographs revealed hip dysplasia (Fig. 7.1). There were no signs of advanced arthritis, and the hip joint was congruent. In order to correct her coverage, improve range of motion, and reduce pain, a peri-acetabular osteotomy was planned.

C. Dowding · P. E. Beaulé (✉)
Division of Orthopaedic Surgery, University of Ottawa, The Ottawa Hospital, Ottawa, ON, Canada
e-mail: pbeaule@toh.ca

R. C. Hamdy, N. Saran (eds.), *Pediatric Pelvic and Proximal Femoral Osteotomies*,
https://doi.org/10.1007/978-3-319-78033-7_7

Preoperative Imaging (see Fig. 7.1)

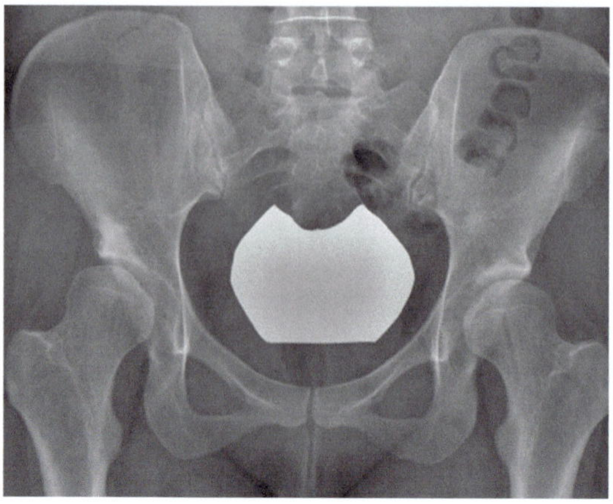

Fig. 7.1 Anteroposterior radiograph showing bilateral hip dysplasia. The right side is more symptomatic. The Tonnis angle is 29° and the center edge angle is 11°

Antero-posterior radiograph showing right hip dysplasia.

Goals of Treatment

The principles of treatment include:

1. Restoring adequate coverage of the femoral head
2. Medializing the hip joint
3. Correcting the version of the acetabulum if required

Treatment Strategy

The treatment strategy for dysplastic cases consists of performing a reorientation of the acetabulum in order to reduce superolateral acetabular inclination, improve femoral head coverage, translate the joint center medially, and restore physiological loading of the anterolateral acetabular rim. This is achieved by performing a series of orthogonal pelvic cuts, which when connected leave the acetabulum within a block of the bone that is free from the rest of the pelvis and can be reoriented in three dimensions. In cases of acetabular retroversion, the version must be corrected to reduce impingement and increase internal rotation. Once the desired correction is achieved, the osteotomy is held in place with two or more fully threaded cortical screws. In cases of concomitant labral pathology or cam lesions, an arthrotomy or arthroscopy can be performed before the peri-acetabular osteotomy (PAO) under the same anesthetic.

Surgical Details

Patient Preparation

A fully radiolucent table is necessary to perform this procedure. Preoperative antibiotics are given as well as tranexamic acid to minimize blood loss. Special sets of osteotomes and pelvic instrumentation are necessary.

Exposure

This procedure is performed in the supine position. The leg on the operative side is free draped, making sure to leave the anterior superior iliac spine (ASIS) exposed. Two types of incisions may be used. In thinner patients, a bikini-type incision is used, whereas larger, more muscular patients require a longitudinal incision extending from the iliac crest into the Smith-Peterson interval. The bikini incision starts 2 cm proximal to the ASIS and follows the direction of the inguinal ligament toward the pubic symphysis (Fig. 7.2). The subcutaneous fat is incised in line with this incision. Once down to the fascial layer, Metzenbaum scissors are used to undermine the fatty layer distally toward the tensor muscle and proximally along the iliac crest. This will reveal the fascia overlying the tensor muscle as well as the abdominal muscles coming off of the iliac crest. Cautery is used to split the insertion of the abdominal and gluteal muscles off of the iliac crest, stopping before the origin of the inguinal ligament at the ASIS is compromised. Distally, the tensor muscle belly is identified, and the fascia overlying it is incised with a scalpel in a lon-

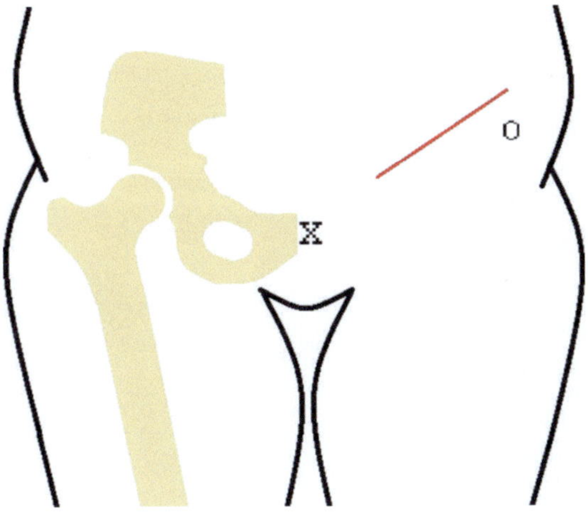

Fig. 7.2 Drawing demonstrating the bikini incision (*red line*) which extends from a point 2 cm proximal to the anterior superior iliac spine (O) toward the pubic symphysis (X)

gitudinal direction. The muscle fibers are released from the underside of the fascia, and the muscle belly is retracted in a lateral direction with a muscle retractor. The fatty interval between tensor and sartorius is developed proximally to the level of the ASIS—keeping in mind that in the distal aspect of the interval, the ascending branch to the lateral circumflex artery is vulnerable. At this point, the main impediment to supra-acetabular access is the attachment of sartorius and the inguinal ligament at the ASIS. As a result, a smaller sliver of bone is taken from the ASIS with the sartorius and inguinal ligament attached is osteotomized in a medial direction using a half-inch broad, flat osteotome. It is important to ensure that a thin wafer of the bone is taken with the soft tissue attachment to facilitate bone-to-bone healing postoperatively. Once the ASIS is mobilized medially, the next step is to expose the inner table of the iliac wing and the interspinous notch. A triangle bump is placed under the knee to relax the psoas tendon. Cautery is then used to release the periosteum along the interspinous notch (between the anterior inferior iliac spine [AIIS] and ASIS). A smooth AVA-type retractor is then passed down the iliac wing to lever the abdominal muscles and iliacus medially and facilitate their reflection off of the inner table, revealing the brim of the true pelvis and the posterior column. Finally, a shield tip elevator is used to perform a subperiosteal release of the tissue off of the lateral aspect of the superior pubic ramus until the pubic root is revealed. The key for the first osteotomy is to get medial to the pubic root. This can be checked on the 30° cephalad view. There is no particular method to avoid bleeding from the obturator foramen; the operator must simply be aware of the location of the neurovascular bundle and take care not to damage it.

Osteotomy

The remainder of this procedure relies heavily upon fluoroscopic imaging and a keen sense of pelvic anatomy.

Superior Ramus Osteotomy The first cut is the superior pubic ramus. A C-arm is brought in perpendicular to the patient from the contralateral side and angled 30° for an outlet pelvic view. Under fluoroscopic guidance, a broad, flat osteotome is inserted on the superior pubic ramus, medial to the roof of the pubis and to the ilioischial line on imaging (Fig. 7.3). The osteotome is advanced with a mallet, taking intermittent X-rays to confirm position. When the inferior cortex is breached, the osteotomy is exaggerated by rotating the osteotome on its axis back and forth with a Farabeuf clamp.

Ischial Osteotomy The next osteotomy is the ischial cut, which is inferior and medial to the cotyloid notch. X-ray is brought back to AP position, and a curved shielded elevator is inserted subperiosteally along the interspinous notch and inserted medially to the direct head of rectus tendon. This is a rectus sparing modification of the original technique. Often there is a bursa overlying the rectus, which can be used as a guide. Using X-ray as a guide, the elevator is advanced inferiorly until it is inferior to the infra-cotyloid groove, centered on the ischium. This technique is heavily dependent on X-ray as the dissection itself is not performed under direct visualization. It should be performed bluntly—avoid any sharp instruments at this point. When position is confirmed, switch the elevator for a forked osteotome, rotate the C-arm 60° away

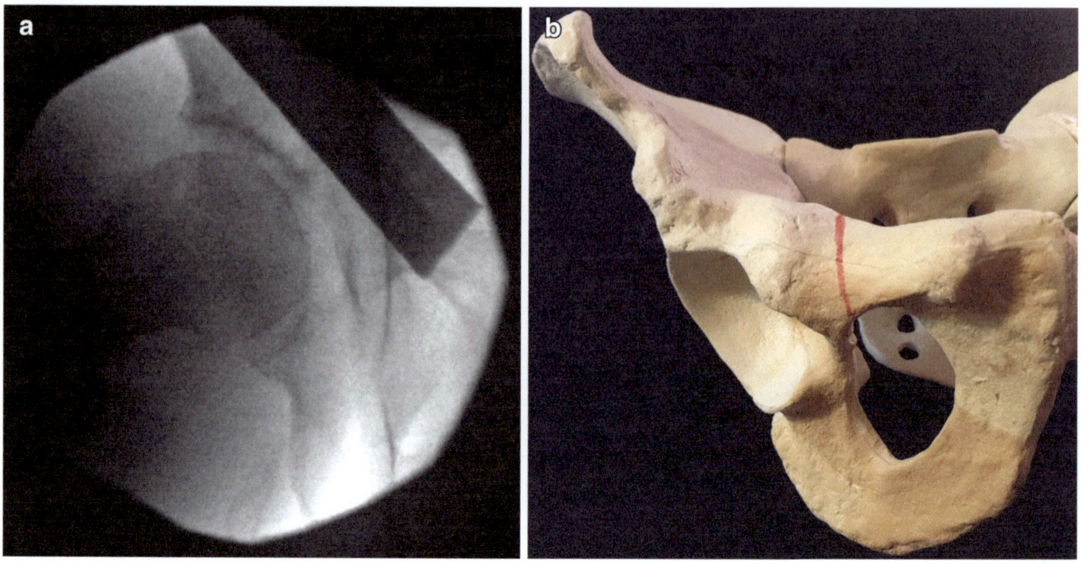

Fig. 7.3 (**a**) Broad osteotome in position for the superior ramus osteotomy. (**b**) Corresponding osteotomy in *red*

from the surgeon (false-profile view), and reconfirm position. The forked osteotome is advanced with a mallet and directed toward the ischial spine. It is important not to disrupt the posterior column, so the osteotomy is stopped at least 2 cm from the ischial spine. The first pass of the osteotome is centered on the ischium; however two more passes must be made centered on the medial and lateral cortices (Fig. 7.4). The leg should be kept in a slightly flexed and abducted position during the ischial and posterior column cuts. Utilize the AP and false-profile shots to ensure the osteotome is centered on the ischium.

Posterior Column and Iliac Osteotomy The final two cuts are oriented to connect the ischial cut to the iliac crest. X-ray is brought back to the AP position, and the AVA retractor is reinserted to visualize the brim of the true pelvis. The posterior column cut must be sufficiently posterior to avoid entering the joint. This is assessed on an iliac oblique view by rotating the C-arm 45° away from the surgeon. A pencil-tip burr is used to start the osteotomy. Starting 1 cm lateral to the brim of the true pelvis, the posterior column is etched with the high-speed pencil-tipped burr heading toward the brim and then obliquely toward the deep extent of the ischial cut (Fig. 7.5a). The intersection between the supra-acetabular and retro-acetabular cuts can be visualized on the 45° fluoro shot. The key here is to stay central within the posterior column. This osteotomy is deepened with a broad osteotome and then completed with a curved, forked osteotome directed toward the ischial cut (Fig. 7.5b). X-ray is brought back to the AP position, and the iliac crest is etched with the burr 1 cm proximal to the ASIS. This is the start point for the iliac cut. An oscillating saw is used to connect the iliac start point with the lateral aspect of the posterior column cut (Fig. 7.6). Care must be taken to leave enough the bone in the posterior column to allow for screw fixation. Finally, a broad osteotome is inserted into the posterior column and iliac cuts and twisted with a Farabeuf to sequentially complete the osteotomies and pry the acetabular block of the bone free from the rest of the pelvis.

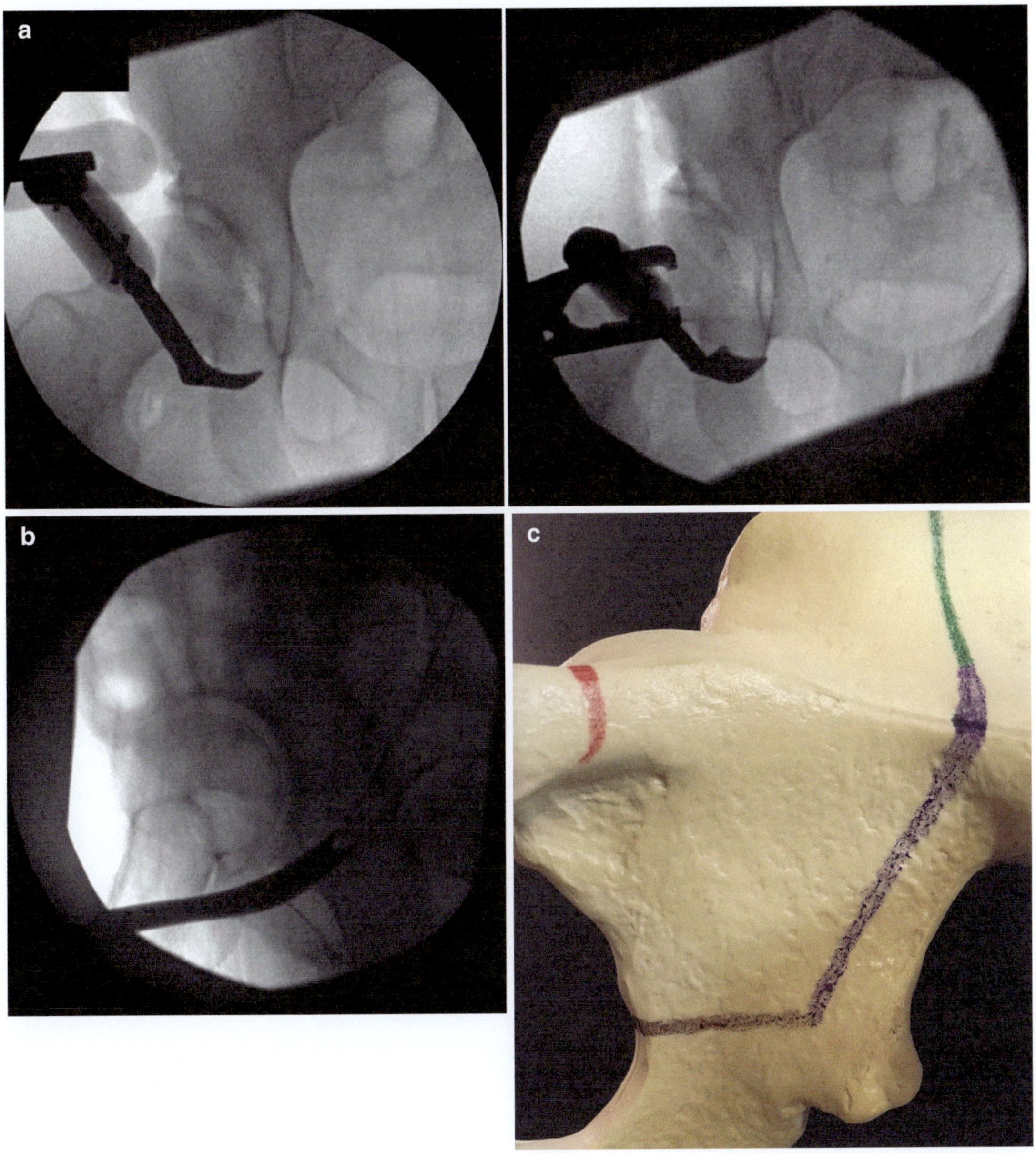

Fig. 7.4 (**a**) Forked osteotome in position for ischial cuts (lateral/medial cortices). (**b**) Oblique view of osteotome heading toward the ischial spine. (**c**) Corresponding osteotomy in *brown, horizontal line*

Reorientation and Fixation

Once the block is mobile, a Shanz pin is inserted into the interspinous notch to aid in reorientation (Fig. 7.7). With dysplastic hips, the fragment is levered down and medial. To deal with acetabular retroversion, the maneuver is to internally rotate the fragment and to dial in the coronal plane alignment as necessary to ensure adequate lateral coverage while improving internal rotation of the hip. This step requires experience to perform properly as it requires a fair amount of intuition to achieve appropriate correction. The most important step is to check on X-ray and adjust the correction as needed. It is important to adequately

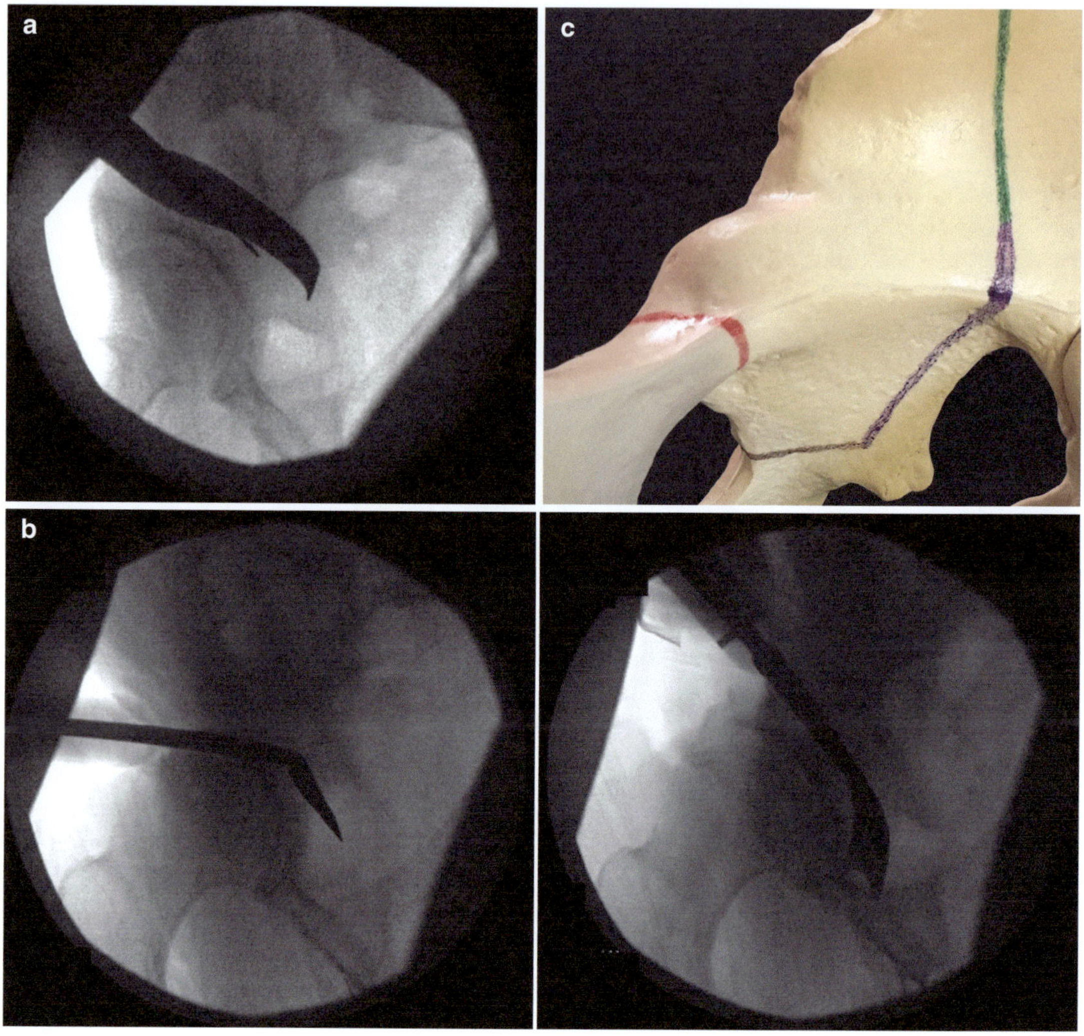

Fig. 7.5 (**a**) A burr is used to etch the planned osteotomy of the posterior column. (**b**) Forked osteotome connects the posterior column osteotomy to the ischial osteotomy. (**c**) Corresponding osteotomy in *purple*

visualize the teardrop—following reorientation, the profile of the teardrop should change. When the desired correction is achieved, the orientation is held with a large, pointed reduction clamp, and a flat-plate AP pelvis image is taken to confirm adequate correction. Assess the center edge angle, the acetabular version, and the Tonnis angle on the AP pelvis image. If the correction is deemed acceptable, fixation is achieved with a 3.5 mm fragment screw inserted through the inner brim into the posterior column, followed by a 70–80-mm-large fragment screw through the Shanz pin hole and also directed toward the sacroiliac joint into the iliac wing. Screw length is checked by rotating the C-arm 60° away from the surgeon.

Closure and Aftercare

After copious irrigation, the ASIS osteotomy is repaired with a 1.0 Vicryl stitch threaded through a 2.5 mm drill hole into the ASIS origin. One Hemovac drain is placed deep to the facia, and then the abdominal/gluteal origin and tensor fas-

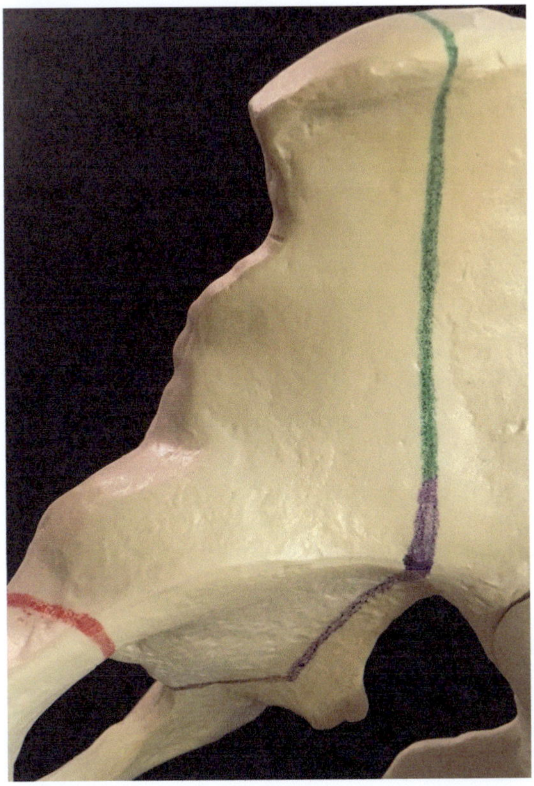

Fig. 7.6 Iliac osteotomy in *green*

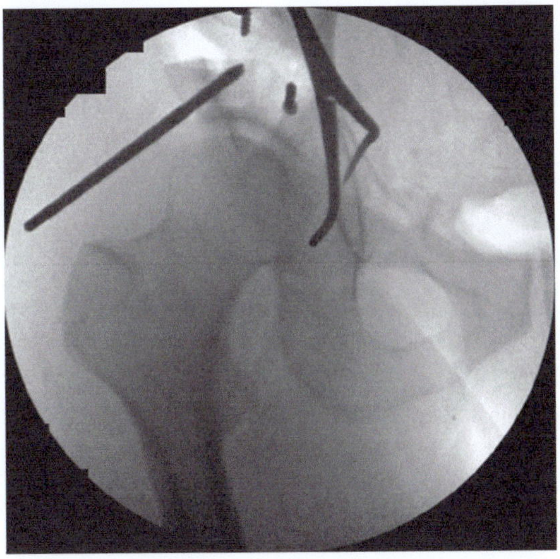

Fig. 7.7 A Shanz pin has been used to reorient the acetabular block. The correction is held provisionally with a large clamp. The first screw has been placed, and the second screw will replace the Shanz pin

cia are repaired with a running 1.0 Vicryl stitch. Local infiltration of anesthetic is done. A second, subcutaneous drain is placed, and then the skin is closed in the typical fashion. Patients are kept toe-touch weight bear until the osteotomy sites heal on follow-up X-rays, usually at around 6 weeks. Oral anticoagulants are taken for 3 weeks starting postoperative day 1 for all patients regardless of age, and patient-controlled anesthesia machines are typically employed in the early postoperative period. Our preference for anticoagulation is oral rivaroxaban, 10 mg daily.

Postoperative Imaging (Fig. 7.8)

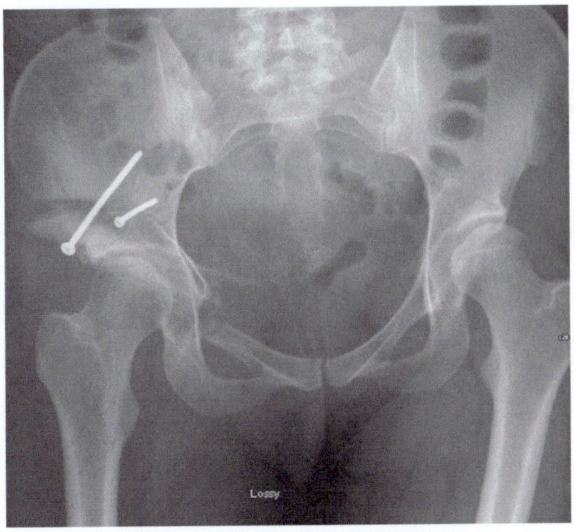

Fig. 7.8 Anteroposterior postoperative radiograph. The postoperative center edge angle measures 39°

Antero-posterior radiograph showing correction with tear drop being flipped ensuring proper medialization.

Pearls and Pitfalls

- This proce.dure requires an intimate knowledge of pelvic anatomy, as well as an understanding of how to utilize fluoroscopy. The incision and exposure are modest, meaning that most of the osteotomy is done under fluoroscopy rather than direct visualization. Having an X-ray technician who is familiar with the procedure is important for efficiency and safety.
- The maneuver for correcting retroversion is to mostly internal rotation of the fragment.
- If the fragment is difficult to reorient, we use a sharp reduction forceps on the pubic ramus to provide counter traction.
- The best way to achieve medialization is to ensure that the fragment is completely free and not hinging on the pelvis at any point.
- Try to achieve as much boney opposition of the fragment on the proximal aspect of the iliac cut.
- There is a balance between maintaining pelvic stability and protecting the acetabulum. While it is vital to avoid disrupting the posterior column, the orthogonal osteotomies must be kept sufficiently extra-articular in order to minimize the risk of avascular necrosis to the acetabular block. Furthermore, joint perforation is a real possibility and must be avoided by regularly checking the path of the osteotomes on fluoroscopy.
- Take great care when completing the osteotomies—especially the ischial and pubic cuts. Levering too much on an osteotome can break the tip of the instrument, and retrieval is extremely difficult and time-consuming.
- Hip arthroscopy is performed first if necessary. Prolonged arthroscopy can result in the extravasation of a large amount of fluid into the soft tissues surrounding the hip. This will make the dissection for the PAO more difficult, so it is helpful to complete the arthroscopy in a timely fashion.

Indications and Contraindications (Table 7.1)

Table 7.1 Bernese peri-acetabular osteotomy: surgical indications and contraindications

Indications
Hip dysplasia
Symptomatic acetabular retroversion
Hip pain
Contraindications
Tönnis grade osteoarthritis >2
Age >35 years
Hip joint incongruency
Open triradiate cartilage
Less than 90 degrees of hip flexion
Less than 30 degree arc of hip rotation

Reference

1. Ganz R, Klaue K, Vinh TS, Mast JW. A new periacetabular osteotomy for the treatment of hip dysplasias. Technique and preliminary results. Clin Orthop Relat Res. 1988;(232):26–36.

Further Reading

Beaulé PE, Dowding C, Parker G, Ryu JJ. What factors predict improvements in outcomes scores and reoperations after the Bernese periacetabular osteotomy? Clin Orthop Relat Res. 2015;473(2):615–22.

Clohisy JC, Schutz AL, St JL, Schoenecker PL, Wright RW. Periacetabular osteotomy: a systematic literature review. Clin Orthop Relat Res. 2009;467(8):2041–52.

Matheney T, Kim YJ, Zurakowski D, Matero C, Millis M. Intermediate to long-term results following the Bernese periacetabular osteotomy and predictors of clinical outcome. J Bone Joint Surg Am. 2009;91(9):2113–23.

Troelsen A, Elmengaard B, Søballe K. Medium-term outcome of periacetabular osteotomy and predictors of conversion to total hip replacement. J Bone Joint Surg. 2009;91(9):2169–79.

8 Periacetabular Osteotomy: Groin Incision-Assisted Approach

Fahad S. Alhuzaimi and Neil Saran

Introduction

Acetabular dysplasia is a common cause of osteoarthritis. The Bernese periacetabular osteotomy (PAO) as described by Ganz is a powerful tool that enables correction of inadequate femoral head coverage due to acetabular dysplasia. In addition to decreasing pressure forces on hip cartilage by increasing contact surface area, it can decrease joint reactive forces through medialization of the hip joint. Also, the osteotomy allows for correction of acetabular version. Since its inception in the mid-1980s, multiple modifications have been described. In this chapter we will highlight a modification that utilizes a groin incision to perform the ischial and pubic cuts.

F. S. Alhuzaimi
Department of Orthopaedic Surgery, Shriners Hospital for Children Canada, Montreal, QC, Canada

N. Saran (✉)
Department of Orthopaedic Surgery, Shriners Hospital for Children Canada, Montreal, QC, Canada

Department of Paediatric Surgery, The Montreal Children's Hospital, Montreal, QC, Canada

Division of Orthopaedic Surgery, Department of Surgery McGill University, Montreal, QC, Canada
e-mail: neil.saran@mcgill.ca

Brief Clinical History

This 27-year-old female presented with a 2-year history of increasing pain in her left groin and abductor region. She was previously known to have mild acetabular dysplasia associated with her underlying diagnosis of fibular hemimelia for which she had been treated with limb lengthening as well as contralateral epiphysiodesis. At the time of discharge from the limb length discrepancy clinic, she was asymptomatic from her hip and functioning well. Her hip pain started shortly after that and until 2 years previous to presentation was controlled with over-the-counter analgesics. In the last 2 years, she started to use a cane and more recently has taken a leave of absence from work because of her hip pain. Currently she is in constant pain and is only able to walk approximately 100–200 m without aid. Her range of motion revealed good flexion (110° on left vs. 105° on right), abduction (35° bilaterally), and external rotation (70° on left, 50° on right). Her internal rotation was normal on the affected side (5° on right and 35° on left). She had positive FADIR (flexion, adduction, and internal rotation) and FABER (flexion, abduction, and external rotation) tests on the left side.

R. C. Hamdy, N. Saran (eds.), *Pediatric Pelvic and Proximal Femoral Osteotomies*,
https://doi.org/10.1007/978-3-319-78033-7_8

Preoperative Imaging

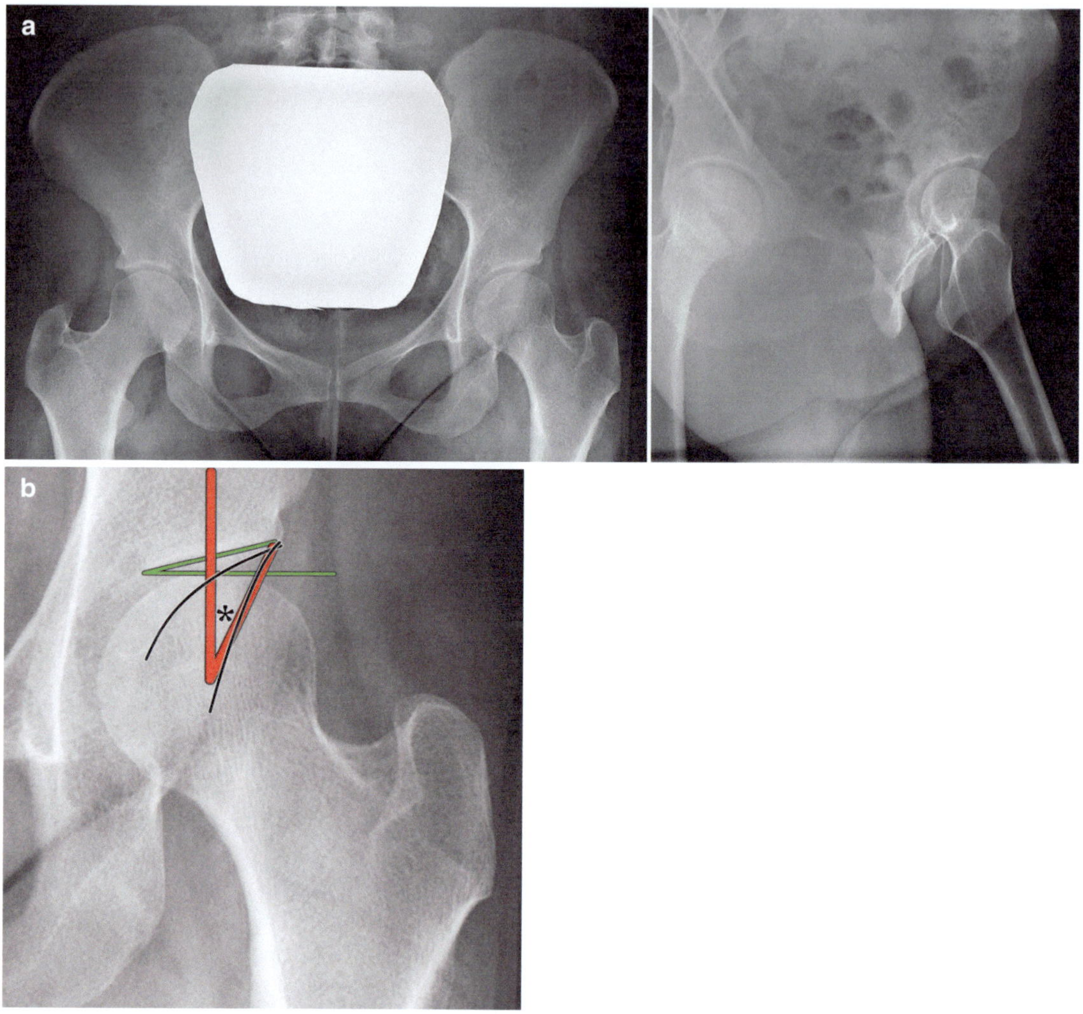

Fig. 8.1 (**a**) Anteroposterior (AP) pelvis and left hip false-profile views showing left acetabulum dysplasia and femoral head uncoverage. (**b**) Left hip AP view showing normal crossover sign. Center-edge angle measuring 24° (*red lines*) and a Tönnis angle of 17° (*green lines*)

Radiological imaging revealed a center-edge angle of 24° and a Tönnis angle of 17° (Fig. 8.1). More interestingly, her magnetic resonance arthrogram showed an inverted labrum (Fig. 8.2), which, once degenerative, is an entity known to be associated with crippling hip pain and deteriorating osteoarthritis unless addressed.

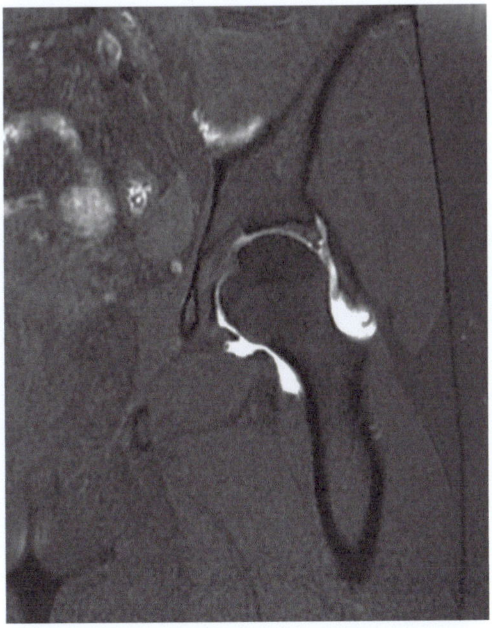

Fig. 8.2 MRI coronal cut showing reduced head to acetabulum contact surface area and an inverted labrum

Goals of Treatment

The main objectives in this case are to offload the inverted labrum by realigning the acetabulum and to decrease the joint reactive forces and force required by the abductors during upright activity by medializing the hip center.

Treatment Strategy

Reorientation of the acetabulum is best performed with a redirectional osteotomy. The Bernese periacetabular osteotomy allows for such reorientation and permits version control as well as medialization. The osteotomy consists of partial cuts of the ischium, ilium, and posterior column as well as a complete cut of the superior pubic ramus (Fig. 8.3). While the original description uses a modified Smith-Petersen approach with takedown of the rectus tendon and full exposure of the hip capsule, the technique highlighted in this chapter is rectus-sparing. The ischial and pubic cuts are made through a medial approach, while the supraacetabular and retroacetabular cuts are made through a standard iliac crest approach. When required, osteoplasty or labral work is typically performed using hip arthroscopy immediately prior to the PAO.

Surgery Details

The patient is positioned supine without bolsters and both arms are abducted 90°. The affected limb and hemipelvis are prepped and draped from the inferior costal margin to the ankle. The medial edge of the drape is at the groin crease. The upper edge of the iliac crest is included in the draping posteriorly.

Medial Approach (Superior Pubic Ramus Osteotomy)

With the leg placed in a frog position, a 5 cm incision is made 1 cm lateral to the groin crease centered on the adductor longus (Fig. 8.4). The fascia over the adductor longus is incised longitudinally, exposing the adductor longus muscle. The fascia is retracted superolaterally, and the adductor longus muscle is bluntly followed to its superior margin where the pectineus muscle is located (Fig. 8.5). The pectineus is then bluntly

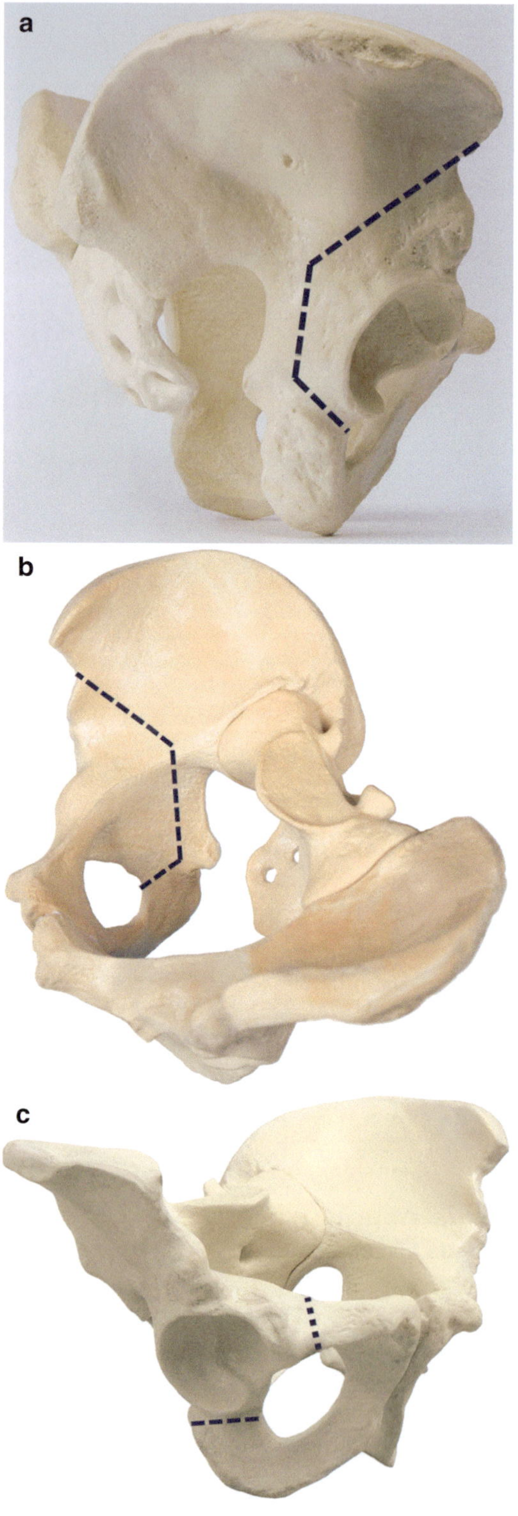

Fig. 8.3 The partial iliac (supraacetabular), posterior column (retroacetabular), and ischial cuts as well as the complete pubic cuts used for the periacetabular osteotomy are drawn on a pelvic saw bone model showing the outer table (**a**), inner table (**b**), and obturator view (**c**)

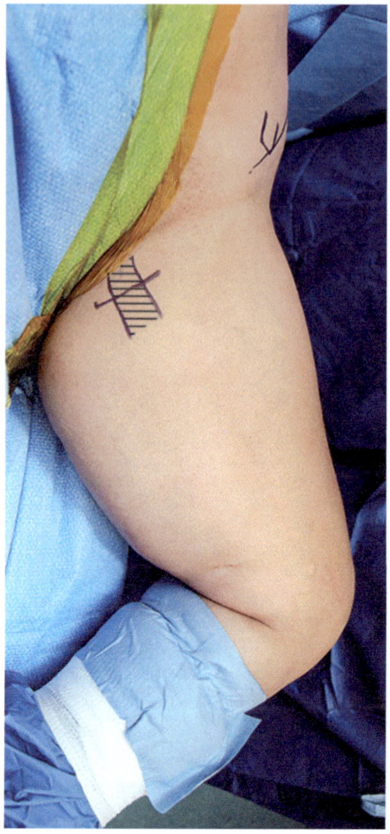

Fig. 8.4 The medial incision made 1 cm distal and parallel to the inguinal crease and perpendicular to the highlighted adductor longus muscle

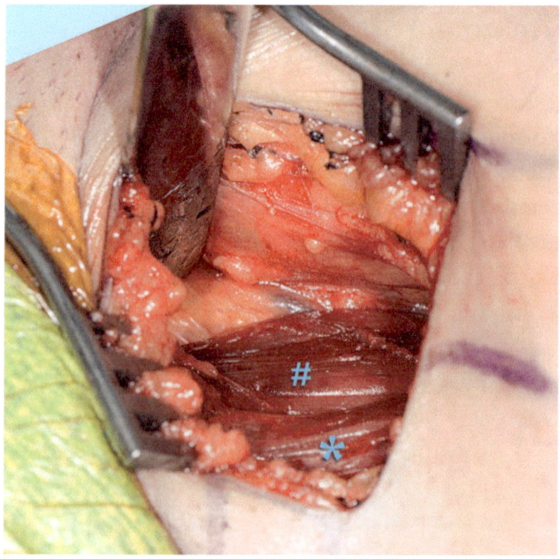

Fig. 8.5 Both the adductor longus (asterisk) and the pectineus (hash) can be visualized once the fascia is incised

followed to its superior margin (see Sect. 8.5) where the superior pubic ramus is located.

The deep floor of the inguinal canal is noted as a yellowish sheath at this level and is retracted superiorly, while the adductor longus and pectineus are retracted inferomedially. Care must be taken to not stray laterally, as the neurovascular bundle is located just lateral to this window.

Once on the ramus, it is subperiosteally dissected using an angled shield-tip elevator. The dissection is continued until the superolateral corner of the obturator foramen is located (Fig. 8.6). If required, fluoroscopy can be useful in making sure that the dissection is in fact over the ramus and not the supraacetabular region, as attempting to strip the bone in this region will result in unnecessary hip joint penetration.

Hohmann retractors are placed around the pubic ramus. A 3–4 mm burr is used to osteotomize the ramus perpendicular to its axis. Alternatively, this can be performed with an osteotome. The small resection facilitates mobilization and medialization of the acetabulum.

Medial Approach (Ischial Osteotomy)

Using the same incision, we shift our attention to the area inferior to the adductor longus muscle while maintaining the frog position. The adductor longus is retracted superolaterally, while gracilis is retracted inferomedially, exposing adductor magnus (Fig. 8.7).

Blunt dissection is carried out between the adductor magnus and gracilis muscles all the way down to the ischial tuberosity. While the ischial tuberosity is generally palpable through this incision, it can be difficult to manually palpate the anterior ischium. This is typically done in blind fashion. An elevator is then placed on the anterior surface of the ischium to sweep the anterior muscles off subperiosteally. Although we do not usually directly visualize the anterior ischium, this is feasible and this approach can also be used when performing a triple pelvic osteotomy (Fig. 8.8).

The infracotyloid groove can be palpated with the elevator marking the site where the ischial cut will begin. A straight osteotome is placed in the infracotyloid groove (Fig. 8.9a), and fluoroscopy is used in anteroposterior (AP) and 45–60° oblique planes to confirm the start point and the

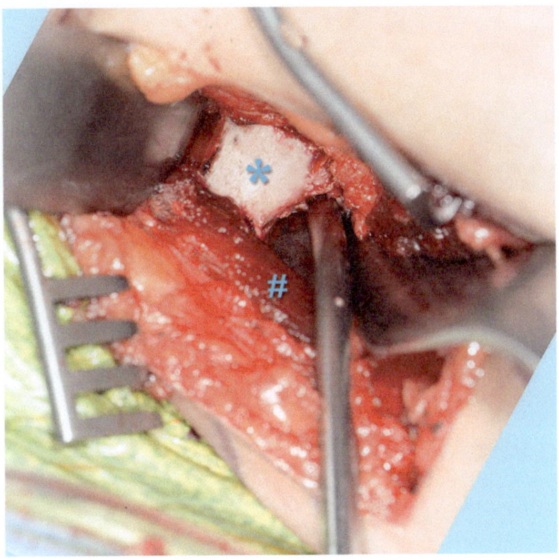

Fig. 8.6 Subperiosteal dissection of the superior pubic ramus (asterisk) is done and is ready for a 3–4 mm resection osteotomy, Adductor longus and pectineus (hash) are retracted inferomedially

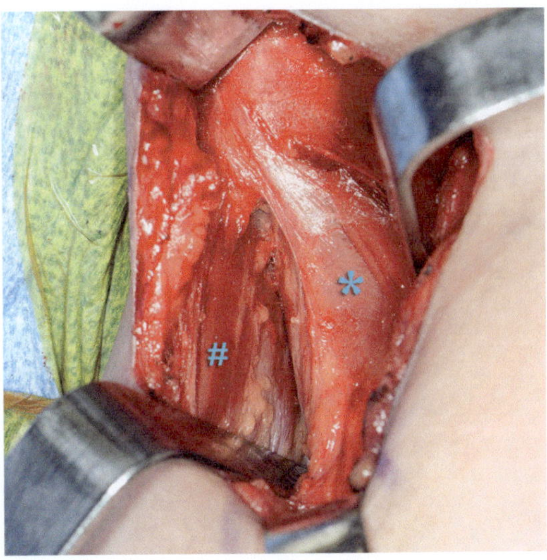

Fig. 8.7 The interval between the adductor magnus (asterisk) and the gracilis (hash) is bluntly dissected all the way down to the ischial tuberosity

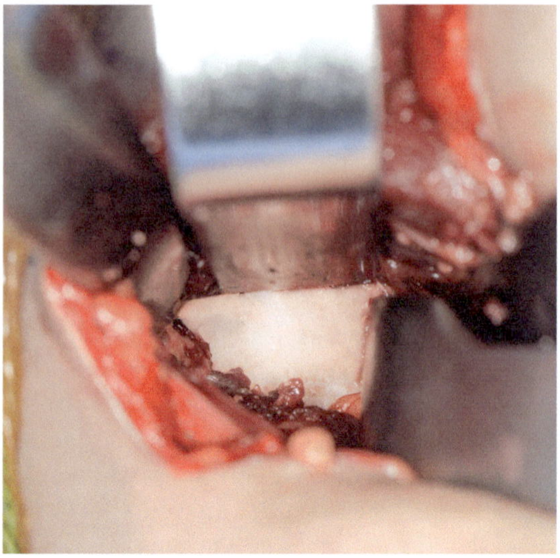

Fig. 8.8 The anterior ischium is not visualized for the Ganz osteotomy; however, an adequate exposure is possible through this incision if a triple pelvic osteotomy is being performed

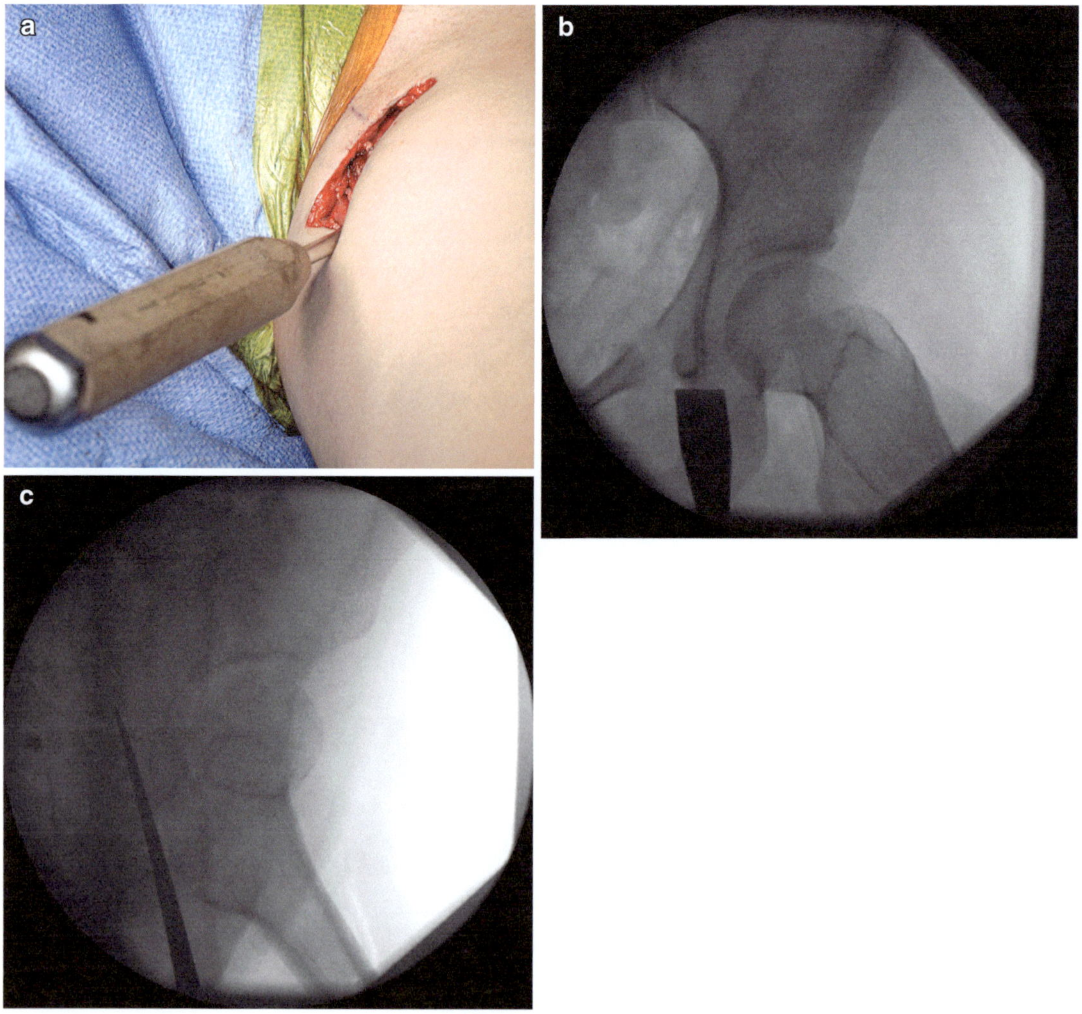

Fig. 8.9 (**a**) A straight osteotome is positioned for the ischial cut. Fluoroscopic image shows the medial cortex cut being performed under fluoroscopy in the anteroposterior (**b**) and *oblique planes* (**c**)

direction of the cut. We typically start with the medial cortex of the ischium on the AP image (Fig. 8.9b) and advance the osteotome toward the ischial spine on an oblique image until the osteotome has just passed the half way mark of the posterior column (Fig. 8.9c). The osteotome is then repositioned for the lateral cortex of the ischium and advanced in a similar manner but only to a depth of about 2–2.5 cm. The osteotome is then positioned centrally on the AP image and advanced under oblique imaging to connect the two previous tracts. It is important to ensure that the tracts are connected and that the partial ischial cut is complete. In order to verify this, the osteotome is inserted into the lateral tract and then walked medially by withdrawing and inserting the osteotome 2–3 mm at a time until one has reached the medial cortex. Of note, during the lateral cut, the hip is slightly extended while maintaining the frog position in order to relax the sciatic nerve, which is vulnerable during this part of the osteotomy.

Smith-Petersen Approach

An oblique incision is made 1 cm below the anterior superior iliac spine (ASIS) and parallel to the iliac crest (Fig. 8.10). The fascia overlying the tensor fascia lata is incised, and the muscle is retracted laterally, while the fascia of the fascia lata and sartorius (and the lateral femoral cutaneous nerve, which is never visualized) are retracted medially. This interval is dissected to the anteroinferior surface of the ASIS. The inner table is exposed by subperiosteally elevating the iliacus muscle off the iliac crest. The sartorius and inguinal canal origin are elevated subperiosteally off the iliac crest and reflected medially along with the iliacus. This allows for full visualization of the inner table and quadrilateral plate. Using fluoroscopy, the projected intersection point between the supra- and retroacetabular cuts is marked in the oblique plane (Fig. 8.11a). The supraacetabular osteotomy is typically planned to start just inferior to the inferior edge of the ASIS and runs perpendicular to the axis of the body. This region of the outer table is then subperiosteally elevated. The supraacetabular osteotomy is performed using an oscillating saw and runs horizontally. The retroacetabular cut is made using a straight osteotome under fluoroscopic guidance (Fig. 8.11b, c). The first pass of the osteotome runs along the inner table and the quadrilateral plate down the posterior column toward the end of the ischial cut under fluoroscopy. While maintaining the start point, each subsequent pass of the osteotome is directed slightly cranially and laterally until the lateral table is cut. The limb is held in an abducted, extended, and externally rotated position during the more lateral cuts to detension the sciatic nerve.

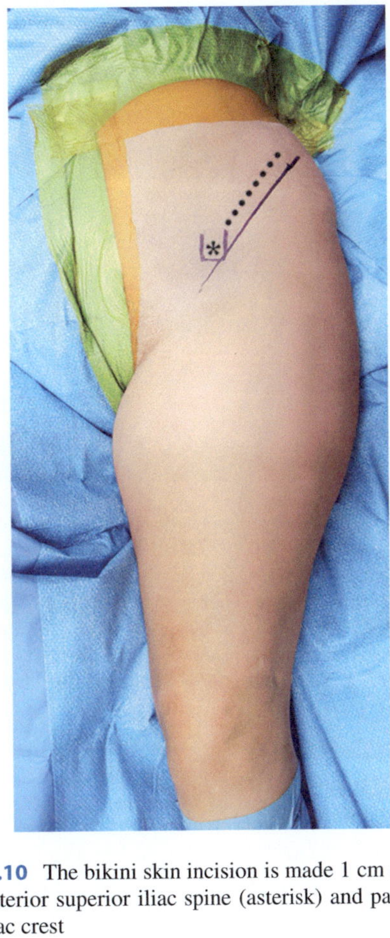

Fig. 8.10 The bikini skin incision is made 1 cm distal to the anterior superior iliac spine (asterisk) and parallel to the iliac crest

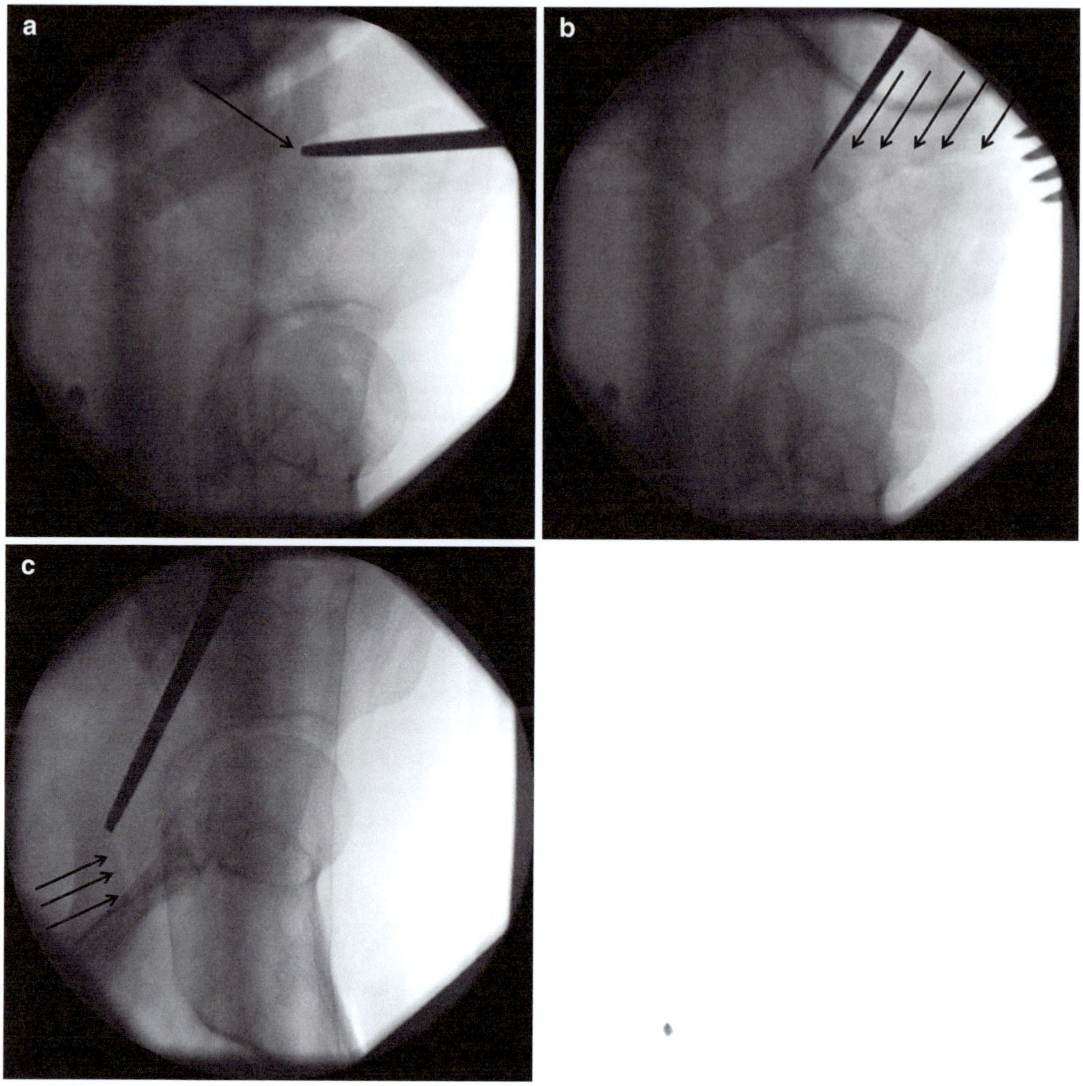

Fig. 8.11 The intersection between the supraacetabular and retroacetabular cuts (*black arrow*) is marked under oblique fluoroscopy as seen by the tip of the osteotome which is positioned just inferior to the anterior superior iliac spine and is held transverse in relation to the pelvis (**a**). A transverse supraacetabular partial iliac cut is made with an oscillating saw and is visible on the fluoroscopic image (*black arrows*), while the retroacetabular cut has been started with the osteotome under fluoroscopy (**b**). The retroacetabular cut runs down the middle of the posterior column, is performed with a straight osteotome, and meets the partial iliac cut (*black arrows*) which can be seen on the fluoroscopic image (**c**). Lateral aspects of the retroacetabular cut do not extend to the partial ischial cut (*black arrows*)

Corrective Maneuver and Fragment Fixation

A 5 mm Schanz pin is inserted in the supraacetabular bone from an anterolateral to posteromedial direction. Often this is placed in the direction of the inner table, starting just below the osteotomy site. This Schanz pin is used to verify that the osteotomy is complete and to further mobilize the fragment. If in doubt, an osteotome placed in the retroacetabular cut can be used to confirm complete mobilization of the acetabular fragment using fluoroscopy by levering on the osteotome and verifying that acetabular fragment disengages from the ischium. The manipulation is carried out under fluoroscopy guidance. Ensure that the fluoroscopy is performed in a perfect AP direction and that the coccyx is aligned with the pubic symphysis. The maneuver involves extension, medialization, internal rotation, and adduction of the fragment, all happening more or less simultaneously. When starting with a retroverted acetabulum, the first Schanz pin is used to internally rotate the hip to correct the version, and a second Schanz pin is then usually placed from directly lateral to medial in the acetabular fragment and used to adduct the fragment until appropriate lateral coverage is achieved. Once the acetabulum has been redirected, the osteotomy is temporarily fixed with 3.2 mm threaded Kirschner wires (Fig. 8.12) and then fixed with 4.5 mm cortical screws. A home-run screw is placed from the anterior inferior iliac spine (AIIS) running posterosuperiorly toward the sacroiliac joint. The spike of the prominent bone just above the AIIS is resected and impacted into the osteotomy site. Two to three additional screws are placed from the iliac crest into the supraacetabular fragment.

Younger patients are kept non-weight bearing, while young adult patients are permitted to be toe-touch weight bearing for 6 weeks, at which point they are weaned off crutches. Range of motion is started immediately postoperatively and strengthening starts at 6 weeks. A return to sports typically occurs between 3–6 months.

At 6 months postoperative, the patient was walking for up to 15 min without a cane and was off all pain medications. Her only complaint was some mild medial incisional pain, on which she is working with physiotherapy. Her hip range of motion is 110° of flexion, 25° of internal rotation, 50° of external rotation, and 35° of abduction.

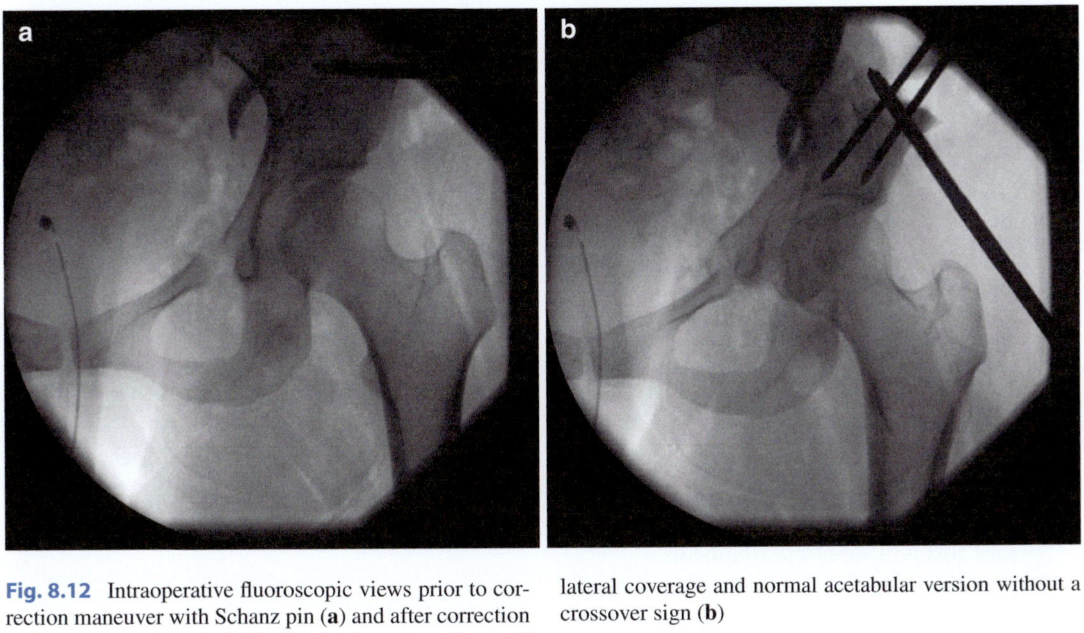

Fig. 8.12 Intraoperative fluoroscopic views prior to correction maneuver with Schanz pin (**a**) and after correction and temporary threaded K-wire fixation showing good lateral coverage and normal acetabular version without a crossover sign (**b**)

Postoperative Imaging

Her postoperative radiographs reveal a good correction with medialization of the hip joint (Fig. 8.13).

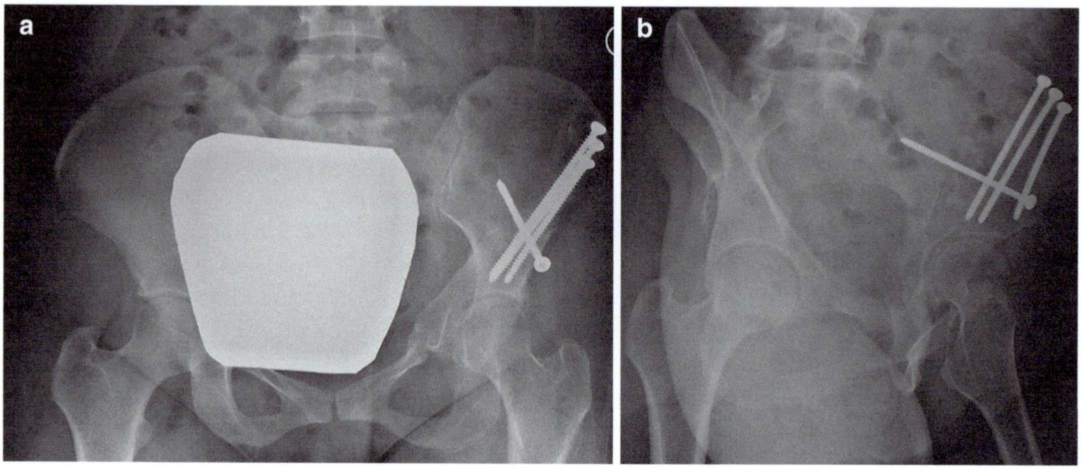

Fig. 8.13 Six-month postoperative anteroposterior pelvic (**a**) and false-profile view (**b**) showing good femoral head coverage, normal acetabulum version, and medialization of the hip joint

Pearls and Pitfalls

- The double approach acquires the same correction as the classical approach. The medialization of the joint is easier with this technique. The exposure of both the pubic and ischial bones is easier.
- Occasionally, the fragment will get caught at the ischial or pubic cuts. Palpation at the pubic cut will confirm this, and a further resection can be performed if it is impinging; another option is to manipulate the ramus with a clamp to make sure it unhinges. Similarly, an osteotome placed in the ischial cut can help to disengage this portion of the fragment.
- Periosteum and muscles can block mobility of the fragment. Some advocate extraperiosteal cut of the pubis, although we do not do this.
- The classic Schanz pin has a tendency to create retroversion, which can be dealt with by internally rotating the fragment. However, when there is significant retroversion, we find that a second Schanz pin can be extremely useful during the corrective maneuver. The original pin is used to correct the version by internally rotating the fragment. Once the version has been corrected, the second pin is placed directly lateral to medial. This pin is then used to adduct the fragment to improve lateral coverage. Alternatively, bone clamps can be used to achieve the same result.
- On the rare occasion that a revision surgery is being performed or the patient is osteopenic due to an underlying disorder, a reconstruction plate can be used to augment fixation and prevent migration of the reoriented acetabular fragment.

Indications and Contraindications (Table 8.1)

Table 8.1 Periacetabular osteotomy: surgical indications and contraindications

Indications
Asymptotic acetabular dysplasia center-edge angle <10°
Symptomatic acetabular dysplasia
Symptomatic acetabular retroversion with retroversion index >30%
Contraindications
Advanced arthrosis (Tönnis grade 2 or 3)
Irreducible hip subluxation
Incongruous hip that may become further incongruous

Further Reading

Clohisy JC, Barrett SE, Gordon JE, Delgado ED, Schoenecker PL. Periacetabular osteotomy in the treatment of severe acetabular dysplasia. Surgical technique. J Bone Joint Surg Am. 2006;88(Suppl 1 Pt 1):65–83.

Ganz R, Klaue K, Vinh TS, Mast JW. A new periacetabular osteotomy for the treatment of hip dysplasias technique and preliminary results. Clin Orthop Relat Res. 1988;(232):26–36.

Leunig M, Siebenrock KA, Ganz R. Rationale of periacetabular osteotomy and background work. Instr Course Lect. 2001;50:229–38.

Li YC, Wu KW, Huang SC, Wang TM, Kuo KN. Modified triple innominate osteotomy for acetabular dysplasia: for better femoral head medialization and coverage. J Pediatr Orthop B. 2012;21(3):193–9.

Periacetabular Osteotomy for Adolescent Neuromuscular Hip Dysplasia: Cerebral Palsy

9

Stephan T. Zmugg and Daniel J. Sucato

Introduction

The adolescent neuromuscular patient with hip instability and dysplasia presents a treatment challenge with little guidance in the literature regarding the optimal treatment. In cerebral palsy, specifically, hip instability is the most common hip disorder and can lead to decreased physical endurance, pain, arthritis, and fixed dislocation. Generally, the pathophysiology is increased contracture of the hip adductors and hip flexor (psoas) which slowly creates an adduction and flexion contracture with slow migration of the femoral head out of the acetabulum. In ambulating cerebral palsy patients, a hip that centers and is congruent can be treated with a redirectional osteotomy with careful attention to maintain posterior coverage while improving lateral coverage. While classically redirection osteotomies are contraindicated in such cases as they typically create retroversion, an appropriately executed periacetabular osteotomy can maintain and even improve posterior coverage.

S. T. Zmugg · D. J. Sucato (✉)
Department of Orthopaedic Surgery, Texas Scottish Rite Hospital, University of Texas at Southwestern Medical School, Dallas, TX, USA
e-mail: stephan.zmugg@tsrh.org; dan.sucato@tsrh.org

Brief Clinical History

This 17-year-old male with right spastic hemiparesis cerebral palsy (CP) presented for the first time to our institution with complaints of right hip pain over the past 5–6 years with a sudden increase in hip pain and difficulty walking secondary to this pain. He normally ambulates without any orthoses and is considered a Gross Motor Function Classification System type I. His current pain is anteriorly, which he states is deep in the groin area and is significantly worse with attempts at weight-bearing. Prior to his recent episode of acute pain, he was having intermittent hip groin pain, which was progressively worsening, requiring more frequent use of anti-inflammatory medications.

He is otherwise healthy with no previous surgical history. He does not take any medications outside of the anti-inflammatory medications.

On physical examination he was noted to have a spastic-type gait on the right. He also had components of a Trendelenburg gait as well as dynamic equinus during the stance phase. He also has a fairly significant antalgic gait in which he really tries to limit time in stance phase on the right side and even uses crutches now for long distance. The right hip was very uncomfortable to any significant range of motion but flexes passively to 85° with 10° of internal rotation and 20° of external rotation. There is a 10° hip flexion contracture. The left hip range of motion was essentially normal.

R. C. Hamdy, N. Saran (eds.), *Pediatric Pelvic and Proximal Femoral Osteotomies*,
https://doi.org/10.1007/978-3-319-78033-7_9

Preoperative Imaging

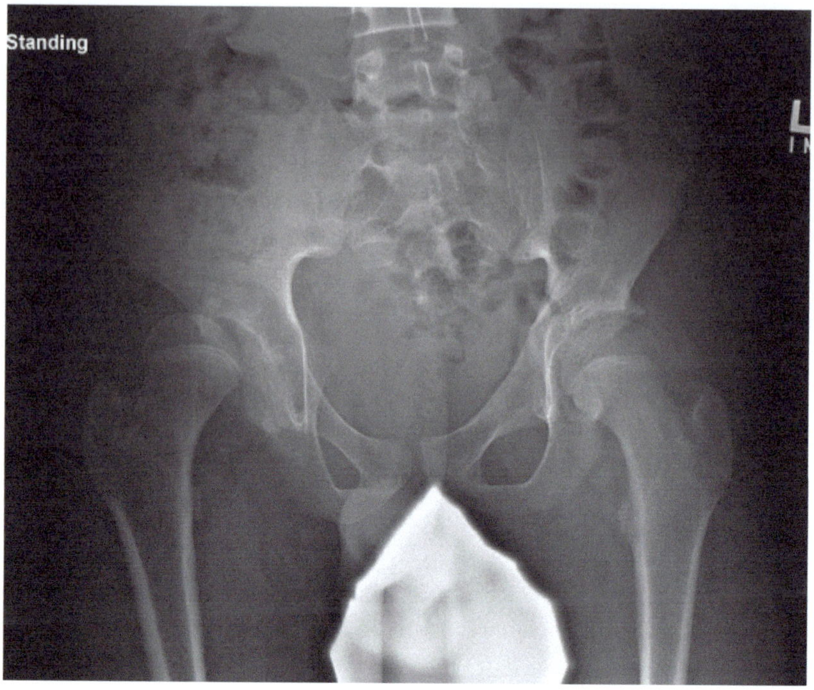

Fig. 9.1 Standing anteroposterior (AP) radiograph demonstrates significant right hip subluxation with a break in Shenton's line, a Reimer's index of 10%, a center-edge angle of −15°, a steep sourcil, and very mild adduction of the left femur. The hip is essentially subluxated

The standing anteroposterior (AP) radiograph demonstrated significant right hip subluxation with a broken Shenton's line, a Reimer's migration index of 10%, a center-edge angle of −15°, a steep sourcil, a large crossover sign, and very mild adduction of the left femur. The hip is essentially dislocated (Fig. 9.1). The false profile demonstrates significantly decreased anterior coverage and a negative anterior center-edge angle (Fig. 9.2). The abduction-internal rotation (AIR or von Rosen) view is an attempt to demonstrate femoral head reduction within the acetabulum, which is not seen in this image (Fig. 9.3). The femoral head on the AIR view appears relatively round without any significant lateral femoral head deformity. The results of the AIR view are not uncommon in CP, especially with a standing radiograph demonstrating hip subluxation as the soft tissue contractures, etc., prevent femoral head reduction. In this situation, when the option of periacetabular osteotomy (PAO) is considered, the AIR view should be obtained in the operating room with the patient completely relaxed under anesthesia, and this often results in a concentric reduction (Fig. 9.4). Occasionally the AIR view is obtained following an adductor release as the hip may reduce better once the soft tissue contractures are released.

After a very lengthy discussion with regard to the goals of surgical treatment to improve the patient's symptoms by providing good femoral coverage, with reduction of the femoral head under the acetabulum and medialization of the hip joint center, the parents provided their informed consent for a soft tissue release (psoas over the brim and a percutaneous adductor release) together with a Bernese periacetabular osteotomy. Since the hip was significantly subluxated preoperatively, a patulous capsule must be present, and a capsulorrhaphy is necessary to assist in the maintenance of hip reduction with time.

The proposal was that this procedure would improve hip mechanics and create a more stable joint with the goals of reducing pain, improving activity endurance, and optimizing the longevity of the native hip joint to prevent or delay development of a painful hip.

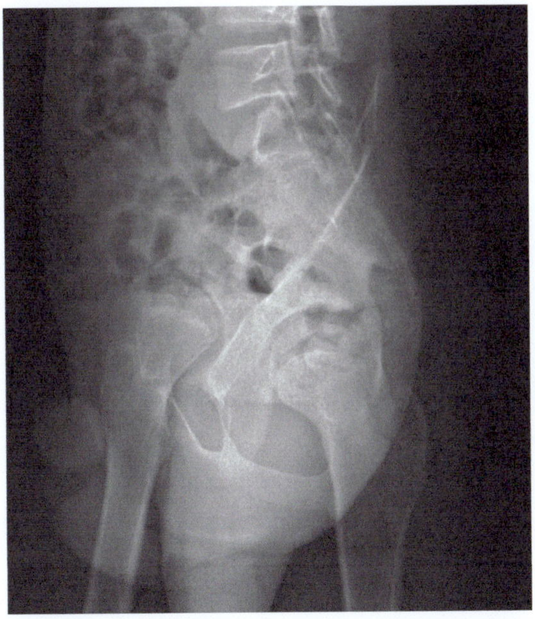

Fig. 9.2 False-profile radiograph showing significantly decreased anterior coverage and a negative anterior center-edge angle

Goals of Treatment

1. To achieve a stable, durable hip
2. To delay development of a painful hip and improve the longevity of the native hip
3. To improve physical endurance by improving hip mechanics and decreasing any symptoms

Treatment Strategy

Introduction

In cerebral palsy, adductor and psoas contractures drive hip subluxation. This results in both acetabular and femoral head deformity. The acetabulum becomes dysplastic and is often hypoplastic with primarily posterior and lateral uncoverage. The tight contracted gluteus minimus muscle causes pressure forces through the joint capsule and onto the lateral femoral head resulting in erosion of the femoral head over this region. Similarly, the contractures increase the force with which the femoral head articulates with the posterolateral edge of the dysplastic acetabulum resulting in arthritic changes to the

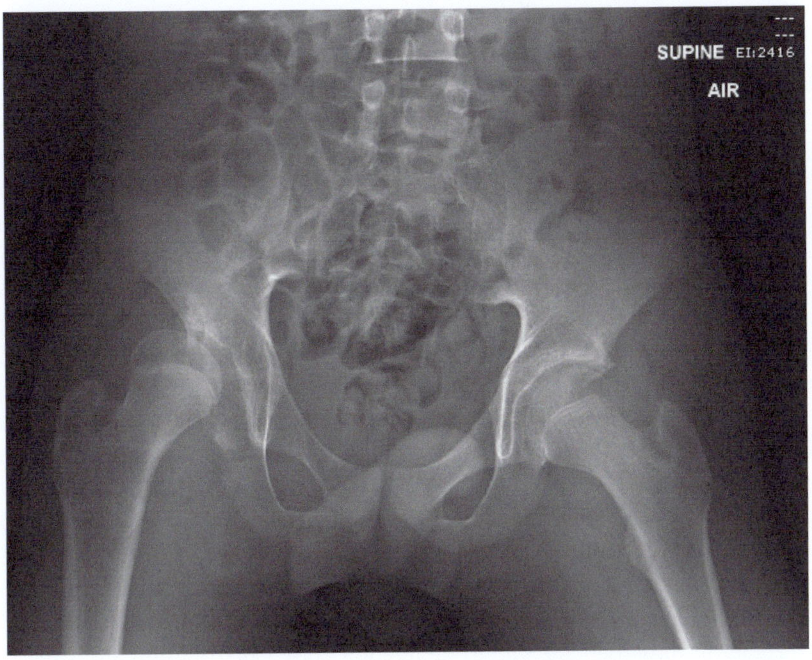

Fig. 9.3 The abduction-internal rotation (or von Rosen) view is an attempt to demonstrate femoral head reduction within the acetabulum, which is *not* seen in this image

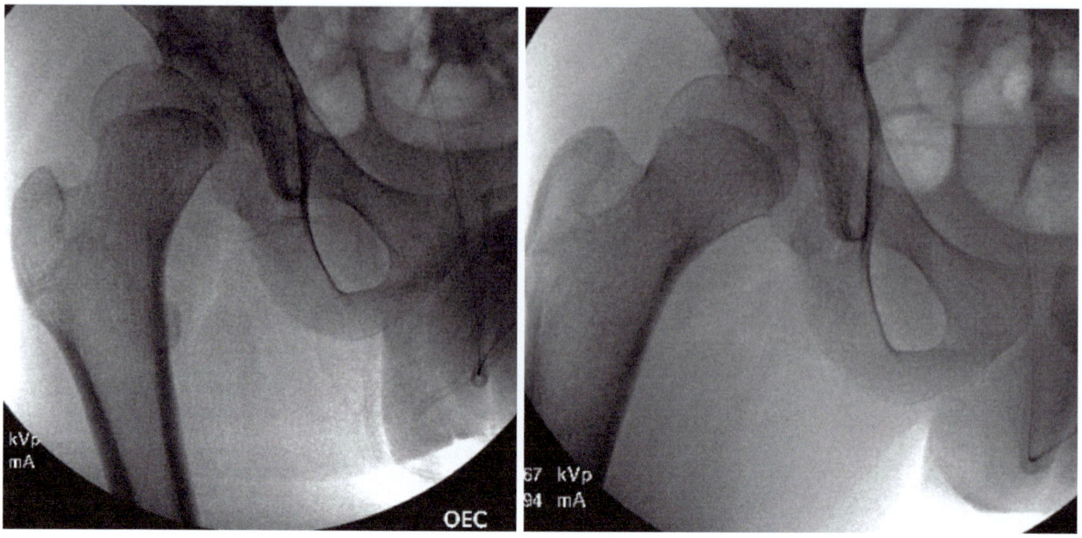

Fig. 9.4 When the patient is under anesthesia and muscle relaxant, the hip appears less subluxated (*left*) and reduces on abduction-internal rotation view (*right*)

labrum and acetabulum. The result is painful hip subluxation.

The literature has shown mixed results with various types of redirectional osteotomies, with general agreement that greater lateral and posterior acetabular coverage is necessary to cover the femoral head. In the young patient with open triradiate cartilage, this is best achieved with a Dega-style or San Diego osteotomy. In the skeletally mature patient, the femoral head is often dislocated at the time of treatment, which can result in pain from direct contact of the femoral head on the lateral aspect of the pelvis. This clinical situation is difficult, and many treatment options have been tried, including a Castle subtrochanteric resection arthroplasty, a Haas proximal valgus osteotomy, or McKale osteotomy, which combines the two previously named procedures. In the setting where the femoral head is reasonably round but is in a dysplastic acetabulum, a periacetabular osteotomy is a very good option to medialize the hip joint center and restore femoral head coverage. The prerequisites are similar as to the patient who is otherwise normal and includes a preoperative evaluation demonstrating a concentric reduction. This is often difficult in these patients due to the tendon contractures restricting motion and often requires a final decision at the time of surgery, while the patient is under general anesthesia to allow muscle relaxation and reduction. The periacetabular (Ganz) osteotomy can be utilized in this patient population, especially if the bone density is robust enough to make the cuts while providing strength to place the Schanz pin to manipulate the acetabular fragment. It is always important to release the hip adductor and hip flexors to limit the continued forces that caused the deformity from the beginning. In addition, control of acetabular version is critical to preventing persistent subluxation.

In this case the treatment strategy is the correction and optimization of the biomechanics of the hip to prevent or delay onset of arthritis, to reduce pain, and to improve the physical endurance of the patient. Specifically, the goals are (1) to medialize of the hip center, which will restore Shenton's line and decrease the joint reaction forces of the hip, (2) to horizontalize the sourcil on the AP and the false-profile radiograph to increase the surface area for articulation of the joint, and (3) to restore or maintain normal acetabular version. Correction of acetabular coverage of the femoral head optimizes load distribution and wear of the joint to prevent premature need for reconstruction. Additionally, thoughtful correction of acetabular version is critical to facilitate an impingement-free range of functional motion and is best judged with confirmation of the anterior and posterior walls meeting laterally on the AP pelvis radiograph.

Surgical Details

Periacetabular (Ganz) Osteotomy

Setup

After a general anesthetic, epidural catheter placement, and Foley catheter insertion, the patient is positioned supine on the operative table with neutral pelvic tilt and rotation. Muscle relaxant is generally utilized throughout the procedure to allow for easier exposure and soft tissue dissection, allowing for easier mobilization and positioning of the acetabular fragment.

Incision

Either a bikini-type incision or an incision just lateral to the iliac crest and carried distally in a Smith-Peterson-type incision can be used for the procedure. In this patient we chose the latter because this patient had more severe deformity, and we planned to perform a capsulorrhaphy, so wide exposure was necessary. In the heavier patient, we prefer the Smith-Peterson-type incision due to concern of wound maceration in the soft tissue cleft that may be present. This approach is also used when it is necessary to look into the joint to address intraarticular pathology.

Inner Table Exposure

The incision is carried down through the subcutaneous tissue to the fascia. The lateral edge of the ilium is incised between the external oblique muscles and the glutei stopping just proximal to the anterior superior iliac spine (ASIS). A subperiosteal dissection of the inner table of the pelvis is performed and continued down into the sciatic notch.

Distal Exposure

To develop the distal exposure, the fascia over the tensor fascia is incised, and the muscle belly of the tensor is retracted off of the septum laterally, while the fascia is retracted medially. This helps to protect the lateral femoral cutaneous nerve, which is not visualized. This interval is dissected proximally to the ASIS.

Anterior Superior Iliac Spine Osteotomy

A 2 cm osteotomy of the ASIS is performed. The depth of this osteotomy is approximately 1–1.5 cm. The ASIS fragment and tensor fascia along with the inguinal ligament and Sartorius muscle are retracted medially, while the tensor muscle is retracted laterally.

Anterior Hip Dissection

Deep in this interval lies the direct head of the rectus femoris, which is left intact. The interval between the medial aspect of the rectus and the iliacus muscle is developed, and with the hip flexed, this dissection allows for identification of the iliocapsularis—an extension of the iliacus as it inserts onto the capsule. This muscle is sharply dissected off the capsule, and the dissection is carried medial between the joint capsule and the psoas. The superior pubic ramus is exposed by connecting the capsular dissection with the inner table dissection and following this past the iliopectineal eminence medially.

Ischial Access

Once the dissection is carried medial to the capsule and visualization becomes difficult, curved Mayo scissors are used to dissect between the capsule and psoas to the level of the ischium just distal to the acetabulum.

Ischial Cut

The Mayo scissors are exchanged for the Ganz osteotome (angled at 50° near its distal end), which is utilized to begin the cut beginning in the infracotyloid groove just below the inferior acetabulum. The cut is visualized under fluoroscopy using both the AP pelvis and especially the false-profile images so that the depth of the cut can go to approximately 2.5 cm (see Fig. 9.5a). It is important to anticipate the fourth posterior column cut to ensure the first cut travels posterior enough to allow for meeting of these two osteotomies.

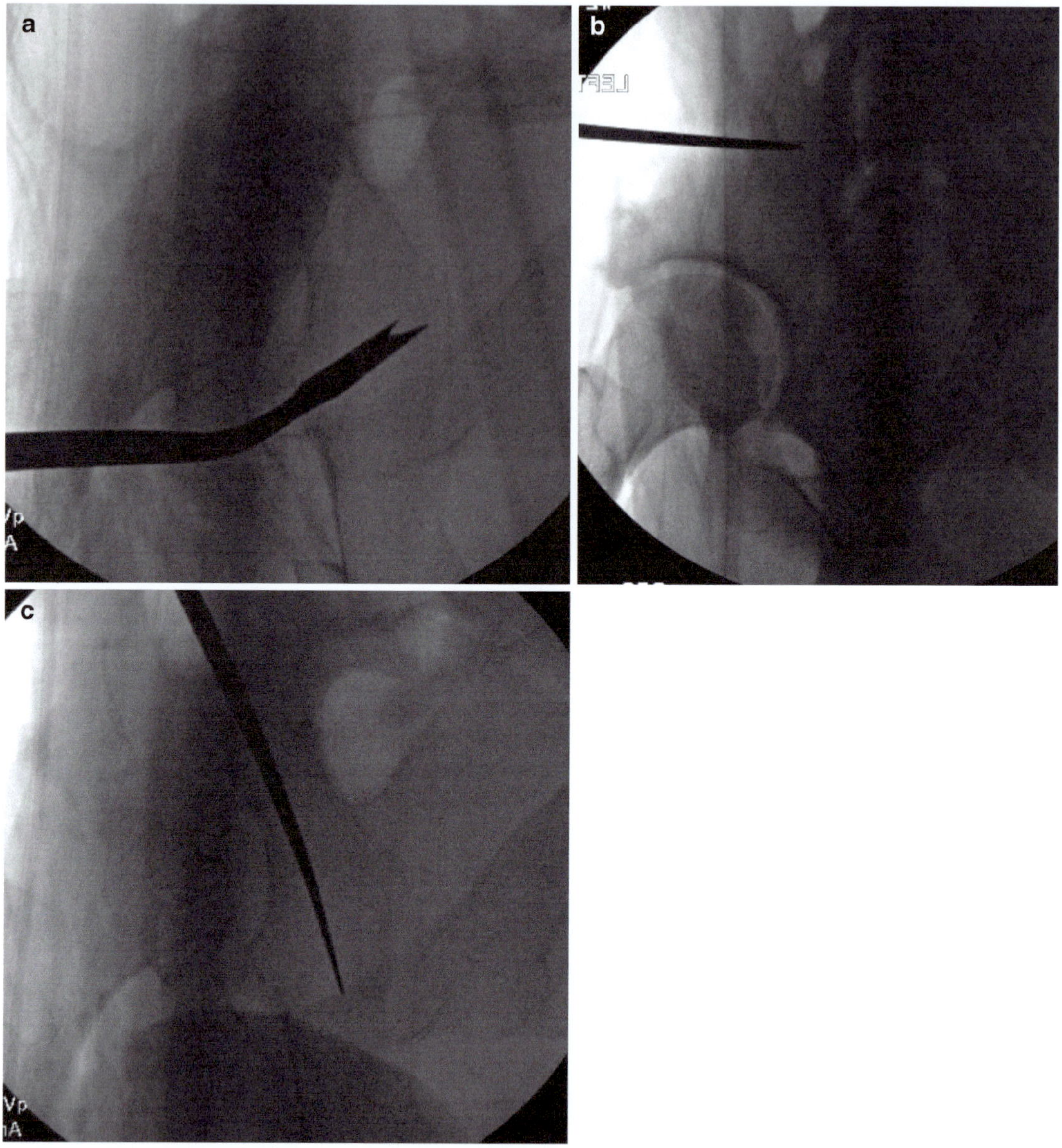

Fig. 9.5 Fluoroscopic image showing the angled forked osteotome starting in the infracotyloid groove and advanced to just past the point of where the posterior column cut will descent (**a**). Fluoroscopy image (taken from another patient) showing the apex between the third (supra-acetabular) and fourth cut (retroacetabular), identified by an osteotome placed just lateral to the pelvic brim on this false-profile image (**b**). The supra-acetabular cut is performed with an oscillating saw and will follow the line of the osteotome used to mark the intersection of the third and fourth cuts. The posterior column or fourth cut is performed with either a slightly curved or straight osteotome and runs down the middle of the posterior column (**c**). The cut should end just beyond where the partial ischial cut had been made to ensure completeness of the osteotomy. This cut takes several passes starting medially and slowly redirecting toward the lateral pelvic wall

Pubic Cut

The second cut is made on the superior ramus beginning just medial to the iliopectineal eminence, angled at approximately 45° into the obturator foramen, and is usually made with a straight osteotome. Care is taken to perform a subperiosteal dissection around the superior ramus to ensure that this does not prevent motion, and Homan retractors are placed within the obturator foramen to protect the obturator neurovascular bundle during the osteotomy. To ensure that the osteotomy is complete, a large osteotome is levered within the osteotomy, and movement should be visualized at the osteotomy site.

Supra-acetabular Cut

Next, attention is turned to the third cut which begins just below the anterior superior iliac spine. To make this osteotomy, a small width of muscle is stripped off the lateral aspect of the pelvis with a Cobb elevator. The cut is made with an oscillating saw and is directed straight toward the floor if the patient is positioned supine and ends just lateral to the pelvic brim. The end point of this third cut is initially visualized with an osteotome placed at the end of this cut using a false-profile fluoroscopy view to ensure that this is in the middle portion of posterior column and will allow for a good starting point for the fourth cut (Fig. 9.5b).

Retroacetabular Cut

The fourth cut is made beginning just lateral to the pelvic brim at the end of the third cut and is usually made with a straight or slightly curved osteotomy, traveling along the posterior column. The osteotomy should bisect the distance between the posterior aspect of the posterior column and the posterior aspect of the acetabulum (Fig. 9.5c). A half-inch osteotome is usually utilized and should be directly visualized as it travels down this posterior column. Several passes of the osteotome are necessary to traverse the posterior column so that, as one completes this cut, the acetabular fragment begins to move laterally. The first pass is along the medial cortex, and with each sequential pass, the osteotome is angled slightly laterally. As this occurs, the osteotomy is propagated through the lateral aspect of the posterior column. Once the osteotomy is complete, a 6.0 mm diameter Schanz pin is placed into the acetabular fragment just proximal to the acetabulum.

Manipulation of the Fragment

Manipulation of the acetabular fragment is the most challenging aspect of this operation. The goal is to achieve optimum coverage without overcovering and to medialize the hip joint to restore Shenton's line while restoring normal acetabular version.

The initial step to reorientation of the acetabulum is to ensure that the superior ramus cut is completely mobile and disengaged. The superior ramus aspect of the acetabular fragment is moved proximal and slightly posterior to the remaining superior ramus by levering the Schanz pin inferomedially. This will allow for continued positioning of the fragment without creating retroversion. Following this, the entire fragment can then be rotated predominantly anteriorly, which will improve both anterior and lateral coverage as posterolateral coverage becomes anterolateral coverage. It is often then necessary to hold onto the superior ramus aspect of the acetabular fragment with a bone reduction forceps and, using this in conjunction with the Schanz pin, to leverage the fragment and provide appropriate rotation. The tendency is to create retroversion as one rotates the fragment anteriorly (this is represented by the crossover sign on the AP radiograph in which the outline of the anterior wall ends more laterally than the posterior wall).

Capsulotomy and Capsulorrhaphy

For those hips in which severe subluxation is present preoperatively, a capsulotomy with capsulorrhaphy may be necessary to tighten the capsule and prevent postoperative subluxation. In general, the author does not perform this as a routine part of the procedure but is indicated when the risk of subluxation is high in the setting of insufficient coverage by the PAO or when excessive valgus is necessary to place the good femoral head into the weightbearing zone.

A T-capsulotomy is created in which the proximal horizontal incision in the capsule is made parallel with the superior aspect of the acetabulum. The lateral aspect of the horizontal cut is made laterally enough to allow this lateral flap to be brought over medially to create tension on the capsule to prevent subluxation. The vertical cut in the capsule is made along the axis of the femoral neck. Generally, tension is placed along the capsule, and a sharp ten-blade scalpel is used to make the cut. The lateral leaflet of capsule is brought over 2–3 cm from its original position and suture in a "pants-over-vest" fashion with #2 Ethibond Excel sutures (Ethicon, Somerville NJ, USA). This suturing of the capsule is done as the final step after the osteotomy has been made and the acetabular fragment has moved. The acetabular incision can then be closed in the normal fashion with the leg held in an abducted position with internal rotation of the leg until the hip spica cast is placed.

Fixation

Following completion of rotation, provisional fixation with 3/32 inch diameter K-wires is performed, and these serve to hold the fragment stable while fluoroscopic images are checked. At this point a fluoroscopic view or an AP pelvic radiograph is utilized to assess the position of the acetabular fragment. Several attempts at positioning the fragment may be necessary to achieve optimal correction in all planes while maintaining normal version (Figs. 9.6 and 9.7). Fixation of the acetabular fragment is varied, depending on the preference of the surgeon and the quality of the bone; however, for the vast majority of the time, we use 3.5 mm diameter stainless steel screws, which provide excellent stability. The screws are generally placed so that they are not close to the acetabular weightbearing surface to avoid interfering with potential future reconstruction options.

Postoperative Imaging (See Figs. 9.6 and 9.7)

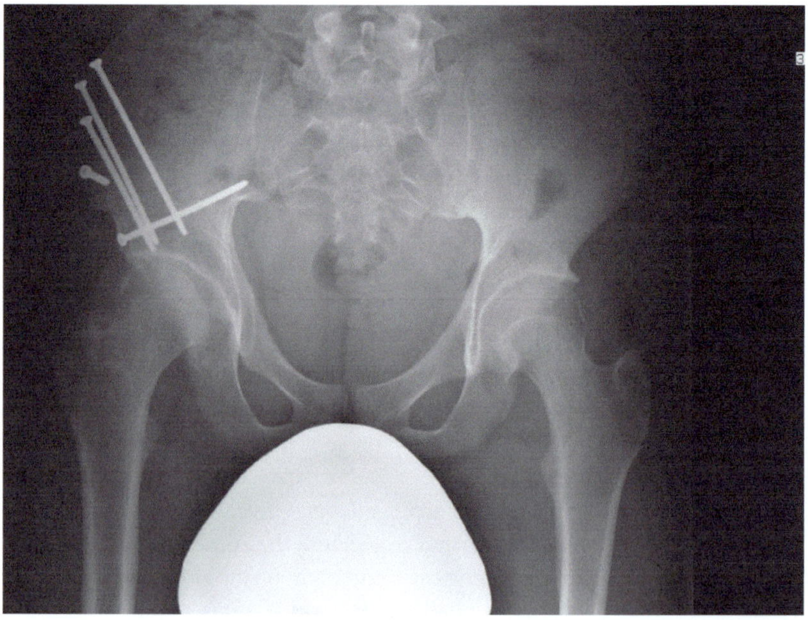

Fig. 9.6 Anteroposterior standing radiograph 9 years following surgery, demonstrating good lateral coverage of the femoral head and some medialization of the hip joint center. There is nice congruency between the femoral head and acetabulum without decreased joint space narrowing or sclerosis with time. Overall, the version of the acetabulum is significantly improved as the crossover sign is much smaller. The patient is ambulating well without pain or external support

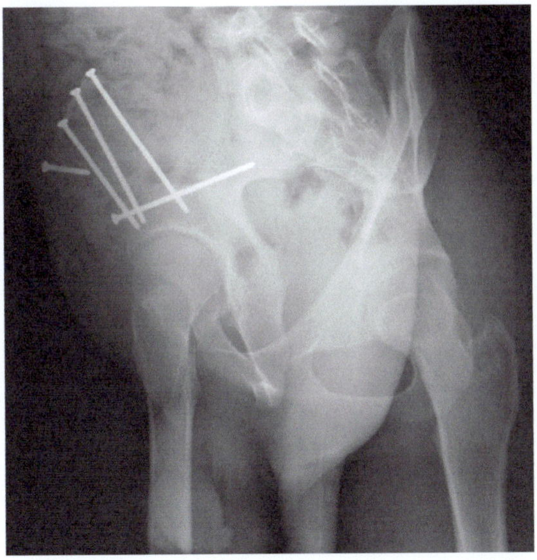

Fig. 9.7 False-profile radiograph 9 years following surgery, demonstrating improvement in the anterior femoral head coverage by the acetabulum

Indications and Contraindications (Table 9.1)

Table 9.1 Periacetabular osteotomy for adolescent neuromuscular hip dysplasia—cerebral palsy: surgical indications and contraindications

Indications
Closed triradiate cartilage
Good joint space (>2 mm)
Reducible hip with good congruency
Either seen on the preoperative abduction-internal rotation view or the fluoroscopy image under anesthesia
Generally an ambulatory patient with good bone density
Contraindications
Wide open triradiate cartilage
Poor bone density making osteotomies and redirection of the fragment with a Schanz pin difficult
Tönnis 2–3 changes—significant joint space narrowing, sclerosis of the subchondral surface
When significant lateral femoral head deformity is present—a valgus with PAO is considered

Pearls and Pitfalls

- Good fluoroscopic imaging is necessary, particularly when making the posterior column cut and during fragment orientation.
- Ensure complete release of the periosteum at the superior pubic ramus cut to allow adequate mobilization of the fragment.
- A good preoperative plan and understanding of the patient's native version and acetabular deficiency are essential to create the appropriate version and coverage during the correction.
- All of the cuts should be aggressive to complete the cut and "pass-point" slightly so that the acetabular fragment will mobilize once all of the cuts are made.
- Epidural usage is critical to allow relative hypotension and decrease blood loss and also affords excellent postoperative pain control.

Suggested Reading

Beck M, Woo A, Leunig M, Ganz R. Gluteus minimus-induced femoral head deformation in dysplasia of the hip. Acta Orthop Scand. 2001;72(1):13–7.

Ganz R, Klaue K, Vinh TS, Mast JW. A new periacetabular osteotomy for the treatment of hip dysplasias. Technique and preliminary results. Clin Orthop. 1988;232:26–36.

Sankar WN. Complete redirectional acetabular osteotomies for neurogenic and syndromic hip dysplasia. J Pediatr Orthop. 2013;33(Suppl 1):S39–44.

Sucato DJ. Treatment of late dysplasia with Ganz osteotomy. Orthop Clin North Am. 2006;37(2):161–71, vi.

10 Hip Instability in Adolescent/Young Adult Down Syndrome

Jill E. Larson and Michael B. Millis

Introduction

The incidence of acetabular dysplasia in the skeletally mature Down syndrome patient population ranges from 8 to 25%, while hip subluxation or dislocation occurs in 1–7%. The morphology of the dysplastic acetabulum in a Down syndrome patient may be similar to idiopathic developmental dysplasia of the hip, with either global or anterior hypoplasia. A distinct subtype of acetabular dysplasia common in trisomy 21 is that of a deficient posterior wall with acetabular retroversion. The instability associated with a dysplastic hip in trisomy 21 is further compounded by generalized hypotonia, ligamentous laxity, and frequently cognitive delays. Untreated hip instability leads to early-onset osteoarthritis and hip pain in young adulthood. With increasing life expectancy in the Down syndrome patient population, the prevention of early osteoarthritis and associated hip pain with maintenance of functional hip range of motion is key to maximizing quality of life. Traditionally, hip instability in Down syndrome has been treated with multiple surgical interventions, including proximal femoral osteotomy, acetabular osteotomies (shelf, innominate, Sutherland, Chiari), and capsular plication with variable results. More recently, a Bernese periacetabular osteotomy (PAO) has demonstrated promising clinical outcomes in treating hip instability in the skeletally mature Down syndrome patient. The following case demonstrates unilateral hip instability in a Down syndrome patient who achieved good functional and radiographic outcomes after PAO.

J. E. Larson
Department of Orthopedic Surgery, Harvard University, Boston Children's Hospital, Boston, MA, USA
e-mail: jill.larson@childrens.harvard.edu

M. B. Millis (✉)
Department of Orthopedic Surgery, Boston Children's Hospital, Child and Adult Hip Program, Boston, MA, USA
e-mail: Michael.Millis@childrens.harvard.edu

Brief Clinical History

A 15-year-old male with Down syndrome (trisomy 21) presented with a 2-month history of right thigh pain and limp. He was previously athletically active. Gait evaluation demon-

R. C. Hamdy, N. Saran (eds.), *Pediatric Pelvic and Proximal Femoral Osteotomies*,
https://doi.org/10.1007/978-3-319-78033-7_10

strated a right abductor lurch and right Trendelenburg sign. Passive hip flexion bilaterally was to 115° without pain. His right hip abducted to only 30° before he experienced discomfort; his left hip abducted painlessly to more than 40°. His right leg measured 1 cm shorter than the left. There was no thigh atrophy. He had no apprehension, impingement, or bicycle sign. His right hip rotation in both flexion and extension was 40°/30° of internal/external rotation compared to 60°/40° of internal/external rotation on the left.

Preoperative Radiographs
(Figs. 10.1, 10.2, 10.3, 10.4, 10.5, 10.6, 10.7, 10.8, 10.9, 10.10)

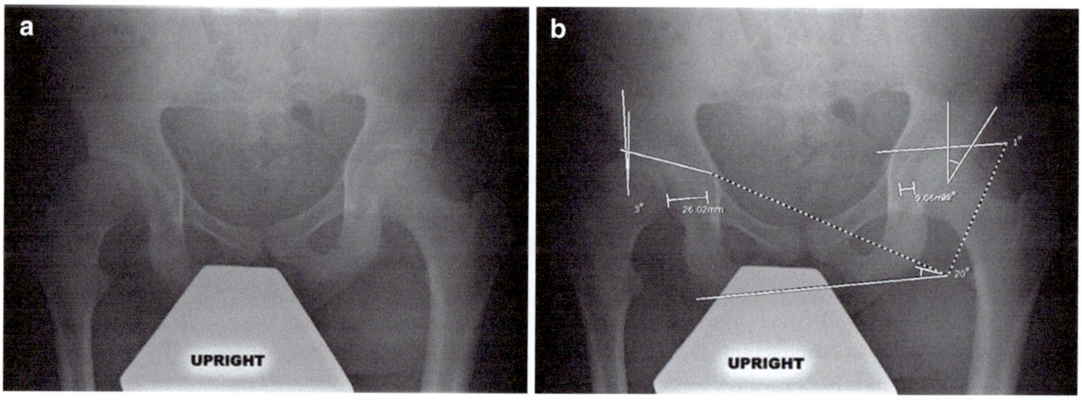

Fig. 10.1 Anteroposterior pelvis standing radiograph without (**a**) and with (**b**) annotation. The lateral center-edge angle of the right hip measured 3°, compared to 32° on the left. The medial clear space was 26 mm on the right side compared to 9 mm on the left. There was increased sclerosis of the weight-bearing zone in the right hip. The Tönnis roof angle measured 20° on the right and 1° on the left

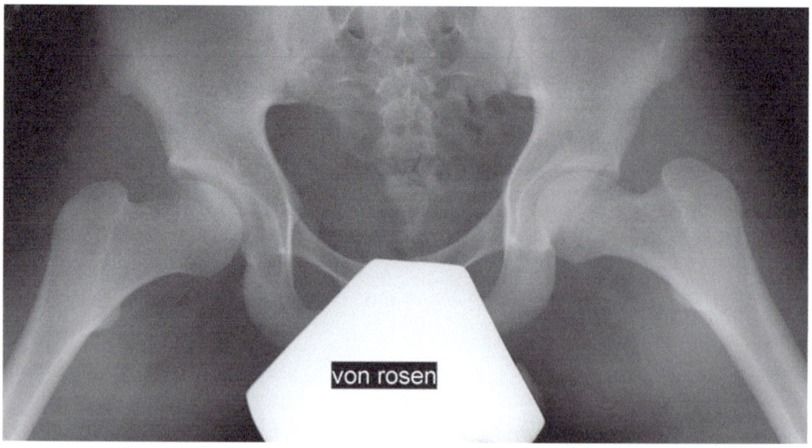

Fig. 10.2 The Von Rosen radiographic view shows a congruous reduction of the right proximal femur into the acetabulum without hinging

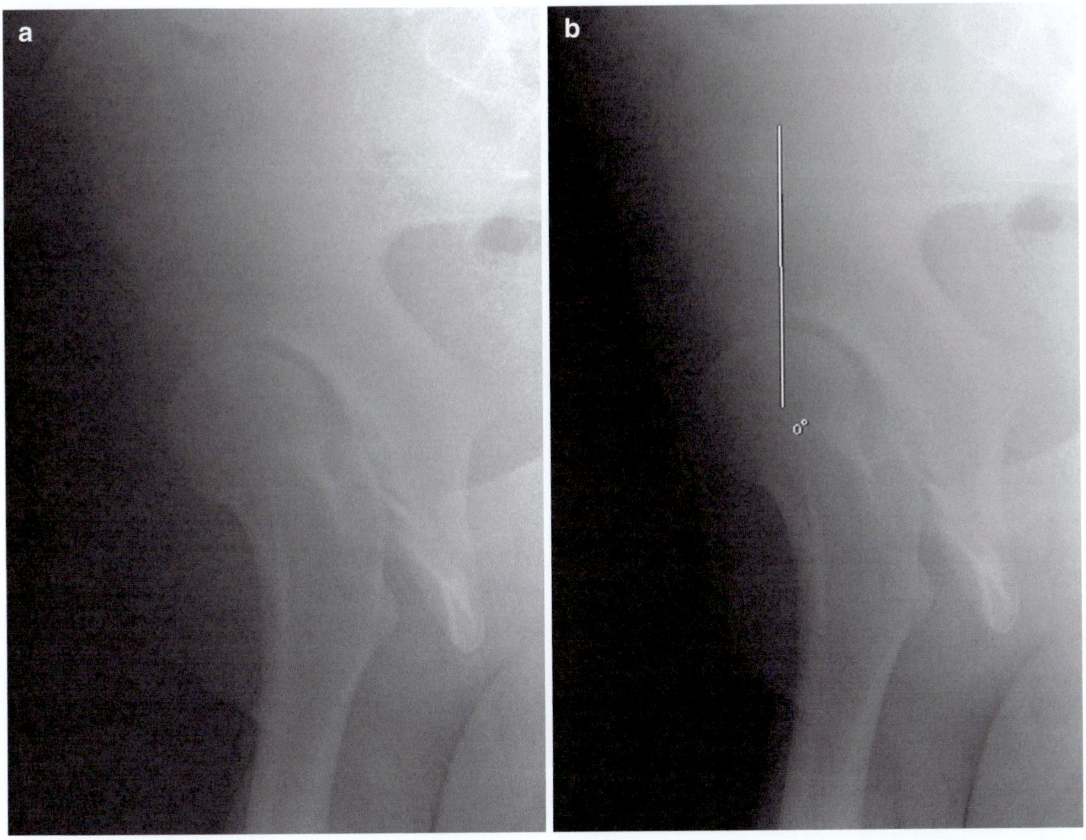

Fig. 10.3 False-profile view right hip without (**a**) and with (**b**) annotation: The anterior center-edge angle was 0° with anterior tilt of the femoral neck, suggesting femoral anteversion. Mild narrowing of the anterior cartilage space and widening of the posterior cartilage space suggest anterior subluxation

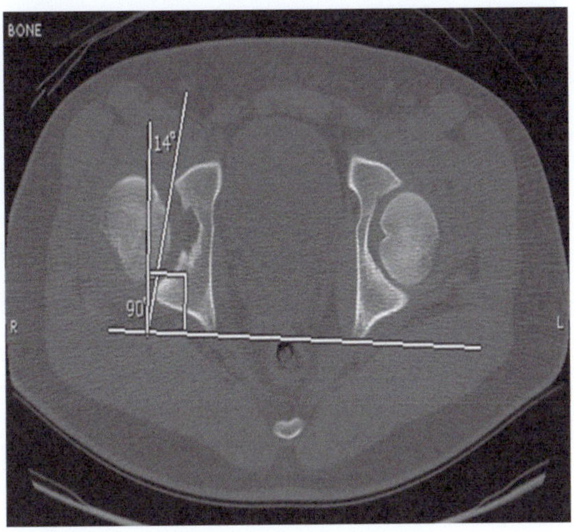

Fig. 10.4 Computed tomography (CT) scan of the pelvis, hips, and knees: axial imaging with CT scan of the pelvis is essential to assess acetabular retroversion in the Down syndrome population. To measure acetabular version, an axial cut with the largest femoral head cross-section is used. The angle is then measured between a line connecting the anterior and posterior acetabular edges and a line tangential to the base of the iliac bones (to account for patient positioning). Although not present in this patient, acetabular retroversion is very common in the Down syndrome patient population and should be preoperatively evaluated with CT scan. A cut through the femoral condyles (not pictured here) is useful to evaluate femoral version

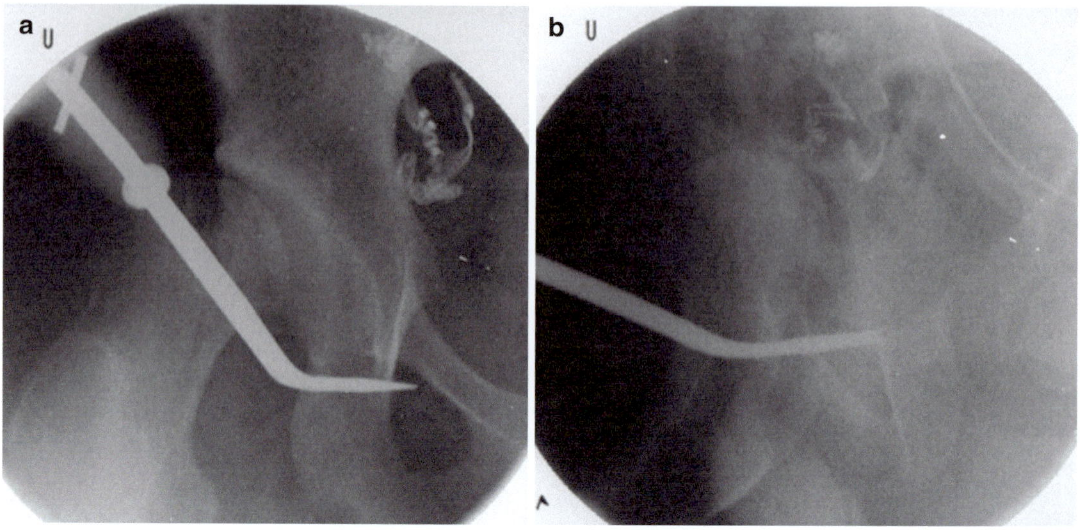

Fig. 10.5 Anteroposterior (**a**) and false-profile (**b**) intraoperative views of the ischial osteotomy

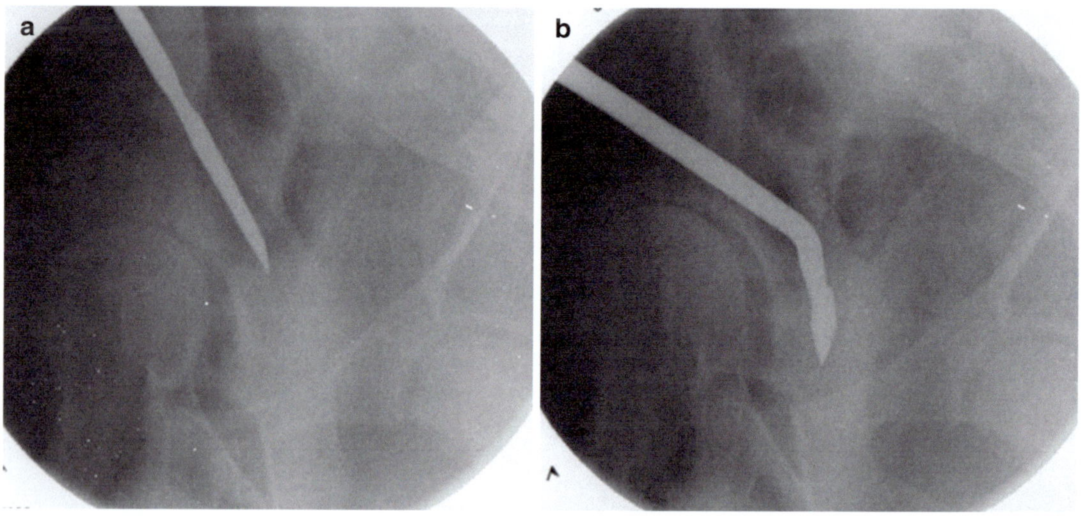

Fig. 10.6 False-profile views of the posterior column osteotomy using a straight osteotome (**a**) and an angled chisel (**b**)

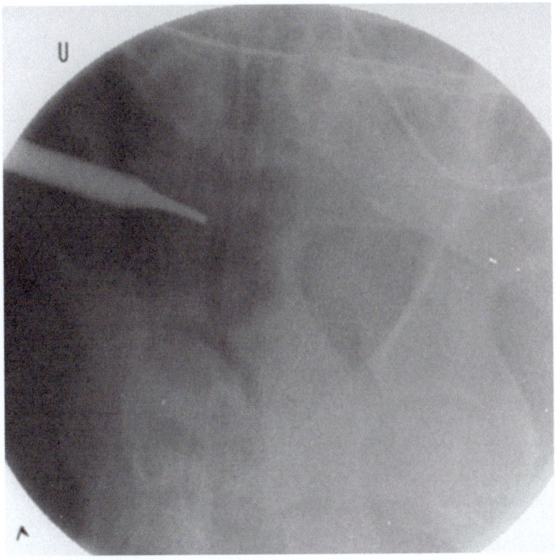

Fig. 10.7 False-profile view of the narrow spiked Hohmann retractor marking the planned course of the supra-acetabular osteotomy

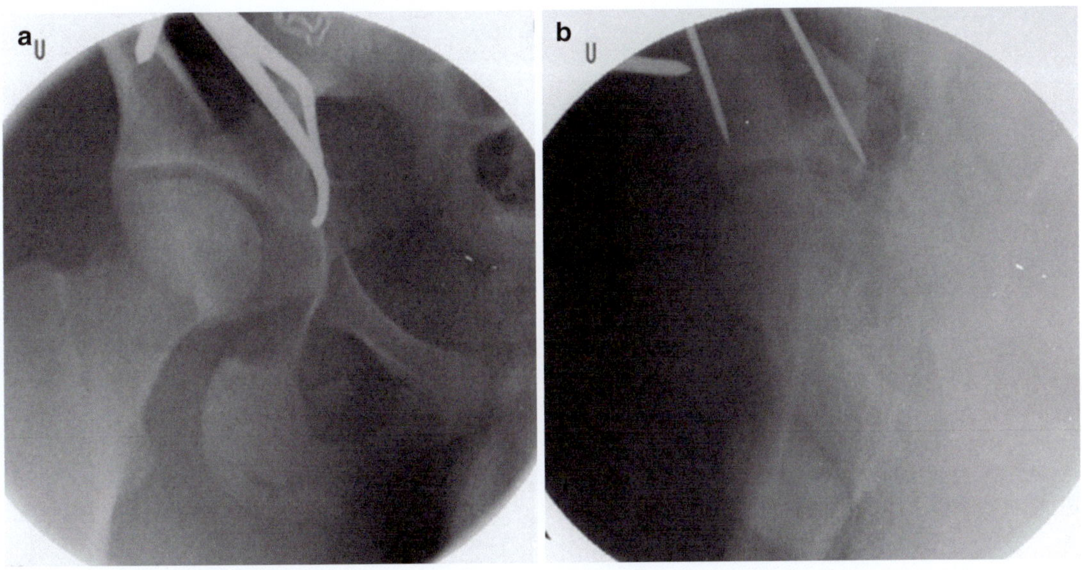

Fig. 10.8 Anteroposterior (**a**) and false-profile (**b**) views demonstrating mobilization of the free fragment with a 5.0 mm Schanz screw and Weber clamp and provisional fixation of the fragment with 3/32 inch K wires

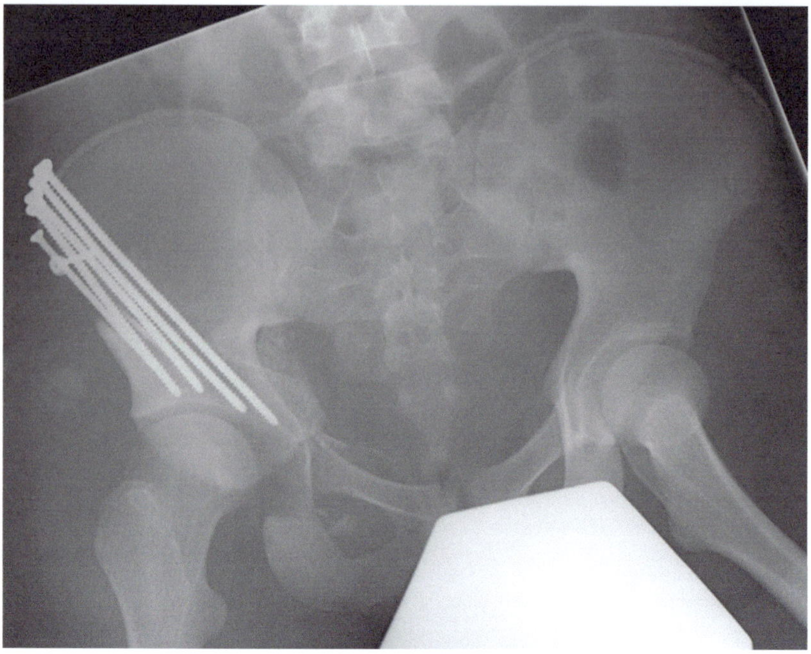

Fig. 10.9 Initial postoperative anteroposterior pelvis

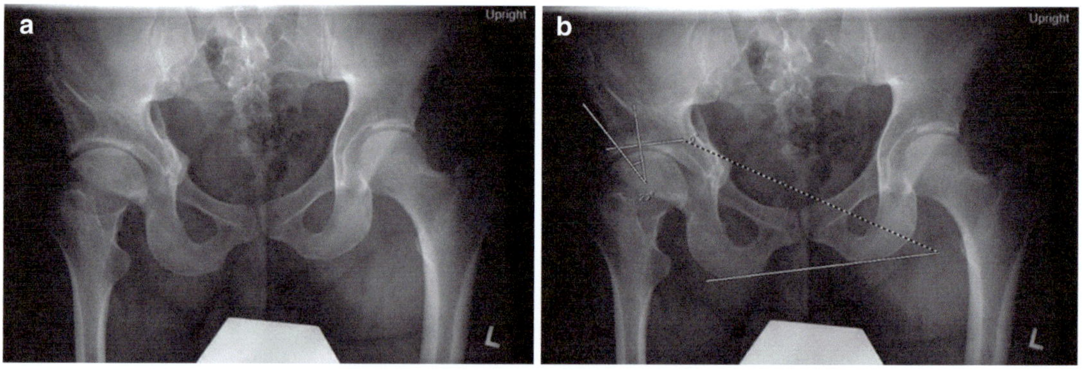

Fig. 10.10 Most recent follow-up at 12 years: patient is asymptomatic and fully active. The anteroposterior pelvis radiograph without (**a**) and with (**b**) annotation: the lateral center-edge angle measured 29° on the right compared to 3° preoperatively. The Tönnis acetabular angle measured 0° on the right compared to 20° preoperatively. Note the hip center has been medialized compared to preoperative images

Goals of Treatment

The goals of surgery are to improve hip function and to improve the long-term prognosis of the hip joint. This includes resolving any associated hip pain due to correctable mechanical abnormalities by improving the stability of the hip joint and delaying the onset of osteoarthritis.

Treatment Strategy

1. To identify pain generators secondary due to correctable anatomic abnormalities.

   In the case of this patient, the pain generators were likely associated with his hip instability, the lateral subluxation, and insufficient anterior and lateral coverage of the femoral head.

2. To devise a careful surgical plan to treat the mechanical abnormality. Based on the patient's interview, physical exam, and preoperative imaging, including computed tomography scan, it was determined that a periacetabular osteotomy was indicated. A periacetabular osteotomy is usually performed without arthrotomy in trisomy 21 patients to avoid aggravating the preexisting capsular laxity. Capsulorrhaphy has not been shown to have consistently positive results in the Down syndrome patient population.
3. To execute the program optimally. This includes (1) preoperative preparation of the patient, family, and treatment team, (2) intraoperative achievement of treatment goals, and (3) appropriate postoperative monitoring with adjustments in post-op activity level as indicated.

Surgical Details

Rectus and Abductor Sparing Periacetabular Osteotomy

The optimal operative plan includes general endotracheal anesthesia supplemented by an intraoperative regional anesthesia (i.e., a unilateral lumbar plexus nerve catheter). No neuromuscular blockade is used intraoperatively, to allow monitoring of nerve function. Any motor nerve irritation can thus be detected by muscle activity.

The patient is positioned in the supine position on the operating room table with the operative leg completely prepped and draped up to the costal margin and medially to the umbilicus. This allows the leg to be placed in various positions during the procedure to optimize exposure and reduce risk to important neurovascular structures. Full intraoperative assessment of hip range of motion is also possible. A direct anterior exposure is utilized (medial portion of the iliofemoral exposure) with an oblique incision just distal and parallel to the iliac wing, crossing the anterior aspect of the hip, just at or below the inguinal crease. The external oblique fascia is lifted to expose the iliac crest. A longitudinal incision is made along the iliac crest. Subperiosteal dissection is carried medially down the inner table of the ilium, coagulating the perforating iliolumbar vessel to achieve hemostasis.

Attention is then turned distally to the interval between the sartorius and tensor fascia lata, protecting the lateral femoral cutaneous nerve. Next, a wafer of bone of is osteotomized off the anterior superior iliac spine (ASIS) after predrilling the fragment; the sartorius and inguinal ligament remain attached to the ASIS.

With the hip flexed and adducted, deep dissection is performed between the iliopsoas and the iliac wing proximally. The sartorius, iliacus, and psoas are mobilized in a medial and distal direction off the AIIS, the straight head of the rectus, and the hip joint capsule. The capsule routinely is not opened in trisomy 21 patients.

Osteotomy #1: Superior Public Ramus

The psoas sheath is opened longitudinally. The hip is flexed and externally rotated, as subperiosteal exposure is carried medially past the iliopectineal eminence to visualize the superior pubic ramus. Dissection is continued subperiosteally anteriorly and posteriorly along the superior pubic ramus and carefully around it circumferentially to reflect obturator membrane off of the superolateral corner of the obturator foramen. Lane or Hohmann retractors are placed around the ramus. The ramus may then be osteotomized under direct vision, protecting the femoral neurovascular bundle, which lies behind the medially retracted psoas, and the obturator neurovascular bundle which lies deep to the ramus. Alternatively, a Statinsky vascular clamp may be passed retrograde under the ramus through the obturator foramen without disrupting the nearby nerve and vessels. Once the tip of the clamp is successfully visualized proximally, it may be used to grasp a suture to which a Gigli saw is attached, to lead the Gigli saw as it is passed antegrade through the foramen. The Gigli saw is then used to make an osteotomy perpendicular to the long axis of the pubic ramus (oriented distal/lateral to proximal/medial as viewed in the frontal plane).

Osteotomy #2: Ischial Incomplete

Safe placement of the angled Ganz chisel is critical for the ischial cut. This is done by first identifying the interval between the medial joint capsule and the iliopsoas, which is located directly distal to the iliopectineal eminence. Sequential dilation of this internal is performed with blunt Lane bone levers whose tips are placed onto the infracotyloid groove of the ischium, just distal to the inferior lip of the acetabulum. Image intensifier control is useful. The tip of a Ganz acetabular chisel is then carefully inserted, with soft tissues protected, through the psoas-capsule interval, and its tip is placed onto the groove. Tactile and imaging confirmation of perfect osteotome position is done. Then the anterior to posterior ischial osteotomy is performed to an appropriate depth, not more than 2 cm, avoiding extension into the lesser sciatic foramen or posterior column. The cut is controlled using the image intensifier in both the anteroposterior and oblique (false-profile) views (Fig. 10.5).

Osteotomy #3: Posterior Column

The posterior column osteotomy may be performed as the third or the fourth step. It is initially performed with a straight osteotome along the medial wall of the pelvis, bisecting the posterior column. Maintain approximately equal width bone bridges between the osteotomy and the posterior margin of the acetabulum and the anterior edge of the greater sciatic notch. The osteotomy is then extended toward the ischial spine, until it is past the point closest approach to the posterior acetabulum. At this point, an angled chisel may be used to divide the small posteromedial ischial bridge remaining. The posterior column osteotomy is initially made through the medial cortex, and into but not through the lateral cortex (Fig. 10.6), which protects the sciatic nerve.

Osteotomy #4: Supra-acetabular Ilium

The supra-acetabular iliac osteotomy may be performed as the third or fourth step. This cut must leave an adequate bridge of bone between the osteotomy and the superior aspect of the acetabulum (>1.5 cm) but must not be so high that the fragment becomes difficult to mobilize. An oscillating saw is used to make a vertical saw cut of the supra-acetabular ilium beginning just distal from the ASIS and directed toward the apex of the sciatic notch (generally, this is perpendicular to the axis of the body in a supine patient). Note that if the acetabulum is severely dysplastic with a high hip center, then the starting point may need to be proximal to the ASIS but is always directed toward the apex of the sciatic notch. The soft tissues are protected medially by a reverse Hohmann retractor. The abductors are protected laterally using a narrow spiked Hohmann retractor placed in a small subgluteal window (Fig. 10.7).

Mobilization of the Acetabular Fragment

Mobility of the acetabular fragment is critical for successful positioning. Adequate mobility may be demonstrated prior to placing the Schanz screw by using a combination of bone spreaders in the iliac osteotomy and posterior column osteotomy, plus pressure with a ball spike pusher on the medial aspect of the fragment.

Positioning and Stabilization of the Acetabular Fragment

A Schanz screw (5.0 mm) is placed from anteriorly to posteriorly in the superior portion of the acetabular fragment, approximately 1–2 cm proximal to the joint. A T-handle chuck is placed on the Schanz screw. A bone spreader may be placed into the iliac osteotomy, and a Weber clamp is placed on the superior ramus to facilitate rotation. Using the T-handle chuck, Schanz screw, Weber clamp, and the bone spreader if needed, the acetabular fragment is reoriented into the desired position—usually first extending and adducting the acetabulum to improve anterior and lateral coverage. The second step of positioning involves rotating the acetabular fragment: internal rotation anteverts the acetabulum, improving posterior coverage but reducing anterior coverage. Conversely, externally rotating the fragment retroverts the acetabulum, improving anterior coverage but reducing posterior coverage. In this patient it was determined that a correction of 25° of adduction and 20° of extension with slight anteversion of the fragment was optimal to optimize coverage and stability and to avoid retroversion and impingement (Fig. 10.8).

Problematic posterior hip instability associated with acetabular retroversion is common in the dysplastic trisomy 21 hip. Such hips require excellent posterior coverage, which usually requires an anteversion component to the correction (internal rotation of the acetabular fragment). Adequate anteversion of the acetabular fragment is usually achieved if on an AP pelvis image, the crossover sign is eliminated and there is no posterior wall sign.

Once the desired reorientation is confirmed fluoroscopically and manually by passive hip range of motion, the fragment is provisionally stabilized with smooth K wires before final fixation is achieved. Final fixation is achieved with several 3.5 mm/4.5 mm fully threaded screws placed through the iliac crest into the acetabular fragment. An anteroposterior homerun screw and/or a medial reconstruction plate may be used for supplemental fixation if bone quality is poor or postoperative compliance is questionable.

The anteriorly protruding anterior spine area is osteotomized and impacted into the anterior osteotomy cleft, and it was fixed with the most anterior screw. Bayonet apposition at the superior pubic ramus is sometimes necessary for adequate medialization and reorientation. In this case the bone edges were trimmed to reduce psoas irritation, and the trimmed bone was used as local graft to facilitate healing.

Postoperative Imaging (Figs. 10.9 and 10.10)

Pearls and Pitfalls

- Ligamentous laxity is universal in this patient population and contributes to hip instability.
  - Persistent subluxation is a known postoperative complication after periacetabular osteotomy in the Down syndrome patient population. It is more common in hips with high Tönnis roof angle (>10°). This should be discussed preoperatively with the family. If subluxation occurs postoperatively, a varus derotational femoral intertrochanteric osteotomy may be considered.
- Intraoperative assessment, both tactile and on imaging, particularly after provisional correction, is essential to monitor for femoral acetabular impingement and instability
  - Over coverage of the femoral head can lead to anterior impingement, intra-articular damage, and posterior instability. This can be mitigated by appropriate intraoperative correction and monitoring for impingement and instability intraoperatively. Taking the hip through a full passive range of motion, especially in flexion and internal rotation, allows for assessment of both anterior impingement and posterior instability. If impingement is noted postoperatively at follow-up and not responsive to nonoperative treatment, consideration can be given to the relief of impingement by either osseous realignment or intra-articular/extra-articular osteoplasty.
- Usual internal fixation methods may not be sufficient in this patient population due to various combinations of ligamentous laxity, poor bone quality, and variable patient compliance.
  - A homerun screw (directed anterior to posterior to stabilize the mobile fragment) or occasionally an additional reconstruction plate placed medially can be helpful in reducing the risk of nonunion in these patients with ligamentous laxity and osteopenia. Consideration should be given to the use of additional bone grafting (both autologous and allogeneic) as well as increased internal fixation in the Down syndrome patient population. Nonunions of the ischium and superior pubic ramus are known complications following periacetabular osteotomy even in patients without ligamentous laxity.
- Expectation management is paramount since outcomes are variable.
  - Preoperative counseling with the young adult patient and the patient's family is very critical in the Down syndrome patient population. It is important to review the goals of surgery, the risks of surgery, and the variable outcomes that can result.

Indications and Contraindications (Table 10.1)

Table 10.1 Periacetabular osteotomy in Down syndrome: surgical indications and contraindications

	Indications	Contraindications
Clinical	Hip, thigh, groin, or leg pain due to mechanical hip instability or dysplasia	Medical comorbidities that preclude surgical intervention
	Gait abnormality (limp, Trendelenburg, lurch, etc.) or decreased functionality due to hip instability or dysplasia	Major cognitive limitations with inability to follow postoperative precautions
		Hip stiffness
Radiographic	Subluxation of the femoral head (break in Shenton's arc, increased medial clear space) and/or lack of lateral coverage of the femoral head	Major incongruity of the hip joint or irreducible subluxation
Additional femoral osteotomy	Persistent hip subluxation or instability after adequate acetabular reorientation with periacetabular osteotomy	

Suggested Reading

Katz DA, Kim YJ, Millis MB. Periacetabular osteotomy in patients with Down's syndrome. J Bone Joint Surg Br. 2005;87(4):544–7.

Murphy SB, Millis MB. Periacetabular osteotomy without abductor dissection using direct anterior exposure. Clin Orthop Relat Res. 1999;364:92–8.

Sankar WN, Schoenecker JG, Mayfield ME, Kim YJ, Millis MB. Acetabular retroversion in Down syndrome. J Pediatr Orthop. 2012;32(3):277–81.

Schrader T, Millis MB. Ganz periacetabular osteotomy. In: Morrissy RT, Weinstein SL, editors. Atlas of pediatric orthopaedic surgery. 4th ed. Philadelphia: Lippincott Williams and Wilkins; 2005. p. 319–27.

11 San Diego Osteotomy (Lateral Acetabuloplasty)

Vidyadhar V. Upasani and Dennis R. Wenger

Introduction

The comprehensive approach to neuromuscular hip disease (dysplasia and dislocation) requires appropriate management of contracted hip flexors, adductors and sometimes distal hamstrings, along with reduction of the hip (with capsulorrhaphy in severe cases) plus proximal femoral and acetabular osteotomies. The San Diego osteotomy (lateral bending acetabuloplasty) allows for better correction of the posterior-superior acetabular deficiency, which is most common in neuromuscular hip disease, resulting in excellent midterm outcomes with low rates of recurrent instability.

Brief Clinical History

This 4-year-old female with cerebral palsy Gross Motor Function Classification System level 5 (GMFCS) and spastic quadriplegia was referred to our orthopedic surgery clinic for evaluation of worsening right hip contracture and expression of pain with prolonged sitting and peroneal care. She was initially treated at an outside facility where a brain magnetic resonance imaging study demonstrated severe cystic encephalomalacia of the cerebrum bilaterally affecting the frontal, temporal, and parietal lobes and the basal ganglia with global cerebral volume loss. She had been followed in the Physical Medicine and Rehabilitation Clinic at our facility and had received physical therapy, occupational therapy, abduction bracing, and botulinum toxin injections to her right hip adductors and bilateral gastrocnemius muscles.

On initial examination she was noted to have global developmental delay with significant cognitive impairment and minimal upper extremity contractures. She had a slight thoracolumbar junctional kyphosis with left-sided pelvic tilt and spinal rotation. She had bilateral hip flexion contractures of 15°, right hip abduction of 10° compared to 40° on the left, 20° bilateral knee flexion contractures with popliteal angles of 130°, and 30° of bilateral ankle dorsiflexion. Radiographs demonstrated a right hip dislocation with right hip adduction contracture and pelvic tilt to the left. We recommend a comprehensive surgical procedure that includes a soft tissue lengthening, hip open reduction and capsulorrhaphy, and proximal femoral plus acetabular osteotomies.

V. V. Upasani (✉)
Rady Children's Hospital San Diego, University of California San Diego, San Diego, CA, USA
e-mail: vupasani@rchsd.org

D. R. Wenger
Department of Orthopedic Surgery, Pediatric Orthopedic Training Program, Rady Children's Hospital San Diego, University of California, San Diego, San Diego, CA, USA
e-mail: dwenger@rchsd.org

R. C. Hamdy, N. Saran (eds.), *Pediatric Pelvic and Proximal Femoral Osteotomies*,
https://doi.org/10.1007/978-3-319-78033-7_11

Preoperative Imaging (Fig. 11.1)

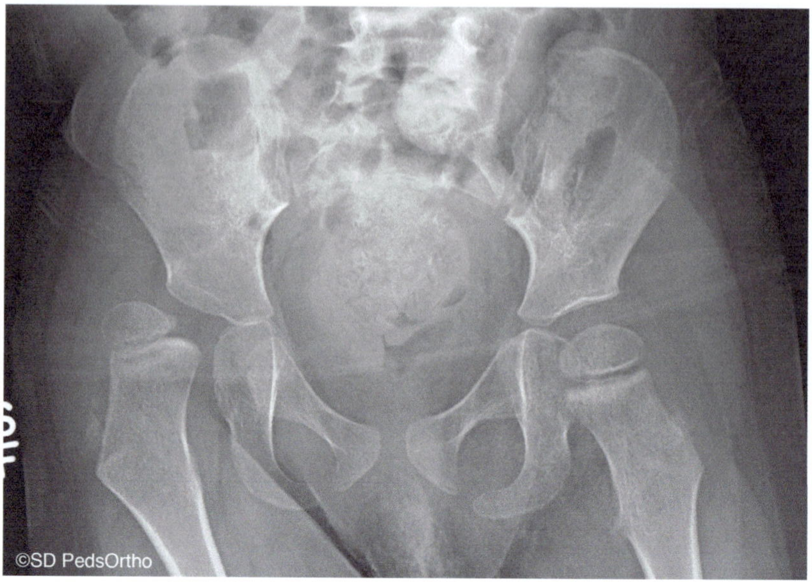

Fig. 11.1 Preoperative anterior posterior radiograph of a 4-year-old female with a right neuromuscular hip dislocation (© San Diego Orthopedics, with permission)

Goals of Treatment

The natural history of the neuromuscular hip in a child with spasticity has been well described. Muscle contractures about the hip and in the thigh result in eventual hip dislocation, femoral head deformity, and degenerative joint disease. Salvage options for a symptomatic dislocated, arthritic spastic hip include proximal femoral resection, interposition arthroplasty, or arthrodesis. In our experience, these patients often have less satisfactory outcomes with recurrent symptoms and worsening pelvic obliquity. We therefore recommend early surgery to prevent this evolution.

The initial approach is to perform soft tissue lengthenings to minimize the spastic forces on the hip (iliopsoas and adductor muscles) followed by prolonged nighttime abduction bracing. If this fails, or the child presents with severe subluxation/dislocation, we recommend the procedure described in this chapter.

The principles of treatment include:

1. Early joint reduction—prior to development of significant femoral head deformity or degeneration
2. Maintaining the reduction with femoral and acetabular osteotomies
3. Minimizing complications including avascular necrosis or recurrent instability/deformity

Treatment Strategy

The San Diego acetabular osteotomy is conceptually similar to the pericapsular osteotomy described by Albee in 1915. The San Diego osteotomy was described by Drs. Scott Mubarak and Dennis Wenger to specifically treat hip dysplasia in patients with neuromuscular disease [1]. The osteotomy aims to improve the superior and posterior acetabular deficiency observed in these patients [2]. The hip deformity observed in neuromuscular patients is thought to be due to spastic hip flexor and adductor muscles which pull the thigh toward the midline causing posterior and lateral subluxation of the femoral head. This constant pressure against the posterior-superior labrum and acetabular anlage results in acetabular deformity, joint instability, femoral head deformation, and eventual joint degeneration. In addition, prolonged sitting adds to the posteriorly directed forces.

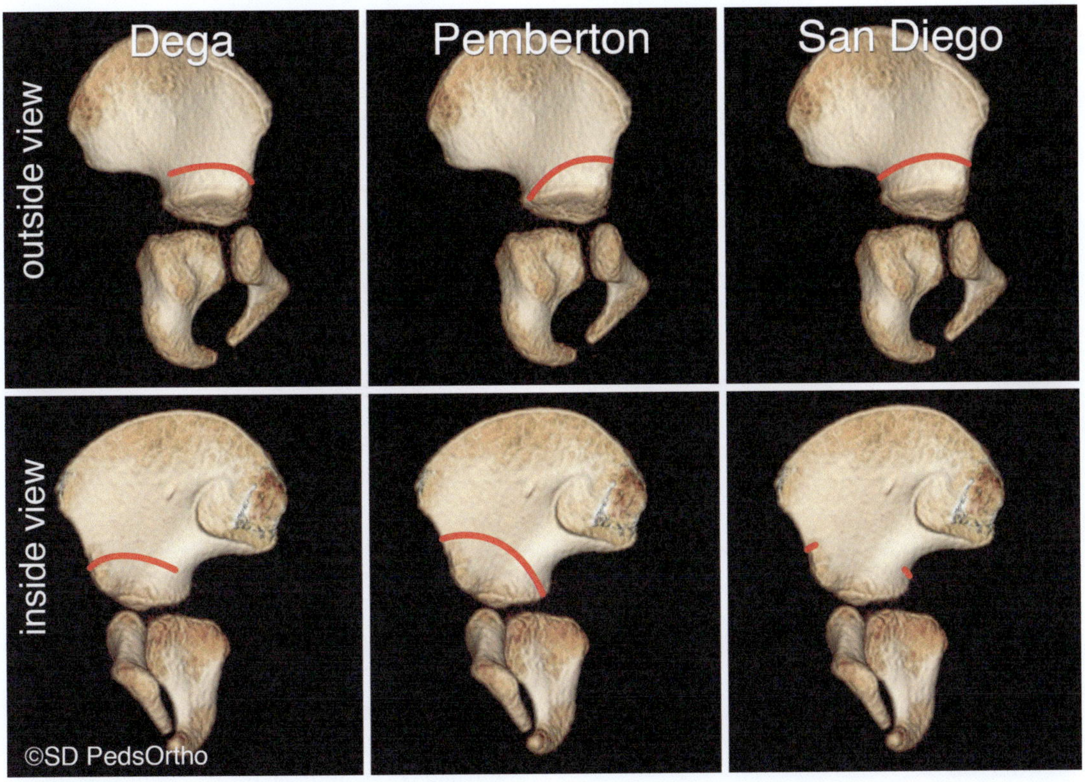

Fig. 11.2 Comparison of the Dega, Pemberton, and San Diego osteotomies demonstrated in the 3D computed tomography reconstructions of a right hemipelvis. The red line depicts the osteotomy visualized from the lateral (*above*) and medial (*below*) view of the hemipelvis (© San Diego Orthopedics, with permission)

The indications for this procedure are patients with neuromuscular hip disease between 2 and 10 years of age with an open triradiate cartilage and acetabular dysplasia (defined as an increased acetabular volume and an acetabular index of greater than 25°).

The comprehensive approach to treating the neuromuscular hip includes soft tissue lengthening procedures of the hip flexors and adductors (primarily the iliopsoas, rectus femoris, adductor longus/brevis, gracilis, and sometimes distal hamstrings), open reduction and capsulorrhaphy if the femoral head is more than 70% subluxated, proximal femoral varus derotation osteotomy (to reduce the neck-shaft angle to about 110° and improve femoral anteversion), and a lateral bending acetabuloplasty (San Diego osteotomy). The correction of anteversion in the non-walking child with cerebral palsy whose limb sometimes turns out 40° remains controversial as the correction will worsen the outward position of the limb.

The San Diego osteotomy is often confused with the Dega or Pemberton osteotomies (Fig. 11.2). The Dega osteotomy cuts through both the medial and lateral cortex of the ilium in the supra-acetabular region and stops about 1 cm short of the sciatic notch. In comparison, the Pemberton osteotomy extends to the posterior limb of the triradiate cartilage between the joint and the sciatic notch. Regardless, both these osteotomies result in improved anterior and superior coverage when the lateral cortex is hinged down through the triradiate cartilage. Unfortunately, the posterior coverage is not improved with the Dega, Pemberton, or Salter osteotomies.

In contrast, the San Diego osteotomy enables acetabular reshaping without disrupting the inner wall of the ilium except at the anterior inferior iliac spine and the sciatic notch. Between these two regions, only the lateral cortex of the ilium is cut. Then, when the supra-acetabular ilium is hinged down through the triradiate cartilage, tri-

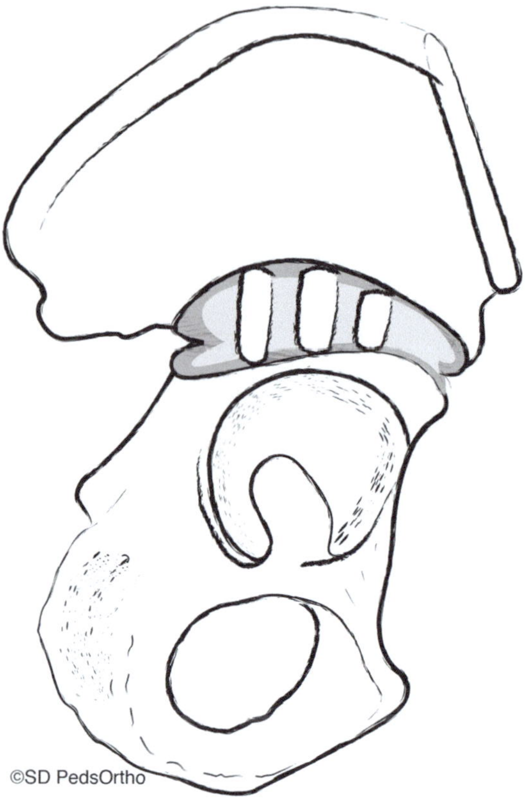

Fig. 11.3 The tri-cortical bone grafts can be optimized to obtain anterior or posterior coverage (© San Diego Orthopedics, with permission)

cortical bone grafts of varying sizes can be inserted from a direct lateral entry, and their size can customize the amount of the acetabular correction achieved (Fig. 11.3). The largest bone graft is placed posteriorly in neuromuscular patients to achieve maximum posterior-superior correction. The elasticity of the osteotomy site holds the triangular grafts in position, and no internal fixation is needed.

Surgical Details

Comprehensive Approach to the Neuromuscular Hip Dislocation

The patient is placed under general anesthesia and positioned supine. Depending on the age of the patient, we often use a caudal block or an epidural for postoperative pain control. A radiolucent bolster is placed under the ipsilateral thorax to elevate the operative hip and pelvis. A bolster behind the hip may disrupt proper draping and imaging. The lower extremity is draped free up to the edge of the rib cage and medially to the umbilicus (Fig. 11.4a).

Step 1 A medial approach is first performed through a transverse incision about 2 cm distal to the groin crease to lengthen the adductor longus, brevis, and gracilis as required.

Step 2 A second incision is then performed parallel to the iliac crest and extending onto the anterior hip using the typical Salter approach. The iliac apophysis is divided to obtain a subperiosteal exposure of the iliac wing down to the sciatic notch both medially and laterally. The hip capsule is then exposed retracting the gluteus medius and minimums. The direct and indirect heads of the rectus femoris muscle are identified and detached. The iliopsoas tendon is identified at the pelvic brim and lengthened, being careful to avoid injury to the femoral nerve. When capsulorrhaphy is indicated, the hip capsule is opened through a T-shaped incision. The femoral head is visualized; femoral anteversion can be approximately calculated by evaluating the rotation between the femoral neck and the posterior femoral condyles. Once the pathologic anatomy is assessed and the degree of shortening or derotation is determined, the wound is packed, and the femoral osteotomy is performed.

Step 3 A third lateral incision is then used to obtain subperiosteal exposure of the proximal femur to perform a varus derotation femoral shortening osteotomy. The femoral neck-shaft angle is decreased to 110°, and the anteversion is partially corrected (extreme or full correction of anteversion often results in a limb/foot that is pointed markedly lateral). One- to two-centimeter segment of the femur can be removed to allow for easy reduction of the femoral head into the acetabulum. The femoral osteotomy is fixed with a 90° angled blade plate.

Step 4 An open reduction of the femoral head is then performed by excising the ligamentum teres, the pulvinar, and the transverse acetabular ligament.

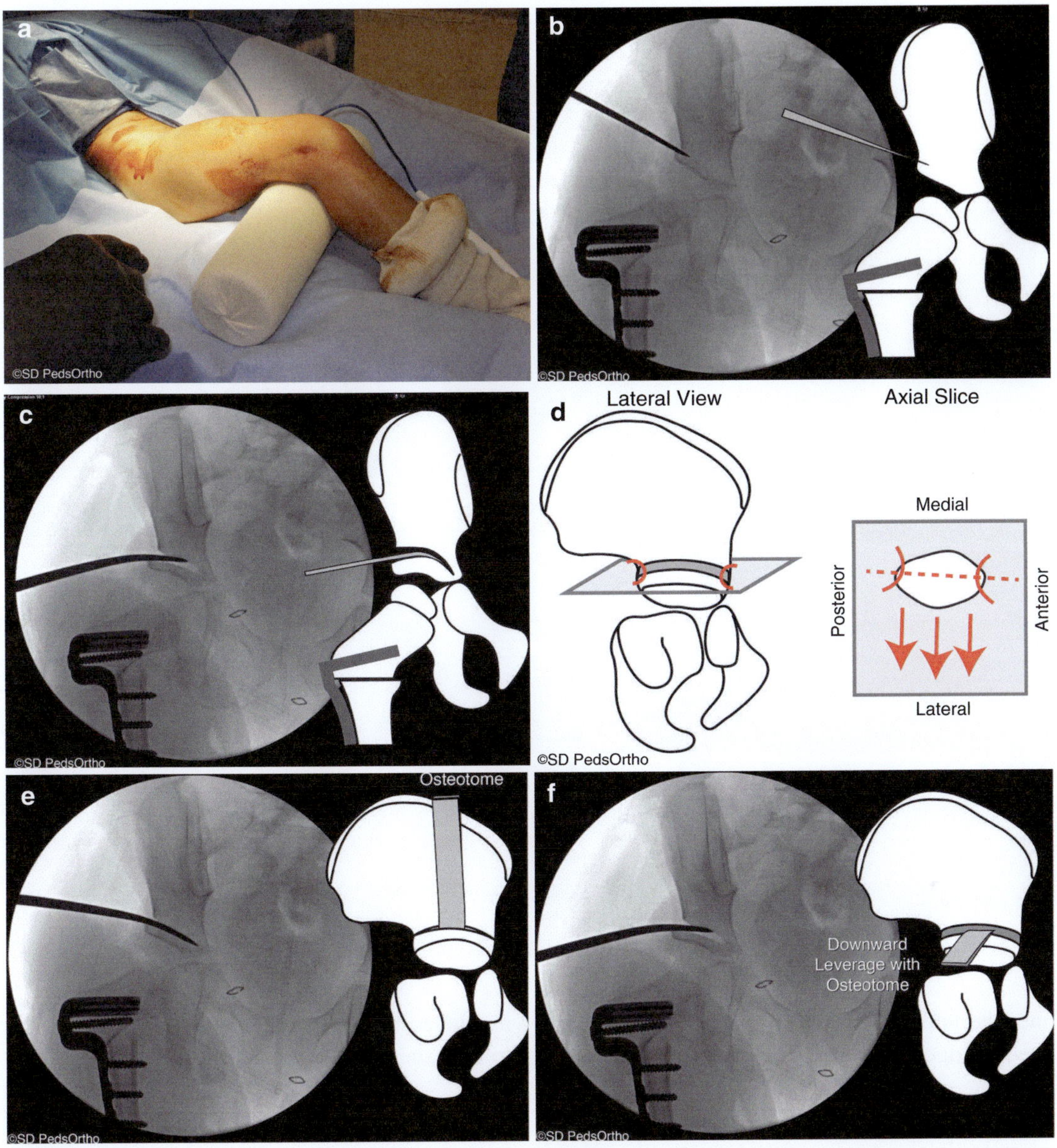

Fig. 11.4 (**a**) The patient is placed in the supine position with the entire lower extremity prepared. (**b**) A straight osteotome is used to first incise the lateral cortex of the ilium just superior to the hip joint. (**c**) A curved osteotome is then advanced to the medial edge of the triradiate cartilage. (**d**) The medial and lateral cortex is cut at the anterior inferior iliac spine and sciatic notch. (**e**) The curved osteotome is then replaced into the osteotomy. (**f**) The curved osteotome is levered down to open the osteotomy. (**g**) Tri-cortical bone grafts are obtained from the iliac wing or femoral shortening osteotomy and positioned to optimized acetabular coverage. (**h**) Image and drawing demonstrating bone grafts in proper position (© San Diego Orthopedics, with permission)

Step 5 Intraoperative fluoroscopy is used to identify the starting point for the lateral acetabuloplasty on the lateral cortex of the ilium. A straight osteotome is placed just superior to the insertion of the hip capsule and directed toward the medial edge of the triradiate cartilage (Fig. 11.4b). This cut is usually about 1 cm above the joint line (documented with an image intensifier view). The lateral cortex of the ilium is cut in a straight line from anterior to posterior (from the anterior inferior iliac spine to the sciatic notch). A curved osteotome is then placed

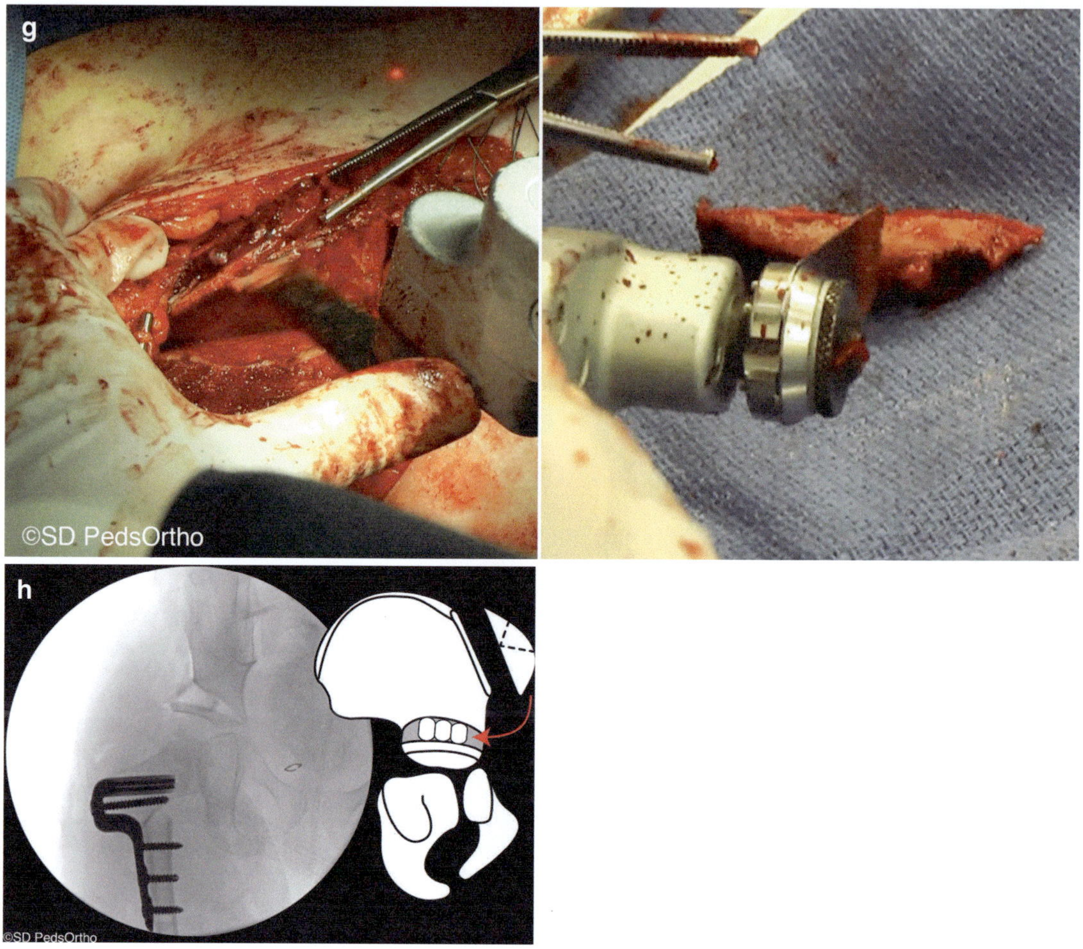

Fig. 11.4 (continued)

into the lateral cortical cut and advanced to the medial edge of the triradiate cartilage using fluoroscopic guidance (Fig. 11.4c). The medial cortex of the iliac wing is then cut at the anterior inferior iliac spine (using a large rongeur) and the sciatic notch using an osteotome, a Lexel rongeur, or a Kerrison rongeur (Fig. 11.4d). Once the anterior and posterior corners of the osteotomy are free (through both medial and lateral cortices), the curved osteotome can be levered down to bend the lateral iliac wing through the triradiate cartilage (Fig. 11.4e, f). Tri-cortical grafts are then prepared, either from the iliac wing or from the femoral shortening osteotomy wedge (Fig. 11.4g). The bone grafts are placed to optimize acetabular correction and often do not require pin stabilization as the medial cortex of the ilium acts as an elastic hinge to hold the grafts in position (Fig. 11.4h).

Step 6 Hip stability is verified with a Barlow maneuver. Nonabsorbable number-1 sutures are placed into the capsule, after excising the redundant capsule. The hip capsule is tightened and closed to ensure that the femoral head is unable to subluxate posteriorly.

Step 7 A hip spica cast is applied for 6 weeks with the hip in 30° of flexion, 30° of abduction, and neutral rotation.

Midterm follow-up for this comprehensive approach to the neuromuscular hip has been documented by McNerney et al. [3].

Postoperative Imaging (Fig. 11.5)

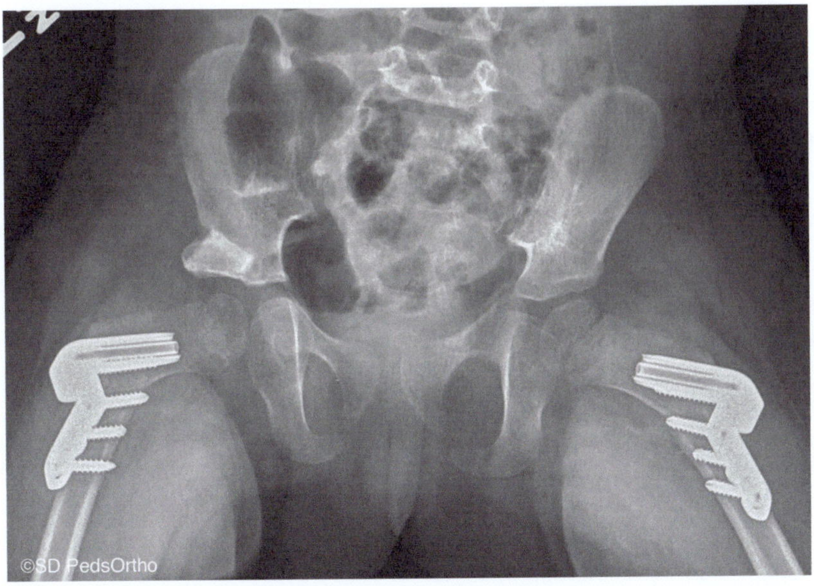

Fig. 11.5 Postoperative anterior posterior radiograph demonstrating hip reduction after open reduction, capsulorrhaphy with femoral and acetabular osteotomy (© San Diego Orthopedics, with permission)

Modification of the San Diego Osteotomy for Developmental Dysplasia of the Hip

The lateral acetabuloplasty can be used in patients with developmental dysplasia of the hip to decrease acetabular volume and correct acetabular dysplasia. As the dysplasia in these patients is noted to be primarily anterior and lateral, the largest bone graft should be placed anteriorly (Fig. 11.6). This is similar to the coverage one may obtain with a Pemberton osteotomy. However, as the medial cortex of the ilium is intact, this osteotomy often does not require pin fixation to maintain the acetabular correction and bone graft position.

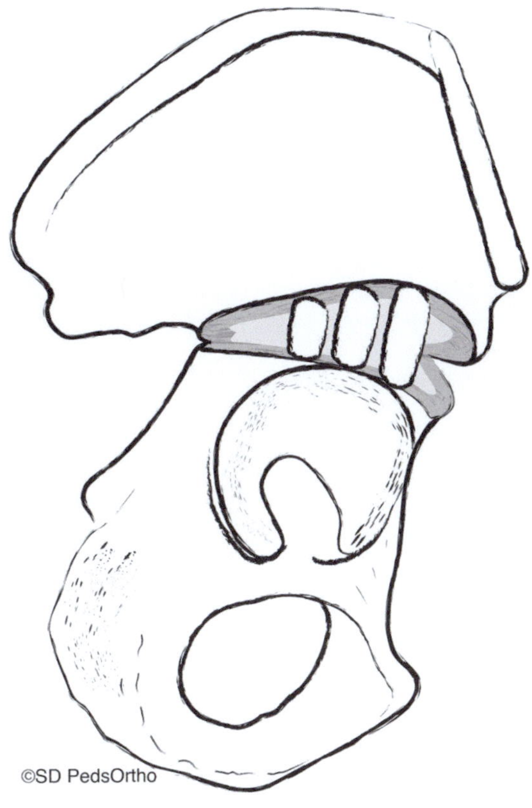

Fig. 11.6 Modification of the San Diego acetabuloplasty that can be used to treat developmental dysplasia of the hip in a normal child who has typical anterolateral acetabular deficiency (This can be used as an alternative for the Pemberton procedure) (© San Diego Orthopedics, with permission)

Pearls and Pitfalls

- Correcting soft tissue contractures (adductors, psoas, often distal hamstrings) is a key to achieving long-term hip stability.
- The osteotomy should be performed relatively close to the joint to optimize free acetabular rotation (bending). However, there should be adequate bone in the supra-acetabular region to ensure that the osteotomy does not propagate into the joint when it is hinged open.
- Excessive correction of the acetabular dysplasia can result in pathologic decrease in acetabular volume and lateral extrusion of the femoral head.
- Appropriate shortening of the femoral osteotomy should be performed to ensure that there is no excessive pressure on the femoral head to decrease the likelihood of postoperative avascular necrosis.
- If the medial iliac cortex is disrupted, a fixation pin may be required to maintain the graft and obtain appropriate acetabular coverage.

Indications and Contraindications (Table 11.1)

Table 11.1 San Diego osteotomy (lateral acetabuloplasty): surgical indications and contraindications

Indications
Ages: 2–10
Open triradiate cartilage
Acetabular dysplasia (acetabular index greater than 25°)
Increased acetabular volume
Contraindication
Skeletally mature

Acknowledgment We want to thank J. D. Bomar, MPH, Research Coordinator and multimedia expert in our orthopedic division, for his extensive effort in compiling this chapter.

References

1. Mubarak SJ, Valencia FG, Wenger DR. One-stage correction of the spastic dislocated hip. Use of pericapsular acetabuloplasty to improve coverage. J Bone Joint Surg Am. 1992;74(9):1347–57.
2. Kim HT, Wenger DR. Location of acetabular deficiency and associated hip dislocation in neuromuscular hip dysplasia: three-dimensional computed tomographic analysis. J Pediatr Orthop. 1997;17(2):143–51.
3. McNerney NP, Mubarak SJ, Wenger DR. One-stage correction of the dysplastic hip in cerebral palsy with the San Diego acetabuloplasty: results and complications in 104 hips. J Pediatr Orthop. 2000;20(1):93–103.

12 Pemberton Osteotomy (Anterolateral Acetabuloplasty)

Ken N. Kuo and Ting-Ming Wang

Introduction

The Pemberton osteotomy was originally described by Pemberton in 1965 as the pericapsular pelvic osteotomy. It is widely recommended for the treatment of acetabular dysplasia, and combined procedure in reduction of hip subluxation, or frank hip dislocation in children. Pemberton acetabuloplasty is characterized by a reshaping of the acetabular roof with hinging on the triradiate cartilage after an incomplete iliac osteotomy. The shape of the acetabulum is modified by rotating the acetabular fragment caudally and anteriorly to improve the anterior and lateral coverage of the femoral head. Two similar modifications of the Pemberton osteotomy, the Dega osteotomy and the San Diego osteotomy, were designed for similar purposes. Most experienced pediatric orthopaedic surgeons can expect the Pemberton acetabuloplasty to yield greater correction of acetabular dysplasia than the Salter innominate osteotomy, without the need of internal fixation for the osteotomy site. The iatrogenic injury to the triradiate cartilage resulting from an incorrectly performed Pemberton osteotomy is a possible serious complication, which may cause premature closure of the triradiate cartilage with a resultant shallow acetabulum. In our previous study, children with developmental dysplasia of the hip who had excessive downward depression of the distal fragment following osteotomy had a higher risk of developing femoral head osteonecrosis because of over reduction of the femoral head.

The Pemberton pericapsular osteotomy has been an effective standard option in our institution in over 20 years for treatment of developmental dysplasia of the hip. This chapter is to demonstrate step-by-step detail of the procedure.

K. N. Kuo (✉)
Department of Orthopaedic Surgery, Taipei Medical University, Taipei, Taiwan

Department of Orthopaedic Surgery, National Taiwan University Hospital, Taipei, Taiwan
e-mail: kennank@aol.com

T.-M. Wang
Department of Orthopaedic Surgery, National Taiwan University Hospital, Taipei, Taiwan
e-mail: dtorth76@yahoo.com.tw

Brief Clinical History

Case 1 The patient is a 7-year-old girl with history right groin pain when walking for some distance or vigorous exercise since 6 months prior to the visit. There was no limitation in usual daily activity. Her birth history and developmental history were completely normal. There was no previous history of hip problem. Her physical examination showed full range of motion in both hips without pain.

Case 2 The patient is a 2-year-old girl who was brought by parents with history of abnormal gait pattern noticed for 6 months and obvious leg

R. C. Hamdy, N. Saran (eds.), *Pediatric Pelvic and Proximal Femoral Osteotomies*,
https://doi.org/10.1007/978-3-319-78033-7_12

length discrepancy noticed for 2 months. There was no known history of hip dysplasia from well-baby checkup. She had no previous treatment. Birth history revealed she was born full term by Cesarean section because of previous section. Birth weight was 3200 g; there was no perinatal problem. Growth and development history was normal. Vaccination was given as scheduled.

Preoperative Imaging

Case 1 Fig. 12.1

Case 2 Fig. 12.2

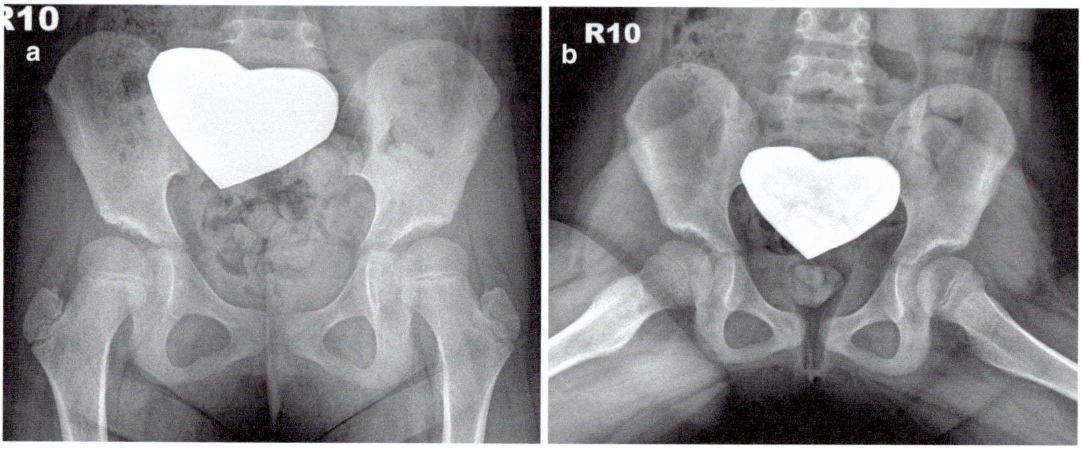

Fig. 12.1 Case 1: A 7-year-old girl, the anteroposterior standing (**a**) and frog lateral view (**b**) showed acetabular dysplasia of right hip. The hips were well located in the acetabulum. The acetabular index measured 30° on the right and 20° on the left. The center-edge angle measured 12° on the right and 22° on the left

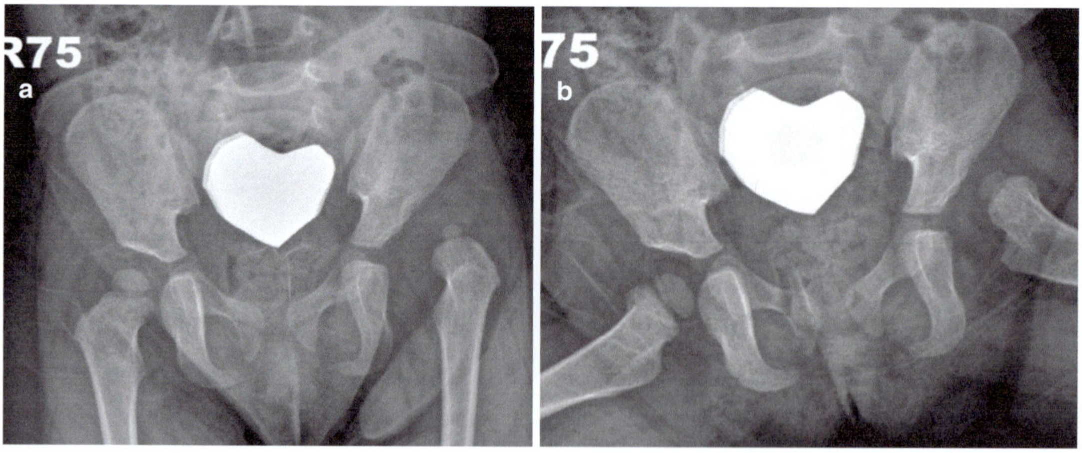

Fig. 12.2 Case 2: A 2-year-old girl, the anteroposterior standing view (**a**) showed dislocated left hip with significant acetabular dysplasia. The frog leg lateral view (**b**) showed unreducible left hip dislocation

Goals of Treatment

Case 1 To improve acetabular coverage of the right hip by Pemberton osteotomy

Case 2 (1) To concentrically reduce the left hip dislocation and (2) to improve acetabular coverage of left hip by Pemberton osteotomy

Treatment Strategy

Case 1 The treatment strategy is to enhance the acetabular coverage by Pemberton osteotomy without opening the joint.

Case 2 The treatment strategy begins with open reduction of femoral head through iliofemoral approach. It is essential to obtain a concentric reduction after cleaning out the obstacles in the acetabulum. With the femoral head reduced in acetabulum under direct vision, test the hip stability in a neutral position as well as in abduction and internal rotation. If the hip is unstable in a neutral position but is stable in abduction and internal rotation, a Pemberton acetabuloplasty is indicated. If hip stability cannot be maintained even in abduction and internal rotation, an additional proximal femoral varus and/or rotational osteotomy should be considered.

Surgical Details

Approach and Exposure

The procedure is performed on supine position with padding under the buttock. An anterior iliofemoral incision is carried out. One should avoid direct cutting on top of the iliac crest. Next, identify the muscle interval between the sartorius and tensor fascia femoris muscles, and isolate lateral femoral cutaneous nerve, which passes distally and laterally beneath the deep fascia in this intermuscular interval. Incise the fascia carefully and retract the lateral femoral cutaneous nerve medially after it is well mobilized proximally and distally. The iliac crest is exposed after releasing the external oblique muscle fibers on the iliac crest. Identify the anterior superior iliac spine. To divide the cartilage at the iliac crest equally, use thumb and index finger to identify the position of the iliac crest, and sharply incise the iliac apophysis exactly in the midline. Strip off medial and lateral half of the iliac apophysis with a periosteal elevator to expose the inner table and outer table of the ilium subperiosteally. Pack a gauze sponge on both tables to facilitate subperiosteal dissection and provide hemostasis. Using a periosteal elevator, elevate the periosteum with the hip abductor muscles from the outer cortex of the ilium until the anterior inferior iliac spine is clearly identified.

Pemberton Osteotomy

Remove the gauze sponge from both inner table and outer table of the iliac bone. Check bleeding from perforating vessels from the iliac wing. Once hemostasis is achieved, proceed with the Pemberton osteotomy. First, locate the sciatic notch with a small periosteal elevator, and protect the soft tissues with a retractor, including the sciatic nerve. Start with medial iliac cut. Outline the cut line with the electrocautery tip. Using a small straight osteotome, start the medial cut line 1–1.5 cm above the superior hip joint line, and curve it inferiorly and posteriorly, pointing toward sciatic notch. The cut line extends halfway to the sciatic notch and ends at the prominent ridge of the pelvic inlet of the ilium (Fig. 12.3). Then, move the attention to the outer table for the lateral cut line; it begins with the same starting point as the medial cut. Using the medial cut line as reference with the same osteotome, make the lateral cut line along the joint capsule (Fig. 12.4). After the cut lines are outlined, use a wider curved osteotome to complete the osteotomy (Fig. 12.5). Starting on the anterior aspect proximal to the upper hip joint capsule, the osteotome cut follows the medial and lateral cut lines. As this cut advances, push the osteotome against the distal fragment to check the degree of downward displacement. If the osteotomy site opens more than 2–3 cm, it means the distal fragment is hinging on the triradiate cartilage, and there is no further advancing necessary.

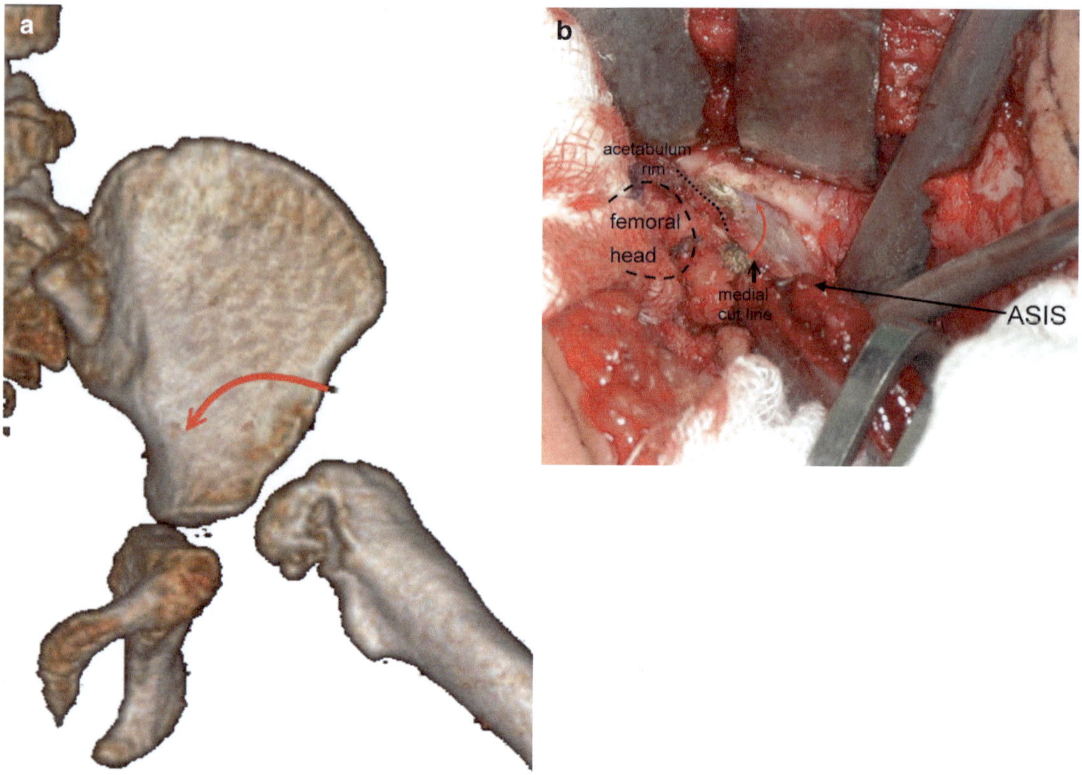

Fig. 12.3 Outline of medial cut line of the left hip. (**a**) Computed tomography shows outline of cut line that extends halfway to the sciatic notch and ends at the prominent ridge of the pelvic inlet of the ilium. (**b**) Actual operation photo showing the direction of the cutting (From Huang et al. 2011, with permission)

Next, we harvest a wedge-shaped iliac crest bone graft (about a 35° wedge) from the ipsilateral iliac wing. A towel roll is placed under the knee to help maintain the hip in an abducted and flexed position. Hold the inferior osteotomy fragment open anteriorly and inferiorly with a towel clip to increase the coverage of the femoral head. Then insert the triangularly shaped bone graft into the osteotomy opening site (Fig. 12.6). Most of the time, the osteotomy bone graft site is stable, and there is no need for internal fixation, especially in younger patients. If the bone graft is not stable, fixation with one or two Kirschner wires may be necessary.

Open Reduction

In those with a dislocated or unstable hip joint, open reduction will be necessary before proceeding with the Pemberton osteotomy. With the same approach, the following detailed procedure is carried out.

Rectus Femoris Tendon and Iliopsoas Tendon

The tendon of the straight head of the rectus femoris muscle is clearly isolated at its origin on the anterior inferior iliac spine. It is desirable to transect the rectus femoris tendon close to the anterior inferior iliac spine but leave a short stump for later tendon reattachment. Bluntly dissect the iliacus muscle belly medial to the ilium, and identify the psoas tendon at the level of the anterior pelvic rim. Be aware of the femoral neurovascular bundle, which is located immediately medial to the psoas muscle and should be retracted and protected with a blunt retractor. Transect the tendinous part of the iliopsoas muscle.

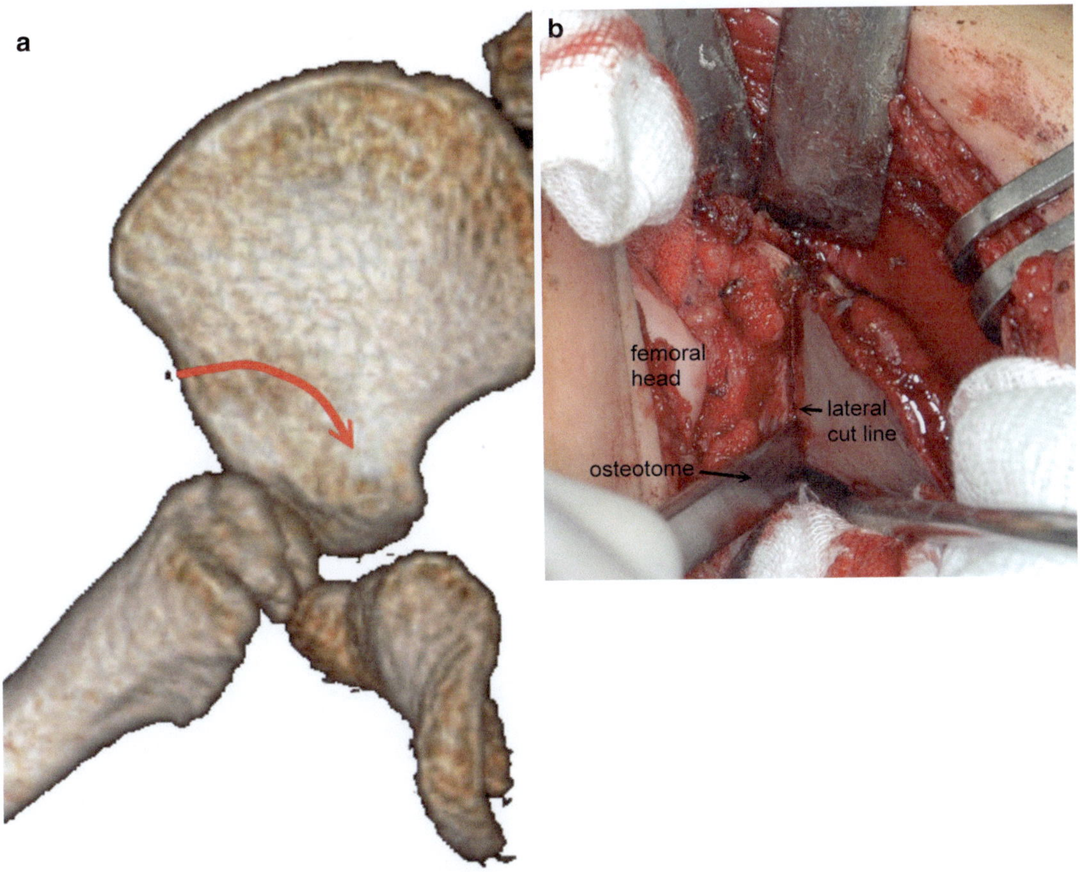

Fig. 12.4 Outline of lateral cut line of the left hip. Use the medial cut line as reference with the same osteotome to make the lateral cut line along the joint capsule. (**a**) Computed tomography outlines the cut and (**b**) shows direction of the cutting in actual operation photo (From Huang et al. 2011, with permission)

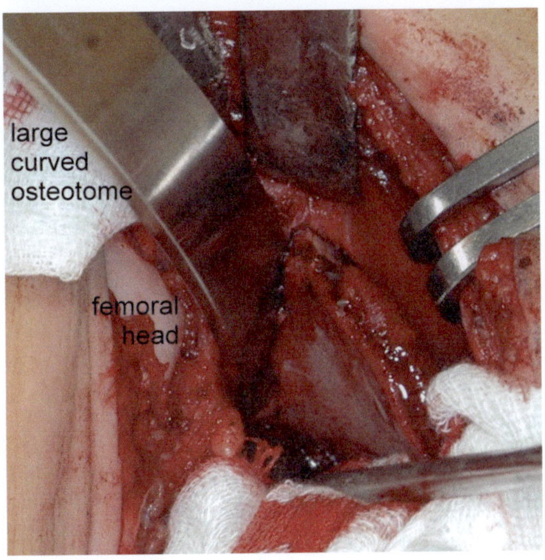

Fig. 12.5 After the cut lines are outlined, use a wider curved osteotome to complete the osteotomy in this photo (From Huang et al. 2011, with permission)

Open Reduction of the Hip Joint

Identify the joint capsule and perform a T-shaped capsulotomy; the horizontal cut should be parallel and near the acetabular rim, including the upper and lower margins of the hip capsule. The stem of the T-shaped capsulotomy should be parallel to the femoral neck and slight superior to avoid a small inferior capsular flap for facilitating the capsulorrhaphy. Divide ligamentum teres sharply at the femoral head, use the ligament teres to trace down to the acetabulum, and remove all of the fibro-fatty tissue (pulvinar tissue) from the true acetabulum. Release the transverse acetabular ligament which can be palpated with finger at the lower margin of the acetabulum. Reduce the femoral head under direct vision, and test the hip stability in a neutral position as well as in abduction and internal rotation.

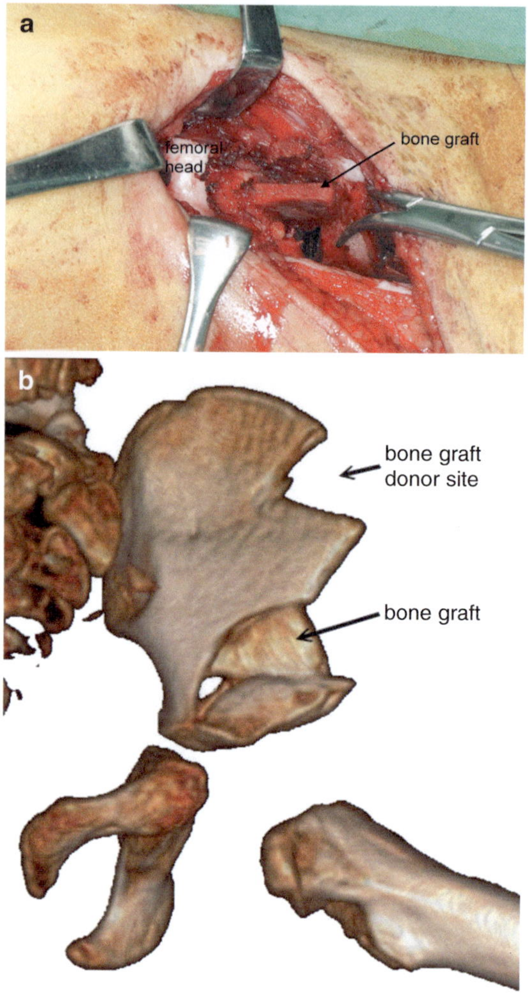

Fig. 12.6 Insert triangularly shaped bone graft into the osteotomy opening site; (**a**) the actual graft insertion and (**b**) computed tomography show graft in the opening space (From Huang et al. 2011, with permission)

Closure

In those who require open reduction, repair the hip capsule by overlapping of the T-capsulotomy flaps. It is not necessary to resect the redundant capsule. Repair the tendon of the straight head of the rectus femoris muscle to the anterior inferior iliac spine. Suture the iliac apophysis over the remaining ilium and close the wound.

Postoperative Care

A hip spica cast is applied after skin closure. The hips should be placed in about 20° of flexion, 30° of abduction, and neutral or slight internal rotation in cast. The spica cast is worn for 4 weeks after a simple Pemberton osteotomy. If a combined open hip reduction procedure is done, we keep the hip spica cast for 6 weeks; this is followed by the use of a hip abduction brace or a bilateral cylinder cast with a spreader bar to hold 30° of abduction of each hip for additional 4 weeks. In those with K-wire fixation, the ends of K-wire are left outside of skin, which can be removed at the same time of cast removal.

Postoperative Imaging

Case 1 Figs. 12.7 and 12.8

Case 2 Figs. 12.9 and 12.10

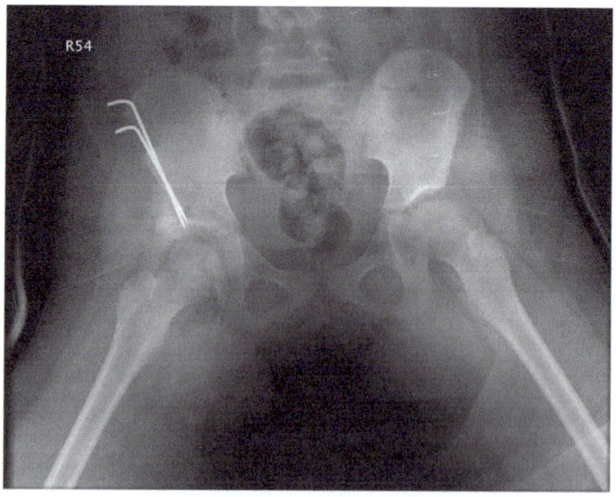

Fig. 12.7 Case 1: Immediate postoperative image in cast. It showed good coverage after osteotomy. Two K-wires were inserted for stability of the bone graft. The ends of K-wires were bend and left outside of skin to facilitate the removal when cast is removed

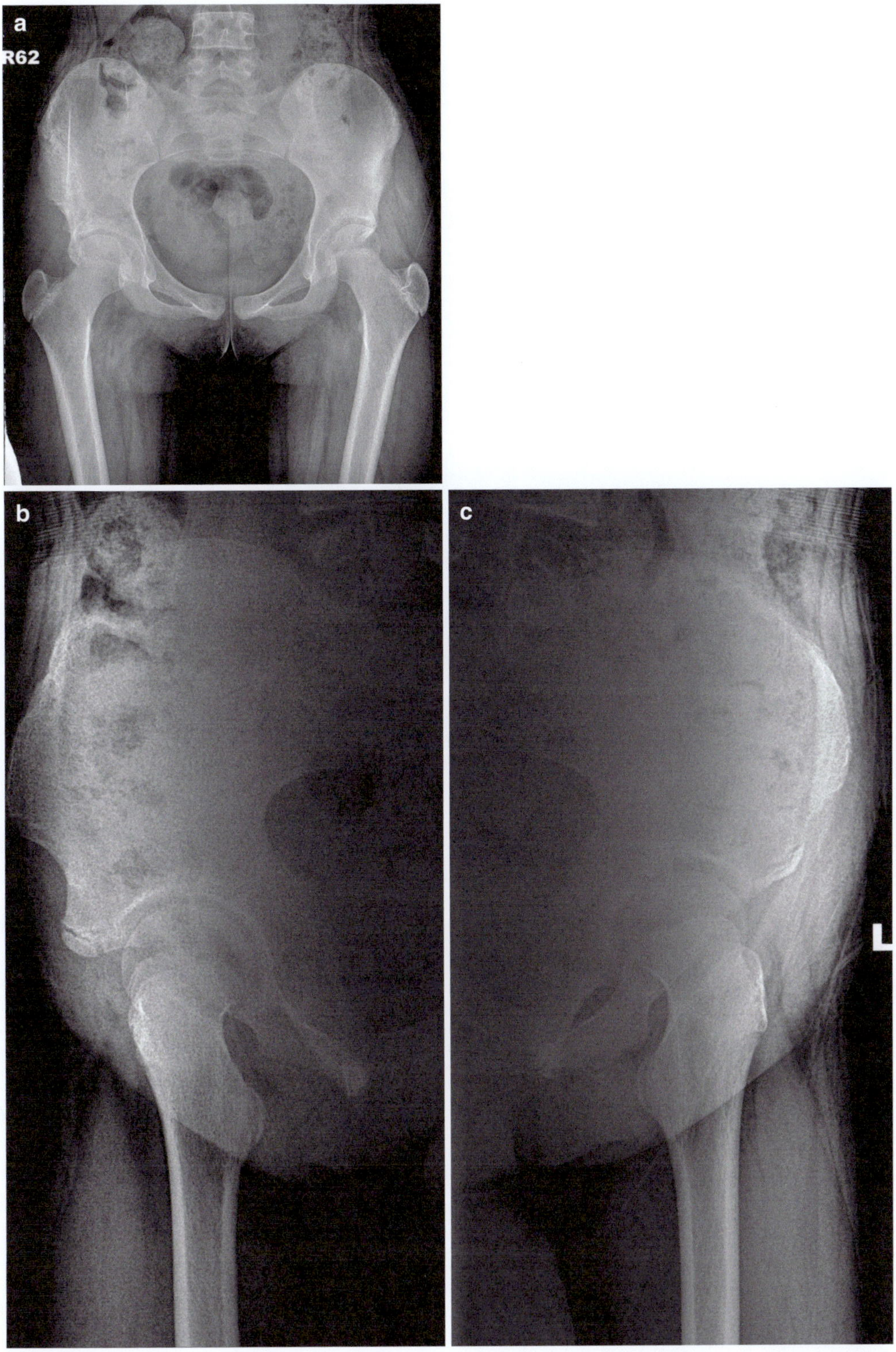

Fig. 12.8 Case 1: Four-and-a-half-year postoperative anteroposterior view in standing position (**a**) and false-profile lateral view of the right hip (**b**) and left hip (**c**). It showed good acetabular coverage in both anteroposterior view and false-profile lateral view, comparable to that of left hip

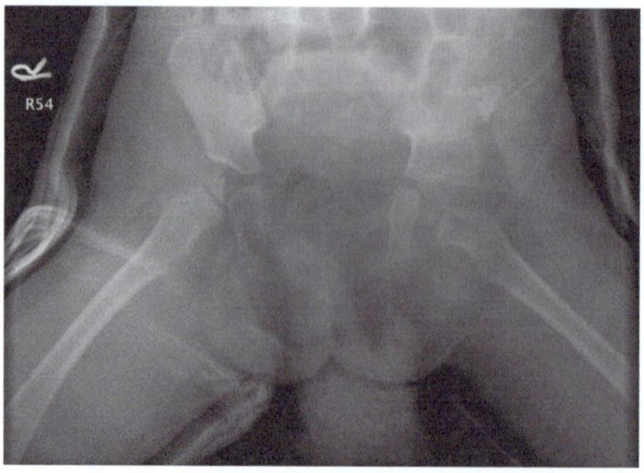

Fig. 12.9 Case 2: Immediate postoperative imaging in cast, the hip reduced with good acetabular coverage

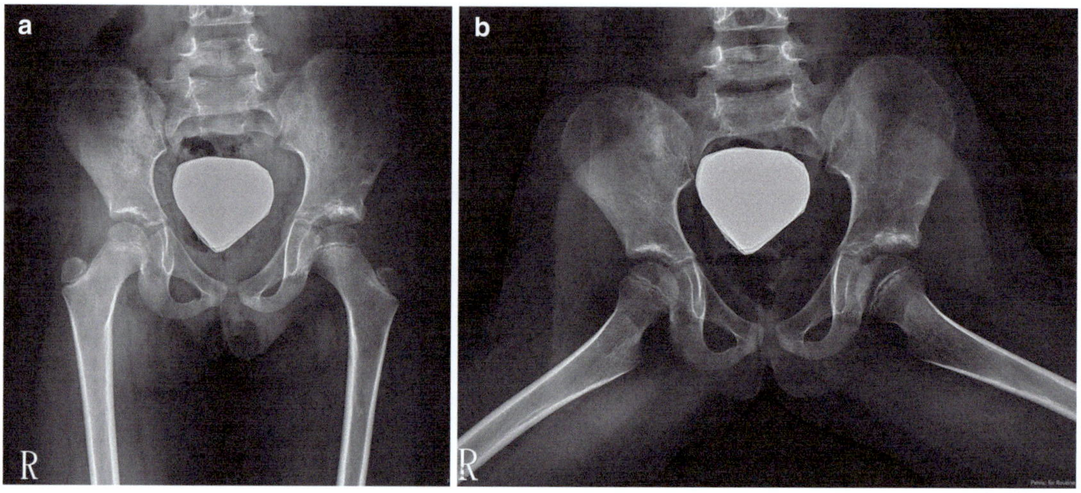

Fig. 12.10 Case 2: 5-year postoperative radiograph showed reduced hip and acetabular coverage well maintained. (**a**) Standing anteroposterior view and (**b**) frog leg lateral view

Pearls and Pitfalls

Pearls

- The thickness of cut is very important, avoiding entering the joint.
- No C-arm fluoroscope is required in our technique.
- We check the opening end point of the iliac osteotomy sequentially by testing the distal fragment for its flexibility as the osteotomy proceeds. This is different from the technique of proceeding straight to the end point at the triradiate cartilage.

Pitfalls

- Bone graft dislodgment.
- Overcorrection may cause femoral head impingement and osteonecrosis.
- Premature closure of triradiate cartilage.
- Trans-iliac lengthening of the ipsilateral limb by opening wedge osteotomy, it usually remodeled in our long-term study.

Indications and Contraindications (Table 12.1)

Table 12.1 Pemberton osteotomy (anterolateral acetabuloplasty): surgical indications and contraindications

Indications
Developmental dysplasia of the hip
Acetabular dysplasia with open triradiate cartilage
Legg-Calvé-Perthes disease with femoral head subluxation/lateral protrusion
Anterosuperior deficiency of the acetabulum secondary to neuromuscular disease
Sequelae of an infected hip with femoral head subluxation
Contraindications
Closed triradiate cartilage
Unreduced femoral head
Deformed femoral head
Small acetabular volume
Active infection/osteomyelitis

Suggested Reading

Coleman SS. The incomplete pericapsular (Pemberton) and innominate (Salter) osteotomies; a complete analysis. Clin Orthop Relat Res. 1974;98:116–23.

Pemberton PA. Pericapsular osteotomy of the ilium for treatment of congenital subluxation and dislocation of the hip. J Bone Joint Surg Am. 1965; 47:65–86.

Huang SC, Wang TM, Wu KW, Fang CF, Kuo KN. Pemberton osteotomy for acetabular dysplasia. JBJS Essent Surg Tech. 2011;1(1):e2. https://doi.org/10.2106/JBJS.ST.K.00003.

Vedantam R, Capelli AM, Schoenecker PL. Pemberton osteotomy for the treatment of developmental dysplasia of the hip in older children. J Pediatr Orthop. 1998;18(2):254–8.

Wu KW, Wang TM, Huang SC, Kuo KN, Chen CW. Analysis of osteonecrosis following Pemberton acetabuloplasty in developmental dysplasia of the hip: long-term results. J Bone Joint Surg Am. 2010;92(11):2083–94.

Pembersal Osteotomy

13

Ayşegül Bursalı and Timur Yıldırım

Introduction

Untreated high dislocation of the hip is a serious cause of physical and psychological disability. It causes premature osteoarthritis, pain, and restricted range of motion. Treatment of developmental dysplasia of the hip should be initiated up to the sixth to seventh week of life in order to provide a painless healthy development of the hip joint. Remodeling capacity of the hip joint may be limited, especially in patients with the treatment initiated after 4 years of age. For older children, treatment options are limited, and generally complex surgical procedures are required. The Pembersal osteotomy is a well-defined surgical technique that provides a significant correction via single osteotomy. Furthermore, a secondary surgery for implant removal is not required because K-wire fixation for the graft is not routinely applied. After the Pembersal osteotomy, just like in the Salter osteotomy, the obturator foramen will be asymmetric on the anteroposterior pelvis. This tells us that there is an acetabular reorientation. In addition to the reorientation, there is a deepening of the acetabulum that takes place just like the Pemberton osteotomy. The differences between the Pembersal osteotomy and the Salter osteotomy are that in the Pembersal osteotomy, the internal table stays intact, the osteotomy is curved, and there is no need for a K-wire fixation. The difference between the Pembersal osteotomy and the Pemberton osteotomy is that in the Pembersal osteotomy, the osteotome cuts through and passes the triradiate cartilage.

A. Bursalı (✉)
Private practice, Istanbul, Turkey

T. Yıldırım
Orthopaedic and Traumatology Department, Baltalimani Bone Diseases Training and Research Hospital, Istanbul, Turkey

Brief Clinical History

The patient was first seen in clinic at the age of 8 years and 6 months and presented for a bilateral limp. Her parents reported that she had already had the diagnosis of developmental dysplasia of the hip (DDH) but did not undergo any treatment. Physical examination revealed positive Trendelenburg sign in both hips and significant restriction of abduction. Tönnis grade 3 DDH on the right side and Tönnis grade 4 DDH on the left were noted according to radiographic evaluation. Acetabular index (AI) angle was measured as 51° on the right hip and 50° on the left. Right femoral head was spherical, but the left femoral head was deformed. The acetabuli were enlarged, shallow, and with a vertical roof on both hips. Open surgical reduction for both hip joints was planned preoperative imaging (Fig. 13.1).

R. C. Hamdy, N. Saran (eds.), *Pediatric Pelvic and Proximal Femoral Osteotomies*,
https://doi.org/10.1007/978-3-319-78033-7_13

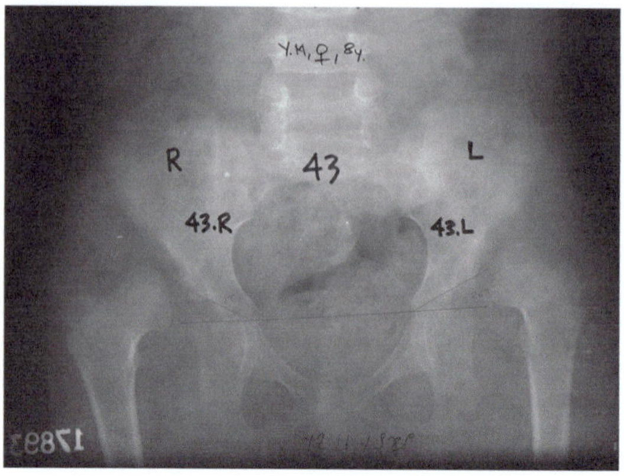

Fig. 13.1 Anteroposterior radiographic image demonstrating bilateral hip dislocation. Tönnis grade 3 developmental dysplasia of the hip on the right side and Tönnis grade 4 on the left

Goals of Treatment

The primary goal of treatment is to obtain a congruent joint surface that is parallel to the ground via correction of the AI angle as much as possible and to provide painless, mobile hip joints with ability to walk without residual limping.

Treatment Strategy

A Pembersal osteotomy allows for deepening of a capacious acetabulum like a Pemberton osteotomy and also reorients the acetabulum like a Salter osteotomy. The AI angle can be corrected about 15° by Salter and Pemberton osteotomies; however, this is often insufficient in older children with moderate to severe dysplasia. Although better angular correction can be obtained by the Steel osteotomy, it can cause femoroacetabular instability due to lack of providing appropriate deepening. Steel osteotomy consists of three incisions and three separate osteotomies. Therefore, it has an increased risk of infection due to number of incisions and osteotomies, longer duration of surgical intervention, and increased blood loss. On the other hand, the Pembersal osteotomy provides correction via a partial or greenstick fracture within the ischium, through the symphysis pubis and the triradiate cartilage as well. Furthermore, it allows for improved congruity by reshaping the acetabulum to better match its shape with the femoral head. Another advantage is that Kirschner (K)-wire fixation for the graft is not necessary.

Surgical Details

Pembersal Osteotomy

Surgical intervention is performed in the supine position. A bikini approach can be used. A Watson-Jones approach can also be performed when concomitant femoral shortening and derotation are planned. A more prominent scar tissue is expected with Watson-Jones technique.

Exposure

The bikini incision starts just proximal to the anterior superior iliac spine (ASIS) and reaches up to the pubic tubercle. After dissection of the subcutaneous tissue, the origin of the rectus femoris muscle is exposed via deepening through the interval between the tensor fascia lata and sartorius muscles. The rectus femoris muscle is suspended by sutures and detached from its origin. Iliocapsularis fibers are removed from the joint capsule, and then the tendon of the iliopsoas muscle is cut at the level of the pelvic brim. The joint capsule is mobilized from the false acetabulum located on the iliac bone and opened with a T-shaped incision. To create this T-shaped incision, the capsule is incised from the posterosuperior aspect to the deepest inferomedial aspect, parallel to the acetabulum. A second incision is made perpendicular to the first one and parallel to the femoral neck. This provides excellent visualization of the hip joint. The femoral head is carefully inspected to note its shape, any chondral lesion, neck anteversion or retroversion, and coxa valga or coxa vara deformities. Acetabular roof and walls with its depth, transverse ligament, and labrum are also evaluated. In untreated older children, the ligamentum teres is generally observed as degenerated and ruptured during the surgical intervention. The pulvinar and the remaining of ligamentum teres are removed. The transverse ligament is incised. The iliac apophysis is split, and the inner and outer tables of the iliac wing are exposed subperiosteally to the sciatic notch. Hohmann retractors are placed in the sciatic notch. At this point, the inner and outer tables of the iliac wing, the superior pubic ramus, and a part of the ischium should be visible. Autograft, which will later be placed in the osteotomy, is harvested from the ilium.

Osteotomy

The osteotomy is performed by using a curved osteotome starting from 1 to 1.5 cm proximal to the ASIS and runs parallel to the acetabulum, ending within the ischium (Figs. 13.2 and 13.3). The osteotomy is kept parallel to the margin of the acetabulum. The osteotomy is kept as close to the inner table as possible to minimize the chance of joint penetration. Furthermore, in cases such as this, a finger can be placed in the acetabulum to further ensure the direction of the osteotome. There is no obligation to distinguish the triradiate cartilage during the osteotomy. The osteotomy is completed once the acetabulum can be easily levered with the osteotome. The acetabulum is reoriented inferiorly, laterally, and anteriorly by using the osteotome and a towel clamp placed in the ASIS. Unlike the Salter osteotomy, there is no need to apply the figure-four position to be able to manipulate the acetabulum. The osteotomy hinges on the greenstick fracture within ischium, the symphysis pubis, and the triradiate cartilage (Fig. 13.4). The lower quarter of the pelvis is reoriented anterolaterally. Intraoperative fluoroscopy and radiographs can be used to verify adequate correction. The bone graft can be positioned to optimize overall coverage. If lateral coverage is needed, the bone graft should be placed in a lateral to medial direction, whereas if more anterior coverage is required, the graft should be placed in an anterolateral to posteromedial direction. Based on the correction desired, the autograft is shaped and wedged into the osteotomy

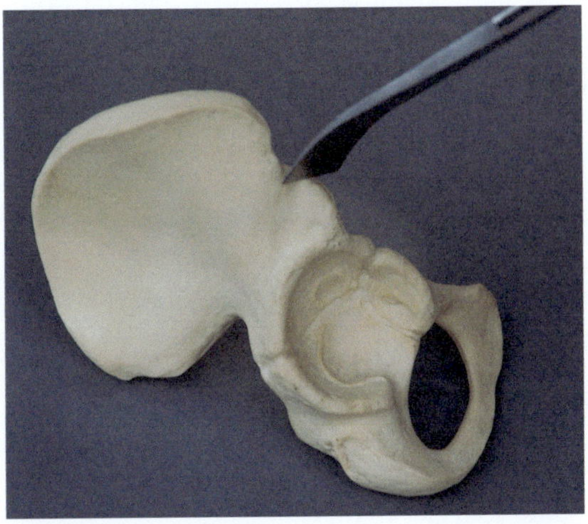

Fig. 13.3 Placement of curved osteotome parallel to the acetabulum

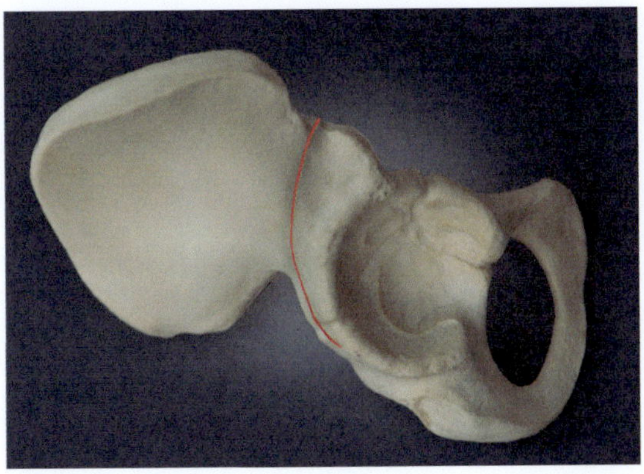

Fig. 13.2 Osteotomy line on the iliac bone of a simulated model of dysplastic acetabulum

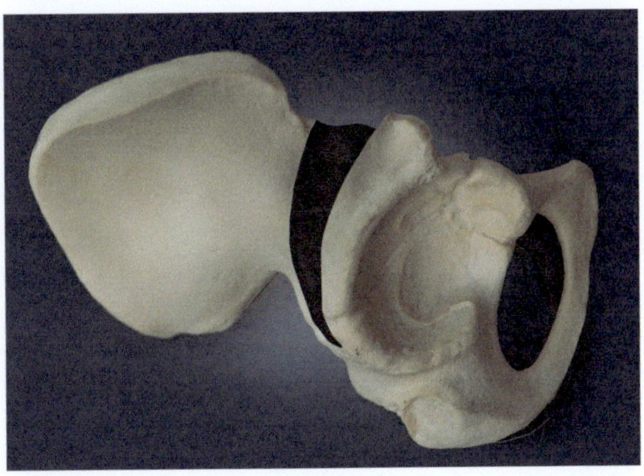

Fig. 13.4 Image of the osteotomy line with the graft placed appropriately

site. Stability is checked. K-wire fixation is not required, as the osteotomy is inherently stable once the graft is wedged in place.

If the femoral head can be reduced easily and stay stable inside the acetabular cavity, the capsule is closed using number 0 or 1 Vicryl sutures following resection of the redundant capsule. The tendon of the rectus femoris is reattached to its origin. Labral resection or release by applying multiple radial incisions to the labrum in order to ease the reduction of the femoral head is never performed. Apophysis of the iliac bone is closed and sutured using number 1 or 2 absorbable suture. Soft tissues are closed and sutured. A hip spica cast is applied.

If the femoral head is easily reduced to the new reoriented acetabulum and is stable, then there is no need for femoral procedures. If a stable reduction cannot be obtained due to increased anteversion or retroversion, coxa valga or coxa vara deformity, or high dislocation of the hip, a femoral osteotomy just below the lesser trochanter is performed in order to achieve shortening and correction of rotational alignment. When shortening is required, a section of bone measuring the distance from the upper border of the acetabulum to the top of the femoral head is resected at the level of the lesser trochanter. Plate fixation is applied postoperative imaging (Figs. 13.5 and 13.6).

Twenty-six years after surgical treatment (Fig. 13.7), degenerative changes are not observed in either of the hip joints. Coverage of the femoral head is sufficient. Femoral neck-shaft angle is 120° in the right hip and 110° in the left. Trendelenburg sign is negative bilaterally; center-edge angle of Wiberg, 30/30; and Tönnis angles, 12/10.

Physical examination: Trendelenburg sign bilaterally negative; hip flexions 90° (*right*)/100° (*left*); abduction 45° bilaterally; internal rotation 30° (*right*)/40° (*left*); impingement sign bilaterally negative; body weight 100 kg. She is now the mother of an 11-year-old girl.

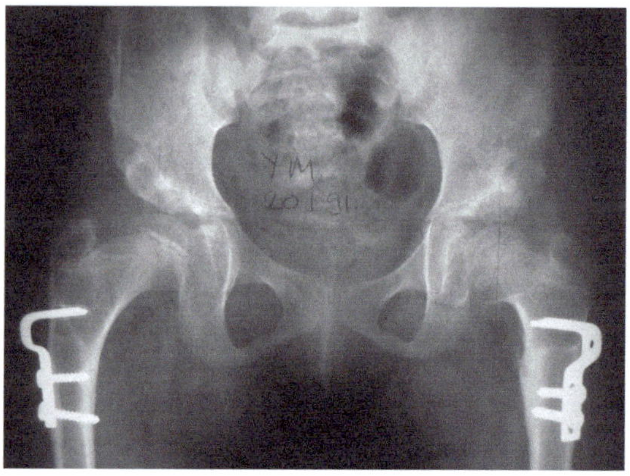

Fig. 13.5 Early postoperative anteroposterior radiographic image. Open surgical reduction combined to Pembersal osteotomy and 3 cm femoral shortening was performed for the right hip first and then the left hip

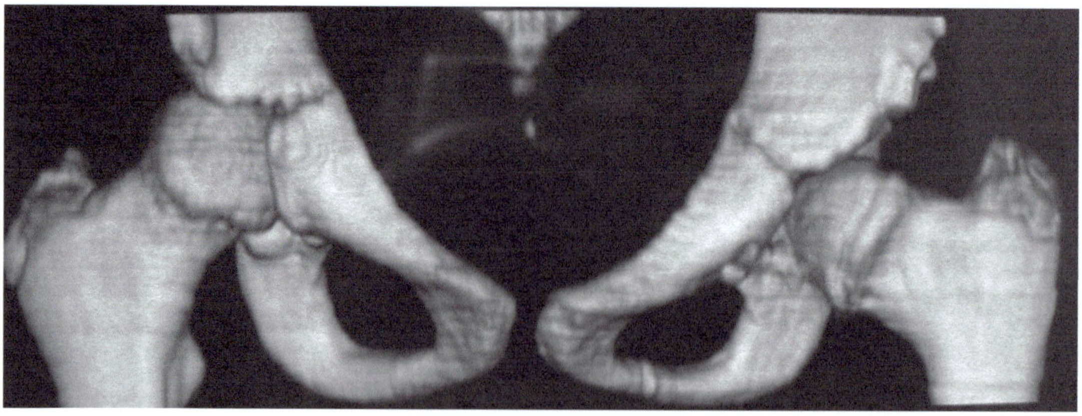

Fig. 13.6 Three-dimensional computed tomography scan of the pelvis 9 years after surgical treatment

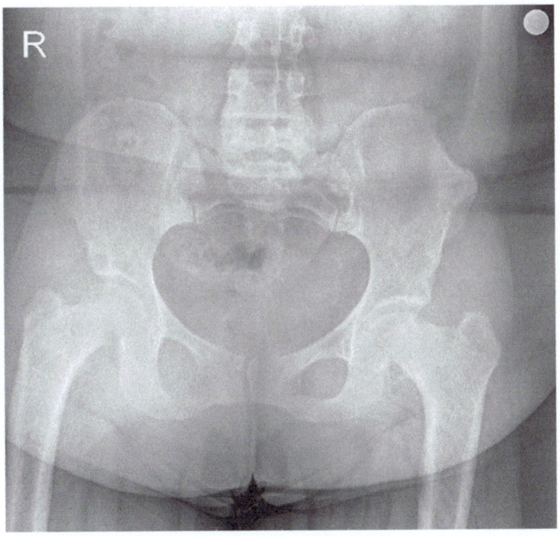

Fig. 13.7 Anteroposterior radiographic image of the pelvis 26 years after surgical treatment

Pearls and Pitfalls

- The Pembersal osteotomy is a suitable technique for patients 4–10 years of age with a dysplastic or dislocated hip joint accompanied by a widened or capacious acetabulum that needs to be reshaped.
- Due to the risk of triradiate cartilage injury, the Pembersal osteotomy is not the first choice in younger children. However, in cases of capacious acetabuli with moderate dysplasia, the Pembersal allows for a redirection of the acetabulum while also allowing the acetabulum to be reshaped.
- Due to decreased elasticity of bone, the procedure may not yield the desired results in children over 10–11 years of age.
- While intraoperative fluoroscopy can be used, it is not absolutely required. In order to avoid joint penetration, one must keep the osteotome close to the inner table. When possible, a finger placed in the acetabulum can also provide additional feedback in terms of directing the osteotome.

Because of the possible change in the acetabular capacity, it may not be the optimum choice in the presence of a large femoral head.

Indications and Contraindications (Table 13.1)

Table 13.1 Pembersal osteotomy: surgical indications and contraindications

Indications
Hip dysplasia and dislocations between 4 and 10 years with capacious acetabulum
Contraindications
Hip dysplasia and dislocations under 4 years old
Lack of congruence
Stiff hip

Suggested Reading

Bursalı A, Tonbul M. How are outcomes affected by combining the Pemberton and Salter osteotomies? Clin Orthop Relat Res. 2008;466(4):837–46.

Marafioti RL, Westin GW. Factors influencing the results of acetabuloplasty in children. J Bone Joint Surg Am. 1980;62(5):765–9.

Perlik PC, Westin GW, Marafioti RL. A combination pelvic osteotomy for acetabular dysplasia in children. J Bone Joint Surg Am. 1985;67(6):842–50.

14 Acetabuloplasty in Closed Triradiate Cartilage

Emily K. Schaeffer and Kishore Mulpuri

Introduction

Hip displacement is a common pathology in neuromuscular conditions, and progressive displacement or dislocation is associated with acetabular dysplasia, pain and decreased function and may lead to the need for hip salvage surgery. The Dega-type pelvic osteotomy is commonly used to correct acetabular dysplasia and maximize coverage of the femoral head in patients with open triradiate cartilages. In older patients, where the triradiate cartilage has closed, more complex peri-acetabular osteotomies are typically indicated. However, the Dega osteotomy can be a simple and effective technique to restore hip stability in patients with neuromuscular conditions, even after closure of the triradiate cartilage. While there are limited reports on the use of this technique in this manner, there are reports that suggest it can be effective in both ambulatory and non-ambulatory patients. In this particular case, the Dega osteotomy in combination with varus derotational osteotomy restored ambulation in a patient with closed triradiate cartilages who had stopped ambulating due to pain from hip displacement.

E. K. Schaeffer · K. Mulpuri (✉)
Orthopaedic Surgery,
British Columbia Children's Hospital,
Vancouver, BC, Canada
e-mail: Emily.Schaeffer@cw.bc.ca;
kmulpuri@cw.bc.ca

Brief Clinical History

This 14-year-7-month-old female is non-verbal, with 22q13 chromosomal deletion, associated autism spectrum disorder, developmental delay and seizure disorder. She is classified at Gross Motor Function Classification System (GMFCS) Level II. She previously underwent a total abdominal colectomy, partial proctectomy and ileostomy for ulcerative colitis at the age of 12 years and 8 months and continues to have a colostomy. She presented with a right dysplastic hip that was 50% uncovered after her parents noted a significantly acute decline in her mobility and gait (Fig. 14.1). As she is non-verbal, her parents had been using decreases in appetite, sleep and mobility as indicators of pain, although she remained independently ambulatory for significant periods of time. It was decided that a varus derotational osteotomy (VDRO) of the right femur, bilateral adductor releases and a Dega osteotomy of the right pelvis were required. At her preoperative appointment, her pain had progressed, and although previously ambulatory, she was now wheelchair-dependent due to pain. She had 40° of internal rotation, 40° of external rotation and 45° of abduction in extension of the right hip compared to 30° of internal rotation, 45° of external rotation and 55° of abduction in extension on the other side. She had popliteal angles of 30° and 50° on the right and left, respectively. The right hip was subluxed posterosuperiorly with cystic changes in the femoral head (Fig. 14.2).

The operative pictures and intraoperative fluoroscopy shown in this case report are from a dif-

R. C. Hamdy, N. Saran (eds.), *Pediatric Pelvic and Proximal Femoral Osteotomies*,
https://doi.org/10.1007/978-3-319-78033-7_14

ferent patient undergoing the same procedure for the left hip. For reference purposes, the pre- and postoperative anteroposterior pelvis radiographs for this patient have also been included (Fig. 14.3). The patient is a 13-year 7-month-old male with spastic quadriplegia and closed triradiate cartilages undergoing a VDRO of the proximal femur and a Dega osteotomy of the left pelvis. The presented case was chosen because complete follow-up for 2 years post-surgery was available, but intraoperative photography was not performed during the procedure.

Preoperative Imaging (See Figs. 14.1, 14.2 and 14.3a)

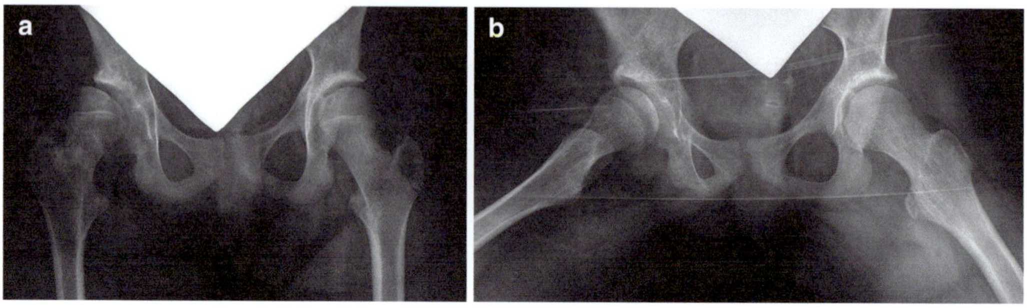

Fig. 14.1 (**a**) Anteroposterior radiograph showing moderate subluxation of the right hip associated with dysplastic remodelling of the right acetabulum. In neutral position, there is lack of bony coverage of the lateral one half of the right femoral head. (**b**) The frog-lateral pelvis radiograph shows that the right hip reduces and aligns with the flattened right acetabulum in this position

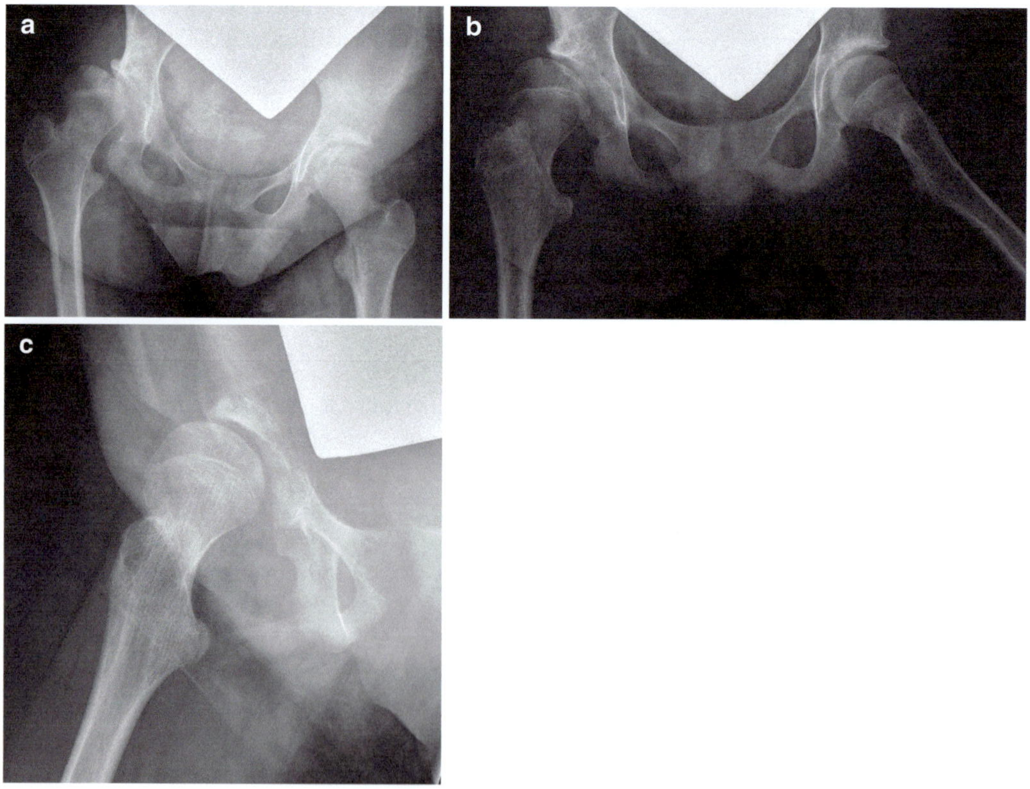

Fig. 14.2 (**a**) Standing anteroposterior, (**b**) supine anteroposterior and (**c**) abduction view radiographs demonstrate continued superior and lateral subluxation of the right hip. The femoral head remains 50% uncovered on abduction views. There is also apparent narrowing of the superior right hip joint space

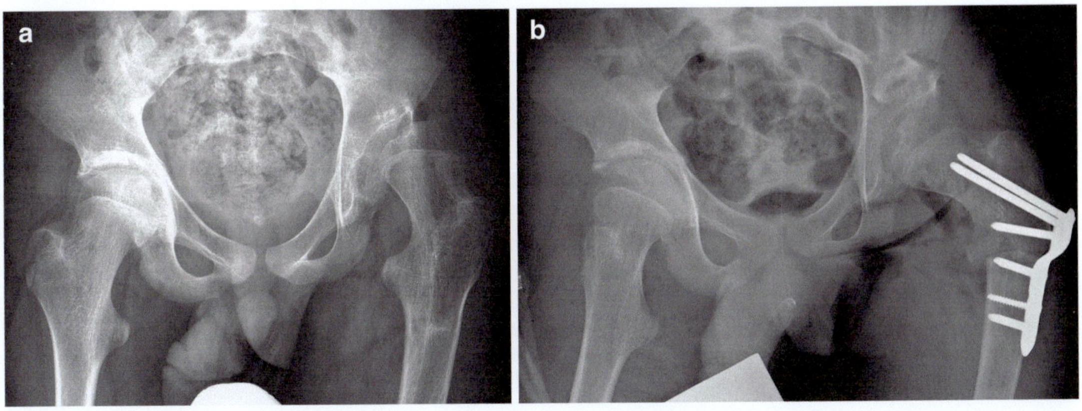

Fig. 14.3 (**a**) Preoperative anteroposterior radiograph of the patient providing operative pictures showing significant superior and lateral displacement of the left femoral head, with less than 50% coverage provided by the upward-sloping left acetabular roof. (**b**) Postoperative anteroposterior radiograph showing the redirection of the left femoral head towards the acetabulum and operative changes of the left acetabular osteotomy

Goals of Treatment

The main goals of treatment include:

Improving coverage of the femoral head
Minimizing shear stresses on articular cartilage to decrease rate of progression to arthritis
Regaining ambulatory ability/potential
Decreasing pain associated with hip subluxation

Treatment Strategy

The treatment strategy consists of realigning the femoral head within the acetabulum by VDRO and maximizing the femoral head coverage and stabilizing the hip by pelvic osteotomy. The Dega osteotomy is a reshaping osteotomy that typically relies on hinging of the fragment through the open triradiate cartilage to provide posterolateral coverage that is often deficient in children with cerebral palsy (CP) with acetabular dysplasia. When the triradiate cartilage has closed, alternative approaches, including the Bernese peri-acetabular osteotomy [1], have been described. However, there is some evidence to suggest that the Dega osteotomy can be used in patients with CP whose triradiate cartilage has closed [2]. Roposch et al. reported on a series of 41 hips with neuromuscular hip dysplasia that underwent a Dega osteotomy [3]. The triradiate cartilage was closed in nine hips in the series. Robb et al. postulated that the easily deformable nature of the peri-acetabular bone in patients with CP makes it possible to use a technique such as the Dega that would normally rely on open triradiate cartilage [4]. The authors report satisfactory outcomes on a series of 47 patients who underwent a Dega-type pelvic osteotomy after closure of the triradiate cartilage together with a varus derotation osteotomy.

Surgical Details

Dega-Type Osteotomy

A VDRO of the right proximal femur was performed prior to the pelvic osteotomy procedure. An incision one fingerbreadth lateral and distal to the iliac crest, curving distally over the anterior superior iliac spine, is made to utilize the Smith-Petersen interval (Fig. 14.4a, b). The top of the iliac crest is exposed by cautery (Fig. 14.4c), and then the interval between the sartorius and the tensor fascia lata is identified. The fascia is incised with a knife, split further with scissors, and the interval developed bluntly. The sartorius is retracted medially and the tensor fascia laterally to allow visualization of the straight head of the rectus femoris muscle tendon inserting on the anterior inferior iliac spine. The tendon is tied and detached. This allows for adequate visualiza-

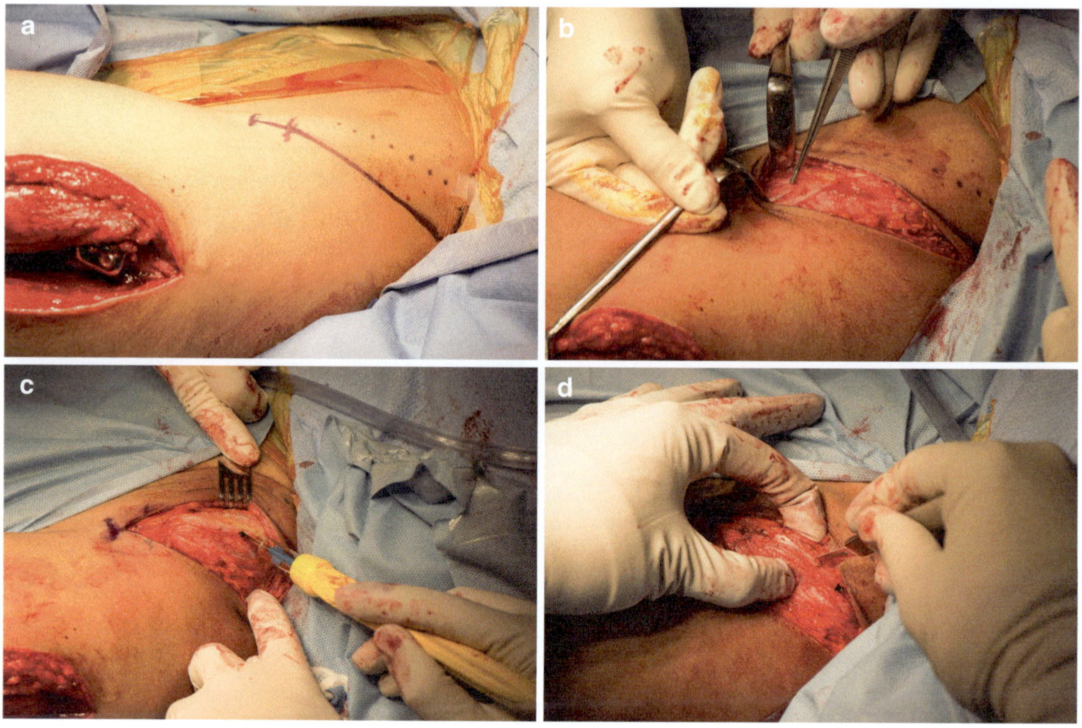

Fig. 14.4 (**a**) Incision site for the osteotomy and (**b**) exposure of the lateral cutaneous nerve of the thigh. (**c**) Exposure of the iliac crest and (**d**) splitting of the iliac crest apophysis

tion of the hip capsule to permit identification of the proximal limits of the reflected head of the rectus femoris. The iliac apophysis is split from posterior to anterior to expose the outer table of the ileum and the top of the hip capsule (Fig. 14.4d). Using a Cobb, the periosteum is teased off distally and posteriorly until reaching the greater sciatic notch. A Rang retractor is placed in the notch to protect the sciatic nerve, and a small notch is then removed from the posterior column using an up-cutting rongeur (Fig. 14.5a). Proceeding anteriorly 2 in., the inner table of the iliac wing is exposed. Under fluoroscopic guidance, the appropriate level for the anterior cut is marked, and then a curved osteotome is used to place a 2 cm cut through the inner and outer tables from an anterior to posterior direction just proximal to the anterior inferior iliac spine. A cautery tip is used to mark the appropriate level for the outer table cut parallel to the top of the acetabulum, approximately 1.5 cm proximal to the existing acetabular lip. The cautery line is deepened with a straight tip burr (Fig. 14.5b), and curved osteotomes are used to complete the cut through the outer table of the iliac wing distally and medially to encounter the inner table at the mid-level of the tear drop (Fig. 14.5c, d). A 1-inch broad osteotome is used to lever the acetabulum down until adequate coverage of the femoral head is achieved. A laminar spreader is then placed anteriorly to hold the fragments apart (Fig. 14.6a, b), while the femoral wedge removed during the VDRO is placed in the largest part of the posterolateral gap (Fig. 14.6c,

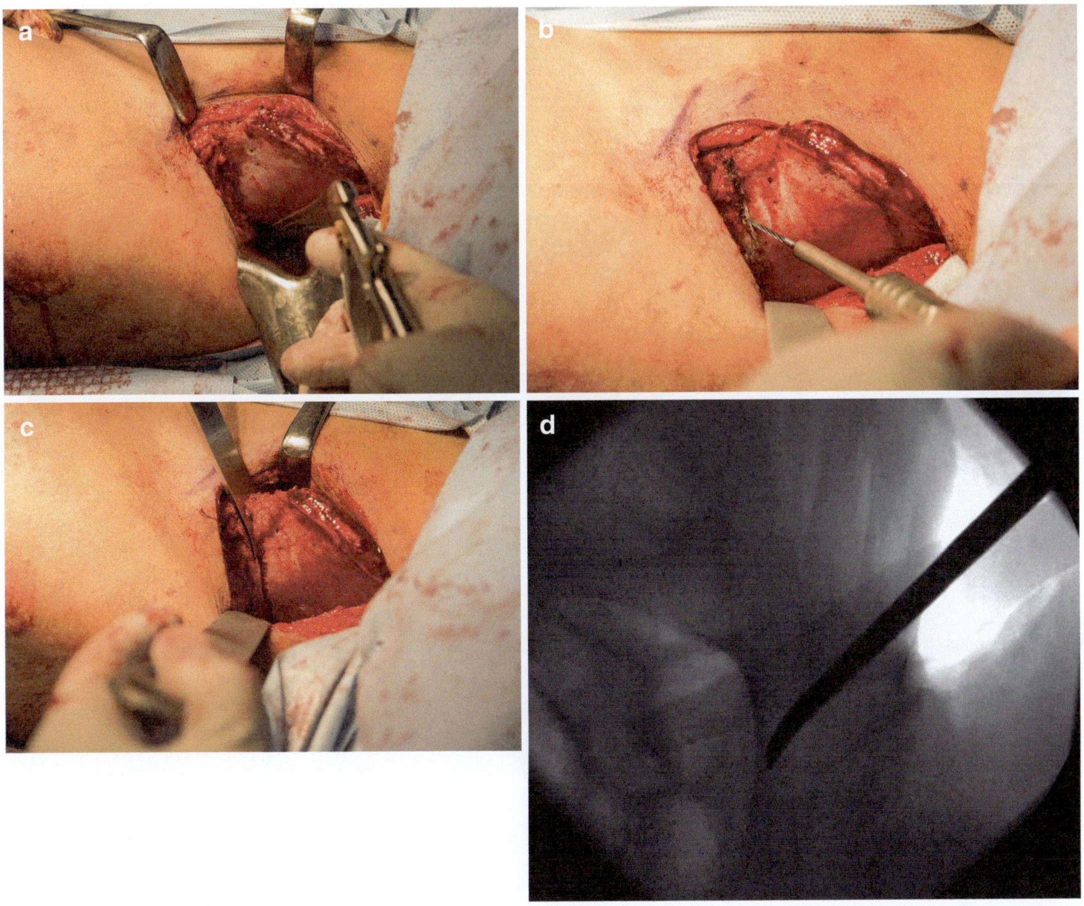

Fig. 14.5 (**a**) Placement of the Rang retractor in the sciatic notch and use of the up-cutting rongeur. (**b**) The straight tip burr is used to deepen the cut through the outer table of the iliac wing parallel to the top of the acetabulum, and (**c**) curved osteotomes complete the cut to both cortices anteriorly, from (**d**) outside to inside of the ileum

d). If a VDRO is not concomitantly performed, an allograft may be used in place. Modifications can be made to the wedge with a saw to optimize fit. Once the wedge is in place, stability of the osteotomy is tested to determine whether there is a need for internal fixation. Smaller bone wedges may then be taken from the iliac crest in order to completely fill the anterior gap of the osteotomy if required. Stability of the osteotomy is once again tested to determine the need for internal fixation. The rectus femoris tendon is then reattached to the anterior inferior iliac spine. The iliac crest apophysis and superficial interval are closed. Application of a hip spica cast or custom hip spica splint is then performed with the hip flexed in mild internal rotation and abduction (Fig. 14.7).

Intraoperative Photographs and Fluoroscopy (See Figs. 14.4, 14.5 and 14.6)

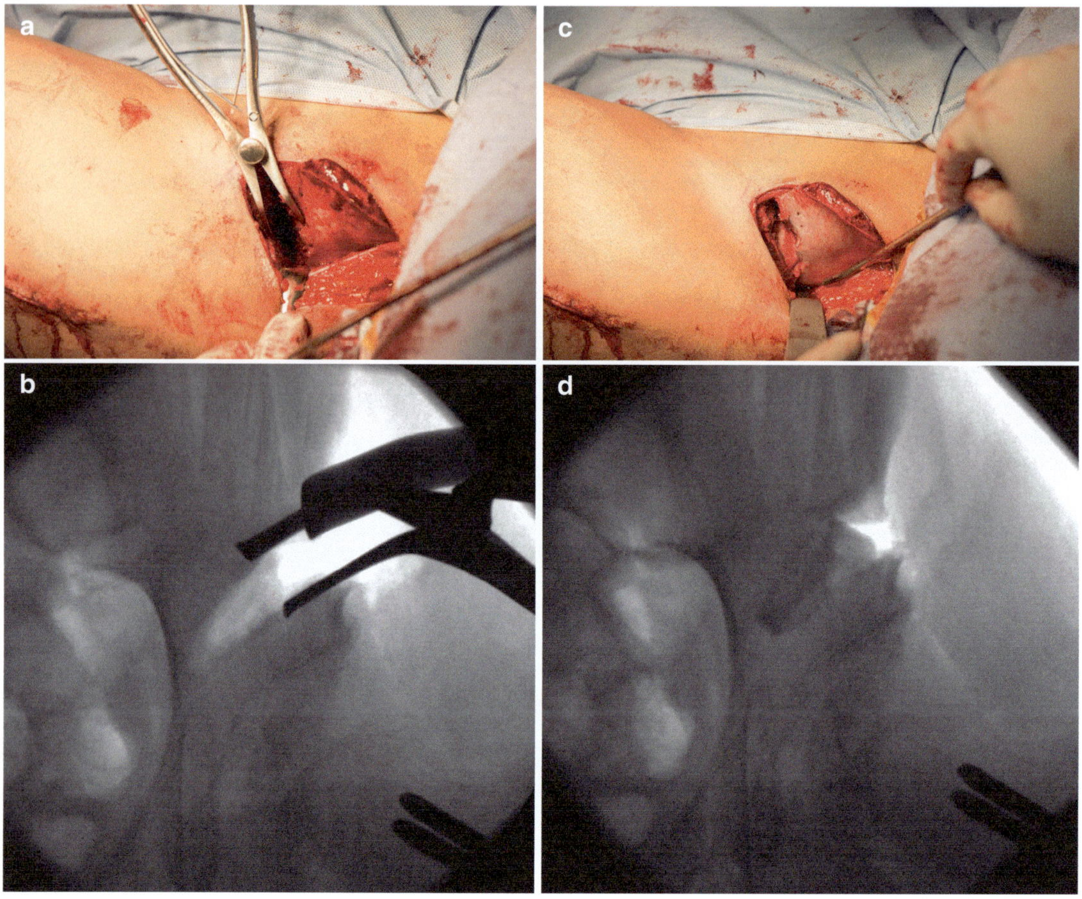

Fig. 14.6 (**a**, **b**) The laminar spreader is used to hold the fragments apart, while the (**c**) and (**d**) bone graft is placed in the osteotomy site

Postoperative Imaging
(See Figs.14.3b, 14.7 and 14.8)

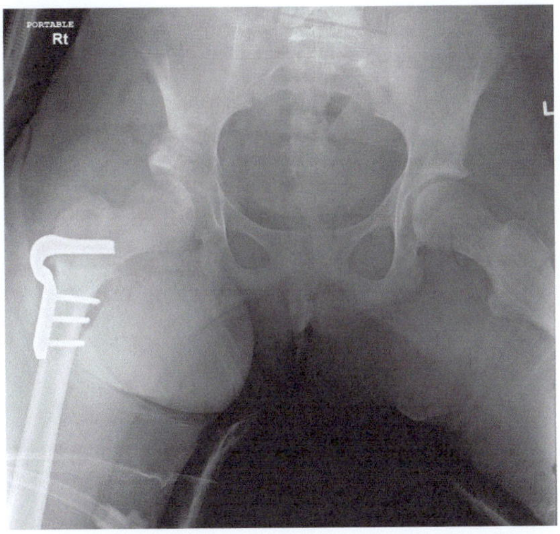

Fig. 14.7 Immediate postoperative supine radiograph obtained in hip spica shows that the right femoral head is now well-positioned with respect to the acetabulum, and the depth of the acetabulum has been improved

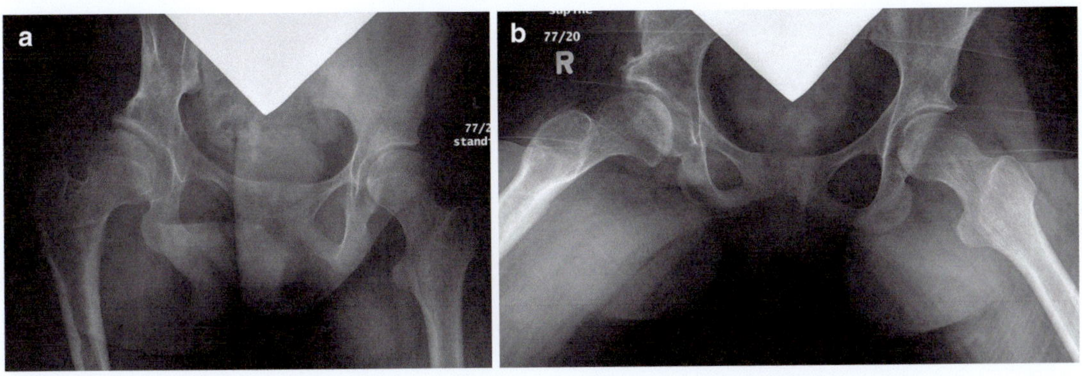

Fig. 14.8 (a) Anteroposterior radiograph showing maintained coverage of the right femoral head 2 year postoperatively. (b) Coverage is maintained in the frog-lateral position. Hardware has been removed, and the patient has returned to independent ambulation as her primary mode of transportation. She has 110° of hip flexion on the right, 115° on the left and 30° and hip abduction on both the right and left

Pearls and Pitfalls

- During the procedure, the surgeon may breach the medial cortex of the ileum; however, should this happen, this is not of great concern as iliac crest reshaping happens through plastic deformation or microfractures.
- The peri-acetabular osteotomy can be used to achieve the same result if a surgeon is more comfortable with that technique.
- Even though the Dega osteotomy is a reconstructive procedure, this surgical technique in this application could be viewed as a salvage surgery because most patients are non-ambulatory. However, as demonstrated in this case, the procedure can also work in ambulatory children.
- There are fewer complications and lower morbidity associated with this procedure in comparison to a peri-acetabular osteotomy.

Indications and Contraindications (Table 14.1)

Table 14.1 Acetabuloplasty in closed triradiate cartilage: surgical indications and contraindications

Indications
Acetabular dysplasia
Increased acetabular volume
Contraindications
Idiopathic developmental dysplasia of the hip (DDH)
Major loss of femoral head shape/cartilage (salvage surgery more appropriate)

References

1. Grudziak JS, Ward WT. Dega osteotomy for the treatment of congenital dysplasia of the hip. J Bone Joint Surg Am. 2001;83-A(6):845–54.
2. MacDonald SJ, Hersche O, Ganz R. Periacetabular osteotomy in the treatment of neurogenic acetabular dysplasia. J Bone Joint Surg Br. 1999;81(6):975–8.
3. Roposch A, Wedge JH. An incomplete periacetabular osteotomy for treatment of neuromuscular hip dysplasia. Clin Orthop Surg. 2005;431:166–75.
4. Robb JE, Brunner R. A Dega-type osteotomy after closure of the triradiate cartilage in non-walking patients with severe cerebral palsy. J Bone Joint Surg Br. 2006;88(7):933–7.

15 Shelf Acetabuloplasty Using Inner Table of Iliac Bone as Graft

Adolfredo Santana, Mehmet Serhan Er, and William G. Mackenzie

Introduction

Shelf acetabuloplasty is a procedure indicated when other redirectional and reconstructive procedures can't be optimally used. All reported techniques have used the outer table of ilium as a graft. Our technique utilizes the inner table of the ilium as a graft and has several advantages over the standard shelf procedure.

The surgical technique as described in this chapter keeps the large, stable, and smooth concave cortical surface of the graft just over the capsule serving as a buttress. There is the option of sparing the elevation of the gluteus from the outer table of the ilium. The abductors do not need to be elevated from their origin on the ilium, and this potentially improves postoperative abductor function.

Brief Clinical History

The patient is a 16-year-old male with Morquio syndrome, who had bilateral tibia/fibula osteotomies for genu valgum. He had hip pain, and it was difficult to walk secondary to pain. He also had pain in multiple joints: ankles, knees, elbows, and disproportionate short stature. There was a positive Trendelenburg, hip flexion to 110° with full extension, and abduction of 45° bilaterally. His popliteal angles are 0°. Foot and ankle exam was normal.

Radiographs of the pelvis (Fig. 15.1) demonstrate bilateral acetabular dysplasia, hip subluxation, and epiphyseal flattening.

In order to relieve pain and improve function, shelf acetabuloplasty was done.

A. Santana · M. Serhan Er · W. G. Mackenzie (✉)
Orthopedic Department, Nemours/Alfred I. duPont Hospital for Children, Wilmington, DE, USA
e-mail: adolfredo.santana@nemours.org; william.mackenzie@nemours.org

R. C. Hamdy, N. Saran (eds.), *Pediatric Pelvic and Proximal Femoral Osteotomies*, https://doi.org/10.1007/978-3-319-78033-7_15

Preoperative Imaging (See Fig. 15.1)

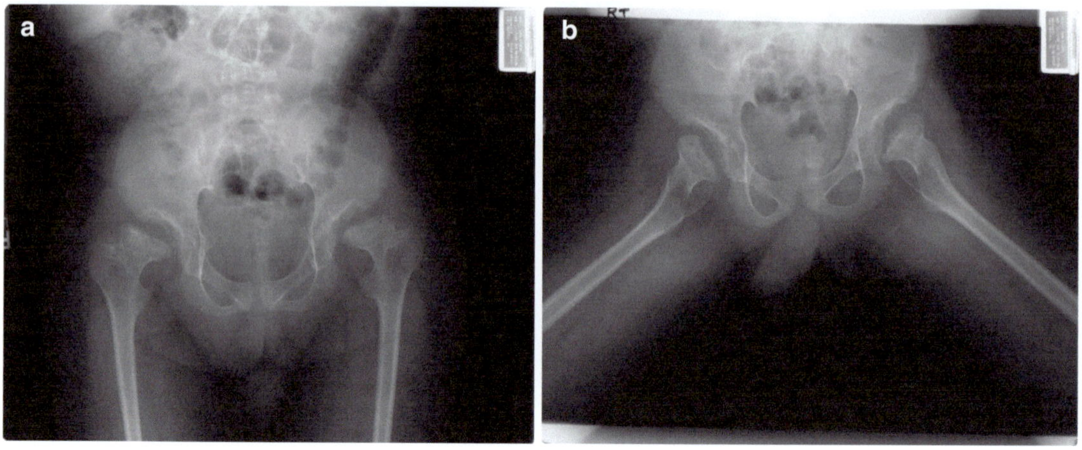

Fig. 15.1 Preoperative radiographs: (**a**) anteroposterior pelvis, (**b**) frog leg pelvis

Goals of Treatment

- Decrease hip pain and maintain range of motion.
- Extend acetabular hip coverage.

Treatment Strategy

The term *shelf acetabuloplasty* applies to a number of procedures in which either a part of the cortical bone of the outer table of the ilium adjacent to the hip is reflected distally over the subluxated femoral head or a free bone graft is used to extend the acetabular roof laterally and anteroposteriorly to augment the dysplastic acetabulum.

All previously reported techniques used the outer table of the ilium as a graft. Our technique utilizes the inner table of the ilium as a graft, which has advantages over the standard shelf acetabuloplasty. It has the option of sparing the elevation of the gluteus from the outer table of the ilium and provides a large cortico-cancellous graft (up to 4 × 5 cm) with a cortical surface that is concave down, matching the acetabular margin.

Reflecting the outer table of the ilium and suturing the bone over the capsule have been a popular technique of shelf acetabuloplasty, as described by Wainwright (1976). Poor results were reported using this technique because fractures of the shelf occur at the site of the hinge just above the dysplastic native acetabular margin.

The surgical technique described here keeps the smooth cortical surface of the graft just over the capsule, serving as a buttress to the capsule, giving a desirable shape and position to the shelf.

Surgical Details

The child is positioned supine on a radiolucent table with a small bump under the involved hip. The hip and leg are prepped and draped to allow wide access to the hemipelvis. A bikini skin incision is then made 1 cm below the anterior superior iliac spine (ASIS), and the interval between the tensor fascia lata and sartorius is developed. This dissection is extended to the origin of the rectus femoris at the anterior inferior iliac spine (AIIS). While the indirect head of rectus femoris can be divided and reflected posteriorly along the lateral edge of the acetabulum, we rarely do this. Abductors do not need to be elevated from their origin on the ilium. A tunnel can be created beneath the abductors to visualize the superior edge of the acetabulum. In children with Morquio syndrome, the abductors are elevated to allow adequate visualization. A 1 cm osteotome is used to create a slot just above the capsule directed slightly (approximately 20° cranially). The direction and location of the cut are monitored under fluoroscopy (Fig. 15.2). The depth of the slot is approximately 1 cm. The slot is then widened with a side-cutting burr. The gluteal fascia is incised at its origin on the iliac apophysis. Utilizing an osteotome, the iliac apophysis is elevated from lateral to medial exposing the inner table of the ilium subperiosteally.

A cortico-cancellous graft (size: approximately 3 × 4 cm in most of our cases) is then harvested from the inner table of the ilium (Fig. 15.3). The graft has a concave cortical surface. The graft is positioned so that the smooth concave cortical surface faces down over the capsule and the curved edge medially fits into the slot (Fig. 15.4). Four holes are put in the graft to suture the graft to the superior surface of the capsule (Fig. 15.5). The holes should be

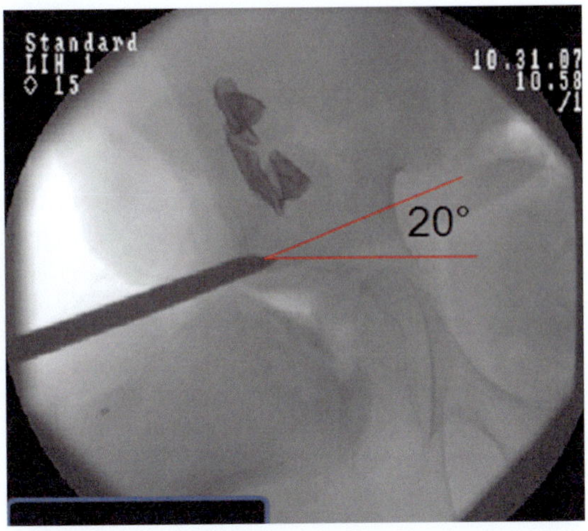

Fig. 15.2 A slot is created just superior to the edge of the acetabulum, angulated 20° cranially

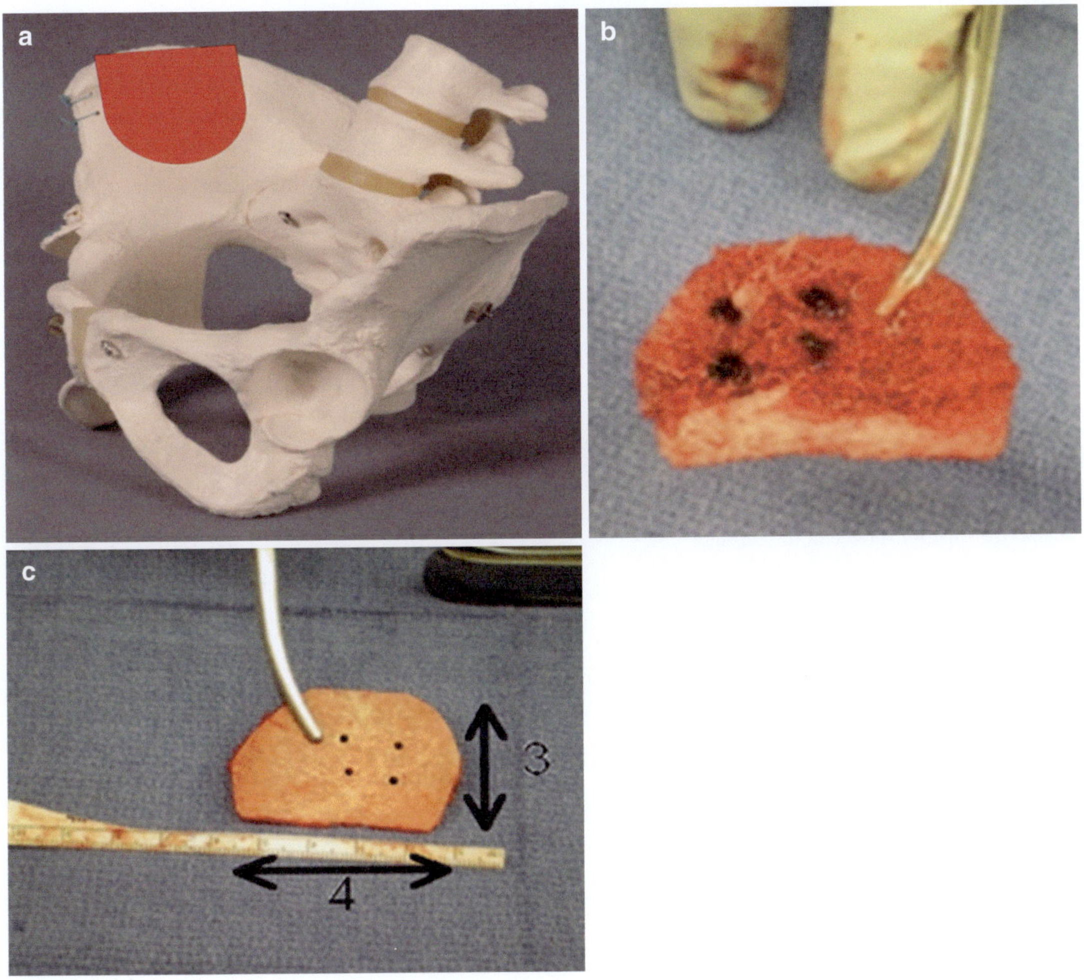

Fig. 15.3 (**a**) Inner table of the ilium. (**b**) *Black arrow* indicates the edge placed into the slot. (**c**) Cortico-cancellous graft (size: approximately 3 × 4 cm in most of our cases) from the inner table of the ilium

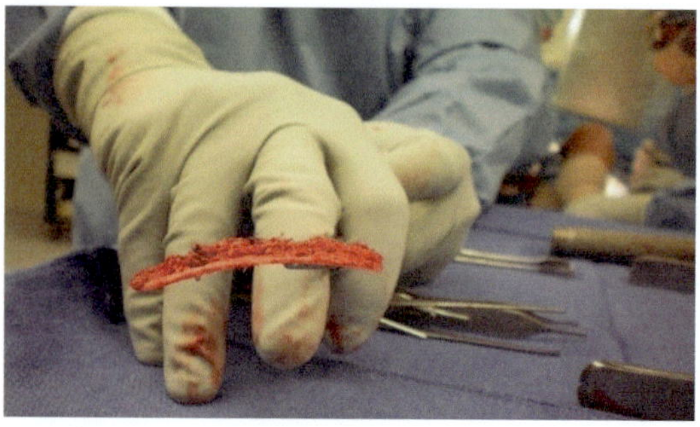

Fig. 15.4 Cortical surface of the graft will cover the capsule, and the cancellous surface will face up

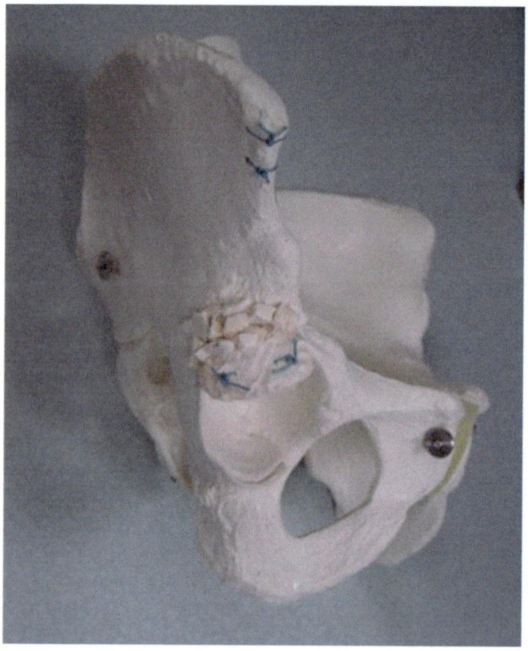

Fig. 15.5 Four holes are put in the graft to suture the graft to the superior surface of the capsule

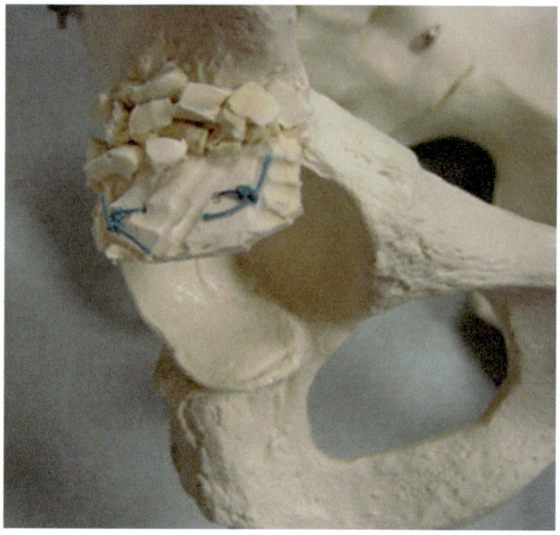

Fig. 15.6 The holes should be placed so as to avoid pulling the graft out of the slot when the sutures are tied

placed so as to avoid pulling the graft out of the slot when the sutures are tied (Fig. 15.6). Two nonabsorbable sutures are placed in the capsule and brought through the holes in the graft. The graft is placed into the domed slot and tamped in. A piece of cortical bone can be wedged above the graft into the slot to stabilize the fixation (shim). The optimal shelf should cover the extruded femoral head, taking care that the lateral outer edge of the graft is not abutting on the neck of the femur or the greater trochanter at terminal abduction. The shelf should not cause any anterior impingement with flexion and internal rotation of the hip.

The hip motion should be assessed at this point, and, if needed, edges of the graft should be trimmed appropriately. The outer wall of the iliac wing just above the slot is roughened with a burr. Subsequently, morselized cancellous bone graft is packed into the gap between the wall of the ilium and the upper cancellous surface of the shelf.

Postoperative Imaging (Fig. 15.7)

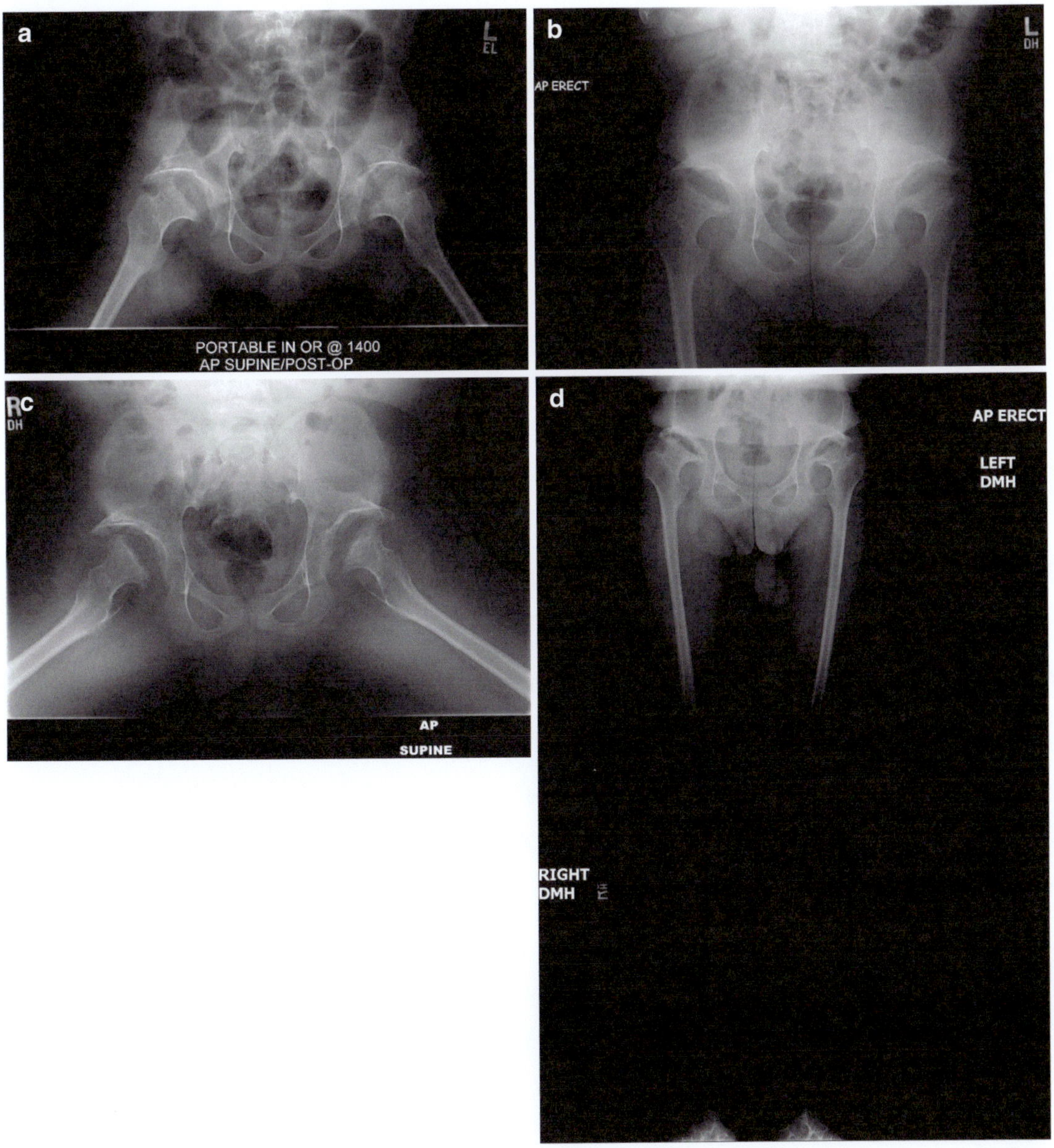

Fig. 15.7 Follow-up radiographs. (**a**) Postoperative: anteroposterior (AP) supine pelvis; (**b**) 1 year after surgery, AP erect; (**c**) 5 years after procedure, AP supine; (**d**) AP erect

Pearls and Pitfalls

- The goal of shelf acetabuloplasty is to achieve a contoured extension of the roof of the acetabulum in order to provide a smooth concave roof over the femoral head and to promote eventual long-term congruence between the uncovered femoral head and the opposing acetabulum. This is a good option in children with a variety of conditions, especially in children with Morquio syndrome.
- An important point in the postoperative care is to apply a single-leg hip spica cast in 20° flexion and 20° abductions for 4–6 weeks, and then full weight bearing is encouraged as soon as it is tolerated by the child.
- The insertion of the cortico-cancellous graft in the slot (approximately 1 cm deep) above the acetabular margin and the suturing of the bone graft to the capsule provide the strength and stability. Elevation of the abductors can be avoided, potentially improving postoperative abductor function.

Indications and Contraindications (Table 15.1)

Table 15.1 Shelf acetabuloplasty using inner table of iliac bone as graft: surgical indications and contraindications

Indications
Acetabular reconstruction when a contoured extension is required; for example, severe acetabular dysplasia when the acetabulum is too small for reorientation
Salvage for a subluxated or dislocated joint
Contraindications
Developmental dysplasia of the hip
When acetabular reconstruction can be achieved by reorientation of the hyaline cartilage surface

Suggested Reading

Dhawale AA, Thacker MM, Belthur MV, Rogers K, Bober MB, Mackenzie WG. The lower extremity in Morquio syndrome. J Pediatr Orthop. 2012;32(5):534–40.

Li WC, Xu RJ. Lateral shelf acetabuloplasty for severe Legg–Calvé–Perthes disease in patients older than 8 years. A mean eleven-year follow-up. Medicine (Baltimore). 2016;95(45):e5272.

Pauwels F. Biomechanics of the normal and diseased hip: theoretical foundation, technique and results 177 of treatment. New York: Springer; 1976. p. 268–9.

Ponseti I. Pathomechanics of the hip after the shelf operation. J Bone Joint Surg Am. 1946;28:229–40.

Wainwright D. The shelf operation for hip dysplasia in adolescence. J Bone Joint Surg Br. 1976;58(2):159–63.

Chiari Pelvic Osteotomy

16

Benjamin J. Shore and Travis Matheney

Introduction

The treatment of hip subluxation, whether from congenital disorders, neuromuscular problems, or acquired disease, remains a challenge. In particular, subluxation of the hip with secondary acetabular dysplasia is particularly difficult when the hip is irreducible and the triradiate cartilage is closed. Chiari in 1974 described a medial displacement osteotomy to be used in children and adults with hip dysplasia and poor joint congruency. Mid- to long-term results demonstrate that this osteotomy remains radiologically effective for at least 25 years. The Chiari osteotomy is an excellent salvage procedure for adolescent and young adults with limited osteoarthritis and hip subluxation and for children with spastic hip subluxation in the setting of closed triradiate cartilage, whose incongruity is not amenable to a re-directional osteotomy.

Brief Clinical History

This 17-year-old male Gross Motor Function Classification System (GMFCS) IV with cerebral palsy presented with progressive right hip pain and decreased functional ability. He was having pain with activities of daily living such as diapering and sitting in his wheelchair. Conservative measures including Botox injections, soft tissue lengthening, and physical therapy had all been previously attempted without relief. Preoperative examination demonstrated a 25° hip flexion contracture on the right. He demonstrates 80° of internal rotation and 10° of external rotation on the right hip. Abduction is limited to 0° in flexion and extension with a mildly positive Galeazzi sign.

B. J. Shore (✉) · T. Matheney
Department of Orthopaedic Surgery, Harvard Medical School, Boston Children's Hospital, Boston, MA, USA
e-mail: Benjamin.shore@childrens.harvard.edu; travis.matheney@childrens.harvard.edu

R. C. Hamdy, N. Saran (eds.), *Pediatric Pelvic and Proximal Femoral Osteotomies*,
https://doi.org/10.1007/978-3-319-78033-7_16

Preoperative Imaging

Radiographs demonstrate hip subluxation, acetabular dysplasia, and incongruity of the hip joint (Fig. 16.1).

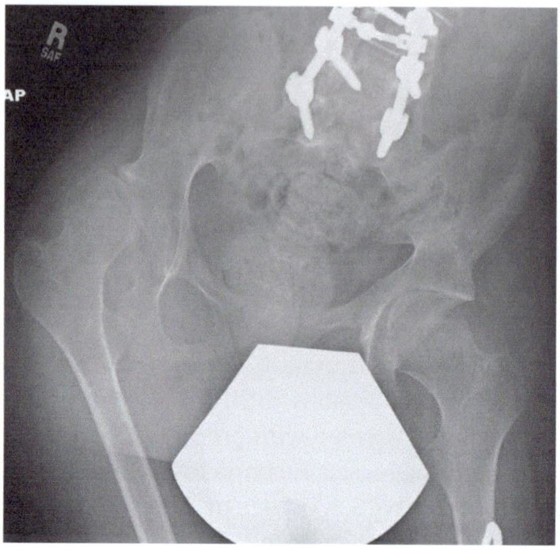

Fig. 16.1 Preoperative radiograph of a 17-year-old male with cerebral palsy, GMFCS IV

Clinical Examination

Examination should begin with observed gait analysis and a careful hip range of motion, in particular internal and external rotation limits, which give information where the damaged portion of the femoral head and possibly acetabulum exist. Imaging studies are designed to document the congruency of the femoral head within the acetabulum, the amount of anterior and lateral acetabular coverage of the femoral head and the reducibility of the femoral head into the native acetabulum. Reconstructed computed tomography (CT) can aid surgeons in the three-dimensional relationship between the acetabulum and femoral head and identify locations of acetabular deficiency (anterolateral vs posterolateral). Radial sequencing magnetic resonance imaging (MRI) can aid surgeons in illustrating the condition and quality of labrum and articular cartilage of the hip joint, during the preoperative assessment. An intraoperative arthrogram is a useful study, which demonstrates the dynamic stability of the hip and the relative congruency of the femoral head and acetabulum. The Von Rosen view can demonstrate the incongruous relationship between the femoral head and acetabulum and demonstrate the reducibility of the femoral head within the acetabulum.

Goals of Treatment

The Chiari pelvic osteotomy is a *salvage* pelvic osteotomy. The main goals are to:

- Relieve pain from a hip joint, which has aspherical incongruity between femoral head and acetabulum.
- Use the ilium to form a "shelf" over the femoral head to stabilize the hip.
- Allow for metaplasia of the interposed hip capsule to form new fibrocartilage.

Treatment Strategy

The treatment strategy consists of performing a single pericapsular osteotomy through the iliac (innominate) bone of the pelvis with associated medialization of the acetabulum and hip joint to improve posterior and lateral femoral head coverage. If additional femoral head coverage is required, the osteotomy can be augmented with a shelf osteotomy where persistent deficiency exists. Additional surgical interventions instead of the Chiari osteotomy include hip arthrodesis, isolated shelf osteotomy, and total hip arthroplasty.

Surgical Details

Positioning

The patient is positioned supine on a radiolucent operating room table. Often a bump is placed under the operative hip to achieve a "sloppy lateral position." The ipsilateral arm is either draped across the chest in small children or in larger patients is forward flexed to 90° and supported on an elevated arm holder. Regional analgesia (Lumbar plexus blockade) and Foley catheterization are inserted preoperatively. Free drape the operative extremity to the level of the costophrenic margin superiorly, medially to the ipsilateral border of the perineum, and laterally to the border of the buttocks. Intraoperative fluoroscopy is employed from the contralateral side of the bed.

Exposure

The ilioinguinal approach is the exposure of choice for this osteotomy (Fig. 16.2a). The incision begins approximately 1–2 cm below the iliac crest and extends medially 1.5–2 cm distal and medial to the anterior superior iliac spine (ASIS). The lateral fibers of the external oblique muscle overhang the lateral ilium and are reflected off the ilium with electrocautery or a #15 blade.

Distally, the interval between the sartorius and tensor fascia lata (TFL) is identified. The TFL fascial compartment is opened, and muscle is stripped directly off the intermuscular septum with a cobb/periosteal elevator. The TFL is retracted laterally, and the intermuscular septum and sartorius muscle are retracted medially (Fig. 16.2b). At this level, the lateral femoral cutaneous nerve (LFCN) of the thigh lies within the sartorial muscle compartment and is not visualized; however, the nerve lies under the fascia between the two muscles and care must be taken to avoid injury during the approach and when closing to avoid a painful neuroma. Blunt dissection of TFL is continued proximally to the ilium and to the level of the anterior inferior iliac spine (AIIS). Continue subperiosteal dissection anteriorly from ASIS inferiorly to the anterior inferior iliac spine (AIIS). Identify the direct head of the rectus femoris inserting into the AIIS, and locate the bifurcation of the indirect head.

At this point, the iliac apophysis is split in the midline, the gluteal muscles are subperiosteally dissected off the outer table ilium, and the iliacus muscle is subperiosteally dissected off the inner table of the ilium; a moist sponge is packed tightly between the ilium and dissected muscles to aid in retraction and hemostasis. A lane bone lever is placed subperiosteally into the greater sciatic notch to give excellent visualization of the acetabular rim (Fig. 16.2c, *arrow*) all the way to the ischial spine. As the periosteum is stripped off the outer table away from the abductor musculature, one encounters

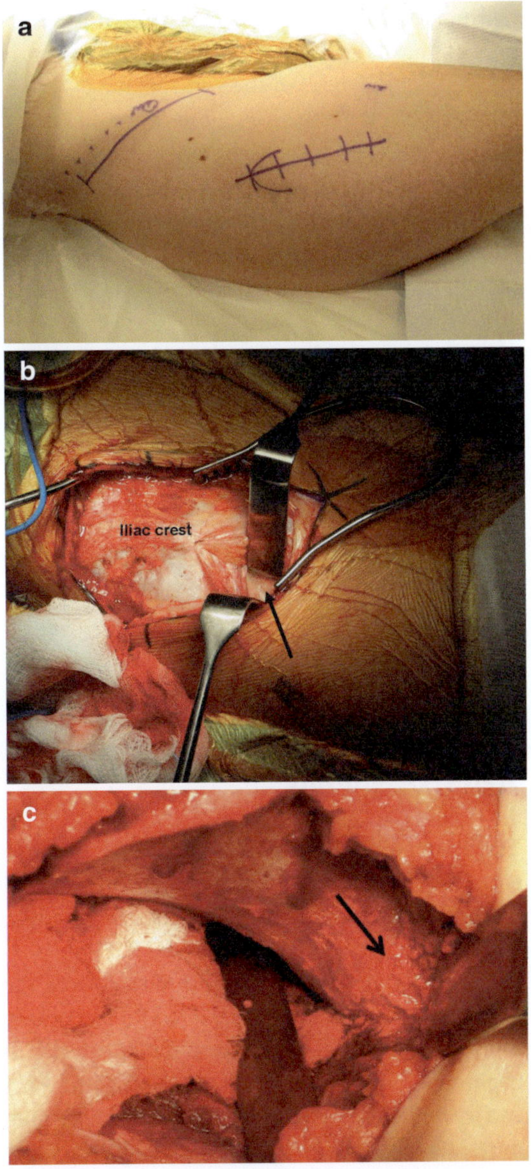

Fig. 16.2 (**a**) Planned incisions for both the ilioinguinal approach and the direct lateral approach to the proximal femur for additional intertrochanteric osteotomy. (**b**) Ilioinguinal approach. Shown are the iliac crest and the direct head of the rectus femoris (*arrow*) deep to the tensor fascia lata (TFL) compartment (TFL retracted posteriorly). (**c**) The outer table of the ilium is exposed. A lane bone lever placed subperiosteally into the greater sciatic notch allows excellent visualization of the acetabular rim (*arrow*) all the way to the ischial spine (From Matheney and Snyder, 2016, with permission)

resistance inferiorly, which indicates the insertion of the indirect head of the rectus femoris on the lateral aspect of the hip capsule.

Return back to the bifurcation of the direct and indirect heads of the rectus femoris tendon. Ligate the indirect head at the bifurcation and follow it posterolaterally to the suspected inserted into the lateral hip capsule. Use a lane retractor to subperiosteally elevate the superior gluteal artery and sciatic nerve away from the apex and anterior margin of the notch. Incise the periosteum along the superior border of the indirect head of rectus femoris. This will allow subsequent release of the abductor minimus off the superior capsule to allow for proper chisel placement for the Chiari osteotomy.

At this point, use fluoroscopy to ensure that you have not been misled by a pseudoacetabulum and your dissection has carried you down to the acetabular margin (Fig. 16.3a). The indirect head of rectus is a key anatomic landmark to the edge of the true acetabulum posteriorly.

Step 1: Osteotomy

Essentially the osteotomy is creating a transverse acetabular "fracture" where both the anterior and posterior acetabular columns are cut and the ilium is displaced either anterolaterally (DDH) or posterolaterally (neuromuscular dysplasia) over the hip joint capsule forming a shelf. The osteotomy is curvilinear in the supra-acetabular region. It begins at the anterior ilium at the level of the AIIS and traverses the capsular edge of the acetabulum to terminate at the sciatic notch. Conventionally the osteotomy is completed with a Gigli saw—which creates a transverse osteotomy (Fig. 16.3b). We use a modification advocated by John Hall, in which the osteotomy is truly curvilinear. The posterior limb of the osteotomy is curved distally aiming a centimeter below the apex of the sciatic notch to increase posterior coverage, thus making the osteotomy more dome-like in appearance with a series of curved or dome-shaped osteotomes, Ganz or Mast chisels (Fig. 16.3c–g). The curvilinear osteotomy is directed cranially and medial 15–20° to facilitate sliding and displacement of the cut surface of the ilium over the hip joint capsule. The inner table of the ilium is often scored to prevent splintering of the inner table at completion of the osteotomy.

Step 2: Acetabular Displacement

Often 100% displacement is required to facilitate appropriate coverage of the hip. The hip is abducted and axial force is applied to the leg as the femoral head is pushed medially to facilitate displacement of the distal fragment. The amount of lateral displacement and relative anterior/posterior displacement is dependent on the degree of coverage that is required for the hip.

When posterior coverage is required, the ilium is displaced posteriorly over the sciatic notch—however, extreme care must be taken to ensure that the sciatic nerve is not entrapped or compressed. It is often necessary to use corticocancellous graft osteotomized from the inner table of the ilium to interpose between the anterior hip joint capsule and the displaced ilium. This graft sits anterolaterally to augment the anterolateral coverage of the femoral head. This anterolateral graft needs to be secured with either a small Ethibond suture (placed through the anterolateral hip capsule and displaced ilium) or a screw/threaded K-wire (similar in trajectory to the screw fixation for transfixing the displaced ilium).

Step 3: Fixation and Closure

The osteotomy is fixed in place with either 3.5 or 4.5 mm cortical screws.

Traditionally, these screws were placed along the iliac crest into the posterior column of the ischium. However, with 100% displacement of the distal fragment, solid screw fixation can be

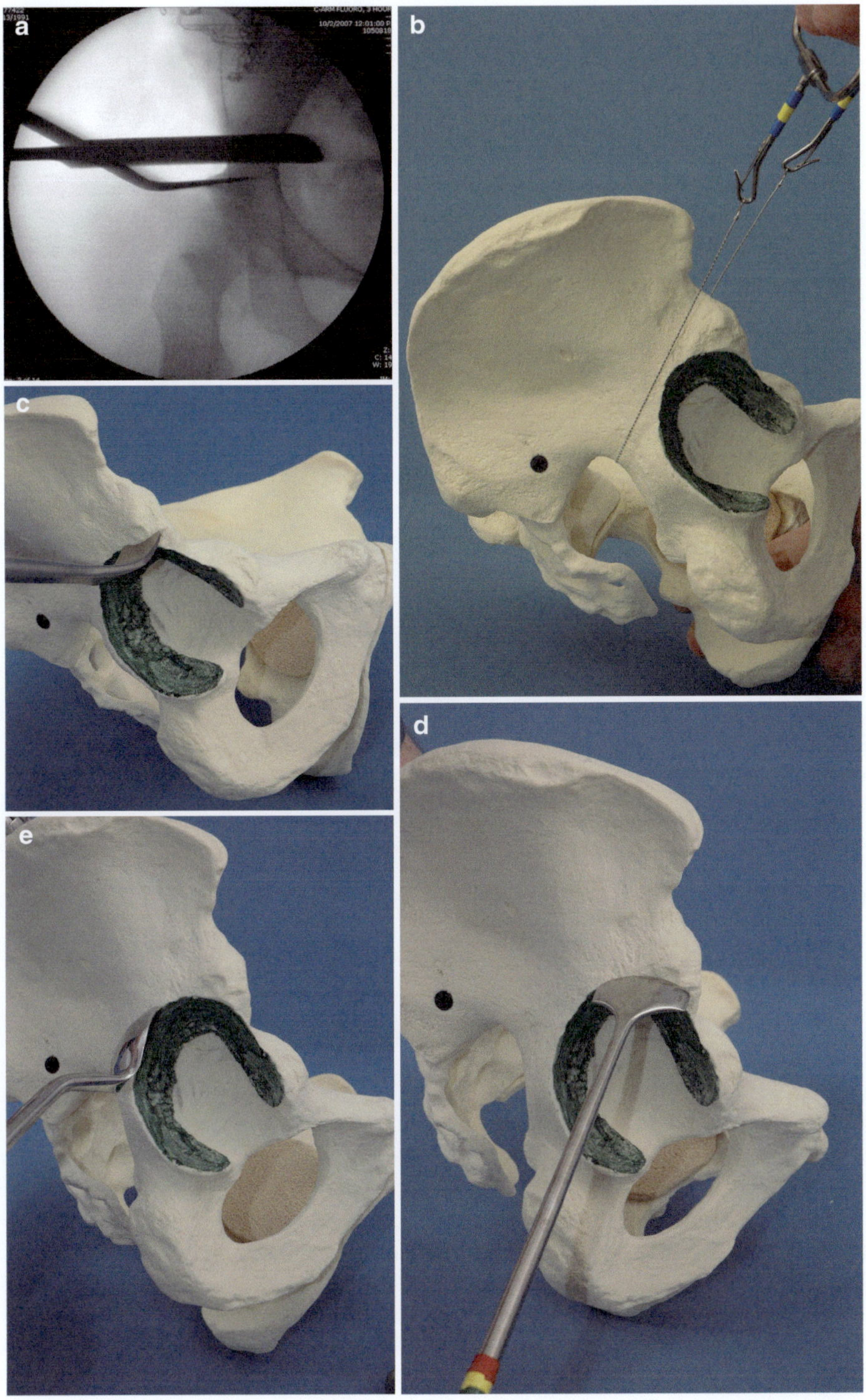

Fig. 16.3 (**a**) Anteroposterior fluoroscopic view of the right during osteotomy. The osteotome enters at the edge of the acetabulum and is directed upward at an angle of about 15° (From Matheney and Snyder, 2016, with permission). (**b**) Sawbones figure demonstrating use of a Gigli saw and path of osteotomy from posterior to anterior. (**c–e**) Bone models demonstrate the planned supra-acetabular osteotomy using a combination of curved and dome-shaped osteotomes (From Matheney and Snyder, 2016, with permission). (**f**) The completed supra-acetabular osteotomy (*arrow*) (From Matheney and Snyder, 2016, with permission). (**g**) Bone model representation of the posterior aspect of the osteotomy. Note the attempt to continue the osteotomy posterior to just above the ischial spine (From Matheney and Snyder, 2016, with permission)

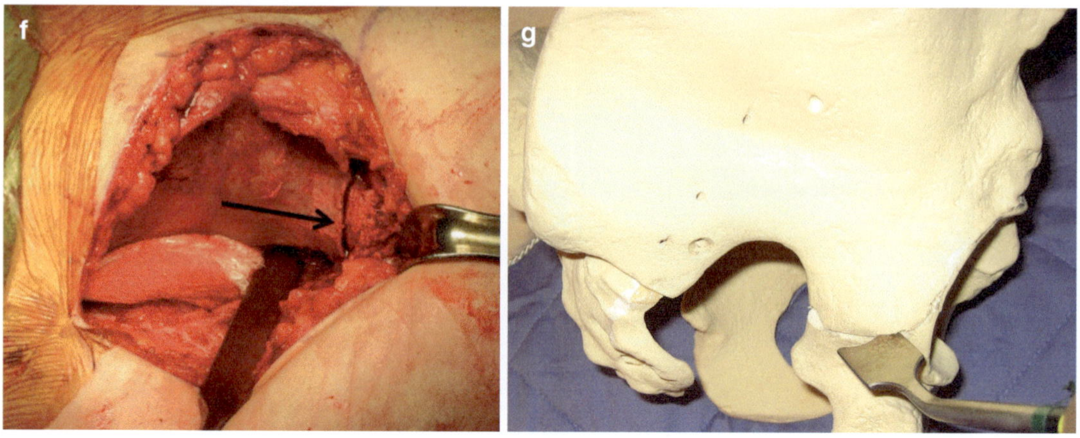

Fig. 16.3 (continued)

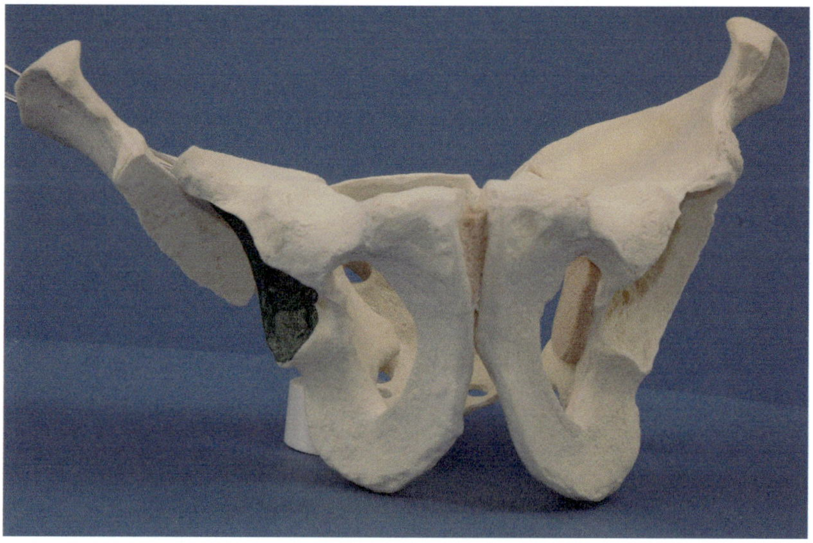

Fig. 16.4 Sawbone representation of the final osteotomy and fixation. Note the displacement of the osteotomy and path of the fixation. We prefer starting fixation off the crest on the lateral aspect of the ilium to obtain the correct trajectory for fixation, especially in cases where the displacement is greater than 50%

challenging. We now prefer screw placement starting inferior from the ASIS on the *outer table* of the ilium and directed medially to facilitate more robust fixation into the ischium and distal fragment (Fig. 16.4). These screws are placed under fluoroscopic guidance, and multiple views are necessary to ensure no penetration into the hip joint. In patients who are not toilet trained, we use Dermabond (2-Octyl cyanoacrylate; Ethicon, Inc., Somerville, NJ) on the skin to provide a waterproof seal. Spica immobilization is not necessary; however, if uncertain about bone quality, fixation or in a neuromuscular patient a one-legged pantaloon spica or a bilateral long leg cast with an A-frame bar is also acceptable if other procedures were preformed simultaneously.

We allow patients to sit up to 90° of hip flexion immediately. The operative leg is kept in approximately 30° of hip abduction with toe-touch weight bearing for 6 weeks (with a foam wedge/long leg casts with a bar). If no immobilization is employed, gentle range of motion from 0° to 70° is permitted.

Postoperative Imaging (Fig. 16.5)

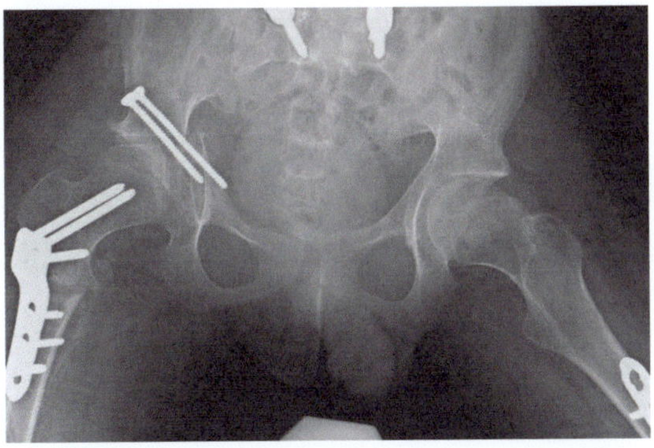

Fig. 16.5 Postoperative radiograph of a 17-year-old male with cerebral palsy, GMFCS IV. This patient underwent concomitant Chiari and femoral osteotomy for shortening and derotation. Note the fixation of the screws for the Chiari starting on the lateral aspect of the ilium

Pearls and Pitfalls

- Recognize significant proximal migration of the femoral head as it can prevent appropriate positioning of the osteotomy, resulting in insufficient translation of the ilium to form a "shelf" to cover the femoral head.
- The indirect head of the rectus femoris is the "lighthouse" to the true acetabulum; follow it posterolaterally to an insertion point on the lateral aspect of the true acetabulum.
- Adequate exposure of the apex and anterior border of the sciatic notch along the posterior column of the acetabulum is necessary for initiating the cut into the posterior column of the acetabulum using a Mast/Ganz chisel.
- Direct the posterior aspect of the osteotomy along the posterior column exiting at the level of the ischial spine into the sciatic notch, rather than at the apex of the sciatic notch. This modification increases posterior coverage and makes the osteotomy more dome shaped.
- Especially in neuromuscular children and those with poor bone quality, splintering of the inner table of ilium is a real concern. Once the lateral cut has been initiated, a K-wire can be inserted into the osteotomy gap and advanced under fluoroscopic guidance to perforate the inner table to create a "postage stamp" series of perforations to minimize splintering of the bone at the inner table of the ilium.
- Use of AO (*Arbeitsgemeinschaft für Osteosynthesefragen*) pelvic/acetabular fracture instruments is helpful. The large pelvic reduction clamp and ball-tipped pushing spike can be useful to facilitate translation of the ilium during the displacement maneuver.
- Multiple orthogonal views of the hip joint are necessary to ensure that no hardware is intra-articular.

Indications and Contraindications (Table 16.1)

Table 16.1 Chiari pelvic osteotomy: surgical indications and contraindications

Indications
Subluxated and irreducible hip
Incongruent dysplastic hip
Patients with dysplasia in whom a re-directional osteotomy is not feasible
Contraindications
Moderate-advanced degenerative joint disease
Severe dysplasia or proximal migration of femoral head where osteotomy and displacement is not technically feasible

Suggested Reading

Bailey TE, Hall JE. Chiari medial displacement osteotomy. J Pediatr Orthop. 1985;5(6):635–41.

Chiari K. Medial displacement osteotomy of the pelvis. Clin Orthop. 1974;98:55–71.

Debnath UK, Guha AR, Karlakki S, Vargese J, Evans GA. Combined femoral and Chiari osteotomies for reconstruction of the painful subluxation or dislocation of the hip in cerebral palsy: a long-term outcome study. J Bone Joint Surg Br. 2006;88(10):1373–8.

Delp SL, Bleck EB, Zajac FE, Bollini G. Biomechanical analysis of the Chiari pelvic osteotomy. Clin Orthop Relat Res. 1990;254:189–98.

Matheney TH, Snyder B. Chiari medial displacement osteotomy of the pelvis. In: Flynn JM, Sankar WN,

Wiesel SW, editors. Operative techniques in pediatric orthopaedic surgery. 2nd ed. Philadelphia: Wolters Kluwer; 2016. p. 923–9.
Ohashi H, Hirohashi K, Yamano Y. Factors influencing the outcome of Chiari pelvic osteotomy: a long-term follow-up. J Bone Joint Surg Br. 2000;82(4):517–25.
Windager R, Pongracz N, Shonecker W, Kotz R. Chiari osteotomy for congenital dislocation and subluxation of the hip: results after 20 to 34 years follow-up. J Bone Joint Surg Br. 1991;73(6):890–5.

Pelvic Osteotomy for Bladder Exstrophy

17

David J. Kirby and Paul D. Sponseller

Introduction

Classic bladder exstrophy is a developmental defect resulting in pubic diastasis and bladder protrusion through the abdominal wall. Within this spectrum of disease is cloacal exstrophy, defined by the development of omphalocele in addition to diastasis and bladder protrusion. This spectrum of diseases is caused by the failure of mesoderm tissue growth around the cloacal membrane during development, resulting in the described midline defects. This may include undergrowth of the pubic rami and external orientation of the anterior and posterior parts of the pelvis, contributing to a diastasis (Fig. 17.1). Patients can also be born with neural tube defects and peripheral defects such as clubfoot. Long-term effects of bladder exstrophy may include incontinence, renal dysfunction, genital and body appearance dissatisfaction, impaired fertility, hip pain, and impaired gait. Treatment involves surgical closure of the bladder, repair of epispadias, and closure of the anterior abdominal wall with subsequent bladder neck reconstruction. The anterior pelvic and abdominal wall closure

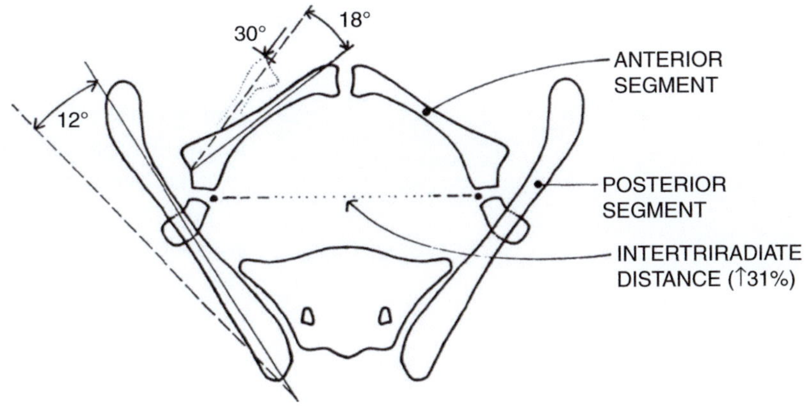

Fig. 17.1 Cross section of pelvis shows outward orientation of iliac and ischiopubic segments and shortening of the ischiopubic segment (From Sponseller et al. 2001, with permission)

D. J. Kirby · P. D. Sponseller (✉)
Division of Pediatric Orthopaedic Surgery, Department of Orthopaedic Surgery, The Johns Hopkins Hospital, Baltimore, MD, USA
e-mail: Dkirby3@jhmi.edu; psponse@jhmi.edu

R. C. Hamdy, N. Saran (eds.), *Pediatric Pelvic and Proximal Femoral Osteotomies*,
https://doi.org/10.1007/978-3-319-78033-7_17

often benefits from bilateral pelvic osteotomies, which allow for improved pubic symphysis approximation. The anterior innominate osteotomy with posterior iliac osteotomy is the corrective osteotomy commonly performed in this procedure. It has been shown to improve initial exstrophy closure success and benefit future urogenital repairs.

Brief Clinic History

Classic Exstrophy

An 11-month-old female born with classic bladder exstrophy presented for exstrophy repair with iliac osteotomy (Fig. 17.2). She was noted to have exstrophy at birth, but her bladder template was too small to allow for repair. She was followed until the bladder template became large enough to allow for closure, at which point orthopedics was consulted to perform the pelvic osteotomy. In addition, she was noted to have congenital clubfoot for which she underwent treatment. On examination, the patient had protrusion of her bladder with the anterior wall defect measuring 2 × 4 cm (see Fig. 17.2a). The umbilicus was low-set and anus anteriorly displaced. Genital exam revealed epispadias with bifid clitoris. Radiographs revealed pubic symphysis diastasis of 3.7 cm. Magnetic resonance imaging revealed pubic ramus length of 2.4 cm, angle of posterior pelvic segment 41°, and angle of anterior pelvic segment 35° (Fig. 17.3). (Table 17.1 provides mean control and diseased values for pelvic measurements.)

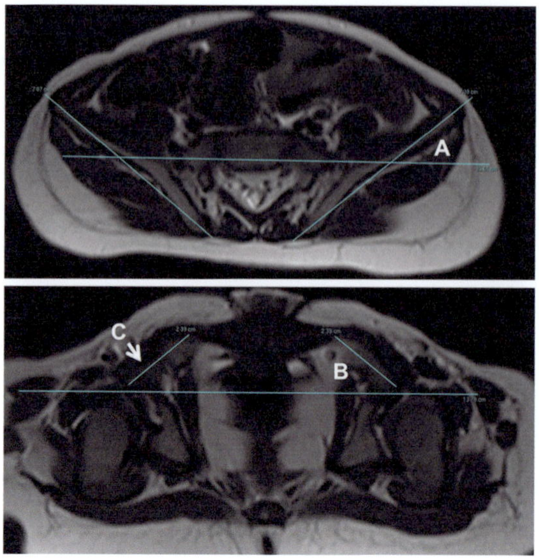

Fig. 17.3 Preoperative pelvic magnetic resonance imaging of a patient with classic bladder exstrophy demonstrating (*top*) a posterior segment angle of 41° *at A*, (*bottom*) anterior segment angle of 35° *at B*, and pubic ramus length of 2.4 cm *at C*

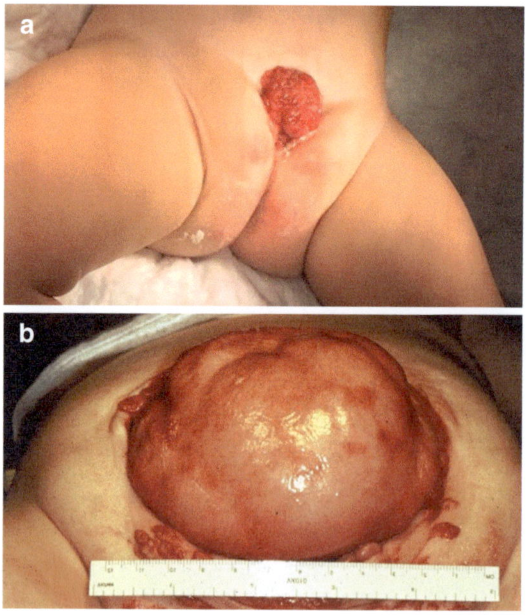

Fig. 17.2 Preoperative abdominal photographs of patients with classic exstrophy (**a**) and cloacal exstrophy (**b**). The patient with classic exstrophy has an anterior abdominal wall defect of 2 cm with bladder protrusion. The patient with cloacal exstrophy has anterior abdominal wall defect measuring 9.5 cm with omphalocele

Cloacal Exstrophy (See Fig. 17.2b)

An 18-month-old male, born genetic 46XY, with cloacal exstrophy, sixth lumbar vertebra, imperforate anus, omphalocele, and ambiguous genitalia presented for exstrophy repair with iliac osteotomy. After birth, the patient underwent a series of procedures, including loop transverse colostomy

Table 17.1 Pelvic measurements in classic exstrophy, cloacal exstrophy, and normal pelvis

	Interpubic distance (cm)	Posterior segment angle (°)	Anterior segment angle (°)	Anterior segment length (cm)
Patients who had classic exstrophy	6	45	33	2
Patients who had cloacal exstrophy	8	32	39	2
Control	1	57	15	3

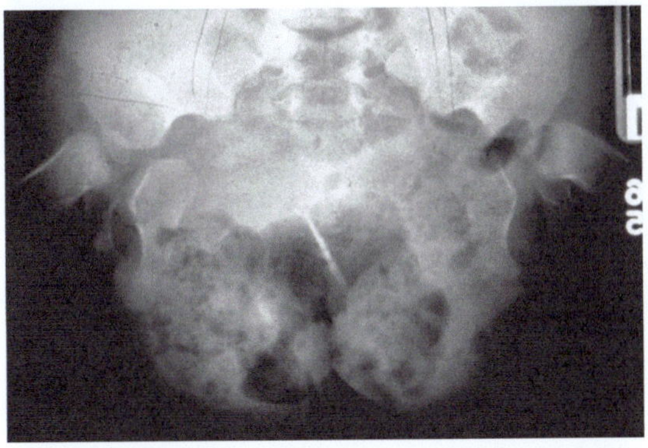

Fig. 17.4 Preoperative pelvic anteroposterior radiograph of a patient with cloacal exstrophy demonstrating 10 cm of pubic symphysis diastasis

and exstrophy repair with subsequent dehiscence and reclosure. On examination, the patient had an anterior abdominal wall defect measuring 9.5 cm with small bowel protrusion and low-set umbilicus. Genitourinary exam revealed epispadias with shortened anterior corporal body. Radiographs revealed pubic diastasis of 10 cm (Fig. 17.4).

Preoperative Imaging (See Figs. 17.2, 17.3, and 17.4)

Goals of Treatment

The goal of the treatment is to assist in the successful closure of the exstrophy. This will allow for timely achievement of urinary continence and maintenance of normal gait. Additionally, closure carries the goal of improving the appearance of the widened perineum and assisting in future urogenital repair.

Treatment Strategy

From an orthopedic viewpoint, the focus of the treatment is to assist successful urologic repair. This can be accomplished by decreasing the degree of pubic diastasis, thereby relieving distracting forces on the anterior abdominal wall. With this in mind, osteotomies on newborns are rarely performed, as ligamentous laxity allows for diastasis reduction and exstrophy repair without great tension. Osteotomies become of benefit in patients older than 1 month, as the transverse anterior osteotomy allows for eased reduction of the pubic diastasis. The additional posterior hinge osteotomy, performed through the same incision, corrects excessive iliac wing external rotation, which decreases distracting forces on the anterior abdominal wall, and is recommended on patients who undergo osteotomy after 2 years of age. Patients are placed in external fixation and light skin traction postoperatively to prevent vesicostomy tube dislodgement and pelvic destabilization. Internal fixation of the diastasis is also advised in patients 8 years or older to maintain correction.

Surgical Details

Anterior Iliac Osteotomy

The procedure is performed with the patient in the supine position under general endotracheal anesthesia (Fig. 17.5). An epidural is often placed for patient comfort. Each step of the osteotomy procedure is performed bilaterally (Fig. 17.6). An oblique incision is made 1–2 cm distal to the anterior superior iliac spine (ASIS), identical to the incision performed for the Salter innominate

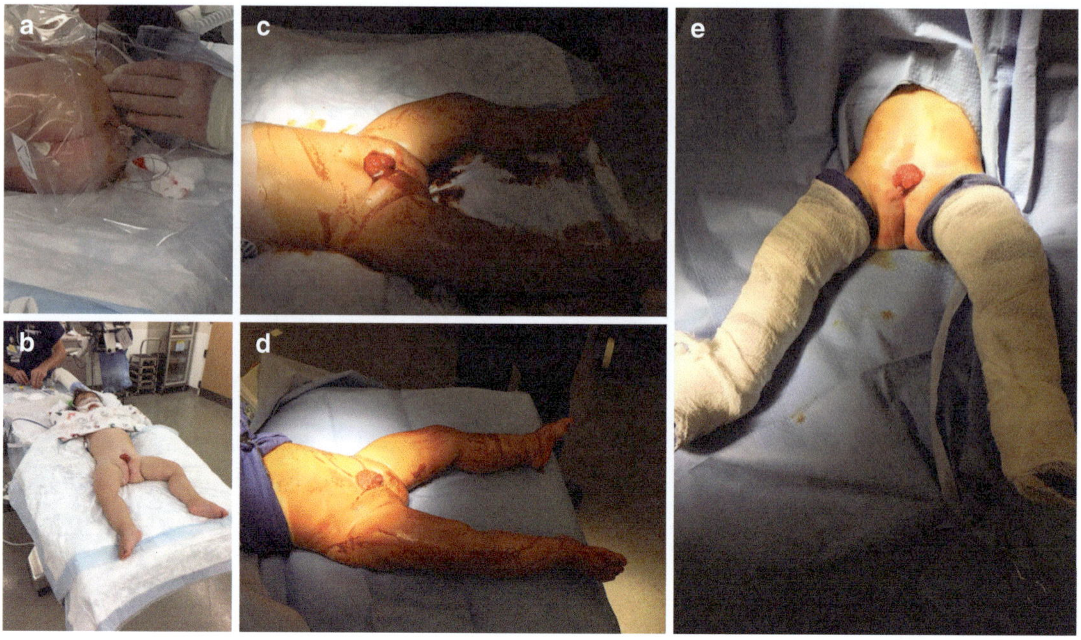

Fig. 17.5 Photographs demonstrating preoperative preparation. (**a**) An epidural is placed. (**b**) The patient is laid supine. (**c**) The skin is prepped with chlorhexidine or povidone-iodine proximally to the midthorax and distally to the toes. (**d**, **e**) The sterile field is then created with placement of two overlapping U-drapes

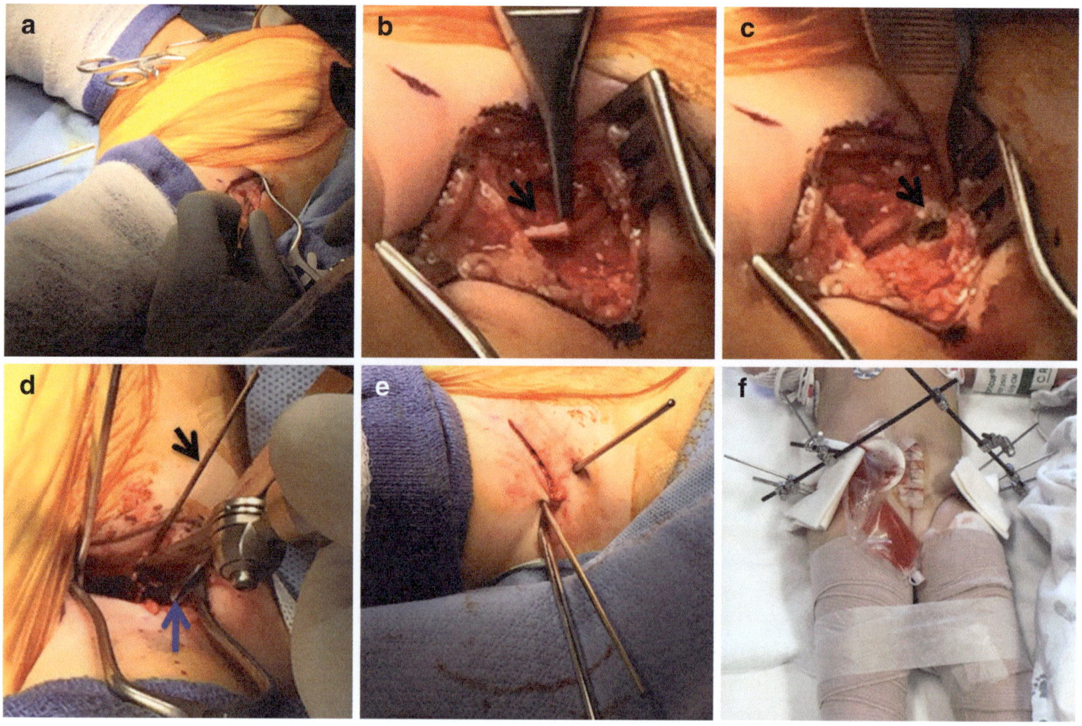

Fig. 17.6 Photographs highlighting key steps of the surgery. (**a**) An oblique incision is made just distal to the anterior superior iliac spine. (**b**) Careful dissection of the lateral femoral cutaneous nerve is performed (*arrow*). (**c**) The iliac apophysis is incised to allow for subperiosteal dissection (*arrow*). (**d**) For the anterior iliac osteotomy, a guide pin is placed (*black arrow*), and an oscillating saw is used to perform the osteotomy (*blue arrow*). (**e**) Pins are placed percutaneously into the proximal and distal pelvic segments, and (**f**) an external fixation device is placed to maintain corrected pelvic positioning

osteotomy (see Fig 17.6a). Care is taken to isolate and preserve the lateral femoral cutaneous nerve, which can be retracted medially (see Fig. 17.6b). Superficial and deep dissection is carried out along the tensor-sartorius interval, freeing the tensor muscle and fascia for lateral retraction. On older children or those with bony anomalies, the femoral nerve may be exposed and protected. The iliac apophysis is then incised for about 1 cm at and posterior to the ASIS to create a small window of exposure of the iliac wing (see Fig. 17.6c). Subperiosteal dissection of the medial aspect of the iliac wing is performed caudally to the triradiate cartilage and posteriorly to the sciatic notch, continuing along to the sacroiliac joint. A nutrient vessel is present on the medial aspect of the iliac wing that should be cauterized to mitigate blood loss. Subperiosteal dissection of the lateral aspect of the iliac wing is then carried out to the sciatic notch. The periosteum of the sciatic notch can then be elevated to provide room for retractors. A guide pin is placed 5–10 mm proximal to the anterior inferior iliac spine, aimed at the most proximal edge of the sciatic notch (Fig. 17.7). This will provide a guide for the anterior osteotomy and will allow the caudal fragment to be large enough for placement of fixation screws. An oscillating saw or Gigli saw is then used to create the transverse osteotomy, using the pins as guides (see Fig. 17.6d). If a portion of the posterior pelvic cortex is left intact, it can be cut with an osteotome. The caudal/distal pelvis should then be separate and mobile relative to the cephalad/proximal iliac wing.

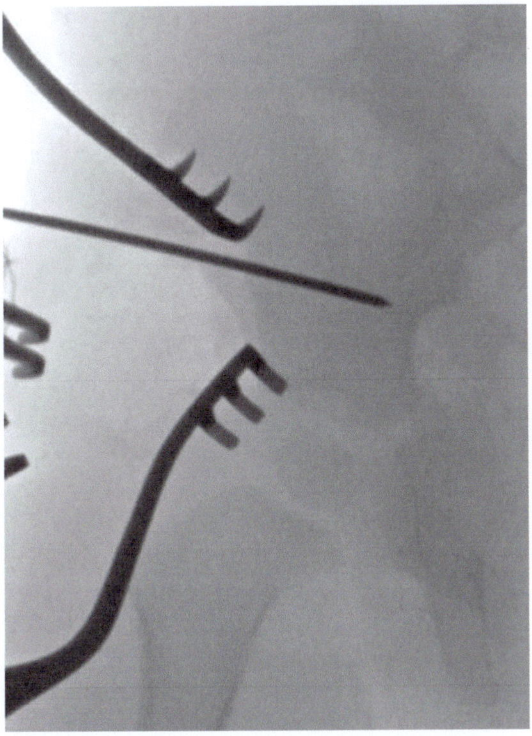

Fig. 17.7 Intraoperative pelvic radiograph demonstrating proper guidance pin placement for the anterior iliac osteotomy

Additional Posterior Iliac Hinge Osteotomy

In children older than 2 years, an additional posterior iliac hinge osteotomy is recommended. This is a vertical closing-wedge osteotomy created with a rongeur or burr at least 1 cm lateral and parallel to the sacroiliac joint. This is started at the sciatic notch where the cortical bone is dense, using a rongeur or burr to create a trough in the bone. The trough can be continued proximally with a rongeur. An osteotome is then used to cut the pelvic outer cortex of the trough. This should be carried out along the distal two-thirds of the trough, leaving the posterior cortex of the proximal one-third intact. This portion of cortex will act as a hinge for the closing-wedge. The iliac wings should now hinge medially.

External Fixation of Osteotomies

One to two threaded pins are placed in the wing of the proximal ilium, and two are placed in the distal pelvic segment (2.5 mm for infants; 4 mm for children; 5 mm for adolescents). The distal segment pins are placed proximally to the acetabular rim and distally to the transverse osteotomy and should have bicortical purchase. The pelvis is then imaged intraoperatively to insure satisfactory pin placement, and urologic repair is performed.

The pelvic ring can then be closed and diastasis reduced by placing horizontal mattress sutures in the pubic rami. The external fixation device is then applied to maintain pelvic positioning (see Fig. 17.6f).

Pubic Diastasis Reduction with Plating

For patients older than 8 years or for those with cloacal exstrophy, supplemental fixation is accomplished through the use of a two-hole plate applied across the pubic symphysis, with screws directed laterally through the superior pubic ramus on each side (Fig. 17.8).

Postoperative Treatment

The patient is to remain supine with light skin traction for 4 weeks. The external fixation device can be removed at 6 weeks when adequate callus has formed.

Postoperative Imaging (See Fig. 17.8)

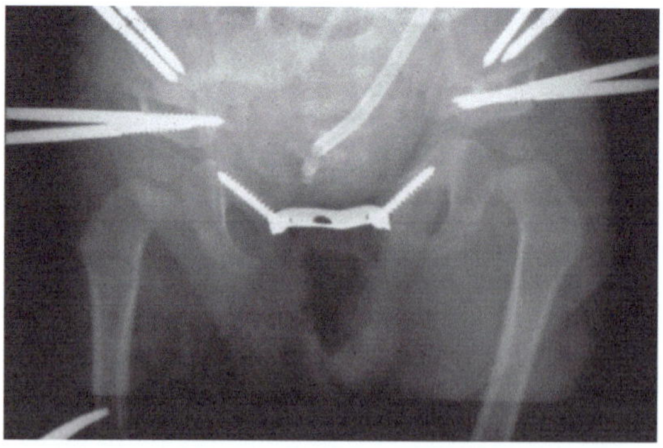

Fig. 17.8 Postoperative pelvic anteroposterior radiograph of a patient with cloacal exstrophy. Proximal and distal segment pins for external fixation are in the proper locations, diastasis is reduced, and iliac wings have been internally rotated. This patient underwent pubic symphysis fixation with the two-hole plate across the pubic symphysis and screws driven laterally through the pubic rami

Pearls and Pitfalls

- Femoral nerve palsy has been noted as a complication to the anterior iliac osteotomy. This complication is thought to be due to increased inguinal ligament tension after pubic apophysis approximation. The posterior iliac osteotomy reduces this tension and is associated with a decreased rate of femoral nerve palsy. Additionally, the femoral nerve should be isolated and protected during the operation in larger children.
- Bony complications, including nonunion, have been observed. Bony union should be verified radiographically before allowing unrestricted activity.
- During posterior iliac osteotomy, damage to the sacroiliac joint has been observed. This is due in part to difficult visualization of the osteotomy site. Vessel coagulation and bone wax are of help for controlling bleeding within the field and improving visualization. Additionally, the posterior osteotomy should be created no more medial than 1 cm lateral to the sacroiliac joint.

Indications (Table 17.2)

Table 17.2 Anterior osteotomy and posterior osteotomy: surgical indications

Anterior osteotomy is indicated for patients with bladder exstrophy: Who have failed pubic diastasis reduction without osteotomy Who are 1 month old or older Who have undergone bladder closure but fail to achieve continence at the appropriate age Whose perineal reconstruction would benefit from pelvic osteotomy Who develop acetabular dysplasia
Posterior osteotomy is recommended in any patient 2 years or older undergoing anterior osteotomy

Suggested Reading

Okubadejo G, Sponseller P, Gearhart J. Complications in orthopedic management of exstrophy. J Pediatr Orthop. 2003;23(4):522–8.

Sponseller P, Bisson L, Gearhart J, Jeffs R, Magid D, Fishman E. The anatomy of the pelvis in the exstrophy complex. J Bone Joint Surg Am. 1995;77(2):177–89.

Sponseller P, Jani M, Jeffs R, Gearhart J. Anterior innominate osteotomy in repair of bladder exstrophy. J Bone Joint Surg Am. 2001;83(2):184–93. https://insights.ovid.com/pubmed?pmid=11216679

Wild A, Sponseller P, Stec A, Gearhart J. The role of osteotomy in surgical repair of bladder exstrophy. Semin Pediatr Surg. 2011;20(2):71–8.

18 Pelvic Osteotomy for Spinal Deformities

Panagiotis Peter Glavas and Stefan Parent

Introduction

Much like lower limb axes are important in the planning and correction of limb deformity, sagittal spinal alignment parameters are key in the assessment and treatment of spinal deformity. They include the standard sagittal spinal alignment parameters (thoracic kyphosis and lumbar lordosis), sagittal sacropelvic alignment (pelvic incidence, pelvic tilt, and sacral slope), and global sagittal balance parameters such as the C7 plumb line, spinal sacral angle, and spinal tilt. In patients with an abnormal sagittal spinal alignment, vertebral osteotomies such as pedicle subtraction osteotomies and fusion can be employed to correct the alignment. However, this can be technically very demanding, be prone to significant neurologic complications, and decrease spinal mobility. Alternatively, pelvic osteotomies can also be used to restore sagittal alignment, thus preserving lumbar mobility and positively impacting the patient's quality of life and function.

P. P. Glavas (✉) · S. Parent
Sainte-Justine University Hospital Center, University of Montreal, Montreal, QC, Canada
e-mail: peter.glavas.hsj@ssss.gouv.qc.ca

Brief Clinical History

This is a 17-year-old female with Langer-Giedion syndrome, also known as trichorhinophalangeal syndrome type 2. It is characterized by numerous abnormalities including dwarfism, brachydactyly, multiple exostoses, and spinal deformities. This patient exhibited progressive worsening of sagittal balance: increasing thoracic kyphosis and lumbar lordosis (Fig. 18.1). In addition, she had multiple exostoses in the upper and lower limbs. She had worsening pain in the lower back, decreased endurance, and limited range of motion in the lumbar and cervical spine. It was decided that performing a pelvic osteotomy would improve the overall sagittal alignment and obviate the need to fuse the spine.

Preoperative Imaging (See Fig. 18.1)

Preoperative anteroposterior (AP) and lateral views of the entire spine. Sagittal and coronal measures are shown. Pelvic incidence (PI) is the angle subtended by a line drawn from the center of the femoral head to the midpoint of the S1 endplate and a line perpendicular to the S1 endplate. Normal values are 46.9 ± 11.4° in the 10–18-year-old age group [1]. Global sagittal balance is shown by the C7 plumb line. Note that the C7 plumb line is passing much anterior to the femoral heads.

R. C. Hamdy, N. Saran (eds.), *Pediatric Pelvic and Proximal Femoral Osteotomies*,
https://doi.org/10.1007/978-3-319-78033-7_18

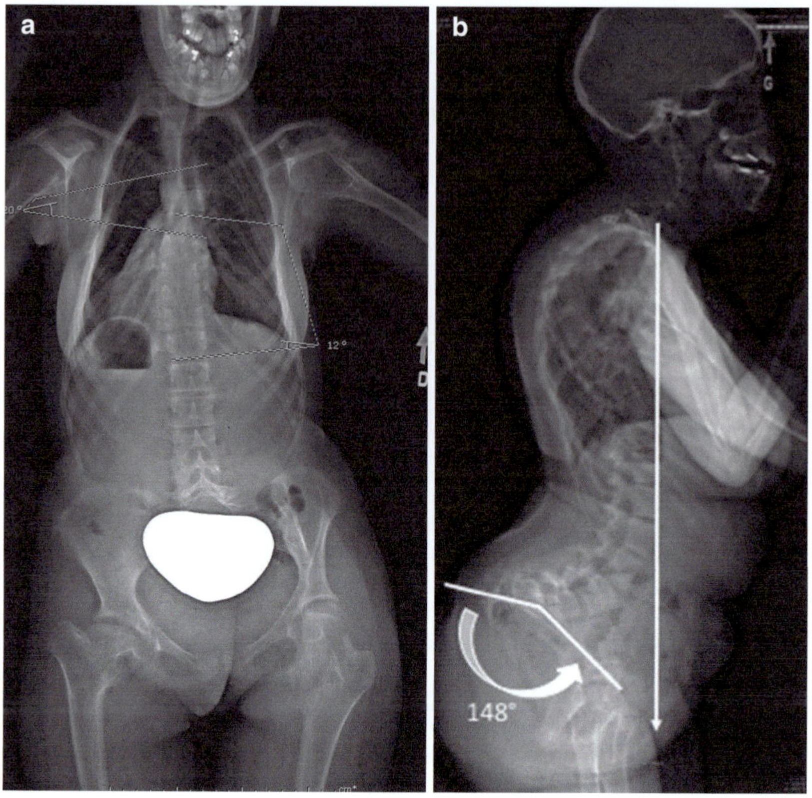

Fig. 18.1 Preoperative (**a**) anteroposterior and (**b**) lateral views of the spine. The coronal plane alignment shows a mild curvature in the thoracic and lumbar spine. The sagittal sacropelvic alignment is given by the pelvic incidence which measures 148°. Global sagittal balance is given by the C7 plumb line (see text for details)

Goals of Treatment

1. Improve sagittal balance.
2. Preserve lumbar motion.
3. Avoid spinal fusion to the pelvis.

Treatment Strategy

The strategy consists of employing a modified double Salter anterior open-wedge osteotomy through bilateral modified Smith-Peterson bikini-type incisions. The net effect of double Salter osteotomies is to open the pelvis anteriorly. This will improve sagittal alignment and has been shown to be as efficient as the more technically demanding and complication prone alternative of sacral subtraction osteotomy [2].

Surgical Details

The procedure is performed in the supine position on a Jackson table. A sandbag can be placed behind the sacrum. Both sides are prepped and draped. A bikini-type incision is made starting 2.5 cm below the anterosuperior iliac spine, AIIS, on the right and left sides (see Chap. 3, Salter Innominate Osteotomy, for details). The sartorius-tensor fasciae latae (TFL) interval is identified and incised. The direct head of the rectus femoris is identified at its origin on the anterior inferior iliac crest. It is divided about 1 cm distal to its origin. A stay suture can be placed in the tendon. The anterior inferior iliac spine (AIIS) is then fully exposed. Care is taken to identify and protect the lateral femoral cutaneous nerve. The iliac crest apophysis is split, and the inner and outer tables are exposed down to the sciatic notch. Rang retractors are placed in the notch to help with exposure and protect the neurovascular bundle during the osteotomy.

Next, an oscillating saw is used to perform the osteotomy. The cut is started just superior to the AIIS and is directed toward the notch. The cut is stopped 1 cm superficial to the notch. It is imperative that a hinge be left posteriorly. Before the osteotomy is opened, the contralateral side is prepared in identical fashion. Once the osteotomy is complete bilaterally, both sides are opened simultaneously using lamina spreaders. This is done progressively to keep the posterior hinge intact.

A wedge of bone is then harvested from each iliac crest and placed in the respective osteotomy sites. We prefer stabilizing each of the osteotomy sites with pins. Wound closure is done in the usual manner. A drain is placed as needed. A full spica cast is then placed with the hips at 80°–90° of flexion, 30° of abduction, and 20–30° of external rotation. The spica cast is kept for 6 weeks or until the osteotomy is healed.

Postoperative Imaging (Fig. 18.2)

Although the PI remains above the normal values, it has decreased compared to the preoperative X-rays. The decrease in PI effectively improved the global sagittal balance as shown by the C7 plumb line.

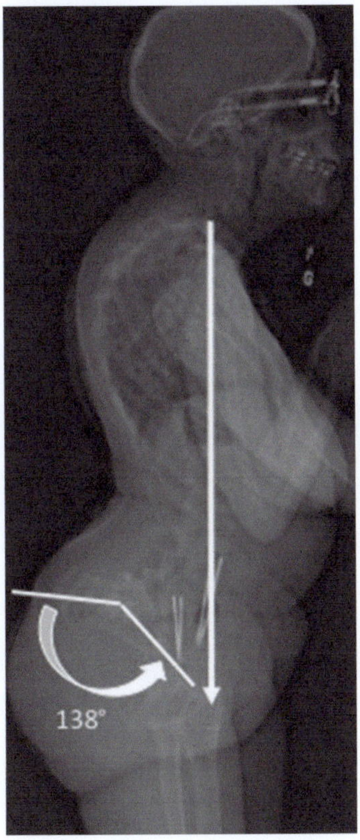

Fig. 18.2 Postoperative lateral view shows an improved pelvic incidence and C7 plumb line (see text for details)

Pearls and Pitfalls

- Care must be taken to preserve the posterior hinge such that the osteotomy site opens anteriorly. Otherwise, the posterior part of the osteotomy will distract and may hinder the correction. In younger children, a thick periosteum may help limit the distraction when the hinge is not preserved.
- If the osteotomy propagates through the notch, we recommend distracting less in order to maintain stability and compromise on the degree of correction.
- Proper imaging prior to surgery should be done. A standing AP and lateral X-rays of the spine should be performed making sure the femoral heads are visible in order to calculate the sagittal balance parameters.
- If available, a three-dimensional print of the patient's pelvis and lumbar spine can help with the preoperative planning.

Indications and Contraindications (Table 18.1)

Table 18.1 Pelvic osteotomy for spinal deformities: surgical indications and contraindications

Indications
Sagittal spinal deformity
As an alternative to sacral subtraction osteotomies
To avoid fusion of spine to the pelvis
Contraindications
Severe spinal deformity in the coronal and/or axial planes
Pelvic dysmorphism that precludes osteotomies
Deficient acetabular coverage

References

1. MacThiong JM, Labelle H, Roussouly P. Pediatric sagittal alignment. Eur Spine J. 2015;20(Suppl 5):S586–90.
2. Bodin A, Roussouly P. Sacral and pelvic osteotomies for correction of spinal deformities. Eur Spine J. 2015;24(Suppl 1):S72–82.

Suggested Reading

Gutman G, Labelle H, Barchi S, Roussouly P, Berthonnaud É, Mac-Thiong JM. Normal sagittal parameters of global spinal balance in children and adolescents: a prospective study of 646 asymptomatic subjects. Eur Spine J. 2016;25(11):3650–7.

Part II

Pediatric Proximal Femoral Osteotomies

19 Varus Derotation Osteotomy

Ryan M. O'Shea and Unni G. Narayanan

Introduction

The varus derotation osteotomy (VDRO) of the proximal femur is a procedure to redirect the femoral head toward the center of the acetabulum. The varus osteotomy reduces the neck shaft angle, while derotation of the shaft addresses femoral anteversion. This procedure is most frequently utilized in neuromuscular patients with hip displacement. Other indications include the treatment of coxa valga, and for containment of the femoral head in Perthes disease, as an alternative to, or in combination with, an innominate osteotomy. Simultaneous correction in the sagittal plane (flexion-extension) can also be achieved.

Brief Clinical History

A 9-year-old boy with bilateral spastic cerebral palsy (CP) functioning at a Gross Motor Function Classification System (GMFCS) level IV presented with increasing adduction contracture of the right hip interfering with care, including diapering, toileting, and dressing. More recently, he was showing evidence of discomfort during these activities as well as with the use of his stander. Examination revealed a hip flexion contracture of 20°, 15° of hip abduction with the knee flexed, and only 5° of abduction with the knee extended. Femoral anteversion assessed via trochanteric palpation was 45°. Anteroposterior (AP) radiograph of the pelvis revealed a subluxated right hip with increased neck shaft angle and a Reimer's migration percentage (MP) of 35% and mild acetabular dysplasia. The left hip was well contained, with an increased neck shaft angle, but intact Shenton's arc, and normal acetabulum. Frog-leg lateral views revealed that the right hip reduced within the acetabulum.

R. M. O'Shea
Department of Orthopaedic Surgery, Kaiser Permanente San Diego, San Diego, CA, USA

U. G. Narayanan (✉)
The Hospital for Sick Children, University of Toronto, Toronto, ON, Canada
e-mail: unni.narayanan@sickkids.ca

R. C. Hamdy, N. Saran (eds.), *Pediatric Pelvic and Proximal Femoral Osteotomies*,
https://doi.org/10.1007/978-3-319-78033-7_19

Preoperative Imaging (Fig. 19.1)

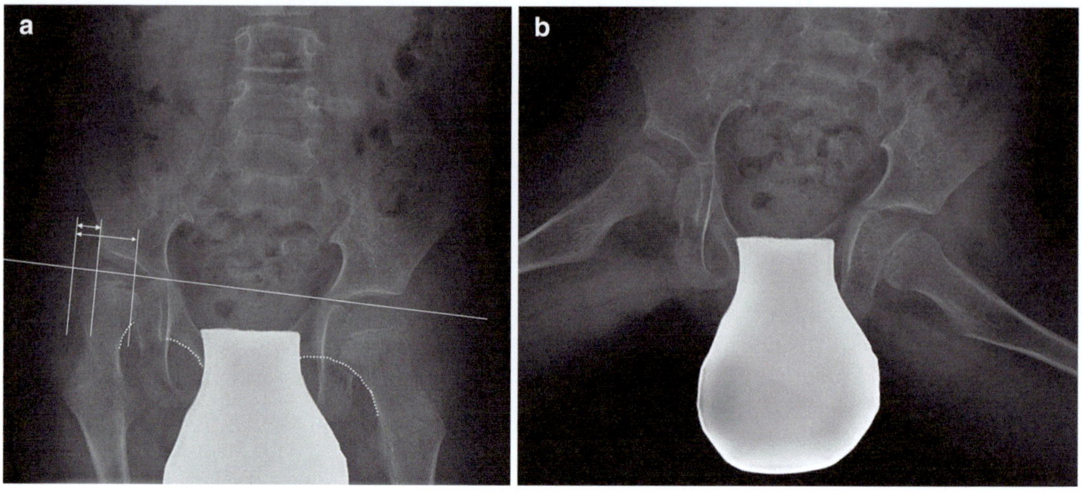

Fig. 19.1 (a) Anterior-posterior and (b) frog-leg lateral radiographs demonstrating right hip subluxation with a Reimer's migration index of 35% and associated acetabular dysplasia

Goals of Treatment

The objective of the procedure is to reduce or contain the femoral head within the acetabulum, in order to achieve the ultimate goals, which are to:

(a) Improve range of motion of the hip, particularly abduction, to facilitate ease of care (dressing, toileting, perineal hygiene, etc.).
(b) Eliminate current pain and minimize the risk of future pain.
(c) Minimize the risk of recurrence and need for repeated interventions.

Treatment Strategy

Surgical reconstruction of hip displacement in patients with CP consists of four sequentially performed components, not all of which might be necessary:

1. The adduction (and flexion) contracture of the hip that is typically associated with hip displacement requires releases of the adductors, which include the adductor longus, the adductor brevis, and the gracilis. Hip flexion contracture can be addressed by iliopsoas tenotomy at the insertion of the lesser trochanter in nonambulatory patients or an intramuscular tenotomy of the psoas alone over the pelvic brim in ambulatory patients.
2. The VDRO of the proximal femur addresses both the coxa valga that is commonly present and the increased femoral anteversion. The osteotomy is stabilized with a 90° blade plate or equivalent implant.
   (a) The amount of varus correction is determined intraoperatively. Following the adductor releases, the hip is examined under fluoroscopy to determine the magnitude of abduction (in degrees from neutral) required to direct the femoral head and neck toward the triradiate cartilage in the center of the acetabulum. The amount of abduction is equivalent to the amount of varus correction necessary to ensure that the head remains reduced even when the hip is in neutral abduction. The resulting neck shaft angle (NSA) after VDRO is usually between 100° and 120° (Fig. 19.2).
   (b) The amount of (external) derotation required is also determined intraoperatively.

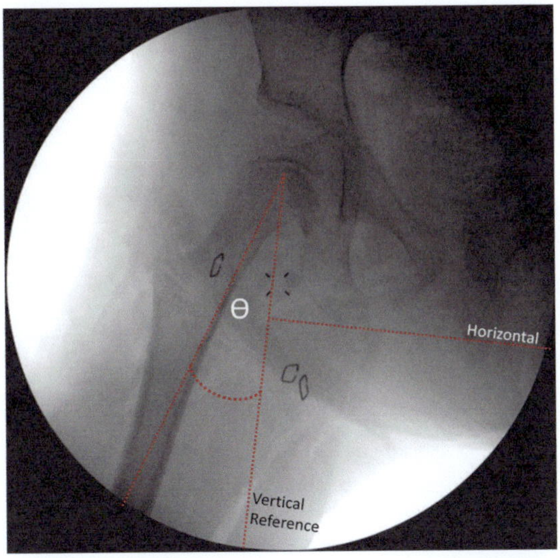

Fig. 19.2 θ represents the degrees of hip abduction from neutral required to direct the femoral head and neck toward the triradiate cartilage and to restore Shenton's arc. This angle determines the amount of varus to be created with the VDRO

In nonambulatory patients, the objective is to reduce the anteversion to approximately 10°. In ambulatory patients, the magnitude of correction is determined preoperatively based on the foot and knee progression angle noted during the gait assessment or motion lab analysis and the torsional profile on the physical examination.

3. An open reduction of the hip is indicated only when the VDRO fails to achieve an adequate reduction. This is seldom necessary except in the management of some dislocated hips.
4. Following the VDRO, some patients require a periacetabular pelvic osteotomy to address the acetabular dysplasia that may be present. The addition of the pelvic osteotomy is influenced by the adequacy of the hip coverage and the stability of the hip following the VDRO, which can be evaluated fluoroscopically or by arthrogram. Following a VDRO, mild acetabular dysplasia might be expected to remodel over time in younger children but is unlikely to do so in children much over 5 years old. Regardless of the age, an isolated proximal femoral osteotomy should probably be augmented with a pelvic osteotomy in the presence of significant acetabular dysplasia [1, 2].

Surgical Details

Setup, Positioning, and Intraoperative Assessment

- Supine position on a radiolucent table permits all components of the hip reconstruction and any other simultaneous lower extremity surgery to be performed without changing patient position. (A bump under the ipsilateral flank facilitates the pelvic osteotomy.)
- The image intensifier is set up perpendicular to the table from the contralateral side. Confirm that good-quality AP and frog-leg lateral images of the hip can be obtained. In bilateral cases that are being performed concurrently by two teams, the image intensifier can be brought in at an angle from the lower (or upper) end of the table to allow both hips to be visualized, by adjusting the C-arm boom, without interfering with either surgical team.
- After performing the hip adductor and flexor release, evaluate fluoroscopically that the femoral head is reduced or reducible. Starting from the neutral position, abduct the hip until the femoral head is centered in the acetabulum and Shenton's arc is restored. The number of degrees of abduction from neutral corresponds to the amount of varus angular correction necessary to ensure that the hip remains well centered, when the hip is in neutral (see Fig. 19.2).

Exposure

- Lateral approach to the proximal femur is performed through a longitudinal incision from the tip of the greater trochanter for 10–12 cm distally in line with the femur.
- The fascia lata is incised in line with the skin incision to expose underlying vastus lateralis.

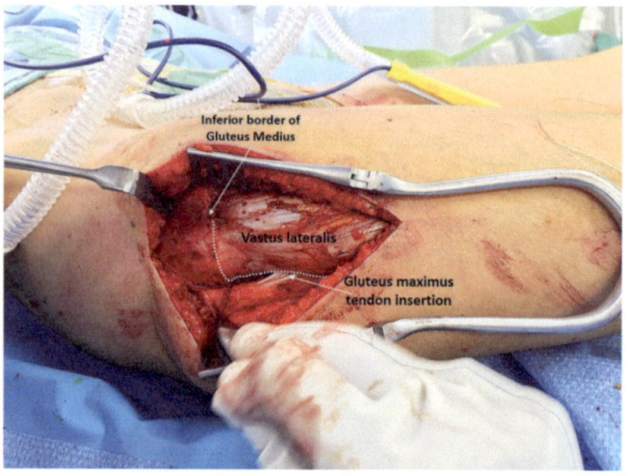

Fig. 19.3 Surgical exposure of the vastus lateralis deep to the fascia lata

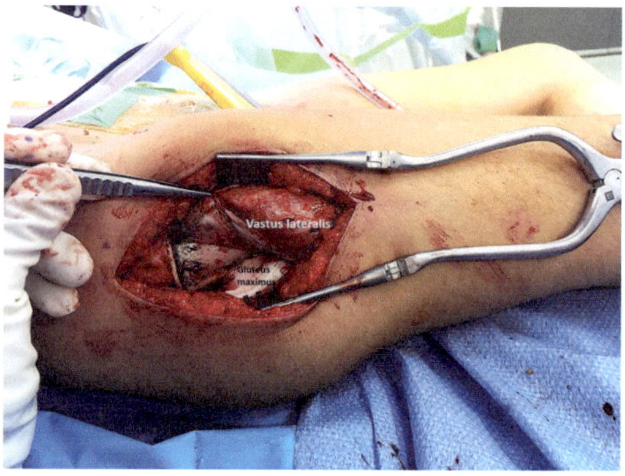

Fig. 19.4 Sub-vastus lateralis approach to expose subperiosteal surface of proximal femur

- The inferior border of the gluteus medius is identified anteriorly as it inserts on the greater trochanter (Fig. 19.3) and serves as landmark for the detachment of the vastus lateralis at the level of the trochanteric ridge.
- Vastus lateralis and its underlying periosteum are incised down to the femur at the level of the trochanteric ridge by electrocautery from anterior to its posterior margin. This is continued distally at right angles along the posterior margin of the vastus lateralis and just anterior to the insertion of the gluteus maximus (Fig. 19.4).
- Distal to the gluteus maximus, the vastus lateralis is elevated off the intermuscular septum. Identify and prophylactically cauterize perforators that emerge through the intermuscular septum.

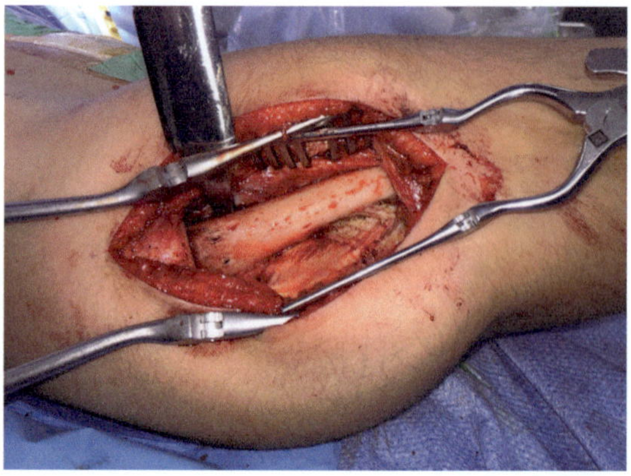

Fig. 19.5 Subperiosteal exposure of the lateral aspect of proximal femur with Hohmann retractor proximal to lesser trochanter

- The vastus lateralis is then elevated subperiosteally to expose the lateral aspect of the proximal femur for sufficient length to accommodate the length of the blade plate.
- The periosteum is elevated circumferentially primarily at the level of the proposed osteotomy, which is proximal to the lesser trochanter. A Hohmann retractor is placed anteriorly (Fig. 19.5).

Guidewire Insertion and Placement of Seating Chisel

- The ideal position of the blade is in the inferior half of the femoral neck just proximal to the calcar.
- For a 90° blade plate, the guidewire is directed proximally at an angle equivalent to the degree of varus correction required. For example, if 30° of varus is required, the guide pin is placed at an angle of 30° from the perpendicular or at $90° - 30° = 60°$ from the long axis (side) of the femur. An osteotomy triangle of 60° placed along the side of the femur will provide the angle of placement (Fig. 19.6).
- For non-cannulated blade plates, the guidewire is inserted in the superior part of the femoral neck to allow space for the blade plate inferior to the guidewire. In cannulated blade plate systems, the guidewire must be in a per-

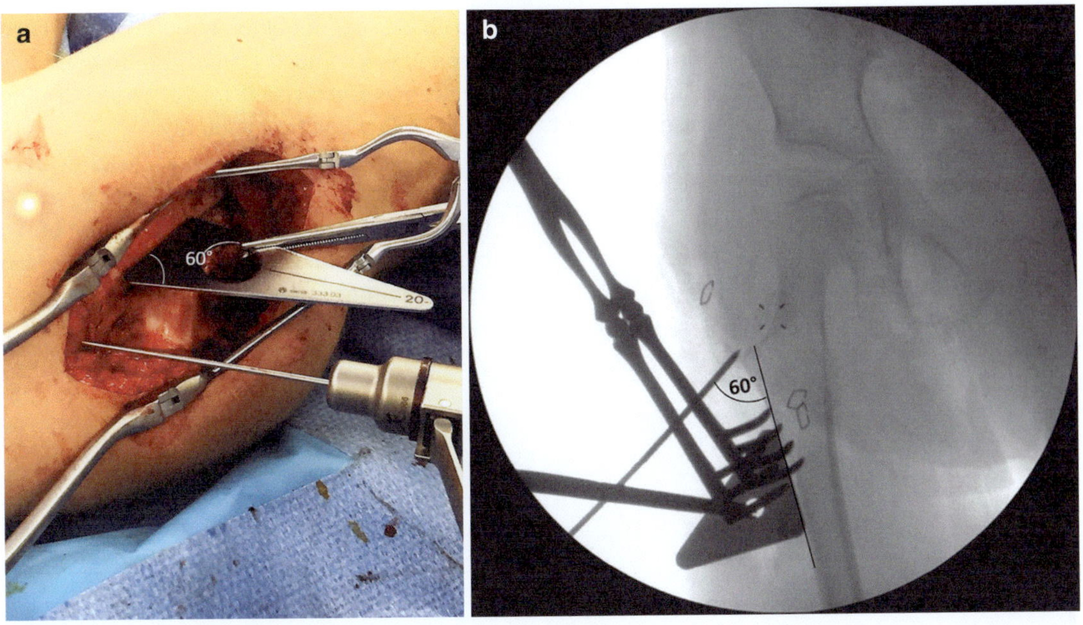

Fig. 19.6 (**a**) 60° triangle guide placed on the lateral aspect of femoral shaft to orient insertion of guidewire (**b**) and corresponding fluoroscopy image

fect position, which will determine ultimate position of the blade.

- The starting point is also in line with the middle of the femoral shaft from anterior to posterior to ensure the plate will lie along the lateral surface of the proximal femur.
- The guide pin must also be in line with the femoral anteversion in the transverse plane. This is facilitated by internal rotation of the leg until the femoral neck is horizontalized by palpation and direct visualization. With the leg held in this position, the guidewire is inserted parallel to the table top/floor (Fig. 19.7).
- The position of the guide wire is checked on the AP and frog-leg lateral view to ensure it lies in the appropriate position (Fig. 19.8). Avoid bending the guidewire when obtaining the frog-leg lateral image.
- Next, the seating chisel is used to create a path for the blade plate. The seating chisel along with plate guide is inserted parallel and inferior to the guidewire. In cannulated systems, the cannulated seating chisel is inserted over the guidewire.
- The face of the chisel must be aligned with the lateral surface of the proximal femur to pre-

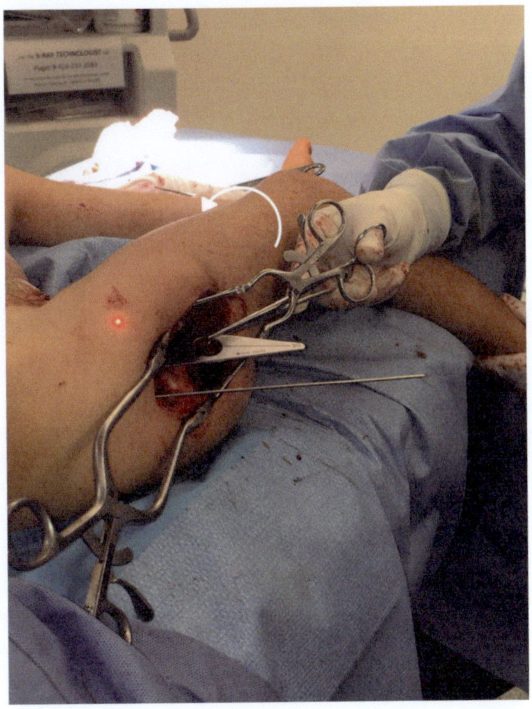

Fig. 19.7 Internal rotation of the lower extremity places the femoral neck in a horizontal position to aid guidewire placement

vent unintended flexion or extension built into the osteotomy (Fig. 19.9). The plate extension guide on the seating chisel helps confirm this.

- Advance the seating chisel with a mallet, and confirm its advancement on AP and frog-leg lateral views. The seating chisel is advanced up to the desired depth corresponding to the blade length selected.
- In patients with good bone health (e.g., ambulatory patients), it is important to disimpact the chisel intermittently and after it has been inserted to its final position. Failure to do this might make it difficult to extract the seating chisel following the osteotomy.
- Final position of the seating chisel is confirmed on AP and frog-leg lateral views (Fig. 19.10). This sets the final position of the blade plate and is crucial to achieving the desired coronal plane correction for any given angled blade plate.

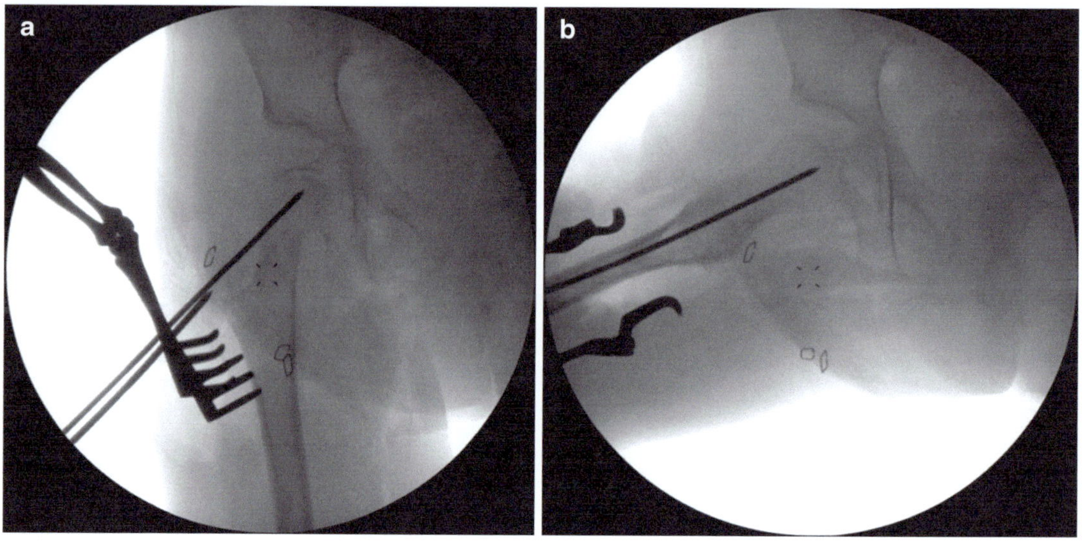

Fig. 19.8 (**a**) Anterior-posterior and (**b**) frog-leg lateral fluoroscopy images demonstrating ideal guidewire placement

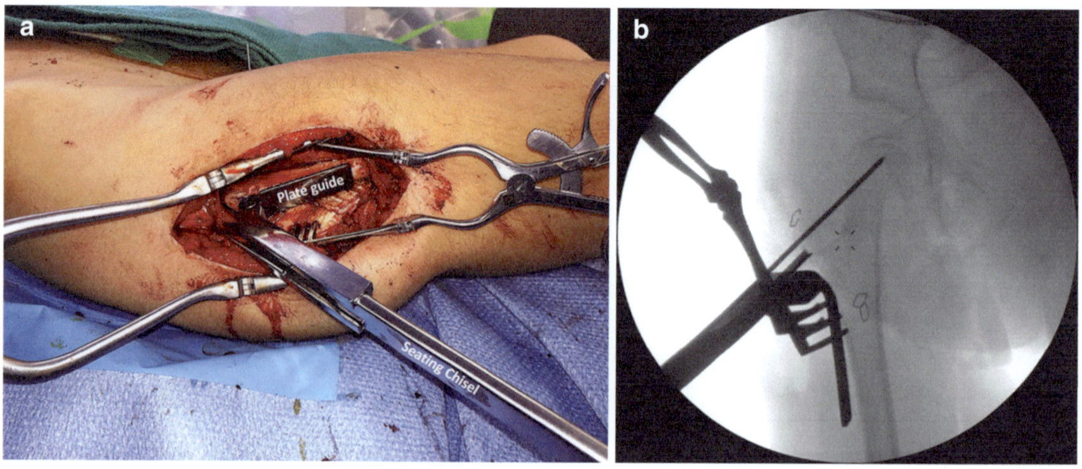

Fig. 19.9 (**a**) The seating chisel is inserted inferior and parallel to the guidewire above. The plate guide should be in line with the femoral shaft to prevent undesired flexion or extension of the osteotomy. (**b**) Fluoroscopy image with the seating chisel and guide confirming appropriate trajectory of the chisel

Proximal Femoral Osteotomy

- The proposed level of the transverse osteotomy is demarcated on the bone at a level at the upper level or just proximal to the lesser trochanter, which is approximately 1.0–1.5 cm below the seating chisel.
- The periosteum is elevated circumferentially at this level (previously done just anteriorly).
- Two parallel 2.4 mm K-wires are placed perpendicular to the long axis of the proximal femur from anterior to posterior on either side of the proposed osteotomy site. These pins act both as a useful retractor of the vastus lateralis anteriorly and also gauge the degree of derotation required following the osteotomy (Fig. 19.11).

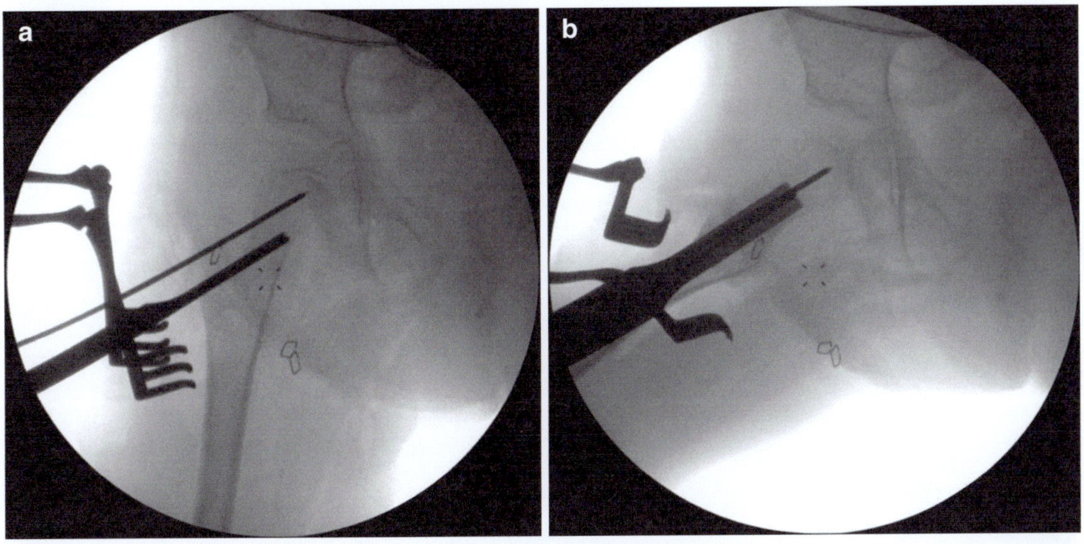

Fig. 19.10 (**a**) Anteroposterior and (**b**) lateral fluoroscopy images demonstrating appropriate position of the seating chisel

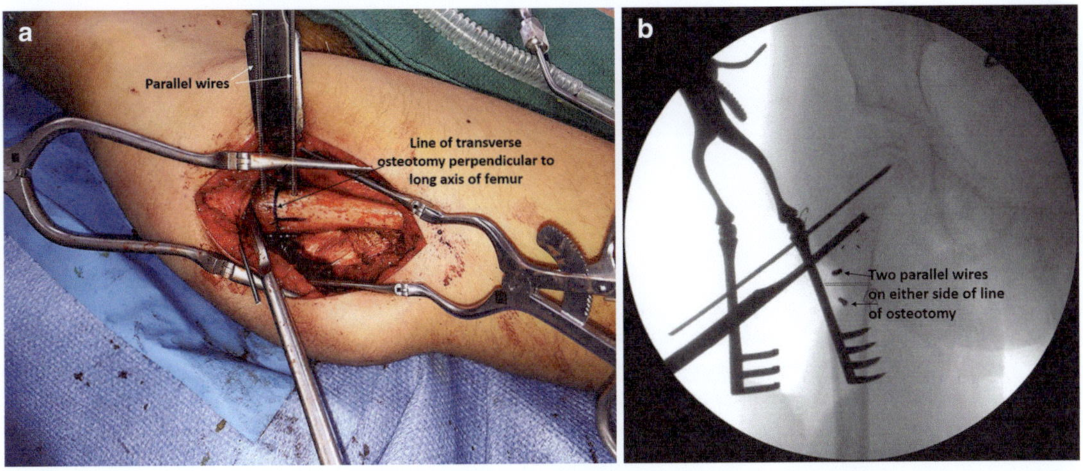

Fig. 19.11 (**a**) Parallel K-wires help gauge derotation of the femur after the osteotomy and serve as anterior retractors of the vastus lateralis. The transverse solid marking on the bone represents the first cut of the planned osteotomy. (**b**) An anteroposterior fluoroscopy image confirms parallel vertical placement of derotation wires above and below the site of proposed osteotomy

- The first osteotomy is a transverse cut, perpendicular to the long axis of the femur, between the two derotation pins.
- Following the first osteotomy, the leg is adducted to allow access to the cut surface of the proximal bone fragment (Fig. 19.12). Elevate the periosteum medially and posteriorly.
- The second bone cut is made at an angle parallel to the seating chisel above to remove a wedge from the medial 50% of the cut surface of the proximal femur fragment (Fig. 19.13). This results in a neutral wedge osteotomy (closing wedge in the medial half and opening wedge in the lateral half). This allows cut surfaces to be opposed for compression. Starting the second cut more laterally (com-

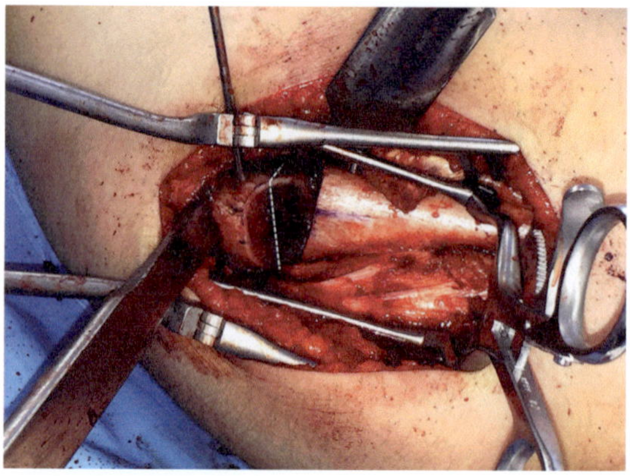

Fig. 19.12 The cut surface of the proximal fragment is exposed by adducting the leg. The dotted line parallel to the seating chisel above represents the plane of the second osteotomy to remove a 50% medial wedge

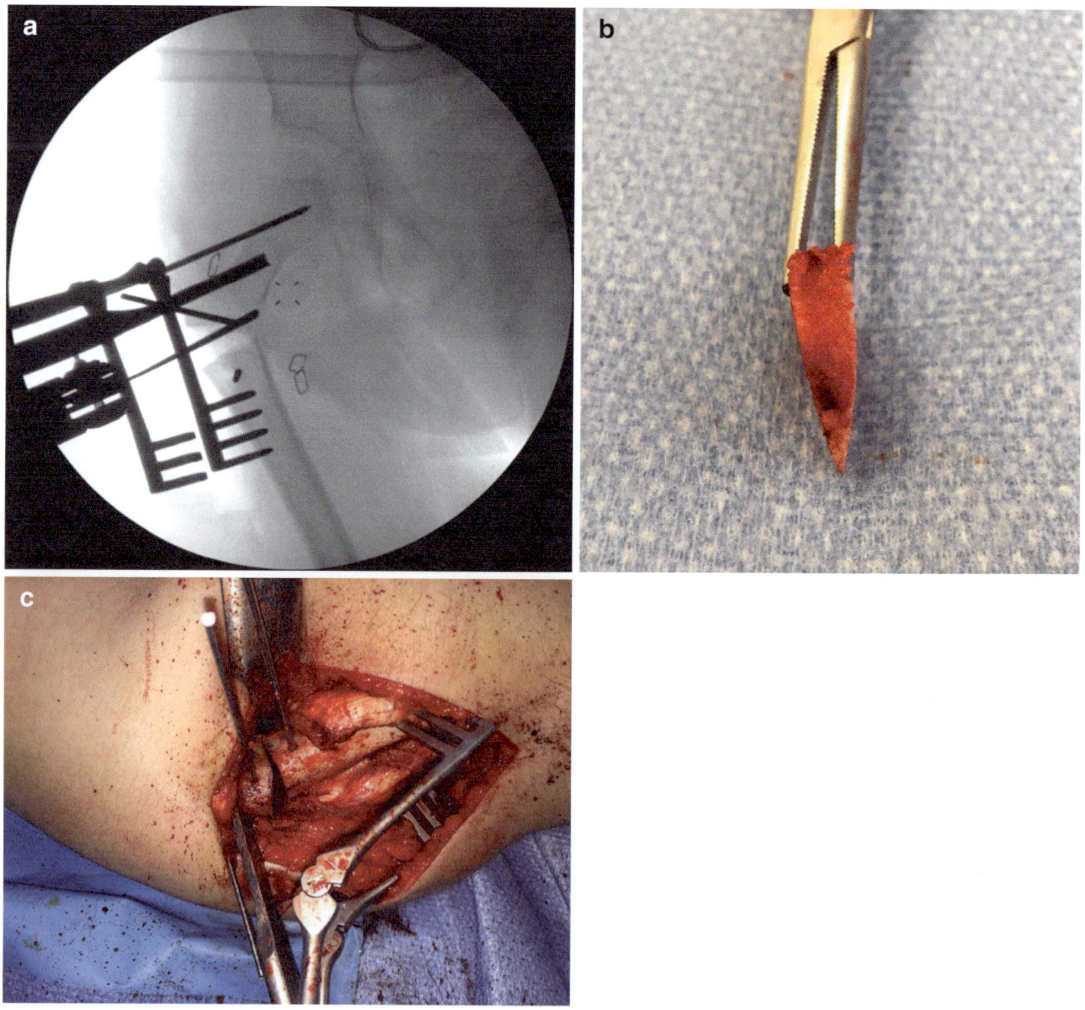

Fig. 19.13 (**a**) A fluoroscopy image demonstrates the saw blade is parallel to the seating chisel. (**b**) A wedge of bone is removed from the medial aspect of the proximal femur, (**c**) and the osteotomy surfaces opposed

plete closing wedge) carries the risk of extending the wedge into the femoral neck and head. Alternatively, just a transverse cut will allow opening wedge, which creates less contact of the cut surfaces at fixation.

- The wedge of bone is then removed and may be utilized as additional bone graft for a periacetabular pelvic osteotomy if necessary.
- Varusization is accompanied by shortening, the extent of which depends on the type of wedge removed. Additional shortening is best achieved by removing additional segment of bone from the proximal end of the distal fragment.

Fixation: Inserting the Blade Plate

- The seating chisel is removed using the slotted hammer, and the blade plate held by its handle is inserted in the path created by the chisel following. The retained guidewire is helpful to ensure that the blade is not being inserted in a different trajectory, particularly in osteoporotic bone.
- The position of the blade plate is verified under fluoroscopy, and the mallet used on the blade plate handle to advance the blade until the side plate is nearly in contact with the lateral surface of the femur.
- The plate is provisionally held against the distal fragment with a Verbrugge clamp (Fig. 19.14).
- The clamp is loosened to allow external (de) rotation of the distal femur. If the guidewire or handle of the blade plate is held parallel to the ground, the femoral neck is lying horizontally. The distal femoral segment can then be derotated until the patella is facing just anteromedially by 10°. The angle between the distal and proximal derotation pins is the amount of derotation achieved (Fig. 19.15).
- During the derotation, the proximal end of the distal fragment might have to be supported with an elevator to prevent it from sagging posteriorly. This will help obtain good contact between the cut surfaces of bone, before securing the Verbrugge clamp.
- The plate is secured with cortical screws. Two of the three screws can be placed eccentrically to compress the osteotomy.
- The blade plate handle is removed and the impactor used with a mallet to advance the blade to its full depth. The 90° blade plate has a medial offset. This medializes the distal femoral segment, which will correct the medial mechanical axis deviation that occurs with varus producing osteotomies. (Fig. 19.16)
- Confirm the position of internal fixation on AP and frog-leg lateral views.

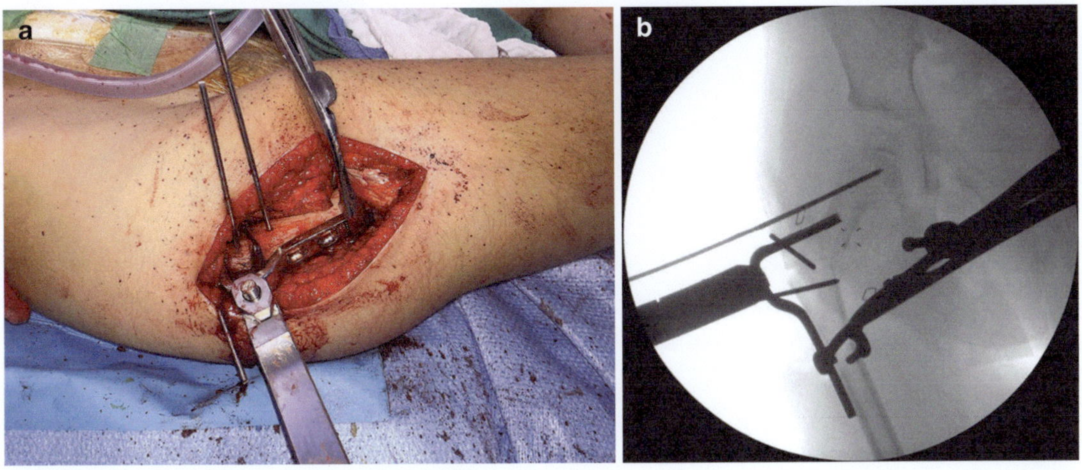

Fig. 19.14 (**a**) Intraoperative photograph and (**b**) corresponding fluoroscopy image after the seating chisel has been removed and the blade plate inserted in its tract. A Verbrugge clamp is applied to hold the plate against the distal femoral shaft

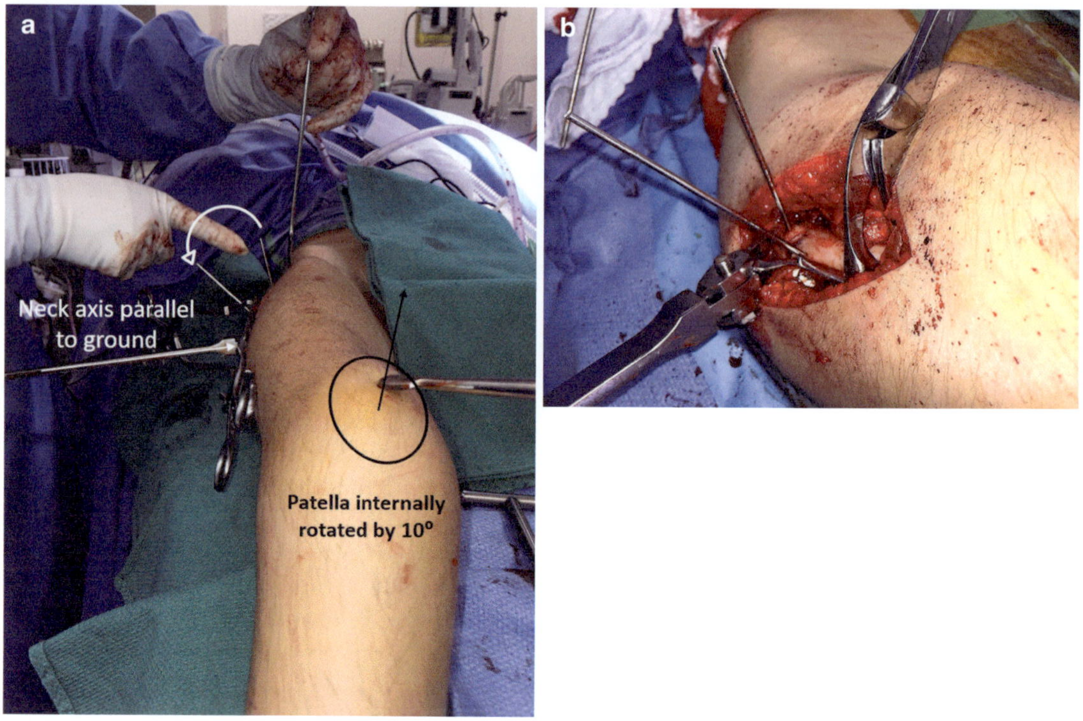

Fig. 19.15 (**a**) The proximal femoral segment (neck axis) is held horizontal, while the distal femoral segment is externally rotated until the patella is pointing 10⁰ internally. (**b**) The angle between the guide wires corresponds to the amount of correction of the femoral anteversion

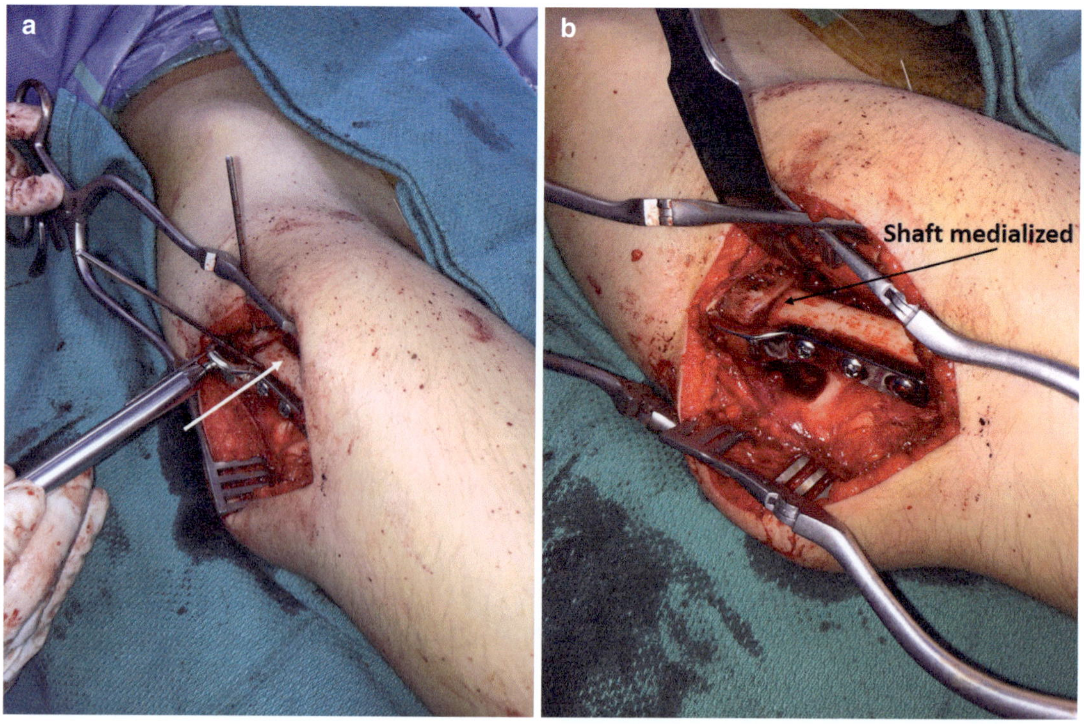

Fig. 19.16 (**a**, **b**) Once the plate has been fixed to the femur, an impactor is used to advance the blade plate to its full depth. The medial offset of the blade plate will therefore medialize the femoral shaft correcting the mechanical axis that would have altered due to the varusization

Closure

- The vastus lateralis is repaired to its origin at the trochanteric ridge with heavy (# 1) absorbable suture (Fig. 19.17). This will completely cover the plate.
- The fascia lata is closed with heavy (# 1) absorbable suture.
- The subcutaneous and subcuticular closure is completed in layers.

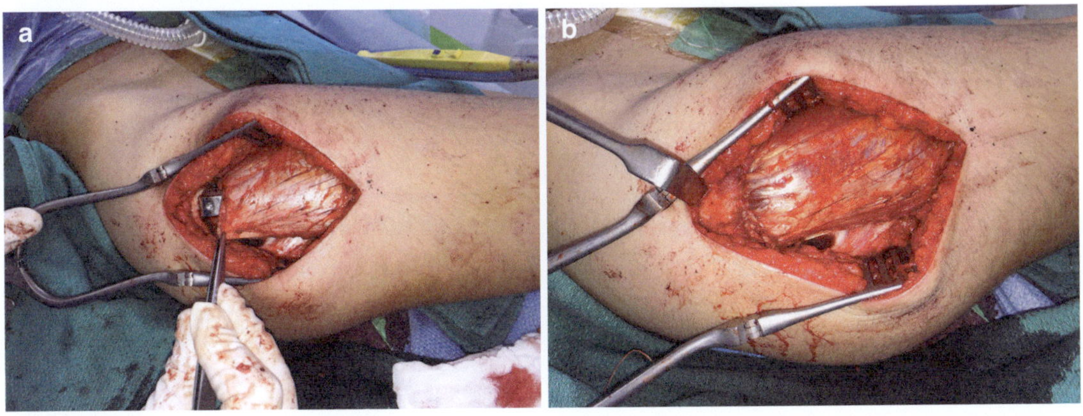

Fig. 19.17 (**a**, **b**) The vastus lateralis is repaired back to its origin over the plate

Postoperative Imaging (Fig. 19.18)

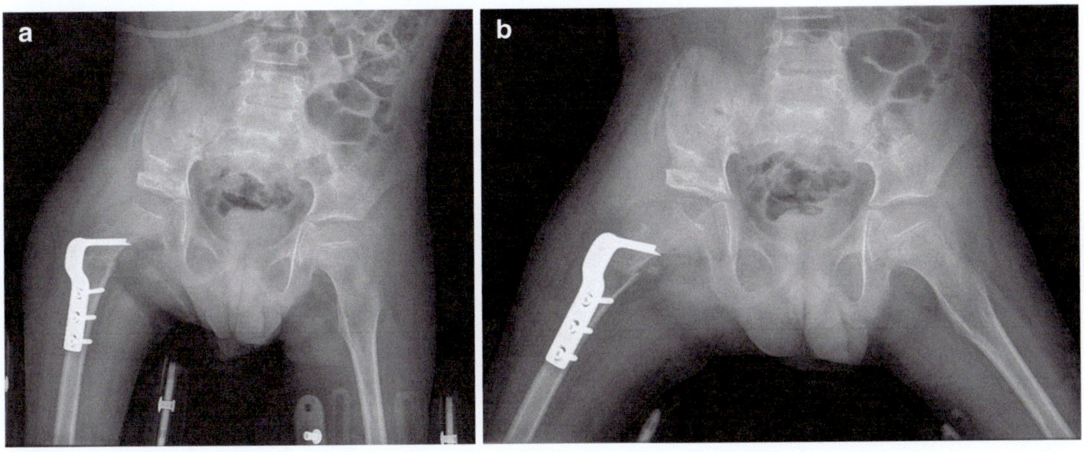

Fig. 19.18 Postoperative anteroposterior (**a**) and frog-leg lateral radiographs (**b**) of the pelvis after the varus derotation osteotomy and pelvic (Dega) osteotomy

Pearls and Pitfalls

- Appropriate guidewire placement facilitates subsequent steps while performing a VDRO. Internally rotating the leg to make the femoral neck horizontal is helpful while placing the guidewire. To identify the optimal guide wire entry point in the anterior-posterior plane, reference the proximal aspect of the femoral diaphysis instead of the greater trochanter, as the latter is usually a slightly posterior structure. Subtle malpositioning of the guidewire can be corrected when placing the seating chisel in non-cannulated systems.
- After provisionally reducing the osteotomy and securing the blade plate, do not overestimate the temporary fixation achieved with a Verbrugge clamp. The assistant must maintain the rotational correction prior to fixing the plate with screws or the correction will be lost.

Indications and Contraindications (Table 19.1)

Table 19.1 Varus derotation osteotomy: Surgical indications and contraindications for varus derotation osteotomy

Indications
Hip subluxation or dislocation with a spherical femoral head
When acetabular dysplasia is present, the acetabulum should be reconstructed
Relative contraindications
Very deformed femoral head
Absolute contraindications
Long-standing hip dislocation with a high-riding deformed femoral head
Severe acetabular dysplasia not amenable to reconstructive osteotomies

References

1. Huh K, Rethlefsen SA, Wren TA, Kay RM. Surgical management of hip subluxation and dislocation in children with cerebral palsy: isolated vdro or combined surgery? J Pediatr Orthop. 2011;31(8):858–63.
2. Shore BJ, Zurakowski D, Chantal D, Powell D, Matheney TH, Snyder BD. Proximal femoral varus derotation osteotomy in children with cerebral palsy: the effect of age, gross motor function classification system level and surgeon volume on surgical success. J Bone Joint Surg Am. 2015;97(24):2024–32.

Suggested Reading

Chang FM, Ma J, Pan Z, Ingram JD, Novais EN. Acetabular remodeling after varus derotational osteotomy in children with cerebral palsy. J Pediatr Orthop. 2016;36(2):198–204.

Reimers J. The stability of hip in children: a radiological study of results of muscle surgery in cerebral palsy. Acta Orthop Scand Suppl. 1980;184:1–100.

20 McHale Procedure in Patients with Neglected Hip Dislocation

Mark Eidelman

Introduction

Most severely involved, nonambulatory patients with neuromuscular problems develop hip dysfunction. Some patients appear with neglected hip dislocation that causes pain, limitation of hip motions, and hygiene care problems. When surgical hip reconstruction is not possible, hip arthrodesis, femoral head resection, and subtrochanteric valgus osteotomy might be effective salvage procedures. In 1990, McHale and coauthors published their technique of subtrochanteric osteotomy with femoral head resection that became a popular salvage procedure [1]. The McHale procedure is widely used due to its effectiveness in achieving the goals of pain relief, increased range of motion, and improved seating ability. This technique has proved to be safe with few complications compared to other salvage procedures.

Brief Clinical History

A 15-year-old boy with cerebral palsy, total body involvement (Fig. 20.1a), Gross Motor Function Classification System (GMFCS) 5, was referred due to severe restriction of hip motions that, according to his caregiver, caused pain on every diaper change. His sitting position was limited and apparently caused more pain. On physical examination, we found severe scissoring, right hip flexion 45°, left hip flexion 60°, right hip abduction 10°, and left hip abduction 15°. Hip rotation bilaterally was severely limited and provoked pain grimace. X-rays revealed bilateral hip dislocation (Fig. 20.1b). There was a skin sore due to pressure of the dislocated femoral head on the left upper thigh (Fig. 20.1c).

M. Eidelman
Pediatric Orthopedics, Ruth Children's Hospital, Technion Faculty of Medicine, Haifa, Israel
e-mail: m_eidelman@rambam.health.gov.il

R. C. Hamdy, N. Saran (eds.), *Pediatric Pelvic and Proximal Femoral Osteotomies*,
https://doi.org/10.1007/978-3-319-78033-7_20

Preoperative Imaging (See Fig. 20.1a–c)

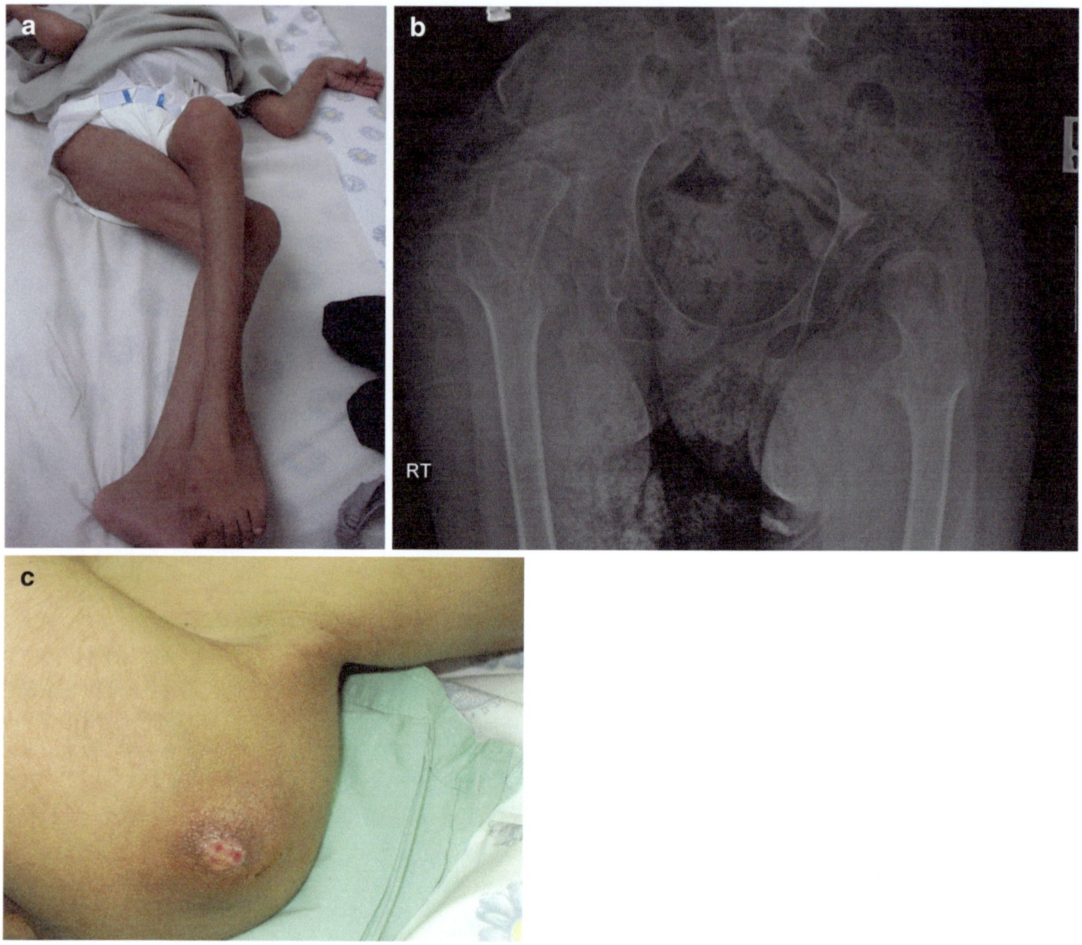

Fig. 20.1 (**a**) Severe scissoring posture and adduction contractures. (**b**) Bilateral neglected hip dislocation (From Eidelman et al. [2], with permission). (**c**) Pressure skin sore of the left dislocated hip (From Eidelman et al. [2], with permission)

Goals of Treatment

To improve abduction and increase hip flexion and eliminate pain and pressure sores

Treatment Strategy

Treatment strategy consists of subtrochanteric valgus osteotomy that reorients the hip joint and eliminates the block for flexion and abduction due to hip dislocation. Creating valgus and tying of the ligamentum teres to the iliopsoas tendon prevents migration of the femur, as usually happens after proximal femoral resection performed in cases of neglected hip dislocation. The use of the locking plate increases fixation stability and avoids using additional spica cast immobilization [2].

Surgical Details

A bump should be placed under the sacrum in order to improve access to the affected hip joint. Anterolateral Watson-Jones approach gives excellent exposure to the hip joint and proximal femur (Fig. 20.2a). Draping should allow full movement of the hip and knee. Tensor fascia lata is identified

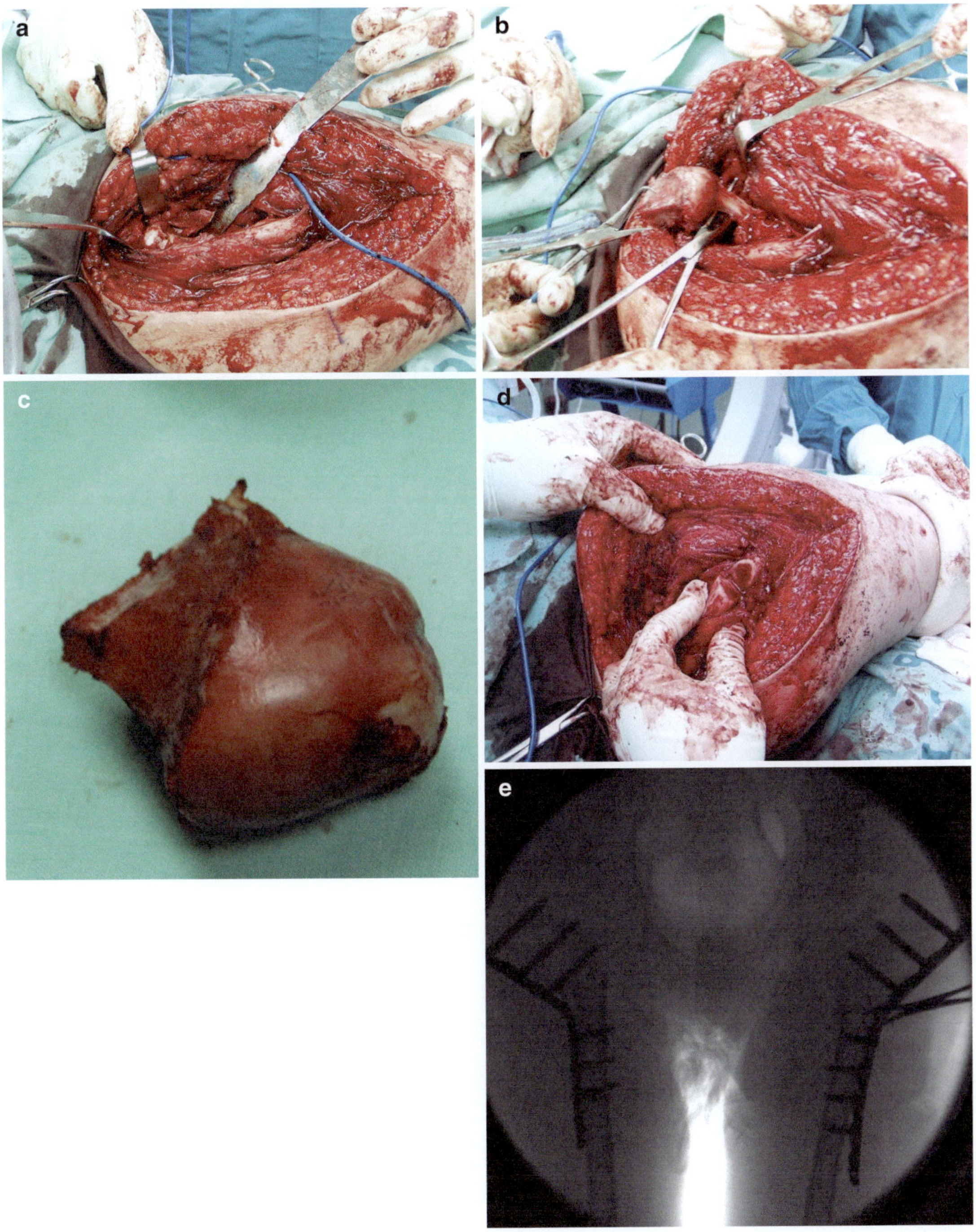

Fig. 20.2 (**a**) Exposure of the hip through the Watson-Jones approach (From Eidelman et al. [2], with permission). (**b**) Osteotomy of the femoral head and release of the ligamentum teres for further attachment to the iliopsoas tendon (From Eidelman et al. [2], with permission). (**c**) Deformed femoral head after excision. (**d**) Subtrochanteric valgus osteotomy. (**e**) Intraoperative X-rays after bilateral McHale operation (From Eidelman et al. [2], with permission)

and reflected anteriorly reveals the anterior border of the gluteus medius retracted posteriorly. After retraction of the rectus femoris and incision of the reflected head of the rectus femoris, the hip capsule is incised in line with the femoral neck. The proximal femoral shaft is exposed, using diathermy to decrease bleeding. Resection of the femoral head is performed, while the ligamentum teres is preserved for further attachment to the iliopsoas tendon (Fig. 20.2b, c). Subtrochanteric open wedge valgus osteotomy (Fig. 20.2d) is performed distal to the lesser trochanter, taking into account that three holes of the Locking Compression Plate™ (LCP) (Depuy Synthes, Warsaw IN, USA) should be proximal to the created osteotomy. After attachment of the ligamentum teres to the iliopsoas tendon, as originally described by McHale [1], a 4.5 mm LCP is prebent and contoured to accommodate the created shape of the femur after the osteotomy. At least three locking screws (Fig. 20.2e) should be inserted in each bone fragment above and below the osteotomy. The wound is closed over the drains above the fascia lata.

Patients with severe cerebral palsy frequently suffer from osteopenia, disuse osteoporosis, and bone fragility. In the original description by McHale et al. [1], most patients were immobilized in hip spica casts, which increased disuse osteopenia even more, with subsequent risk of postoperative fractures. Locking plate technology prevents using additional immobilization. Epidural anesthesia is an important part of the procedure, allowing pain-free management a few days after surgery. An abduction pillow is used for the first 3 weeks after surgery. Gentle passive range of motion and sitting in a wheelchair is allowed immediately following surgery.

Pearls and Pitfalls

- The amount of subtrochanteric valgus osteotomy is crucial for the success of the operation. Osteotomy should be performed as close as possible to the level of the lesser trochanter but must accommodate three locking screws for sufficient plate fixation.
- Accurate prebending of the locking plate is important: at the end, created curvature of the plate will dictate correction.
- In order to fix the plate close enough to the level of the osteotomy, usually the most proximal screw starts at the level just below the top of the greater trochanter.
- Despite the fact that we tie the ligamentum teres to the iliopsoas (as advised in the original description), it seems that valgus osteotomy is the main factor for preventing proximal femoral migration.

Indications and Contraindications (Table 20.1)

Table 20.1 McHale operation in patients with neglected hip dislocation. Surgical indications and contraindications

Indications
Neglected hip dislocation when reconstruction impossible
Stiff and painful hip joint
Contraindications
Painless hips
High risk anesthesia patients

References

1. McHale KA, Bagg M, Nason SS. Treatment of the chronically dislocated hip in adolescents with cerebral palsy with femoral head resection and subtrochanteric valgus osteotomy. J Pediatr Orthop. 1990;10(4):504–9.
2. Eidelman M, Katzman A, Zaidman M, Keren Y. McHale operation in patients with neglected hip dislocations: the importance of locking plates. Adv Orthop Surg. 2014;2014:6. https://doi.org/10.1155/2014/813719.

21 Valgus Osteotomy (Without Head Resection) for Chronic Neuromuscular Hip Dislocation

Thierry E. Benaroch and Fahad S. Alhuzaimi

Introduction

The chronically painful dislocated hip in the non-ambulatory spastic adolescent presents a difficult treatment dilemma. This may lead to intractable pain, decreased sitting tolerance, problems with perineal hygiene, and decubitus ulcers. Ideally, a hip reconstruction consisting of a varus shortening derotation femoral osteotomy along with a pelvic osteotomy and an open reduction of the hip would achieve adequate anatomy, but the femoral head in a long-standing hip dislocation has often destroyed cartilage surface and is grossly misshapen, thereby precluding any type of successful reconstruction.

Most would agree that pain is the primary surgical indication for these hips, but not every dislocated hip is painful. The incidence of pain in a chronic spastic hip dislocation ranges from 18 to 55%. Conservative measures such as muscle relaxant medication, modifying wheelchair positioning, botulinum toxin injection, and intrathecal baclofen should first be attempted. Should these measures fail to alleviate the pain, then a salvage surgical solution must be addressed.

Many surgical procedures have been reported to treat this condition with various success rates. These procedures include proximal femoral resection arthroplasty, subtrochanteric valgus osteotomy with or without femoral head resection, and prosthetic replacement. The aim of this chapter is to describe the technique of the modified Hass subtrochanteric valgus osteotomy popularized by Hogan in which the femoral head is not resected.

Brief Clinical History

This is a 17-year-old known case of cerebral palsy, Gross Motor Function Classification System (GMFCS) 5. He requires assistance in all of his daily activities. For the past 2 years, he is complaining of exquisite right hip pain, and his caregiver is having difficulty with positioning, both in the wheelchair and in bed. His past medical and surgical history includes multiple hospital admissions for pneumonia and insertion of a baclofen pump. On examination, he has no bedsores. The right hip is fixed in 30° of adduction, and any abduction movement is painful and limited. He has a 30° hip flexion contracture, and any flexion past 70° is painful. There is limited painful rotation.

T. E. Benaroch (✉) · F. S. Alhuzaimi
Division of Paediatric Orthopaedic Surgery, Department of Paediatric Surgery, Montreal Children's Hospital, McGill University Health Centre, Montréal, QC, Canada

Department of Orthopaedic Surgery, Shriners Hospital for Children-Canada, Montréal, QC, Canada
e-mail: tbenaroch@shrinenet.org

R. C. Hamdy, N. Saran (eds.), *Pediatric Pelvic and Proximal Femoral Osteotomies*,
https://doi.org/10.1007/978-3-319-78033-7_21

Preoperative Imaging (Fig. 21.1)

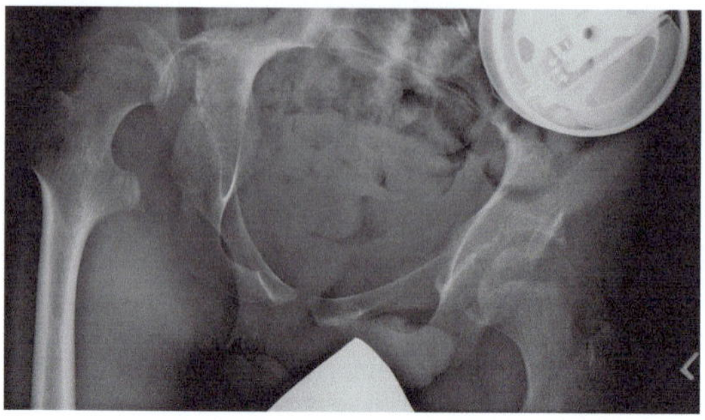

Fig. 21.1 Preoperative anteroposterior (AP) view of the pelvis showing high right hip dislocation, right acetabular dysplasia, and pelvic tilt

Goals of Treatment

In these difficult cases, our aim is to achieve a painless mobile hip to improve the quality of life and to facilitate the positioning of the patient in the wheelchair.

Surgical Details

The procedure is performed with the patient placed supine on the radiolucent table. A bump is placed under the affected hip allowing the buttock of the operative side to be free. A 15-20 cm curvilinear incision is performed just proximal to the tip of the dislocated femoral head coursing slightly posterior to the greater trochanter and extending distally along the lateral aspect of the femur. After cutting through the iliotibial band, a thorough subperiosteal dissection of the subtrochanteric region of the femur is performed. The iliopsoas tendon is identified and subsequently cuts off the lesser trochanter. The hip joint is exposed by making a longitudinal cut in the capsule, and a "T" incision is made parallel to the acetabulum to fully expose the femoral head. The proximal femoral valgus osteotomy is performed using a laterally based wedge of 45–60° (Fig. 21.2). The transverse superior cut should be made at the level just inferior to the lesser trochanter. A second oblique cut 2–2.5 cm below the proximal superior transverse cut should be performed. The longer the laterally based wedge, the larger the correction. A 7-hole 3.5 mm small fragment dynamic compression plate (DCP) is then contoured and placed laterally on the femoral shaft (Fig. 21.3). A 6-hole 3.5 small fragment DCP is then placed anteriorly across the osteotomy site at approximately 90° to the first plate. This adds additional stability to the osteotomy (Fig. 21.4). Postoperatively early range of motion is instituted. A hip abduction pillow can be used to keep legs abducted, and early physical therapy is instituted to work on range of motion and stretching exercises.

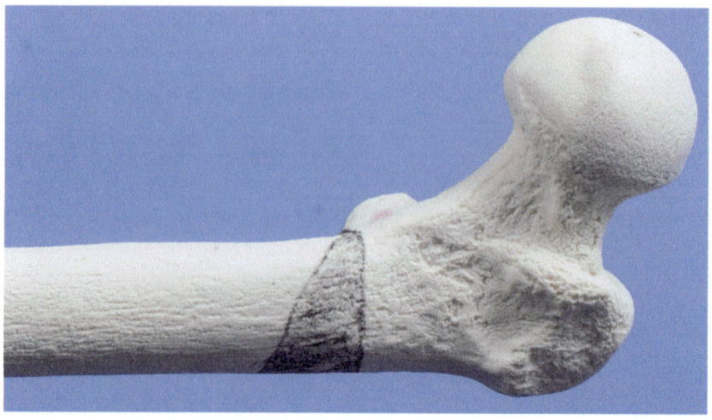

Fig. 21.2 The lateral closing wedge osteotomy shown on a saw bone, keeping in mind the larger the lateral limb of the osteotomy, the greater the valgus achieved

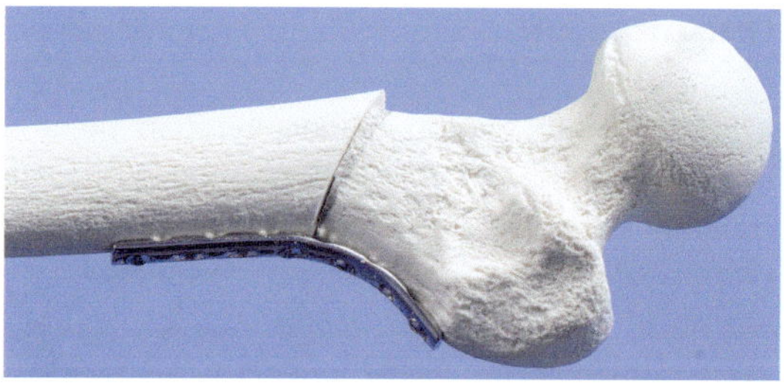

Fig. 21.3 The osteotomy is performed and fixed in place using a laterally pre-contoured 3.5 mm small fragment dynamic compression plate

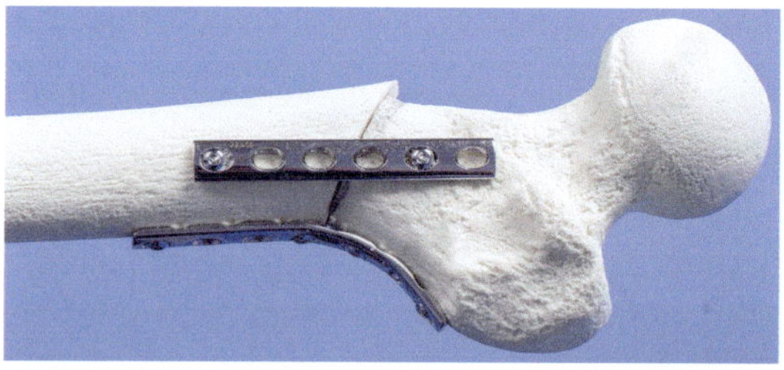

Fig. 21.4 The fixation is augmented with an anteriorly placed 3.5 mm small fragment dynamic compression plate

Postoperative Imaging (Fig. 21.5)

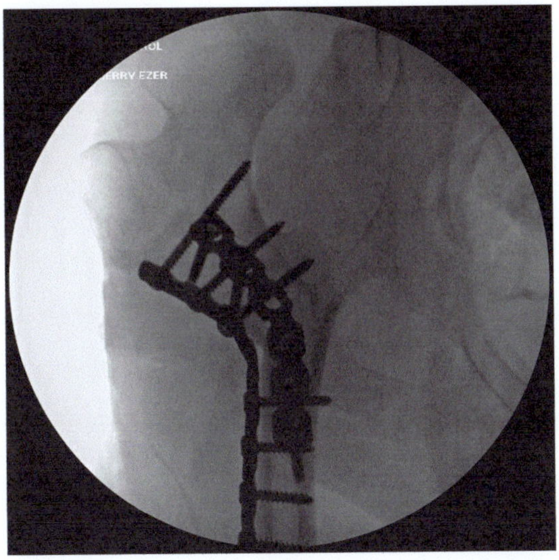

Fig. 21.5 Postoperative anteroposterior (AP) view showing the subtrochanteric valgus osteotomy with the femoral head directed away from the acetabulum

Pearls and Pitfalls

Pearls

- A thorough circumferential subperiosteal dissection of the proximal part of the femur is necessary to identify the lesser trochanter to facilitate the osteotomy.
- Iliopsoas tenotomy off the lesser trochanter will allow easier mobilization of the femoral fragments after the osteotomy.
- Proximal transverse osteotomy cut should be just inferior to the lesser trochanter.
- Do not underestimate size of wedge to be removed. Typically the lateral base should be at least 2.5 cm wide.
- To avoid hardware failure, two plates perpendicular to each other should be used. As well, the 3.5 mm or recon plates should be used to facilitate contouring of the plates.

Pitfalls

- Omitting to do a capsulotomy to visualize femoral head
- Using one plate instead of two
- Underestimating the size of the wedge to be removed

Indications and Contraindications (Table 21.1)

Table 21.1 Valgus osteotomy (without head resection) for chronic neuromuscular hip dislocation: surgical indications and contraindications

Indications
Painful
Long-standing dislocation
Nonambulatory (preferably)
Severe global acetabular dysplasia and misshapen femoral head precluding a successful anatomic reconstruction
Contraindication
Asymptomatic hip dislocation in a nonambulatory spastic child/adolescent

Suggested Reading

Baxter MP, D'Astous JL. Femoral resection-interposition arthroplasty: salvage hip surgery for the severely disabled child with cerebral palsy. J Pediatr Orthop. 1986;6(6):681–5.

Castle ME, Schneider C. Proximal femoral resection-interposition arthroplasty. J Bone Joint Surg Am. 1978;60(8):1051–4.

Hass JA. Subtrochanteric osteotomy for pelvic support. J Bone Joint Surg Am. 1943;25:281–91.

Hogan KA, Blake M, Gross RH. Subtrochanteric valgus osteotomy for chronically dislocated, painful spastic hips: surgical technique. J Bone Joint Surg Am. 2007;89(2):226–31.

Leet AI, Chhor K, Launay F, Kier-York J, Sponseller PD. Femoral head resection for painful hip subluxation in cerebral palsy: is valgus osteotomy in conjunction with femoral head resection preferable to proximal femoral head resection and traction? J Pediatr Orthop. 2005;25(1):70–3.

McCarthy RE, Simon S, Douglas B, Zawacki R, Reese N. Proximal femoral resection to all adults who have severe cerebral palsy to sit. J Bone Joint Surg Am. 1988;70(7):1011–6.

McHale KA, Bagg M, Nason SS. Treatment of the chronically dislocated hip in adolescents with cerebral palsy with femoral head resection and subtrochanteric valgus osteotomy. J Pediatr Orthop. 1990;10(4):504–9.

22 Percutaneous Proximal Femoral Osteotomy with External Fixator for Chronically Dislocated Hips in Patients with Cerebral Palsy

Yaroslav Basyuk and Sanjeev Sabharwal

Introduction

Hip subluxation and dislocation is common in nonambulatory patients with cerebral palsy (CP), especially in more severe forms such as those with Gross Motor Function Classification System (GMFCS) level V. Pain, discomfort, and deformity causing difficulty with positioning and perineal care are frequent concerns among the patient's caregivers. In the adolescent patient with CP who has a chronic dislocation and loss of femoral head sphericity, relocating the deformed head into a dysplastic acetabulum is not indicated. In such patients, salvage procedures such as hip arthrodesis, proximal femoral resection, hip arthroplasty, and proximal femoral valgus osteotomy have been reported. Subtrochanteric valgus osteotomy (SVO) has been described primarily with an open technique, but complications are common. Percutaneous SVO using an external fixator for stabilization may provide a sustained correction deformity as well as improve quality of life measures while minimizing morbidity.

Brief Clinical History

A 14-year-old male presented with history of cerebral palsy, spastic quadriplegia, GMFCS level V with chronic right hip dislocation. Despite receiving physical therapy and frequent turning, he had recently developed a superficial pressure sore overlying the right-sided greater trochanter which was healing. In addition, the parents stated that he had considerable pain and discomfort around the right hip when attempting transfers. Physical examination revealed a positive Galeazzi sign with the right knee being lower than the left side. The right hip had a 30° flexion contracture with abduction of 5° (Fig. 22.1a, b). Radiographs (Fig. 22.1c) and computed tomography scan (Fig. 22.1d) revealed a dislocated right hip with a dysplastic acetabulum as well as loss of sphericity of the femoral head.

Y. Basyuk, MD
Orthopaedics, University Hospital, Newark, NJ, USA
e-mail: basyukya@njms.rutgers.edu

S. Sabharwal, MD, MPH (✉)
Department of Orthopedics, University of California, San Francisco, CA, USA

Division of Pediatric Orthopedics, University of California, San Francisco, CA, USA

Department of Orthopedic Surgery, Benioff Children's Hospital of Oakland, University of California, San Francisco, Oakland, CA, USA

R. C. Hamdy, N. Saran (eds.), *Pediatric Pelvic and Proximal Femoral Osteotomies*,
https://doi.org/10.1007/978-3-319-78033-7_22

Preoperative Imaging (See Fig. 22.1)

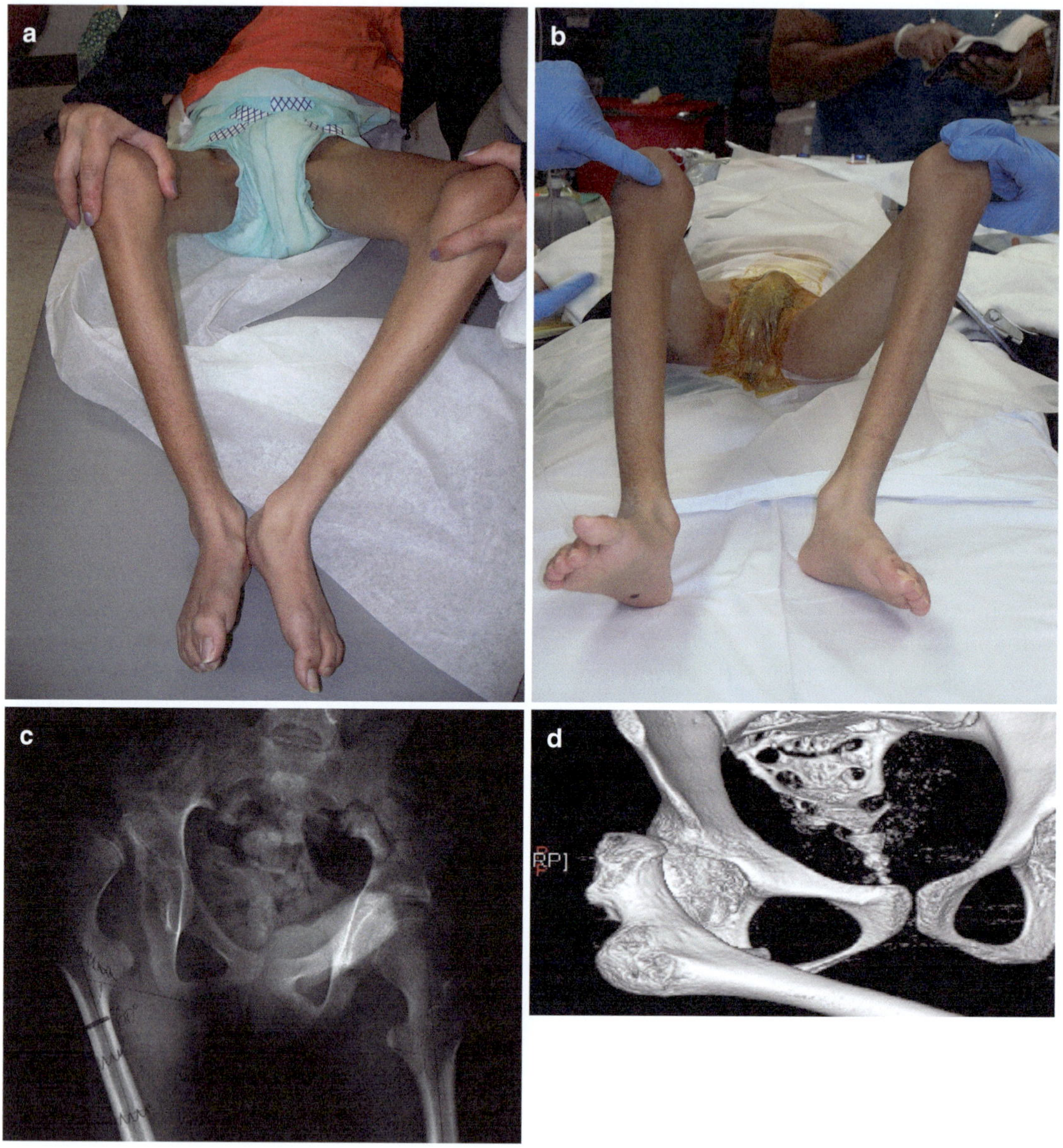

Fig. 22.1 Preoperative examination of a patient with cerebral palsy (Gross Motor Function Classification System V). (**a**) Patient's maximum abduction awake. (**b**) Patients maximum abduction under general anesthesia. (**c**) Preoperative pelvis X-ray showing a chronically dislocated right hip. (**d**) Preoperative three-dimensional (3D) computed tomography reconstruction showing significant femoral head wear and loss of femoral head sphericity as well as a dysplastic acetabulum

Goals of Treatment

The principles of treatment include:

1. Relieve pain and improve sitting tolerance, ease of transfers, and perineal care.
2. Correct deformity and improve the dislocated hip caused by abduction.
3. Minimize complications.

Treatment Strategy

The treatment strategy consists of treating a chronically dislocated hip and its associated adduction deformity in patients with cerebral palsy with a percutaneous proximal femoral subtrochanteric valgus osteotomy stabilized with an external fixator. The goal of treatment is to improve quality of life, caregiver satisfaction, and hip abduction as well as provide deformity correction while minimizing the morbidity associated with an open approach in these patients.

Surgical Details

Placement of External Fixator Pins and Frame

After induction of general anesthesia, the patient is placed supine on a radiolucent Jackson Table™ with a folded sheet placed in the midline under the sacrum. The affected extremity is brought to the edge of table, prepared, and free draped. An open adductor longus tenotomy is performed via a medial incision overlying the taut tendon. Next, the hip is brought into a "hip neutral" position, with an appropriate amount of adduction approximating the planned magnitude of valgus correction, and an AP view of the proximal femur is visualized with fluoroscopy (Fig. 22.2a). This is the way the hip should appear after the corrective osteotomy is performed. In addition, placing the proximal half-pins in this position avoids the need for more extensive skin and soft tissue release around the pins after the corrective osteotomy. Next, with the limb in the "hip neutral" position, a 1.8 mm Ilizarov wire is initially inserted by hand, starting at the palpable proximal tip of the greater trochanter and is then advanced using a wire driver toward the center of the femoral head. In children, the starting point can be cartilaginous and proximal to the ossified portion of greater trochanter that can be visualized with fluoroscopy. Using this reference guide and staying parallel and distal to this temporary reference wire, a 3.8 or 4.8 mm drill bit is used to drill a hole from the base of the greater trochanter to the lesser trochanter. A 5 or 6 mm hydroxyapatite-coated half-pin is placed in the path of the drilled hole, staying parallel to the proximal reference wire (Fig. 22.2b, c). The size of the half-pin is based on the width of the underlying bone and should not exceed more than one-third the diameter of the underlying femoral shaft at the site of pin insertion. Once the half-pin has been inserted by hand, the reference wire can be removed and the leg brought to neutral abduction. A 90 or 120° Ilizarov™ femoral arch is placed onto the half-pin with a pin fixation bolt and kept at 90° to the floor. There should be at least two fingerbreadths between the arch and the underlying skin. In addition, attention must be paid to allow adequate clearance between the proximal arch and the abdomen and the posterior thigh to prevent impingement during sitting and lying down, respectively. After the position of the arc has been secured by tightening the pin fixation bolt, a second half-pin can be added to the proximal arch with the leg adducted as before. With the second pin, the sagittal alignment of the proximal arch becomes fixed.

Next, with the patella facing toward the ceiling, i.e., the "knee neutral position" (with the limb in neutral alignment in the frontal, transverse, and sagittal planes), a half-pin is placed in essentially at a right angle to the femoral shaft. A second femoral arch is mounted to this half-pin, 1–2 cm closer to the skin than the proximal arch in order to allow for lateral translation during osteotomy correction (Fig. 22.2d). A second half-pin is added to the distal arch, often using a Ranch cube™ while maintaining orthogonal position of the frame to their respective femoral segment.

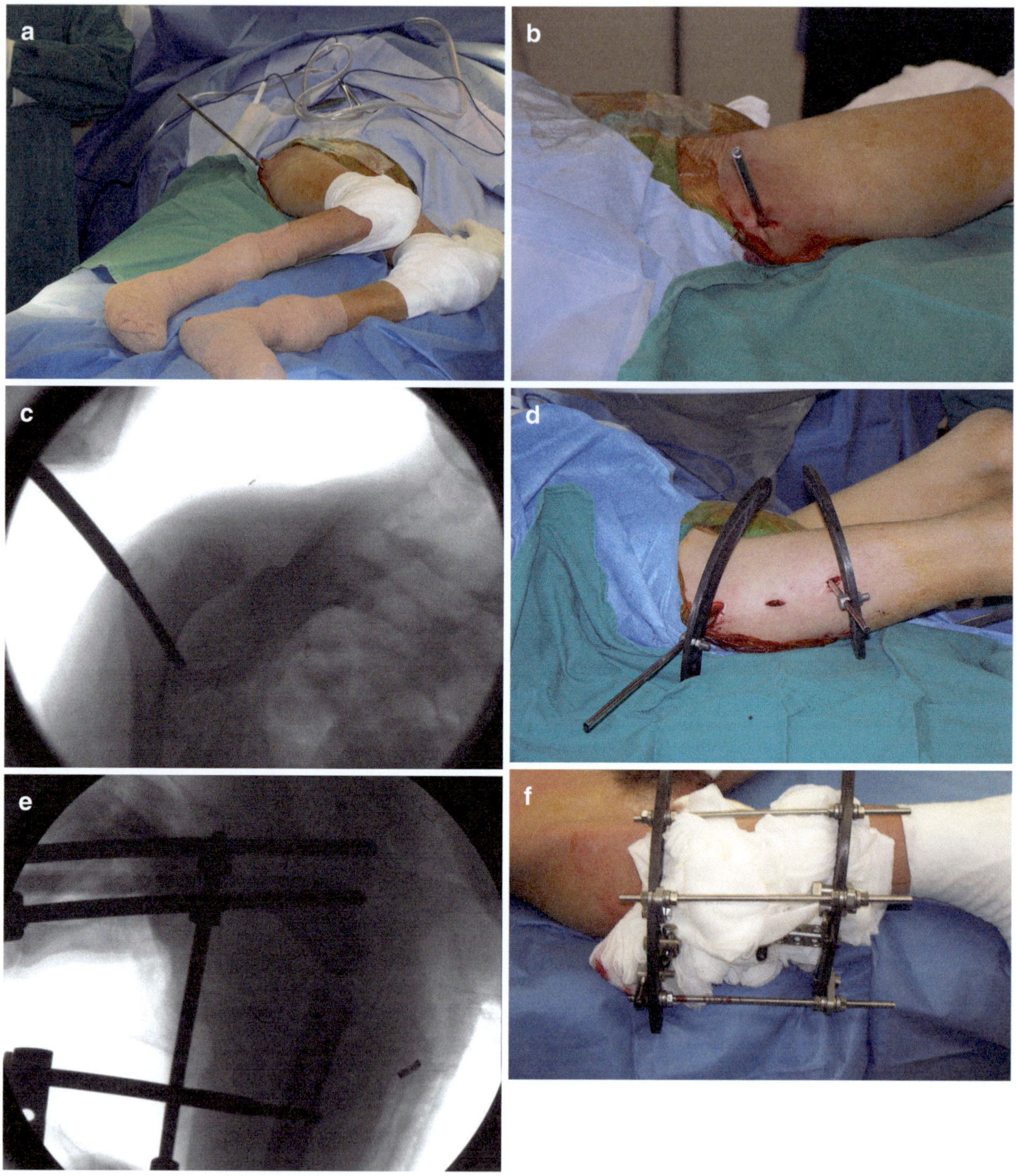

Fig. 22.2 Intraoperative technique and postoperative imaging. (**a**) Positioning shows the proximal pin placement with the "hip neutral" position. (**b**) Side view of "knee neutral" position. (**c**) Placement of the first proximal half-pin from greater to lesser trochanter. (**d**) Placement of the two femoral arches orthogonal to their respective femoral segments. (**e**) Final fluoroscopic view after angular correction using the conical washers to compress between the two femoral arches. (**f**) Clinical photo of the final construct. Note the near parallel orientation of the two femoral arches as well as the three evenly spaced threaded rods. The conical washers at the ends of each rod allow for "fine tuning" the angular correction and translation at the osteotomy site. (**g**) An anteroposterior X-ray showing complete healing. (**h**) Intraoperative photograph showing the incision used for the percutaneous osteotomy. A 5 mm half-pin is seen below the osteotome. (**i**) Intraoperative photograph showing the two femoral arches connected via threaded rods and conical washers (*arrows*) and the occlusive dressing over the osteotomy site

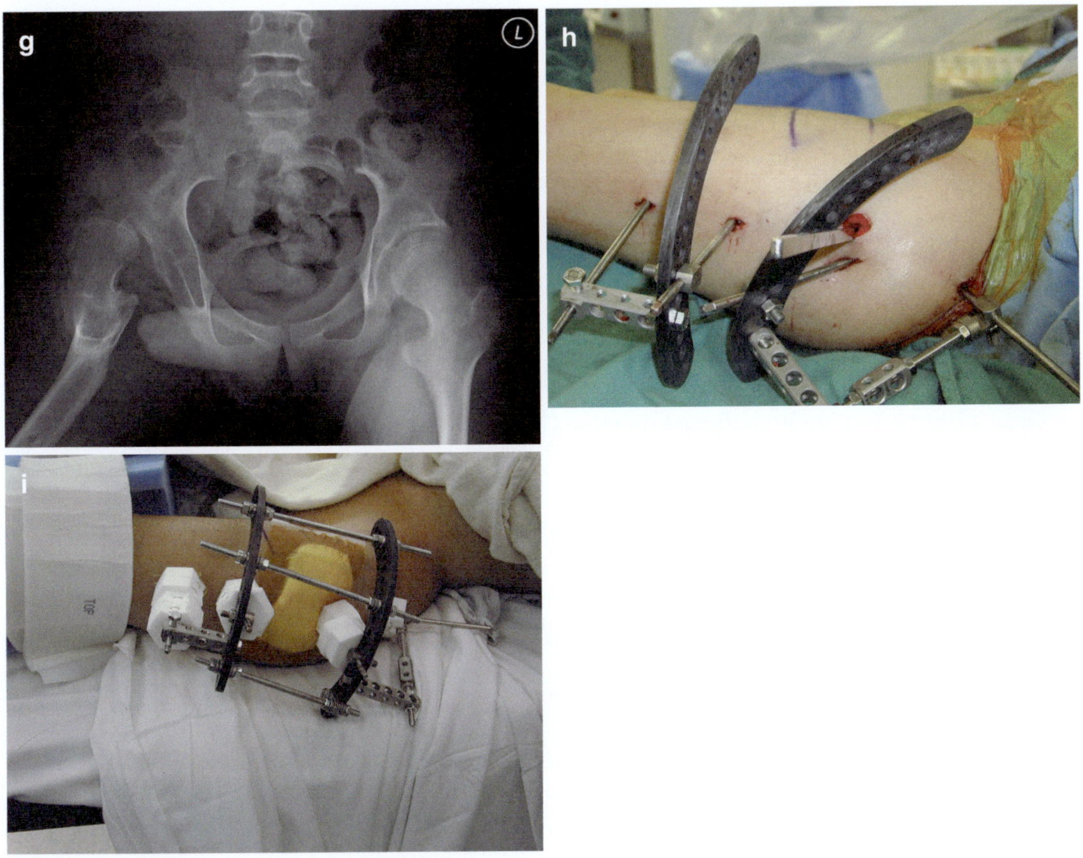

Fig. 22.2 (continued)

Osteotomy and Final Construct Assembly

After the proximal and distal arches have been stabilized with half-pins, a 2 cm longitudinal incision is made at the level of the proposed osteotomy site, just distal to the lesser trochanter, between the two arches. A percutaneous subperiosteal dissection on the lateral cortex at the level of the osteotomy is done with a periosteal elevator. Under fluoroscopy, a 3.8 mm drill bit is used to create one or two drill holes through the lateral cortex and subsequently directed anteriorly and posteriorly to create multiple perforations at the far, medial cortex at right angles to the proximal femoral shaft. Once this is done, a quarter inch or half inch osteotomy is used percutaneously through the same incision to complete the osteotomy by connecting the drill holes. Next, appropriate abduction and lateral translation of the distal fragment is done, with the surgical assistant abducting the leg and the surgeon bringing the proximal and distal arches parallel to each other. An attempt is made to impale the distal end of the proximal fragment into the medullary canal of the distal fragment in order to provide some intrinsic stability to the osteotomy.

Once appropriately realigned, the two arches are connected to each other with three evenly spaced threaded rods and conical washers. The alignment of the osteotomy can be further "fine-tuned" fluoroscopically with differential compression and distraction of the threaded rods, to adjust the frontal and sagittal angulation at the osteotomy site (Fig. 22.2e, f). If any tenting of the skin is present around the half-pins, appropriate skin releases are carried out. The surgical wounds are closed with absorbable sutures, and an occlusive dressing is applied. Care is taken to separate the osteotomy and pin sites under the same dressing to prevent infection.

An abduction pillow is placed. With this percutaneous technique, we do not routinely administer any form of chemical or radiation prophylaxis against heterotopic ossification. A well-padded abduction pillow is placed to help maintain the abduction correction.

Once adequate healing is confirmed on radiographs, usually 3–4 months postoperatively, the external fixator is removed under general anesthesia and the patient placed in a well-padded hip abduction brace for 10–14 days, in order to prevent a fracture through the osteotomy or pin-tract sites (Fig. 22.2g).

Postoperative Imaging (Fig. 22.2g)

Pearls and Pitfalls

- Apply the proximal and distal pins while in "hip neutral" and "knee neutral" positions, respectively. This will help avoid performing extensive skin releases around the half-pins after deformity correction.
- Allow enough space between the proximal arch and skin to prevent impingement on the abdomen and posterior thigh.
- An adductor longus tenotomy should be performed initially in order to improve hip abduction and maximize the valgus correction.
- The half-pin should not be larger than one-third diameter of the femur at the site of pin insertion. Using a pin with a larger diameter may cause an iatrogenic fracture, especially after pin removal. In addition, if available, hydroxyapatite-coated pins should be used in order to enhance fixation to the bone and minimize pin loosening.
- The osteotomy site should be ideally in the proximal meta-diaphyseal portion bone in order to increase the surface area between the proximal and distal bone fragments, thus enhancing bony healing.
- An abduction brace is used in the immediate postoperative period after external fixator removal to help prevent a fracture.

Indications and Contraindications (Table 22.1)

Table 22.1 Percutaneous proximal femoral osteotomy with external fixator for chronically dislocated hips in patients with cerebral palsy: surgical indications and contraindications

Main indication
Chronically dislocated, painful hip with loss of femoral head sphericity in a child/adolescent with cerebral palsy (usually GMFCS level V)
Others indications
Developmental coxa vara [1], severe slipped capital femoral epiphysis [2]
Contraindications
Spherical femoral head (potentially reducible in the native acetabulum) in a child with cerebral palsy
Inability to tolerate or place an external fixator due to social setting, body habitus, decubitus ulcer, etc.
Patient not medically fit to undergo general anesthesia

References

1. Sabharwal S, Mittal R, Cox G. Percutaneous triplanar femoral osteotomy correction for developmental coxa vara: a new technique. J Pediatr Orthop. 2005;25(1):28–33.
2. Sabharwal S, Mittal R, Zhao C. Percutaneous osteotomy for deformity correction in adolescents with severe slipped capital femoral epiphysis. J Pediatr Orthop B. 2006;15(6):396–403.

Suggested Reading

Hogan KA, Blake M, Gross RH. Subtrochanteric valgus osteotomy for chronically dislocated, painful spastic hips. J Bone Joint Surg Am. 2006;88(12):2624–31.

Martinez M, Kim S, Sabharwal S. Percutaneous subtrochanteric osteotomy for painful dislocated hips in patients with cerebral palsy. J Pediatr Orthop. 2017;37(2):111–20.

23 Flexion-Valgus Intertrochanteric Osteotomy for Late-Slipped Capital Femoral Epiphysis Deformity

H. Kerr Graham, Benjamin J. Shore, and Simon P. Kelley

Introduction

Osteotomy of the proximal femur has been used to correct deformity associated with slipped capital femoral epiphysis (SCFE) for more than 50 years. Southwick described an osteotomy "through the lesser trochanter" in 1963 and reported his results in later publications. Current concepts are similar to the flexion osteotomy in the intertrochanteric region, described by Imhauser in 1973. The principal indications are for the management of moderate to severe, symptomatic deformity of the proximal femur, after healing of SCFE. The components of flexion-valgus intertrochanteric osteotomy (FVIT) for SCFE deformity include combinations of flexion and valgus. Biomechanical modelling by Rab [1], axial imaging and clinical studies support flexion as being the key component of deformity correction with a small degree of valgus usually required. The evolution of fixation for FVIT in SCFE has included simple plates, compression plates, blade plates and locking plates. Accompanying procedures may include surgical hip dislocation (SHD) and additional surgery for femoro-acetabular impingement (FAI) at the time of FVIT or as a staged procedure. FVIT for moderate to severe deformity of the proximal femur after healing of a SCFE is a technically demanding procedure. However, FVIT can relieve pain, improve gait and function and preserve the native hip until a more suitable age for arthroplasty.

Brief Clinical History

The candidate for FVIT after SCFE is usually an adolescent with a history of a moderate to severe slip, pinned in situ, when the capital epiphysis has closed. The interval between the slip, pinning and FVIT should be long enough to assess the level of symptoms off a stable baseline and to allow some time for remodelling. It should not be overly prolonged because the metaphyseal bump results in progressive damage to the labrum and acetabular hyaline cartilage, which will not recover after FVIT.

The key symptoms are pain with activities, pain during sitting in high flexion and limping.

H. Kerr Graham (✉)
Department of Orthopaedic Surgery (NHMRC CP-CRE), Royal Children's Hospital, Parkville, VIC, Australia
e-mail: kerr.graham@rch.org.au

B. J. Shore
Department of Orthopaedic Surgery, Harvard Medical School, Boston Children's Hospital, Boston, MA, USA
e-mail: Benjamin.shore@childrens.harvard.edu

S. P. Kelley
Department of Surgery, University of Toronto, Toronto, ON, Canada

The Hospital for Sick Children, Toronto, ON, Canada
e-mail: simon.kelley@sickkids.ca

R. C. Hamdy, N. Saran (eds.), *Pediatric Pelvic and Proximal Femoral Osteotomies*, https://doi.org/10.1007/978-3-319-78033-7_23

Preoperative Imaging

We routinely order three radiographs: an anteroposterior (AP) view of the hips, a lateral view of the affected hip and a prone extension (PE) view of the affected hip. The PE radiograph is performed by positioning the patient prone on the X-ray table to allow the affected hip to be moved into maximal extension, usually between 30° and 50° (Figs. 23.1 and 23.2). This shows the morphology of the femoral head and neck and simulates the flexion that will be incorporated into the correction. Critically it allows the surgeon to visualize the anticipated postoperative appearance of the hip, the restoration of the head-shaft angle, including how the anterolateral impingement lesion moves away from the acetabulum.

It can also be noted on this prone extension view the height of the greater trochanter and the degree of varus, which has the effect of reducing the offset of the hip. It is from this radiograph, rather than the AP radiograph that the magnitude of valgus correction should be calculated, which is designed to again restore head-shaft angle, restore hip offset and thus improve abductor efficiency.

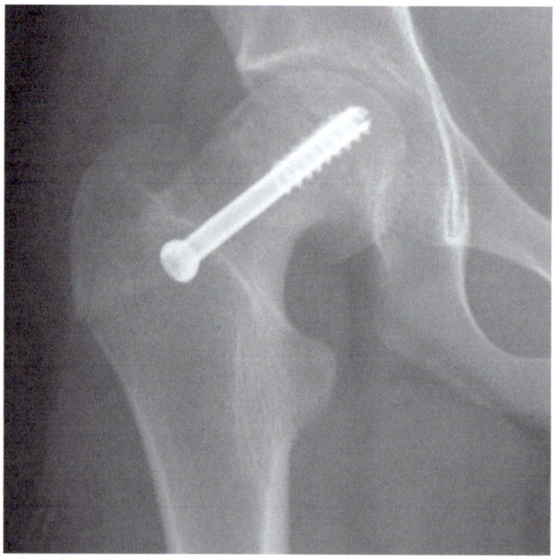

Fig. 23.1 Anteroposterior radiograph of Grade III slip right hip in a 12-year-old girl, pinned in situ. Lateral slip angle 70°

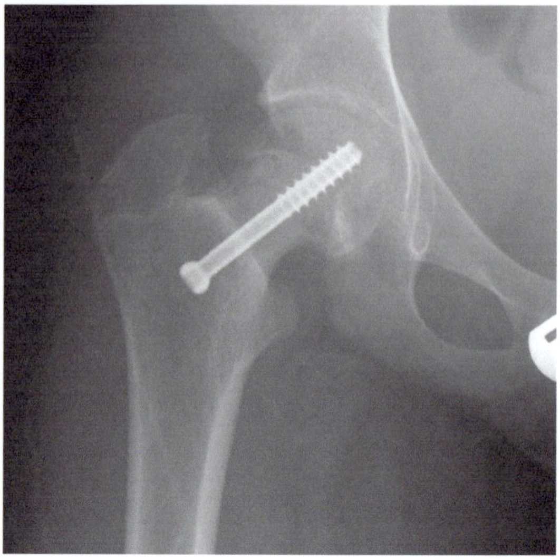

Fig. 23.2 Prone extension radiograph right hip, same patient as Fig. 23.1, right to left reversed to allow comparison. Note that the fixation screw, in the position of extension is now seen "en face". In addition, the lateral border of the superior femoral neck is now concave, whereas it was straight in Fig. 23.1. That is, Fig. 23.1 shows an impingement lesion. In addition, note that in this position which simulates the correction of a pure flexion osteotomy, the greater trochanter is excessively high, indicating that a significant degree of valgus should be incorporated into the osteotomy

Goals of Treatment

The patient's immediate goals are usually the relief of symptoms, pain and limping. It is not unusual for adolescents to exaggerate pain when embarrassment about the cosmesis of gait is the underlying concern. Surgical goals may also include preservation of the native hip by preventing progression of further chondrolabral damage and cartilage loss from FAI.

Treatment Strategy

Preoperative assessment includes evaluation for significant medical comorbidities including obesity, diabetes, metabolic syndrome, smoking and bone health. Healing in adolescents can be slow and smoking is a contraindication. Weight loss is often helpful but difficult. Occasionally bariatric surgery needs to be considered before FVIT. Assessment by a metabolic physician is often helpful.

The primary deformity is extension, in the sagittal plane. Hip flexion is blocked by the proximal metaphysis abutting the anterolateral acetabular rim (Fig. 23.3). As flexion is blocked, there is a corresponding increase in extension, apparent on clinical examination and best appreciated in the prone position.

In the coronal plane, the primary deformity is varus, which reduces the head-shaft angle and thus shortens the affected limb. This has the effect of reducing the available abduction range. In an attempt to prevent lateral impingement, the pelvis tilts up on the affected side. Apparent leg length discrepancy (LLD) is always greater than real LLD (see Fig. 23.3).

In the transverse plane, external hip rotation is marked, and patients often complain that their "leg is turned outwards". Most of external rotation is not fixed but a compensatory mechanism to clear the anterolateral impingement caused by the primary components of the deformity, extension and varus (see Fig. 23.3).

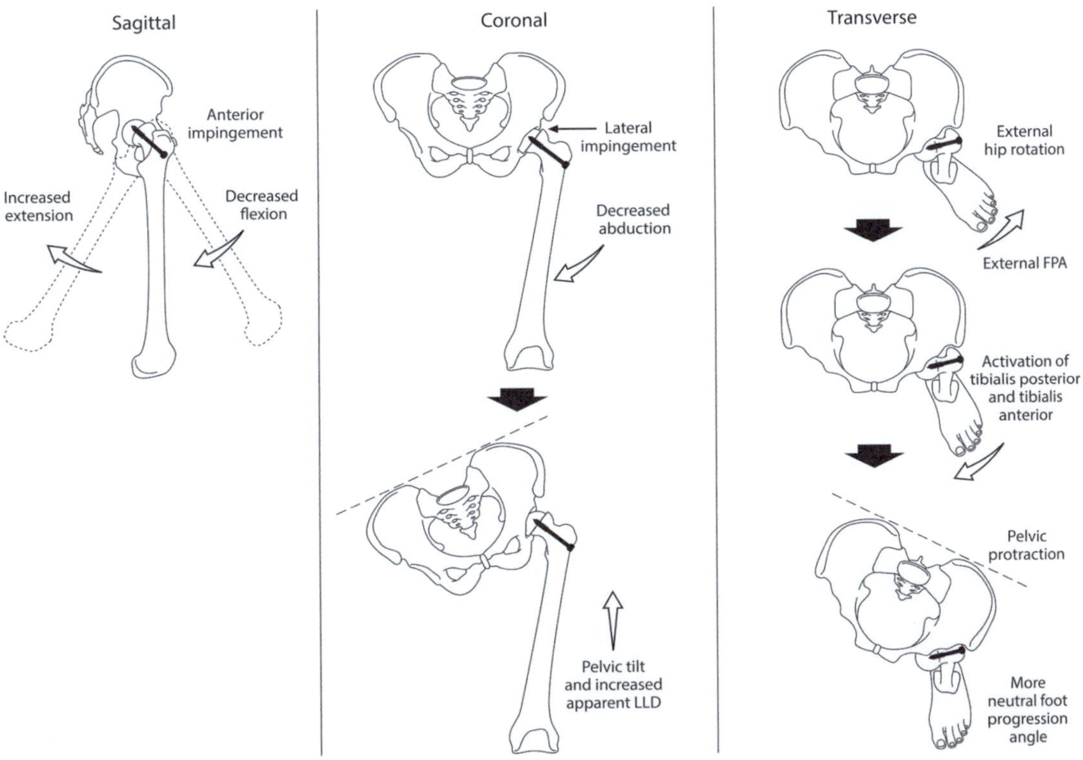

Fig. 23.3 The change in hip motion and gait resulting from a chronic high-degree slip in sagittal, coronal and transverse planes. In the sagittal plane, as flexion increases, extension increases, permitting the prone extension radiograph described above.
In the coronal plane, when the slip is severe, hip abduction range is lost, resulting in upward pelvic tilt on the affected side, increasing apparent leg length discrepancy and resulting in a painful limp
In the transverse plane, the inability to internally rotate at the hip, because of the anterolateral impingement lesion, results in an external foot progression angle (FPA). Most teenagers try to compensate for this by two mechanisms: (1) activation of tibialis posterior and tibialis anterior to improve FPA and (2) ipsilateral pelvic protraction to further neutralize the external FPA

Preoperative Planning: Blade Plate Method (Fig. 23.4)

Step 1 Measure the head-shaft angle on both the AP and lateral radiograph by Southwick's method. This can be compared to the values taken from the contralateral hip, assuming unilateral pathology. In the case of bilateral pathology, 145° on the AP view and 10° on the lateral view are used. Using subtraction, both the varus and exten-

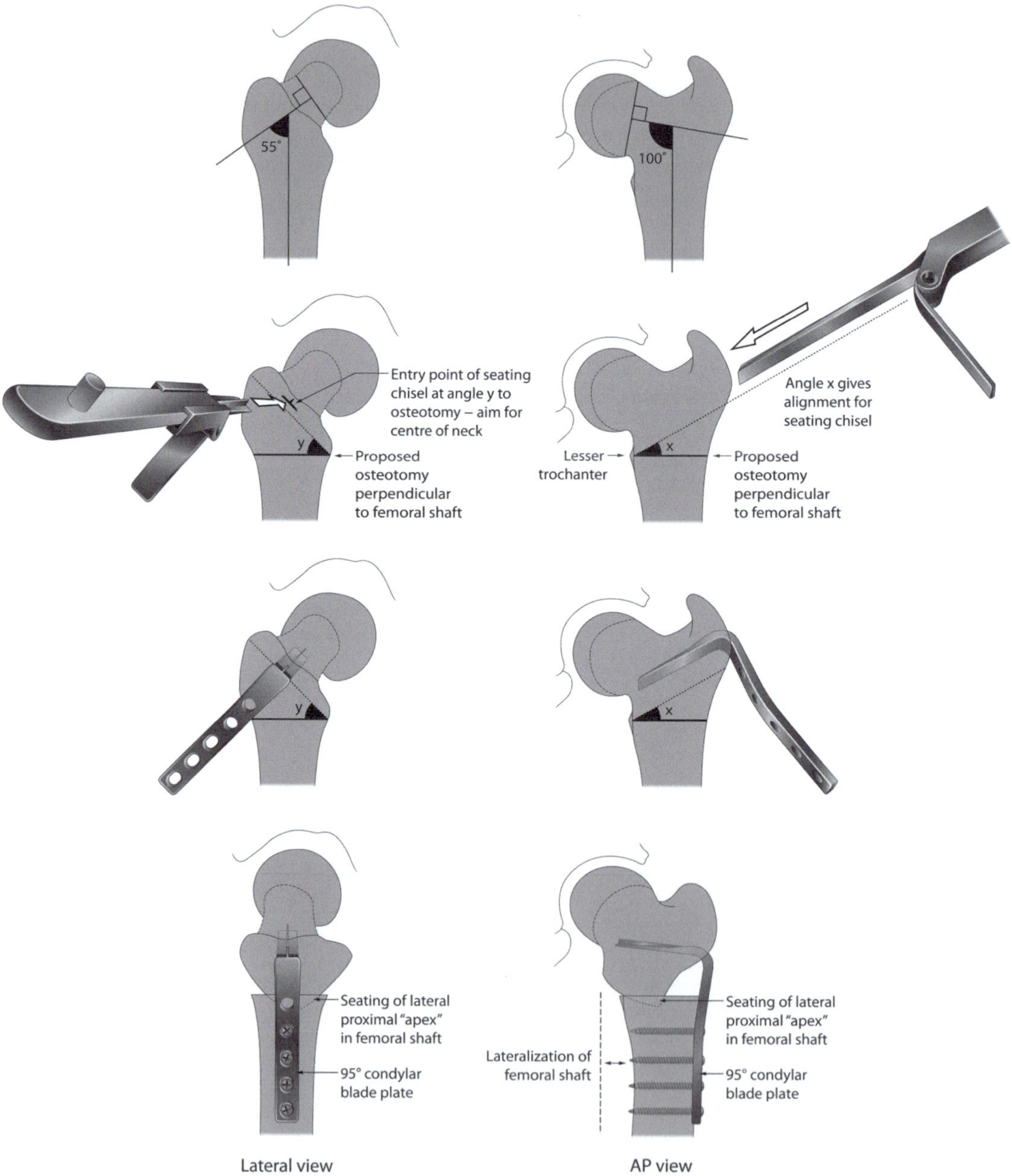

Fig. 23.4 Planning for flexion-valgus intertrochanteric osteotomy is best broken down into lateral (*left-hand column*) and AP views (*right-hand column*). Depicted are schematic representations of the correction utilizing a 95° condylar blade plate. Panels show initial imaging, planning for the entry point of guidewire and seating chisel, insertion of blade plate and final correction incorporating both flexion and valgus. Note the typically larger correction in the sagittal plane

sion deformity of the affected hip can be calculated and thus the amount of valgus and flexion correction to be built in to the osteotomy.

Step 2 The line of the proposed osteotomy is marked on both the AP and lateral radiographs. This is a simple transverse osteotomy, just above the lesser trochanter.

Step 3 On the AP view, a line subtending an angle "x" at the medial extent of the proposed osteotomy equating to that of the proposed valgus correction minus 5° (when using a 95° condylar blade plate). The guidewire, and subsequently the seating chisel, will be inserted superior to this line and parallel to it (Fig. 23.5).

Step 4 On the lateral, a line is marked subtending an angle "y" at the posterior extent of the proposed osteotomy equating to that of the proposed flexion correction. This marks the rotation of the seating chisel required. The blade of the seating chisel will sit parallel and superior to this line, close to the midpoint of the femoral neck (Fig. 23.6).

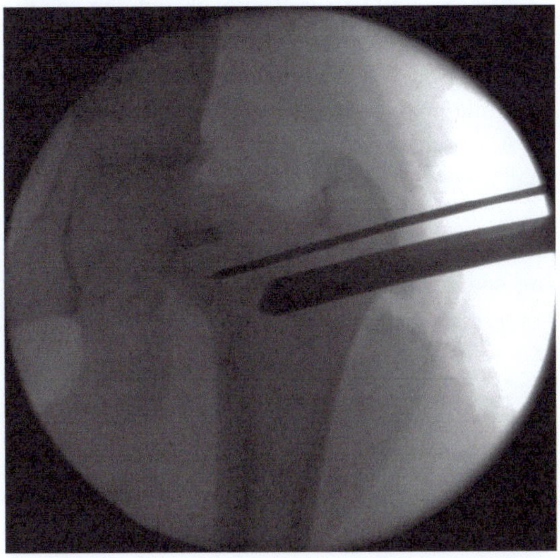

Fig. 23.5 Fluoroscopic images illustrating flexion-valgus intertrochanteric osteotomy for a Grade III stable slip left hip in a 16-year-old boy weighing 126 kg. Note the large anterolateral metaphyseal bump which was causing pain and a severe limp. The remnant of a screw which broke during the early phase of treatment is still present within the femoral head. In the anteroposterior view, the guidewire has been inserted to achieve a 30° of valgus correction, and the seating chisel is being advanced towards the calcar

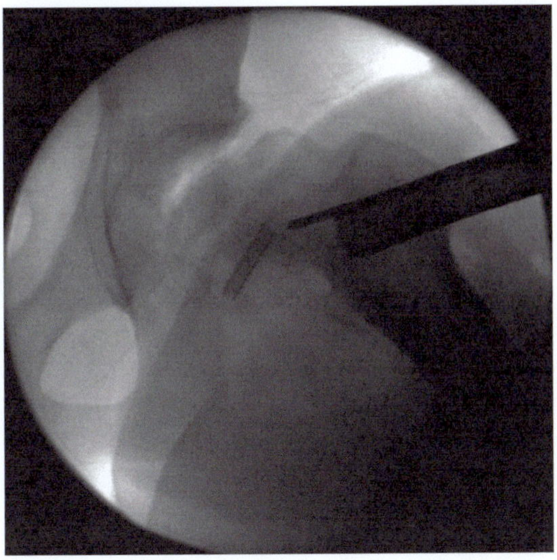

Fig. 23.6 On the lateral view, the large anterolateral bump, with impingement on the lateral acetabular margin, is seen as well as an oblique view of the seating chisel as it is advanced towards the calcar

Step 5 A template of the condylar blade plate can be traced onto the digital AP and lateral radiographs, to identify the size of the implant and length of the blade required.

Step 6 A trial correction can be performed using TraumaCad or on tracing paper by cutting the osteotomy and realigning the fragments to confirm the postoperative position of the implant and bony fragments.

The most useful implants are the fixed-angle blade plate or a proximal femoral locking plate. We aim for stable fixation with compression, sufficient to allow touch weight bearing from postoperative day 1. Expecting an obese adolescent to comply with non-weight bearing is unrealistic and potentially dangerous. Most operative series report hardware failure, which remains a constant risk in this population, following this type of reconstructive surgery.

Postoperative follow-up should be regular and meticulous, for a minimum of 2 years after surgery. The removal of implants at 12–24 months after surgery should be part of the plan because the majority of patients will require an arthroplasty, sometime in the future, and retained femoral hardware has been shown to increase the complications associated with primary hip arthroplasty.

Surgical Details

The patient is supine on a radiolucent operating table. Prior to skin preparation and draping, the hip is examined using fluoroscopy and the operative plan rechecked. It is essential that the hip have adequate range of motion to ensure good-quality lateral views.

A standard lateral approach is performed to expose the proximal femur.

Vastus lateralis is dissected and lifted anteriorly from the intermuscular septum posteriorly for subperiosteal exposure of the femoral shaft. An exposure of adequate length is required to allow correction following osteotomy. The combination of flexion and valgus results in acute lengthening and generates a marked increase in soft tissue tension.

The following surgical description pertains to the use of a 95° condylar blade plate. A 100°, 110° or 120° proximal femoral locking plate may also be used based upon preoperative planning with modifications of the surgical technique reflecting the specifics of that device. The authors routinely use both devices for this procedure.

The insertion of the guidewire is the key step. Each succeeding step and the success of the procedure stem from accurate referencing from a perfectly placed guidewire. The guidewire must be strong enough to avoid bending or breaking when the hip is ranged into position to obtain lateral radiographs. The guidewire is inserted at a point approximately 15 mm distal to the greater trochanter, inferomedially at the predetermined angle to the proposed perpendicular osteotomy for the correction of the valgus (angle x, see Figs. 23.4 and 23.5). This acts as a guide for the seating chisel. When using a 95° condylar blade plate, the angle of the guidewire to the proposed osteotomy site is equal to the desired valgus angle minus 5° (see Figs. 23.5 and 23.6).

The second critical step is cutting the track with the seating chisel. For the flexion component, the angled guide is attached to the seating chisel and rotated away from the operating table towards the ceiling when the patient is positioned supine. Flexing the hip requires absolute stability of the seating chisel within the proximal femur. In practice, this means cutting a single track and having the tip of the blade in the hard bone of the calcar (Fig. 23.7). An appropriate implant for the typical large adolescent patient is the AO Synthes 95° fixed-angle blade plate (Synthes, Westchester PA, USA). We prefer this to the 90° implant because we usually employ a degree of valgus correction and we aim to lateralize, not medialize, the distal fragment, which is obligatory with the medial offset of the 90° blade plate. There is one and only one opportunity to cut a single, strong track with the tip ending in the strong bone of the calcar. Penetration of the calcar and fracture of the femoral neck must be avoided.

It is essential to loosen/back out the seating chisel by 10–15 mm before osteotomizing the femur. Removal of a jammed seating chisel from a mobile proximal femur can be difficult.

A simple transverse osteotomy of the proximal femoral shaft is performed, just above the lesser trochanter and 20 mm distal to the insertion point of the seating chisel, using an oscillating saw. Given the need to control rotation and sometimes make an adjustment intraoperatively, it is wise to make a reference mark using the saw blade on the anterolateral aspect of the femur traversing the site of the osteotomy, before the bone is cut. In many adolescents, the flexion component substantially increases the range of internal rotation, and no further correction is required. In others, a small amount of internal rotation is required to match the contralateral hip, if it has a satisfactory range of rotation. The 20 mm segment is essential to stability of the blade plate within the proximal femur, when subjected to the acute tension forces resulting from acute valgus and flexion correction. With the osteotomy complete, the seating chisel can be replaced by the definitive implant. To increase apposition,

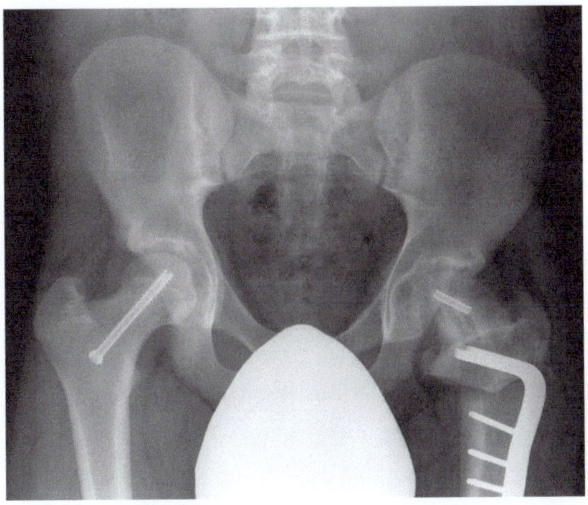

Fig. 23.7 Anteroposterior radiograph of the same patient immediately after surgery showing a good correction of the proximal femur, incorporating both valgus and flexion. Note that the lateral proximal metaphyseal edge has been invaginated into the distal end of the metaphysis, increasing contact and permitting reasonably rapid union despite no wedges being cut

increase stability and maintain length, we try to insert the lateral edge of the proximal fragment inside the metaphyseal surface of the distal fragment (see Fig. 23.7). Reduction requires a lot of effort because this is an acute lengthening osteotomy—the amount of lengthening is the combined amount of flexion and valgus. A minor degree of trimming of the posterolateral aspect of the cut surface of the distal fragment can achieve improved contact and stability, at the expense of losing some length.

At least two of the side plate screws should be inserted using dynamic compression. The most proximal hole is at the level of the osteotomy and is not usually utilized for fixation.

When fixation is complete, the hip is again ranged using fluoroscopy and the correction assessed. At this point, it is usually clear that internal rotation has been restored, and no rotational correction is required.

Flexion should be possible to >90° without impingement.

Evidence of persisting FAI from the anterior or lateral metaphyseal bump should now be assessed. Persistent FAI is an indication for an additional osteoplasty as described by Bali and colleagues [2].

Postoperative Imaging

Apart from the saved fluoroscopic images, a good-quality AP radiograph of the pelvis and cross-table lateral are required. It is important to have both clinical and radiographic confidence in the stability of fixation to not only permit but encourage early weight bearing (Figs. 23.8 and 23.9).

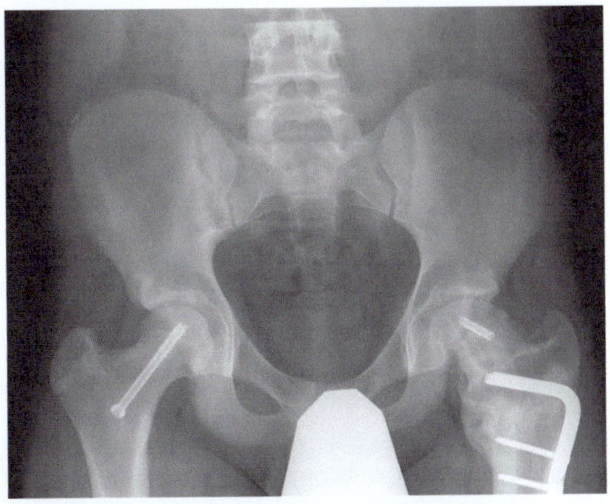

Fig. 23.8 Same patient as Figs. 23.5, 23.6, and 23.7 at 3 months after surgery. Consolidation of the osteotomy is now complete in both anteroposterior and lateral views. Touch weight bearing was permitted from postoperative day 1

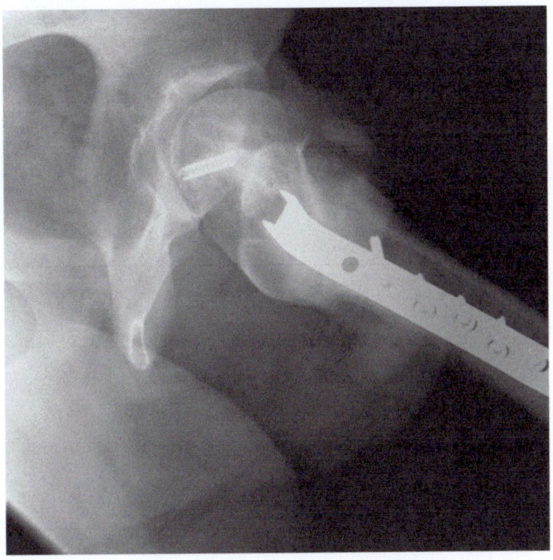

Fig. 23.9 Lateral view of same patient as noted in Figs. 23.5, 23.6, 23.7, and 23.8. The metaphyseal bump has been moved well away from the margin of the acetabulum and impingement has been relieved. By careful positioning of the blade plate, there has been little translational deformity and this hip should be amenable to total hip arthroplasty in due course hopefully, with only limited difficulties for the arthroplasty surgeon

Pearls and Pitfalls

- Plan twice; cut once.
- Use strong implants with the tip of the blade plate in the calcar.
- Have locking plates available in case fixation with a blade plate proves suboptimal (Fig. 23.10).
- The site of correction is centred in the femoral neck, not the femoral head, to avoid transla-

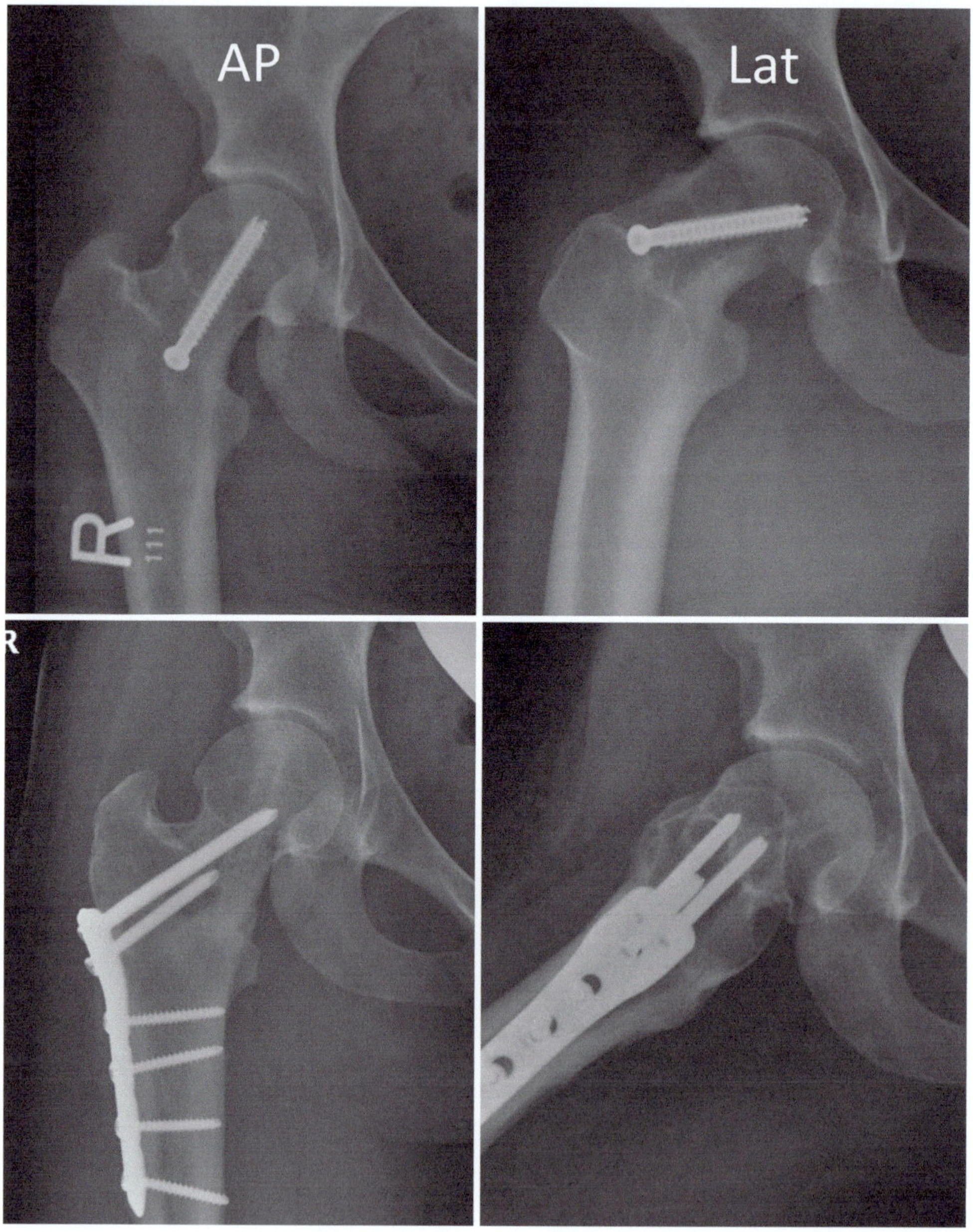

Fig. 23.10 Pre- and postoperative anteroposterior and lateral radiographs of a right hip following flexion-valgus intertrochanteric osteotomy, for moderate extension deformity following in situ pinning of right slipped capital femoral epiphysis. A 120° locking plate provides excellent stability and allows near anatomic correction, including lateral translation of the femoral shaft, thus restoring mechanical axis which may facilitate subsequent total hip arthroplasty. The locking plate is a good method of fixation in this patient population

tional deformity and making greater difficulties for future arthroplasty surgery.

- The deformity in the proximal femur is three-dimensional.
- The gait disturbance is three-dimensional.
- Deformity correction is planned in two dimensions (sagittal/flexion and coronal/valgus).
- The third dimension, rotation, takes care of itself, in most children and adolescents. In a few patients, some additional internal rotation is required.
- A flexion osteotomy has its greatest impact in the transverse plane, increasing internal rotation.
- FVIT is very effective in moving the impingement lesion away from contact with the anterior and lateral acetabulum in most hips. However, this is not always complete, and therefore some surgeons prefer a surgical hip dislocation (SHD) to assess impingement at the time of FVIT. This permits surgical treatment of labral lesions or persistent impingement at the time of the FVIT.
- Impingement can also be dealt with by an anterior approach to the hip at the time of FVIT [2].
- If this opportunity has been missed, some patients may benefit from arthroscopic surgery at the time of removal of the blade plate. What's good for the hip is good for gait, and vice-versa.

Indications and Contraindications (Table 23.1)

Table 23.1 Flexion-valgus intertrochanteric osteotomy for late slipped capital femoral epiphysis deformity: surgical indications and contraindications

Indications
Symptomatic, moderate to severe slipped capital femoral epiphysis: lateral slip angle 30–80°
Post physeal closure and before degenerative arthritis
Good general health
Contraindications
Avascular necrosis
Degenerative arthritis with arthroplasty needed within 5 years
Smoking
Morbid obesity
Poorly controlled diabetes and metabolic syndrome

References

1. Rab G. The geometry of slipped capital femoral epiphysis: implications for movement, impingement, and corrective surgery. J Pediatr Orthop. 1999;19(4):419–24.
2. Bali NS, Harrison JO, Bache CE. A modified Imhäuser osteotomy. An assessment of the addition of an open femoral neck osteoplasty. Bone Joint J. 2014;96-B(8):1119–23.

Suggested Readings

Mac Lean SB, Evans S, O'Hara JN. A comparison of reversed locking compression-distal femoral plates and blade plates in osteotomies for young adult hip pathology. Hip Int. 2013;23(6):565–9.

Sangeux M, Passmore E, Gomez G, Balakumar J, Graham HK. Slipped capital femoral epiphysis, fixation by single screw in situ: a kinematic and radiographic study. Clin Biomech (Bristol, Avon). 2014;29(5):523–30.

Schai PA, Exner GU, Hänsch O. Prevention of secondary coxarthrosis in slipped capital femoral epiphysis: a long-term follow-up study after corrective intertrochanteric osteotomy. J Pediatr Orthop. 1996;5(3):135–43.

24 Combined Osteotomy and Osteoplasty for Healed Slipped Capital Femoral Epiphysis (SCFE) Deformity

Neil Saran

Introduction

Healed deformity of slipped capital femoral epiphysis (SCFE) is known to be associated with acetabular labral and chondral pathology that results in early osteoarthritis of the hip. Furthermore, the metaphyseal bump in addition to proximal femoral anatomy can cause alterations in range of motion of the hip that precludes participation in various activities including some activities of daily living. While mild slips can be treated effectively with a femoral head-neck junction reshaping, moderate to severe deformities require treatment of both the metaphyseal bump (cam lesion) and a proximal femoral intertrochanteric/subtrochanteric osteotomy to further eliminate femoroacetabular impingement and provide a more functional range of motion.

Brief Clinical History

This 14-year 9-month-old male presented with a 9-month history of left groin pain. He had been having difficulty playing sports and would limp for up to a day after gym class. He was treated for a stable SCFE 1.5 years earlier with an in situ pinning. Examination revealed a normal gait and no Trendelenburg sign. He had 90° of flexion, 20° of obligate external rotation at 90° of hip flexion, 80° of external rotation, and 10° of abduction of the left hip compared to 120° of flexion, 30° of internal rotation, 50° of external rotation, and 35° of abduction on the other side. He had groin pain on flexion, adduction, and internal rotation of the hip. Radiographs revealed a cam lesion of the proximal femur along with the typical findings of a moderate slip including coxa vara, decreased articulotrochanteric distance, and femoral head retroversion. It was decided that in order to alleviate the impingement and to improve range of motion, a cam resection and femoral osteotomy were required.

Preoperative Imaging (Fig. 24.1)

N. Saran
Department of Orthopaedic Surgery, Shriners Hospital for Children Canada, Montreal, QC, Canada

Department of Paediatric Surgery, The Montreal Children's Hospital, Montreal, QC, Canada

Division of Orthopaedic Surgery, Department of Surgery McGill University, Montreal, QC, Canada
e-mail: neil.saran@mcgill.ca

R. C. Hamdy, N. Saran (eds.), *Pediatric Pelvic and Proximal Femoral Osteotomies*,
https://doi.org/10.1007/978-3-319-78033-7_24

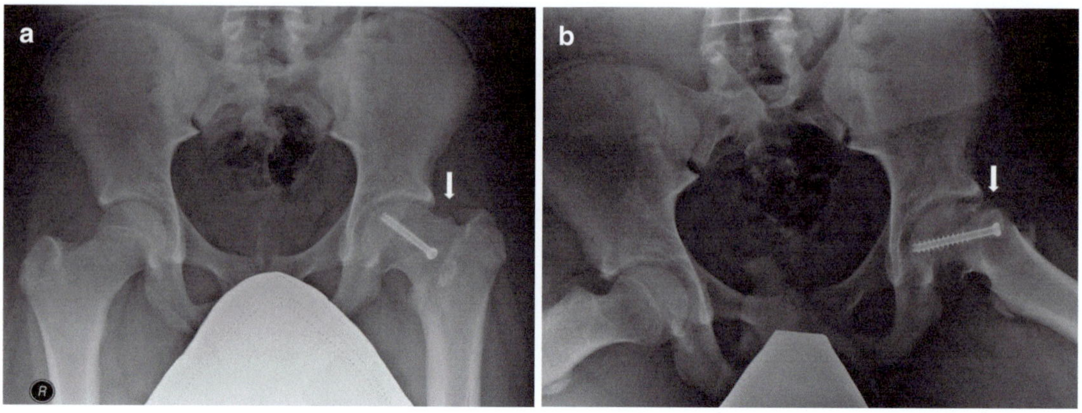

Fig. 24.1 (**a**) Anteroposterior radiograph showing a healed slipped capital femoral epiphysis of the left hip previously treated with an in situ pin. The left hip has a decreased neck shaft angle (110°), decreased articulotrochanteric distance, and a lateral metaphyseal bump (*white arrow*). (**b**) The frog-lateral pelvis X-ray shows 40° of femoral head retroversion and a large anterior metaphyseal bump (*white arrow*) at the femoral head-neck junction that is limiting hip flexion

Goals of Treatment

The principles of treatment include:

Removal of the cam lesion ± labral repair
Improving hip ROM (>100° flexion and >20° of internal rotation)

Treatment Strategy

The treatment strategy consists of treating the impingement and deformity using a femoral head vascular-friendly approach. The surgical hip dislocation [1] allows for a safe approach to the hip and treatment of the femoral cam lesion as well as any labral pathology that may be identified at the time of dislocation. Other options include anterior arthrotomy without dislocation and arthroscopic techniques to remove the bump although if one of these other approaches is utilized, the femoral deformity should be addressed first to facilitate the intra-articular osteoplasty. If after osteoplasty, 100° of flexion and 20° of internal rotation are achieved, then the femoral osteotomy is not performed. If required, the goal of the osteotomy is to improve range of motion by improving the neck shaft angle, articulotrochanteric distance, femoral retroversion, and rotation of the hip.

Surgical Details

Surgical Hip Dislocation

Setup An epidural catheter is placed at the beginning of the case with the catheter taped up towards the contralateral shoulder. A Foley catheter is placed. The patient is positioned in the lateral decubitus position using a bean bag, axillary roll, and well-padded arm holder. The hip and leg are prepped up to the costal margin.

Approach A 20 cm straight incision centered on the greater trochanter is made with the hip flexed 30° (Fig. 24.2). This may need to be extended an additional 5 cm distally for the femoral osteotomy. The iliotibial band and gluteus maximus fibers are split at the midsagittal level along the length of the incision.
The trochanteric bursa is incised at the level of the trochanter and reflected posteriorly. The obturator internus and piriformis tendons are identified. The gluteus medius is located and retracted anterosuperiorly. Doing so will uncover the gluteus minimus muscle.

The inferior edge of the gluteus minimus is typically located deep to the piriformis tendon, and therefore, the piriformis is gently retracted distally allowing identification of the inferior

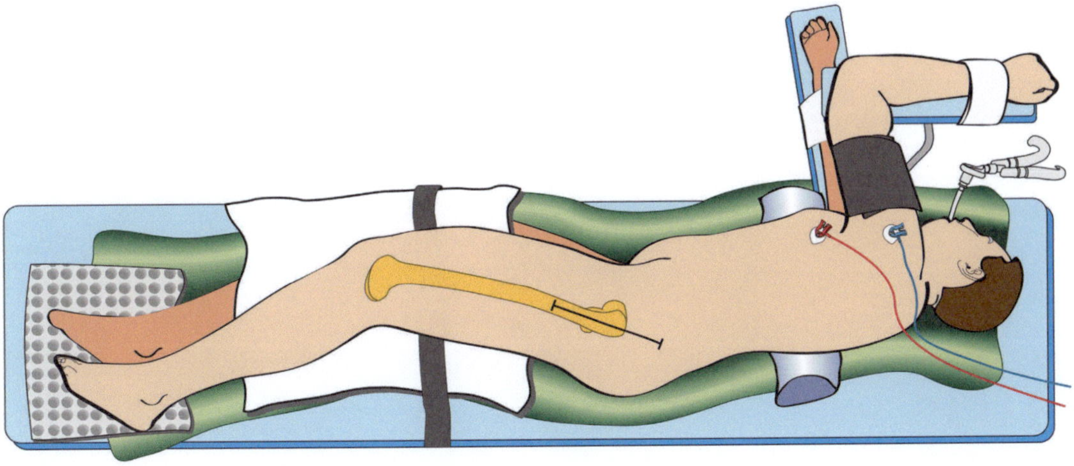

Fig. 24.2 The patient is positioned in the lateral decubitus position with a full-length bean bag holding the patient stable. Other forms of positioners can be used. The incision is typically 15 cm in length centered over the tip of the greater trochanter

edge of the muscle. A Cobb elevator is used to elevate the muscle proximally off the hip capsule. The elevator is replaced with an L-shaped retractor. The superior edge of the piriformis tendon is traced up toward its attachment on the greater trochanter in order to gage the level of the trochanteric osteotomy. Starting anterior to the gluteus maximus insertion on the femur, the vastus lateralis is reflected anteriorly leaving its origin attached to the greater trochanter and is retracted with a Hohmann retractor (Fig. 24.3a).

Trochanteric Osteotomy The trochanteric osteotomy is then marked. It should be large enough for ease of reattachment; however, it should not create a notch in the femur distally, and the piriformis should remain with the stable trochanter. The depth of this cut is typically around 1.5 cm from the lateral aspect of the trochanter. The piriformis insertion on the greater trochanter helps to guide the depth of this cut. The exact insertion point cannot be visualized; however, following the tendon toward the insertion prevents an excessive osteotomy which will jeopardize femoral ahead vascularity. The direction of this osteotomy is from posterior to anterior using the tibia as a guide for direction when the knee is flexed to 90°. The osteotomy is performed with an oscillating saw and can be completed with an osteotome. Often, the piriformis tendon is partially attached to the osteotomized trochanter which is acceptable so long as the tendon is still also attached to the stable trochanter.

Exposure of the Hip Capsule The trochanter is then flipped anteriorly along with the vastus lateralis and gluteus medius and minimus muscles that are attached to it. If the piriformis is partially attached to the trochanter, the fibers are released. Bone wax is applied to the bed of the stable trochanter to prevent it from bleeding throughout the surgery. The remaining attachments of the vastus on the stable trochanter are then released off the femur, and the remaining attachments of the gluteus medius and minimus on the stable trochanter are released off of the hip capsule. The gluteus-vastus sling is then retracted anteriorly, and the gluteal muscles and iliocapsularis are dissected off the hip capsule using a Cobb elevator. The hip will need to be flexed, abducted, and externally rotated to allow the dissection to be carried medially enough to allow for full exposure of the hip capsule. Once the dissection is carried 2 cm past the acetabular rim, short-tipped pointed Hohmanns are hammered into the supra-acetabular bone to act as self-retainers (Fig. 24.3b).

Capsulotomy and Dislocation A Z-shaped capsulotomy is then performed starting with

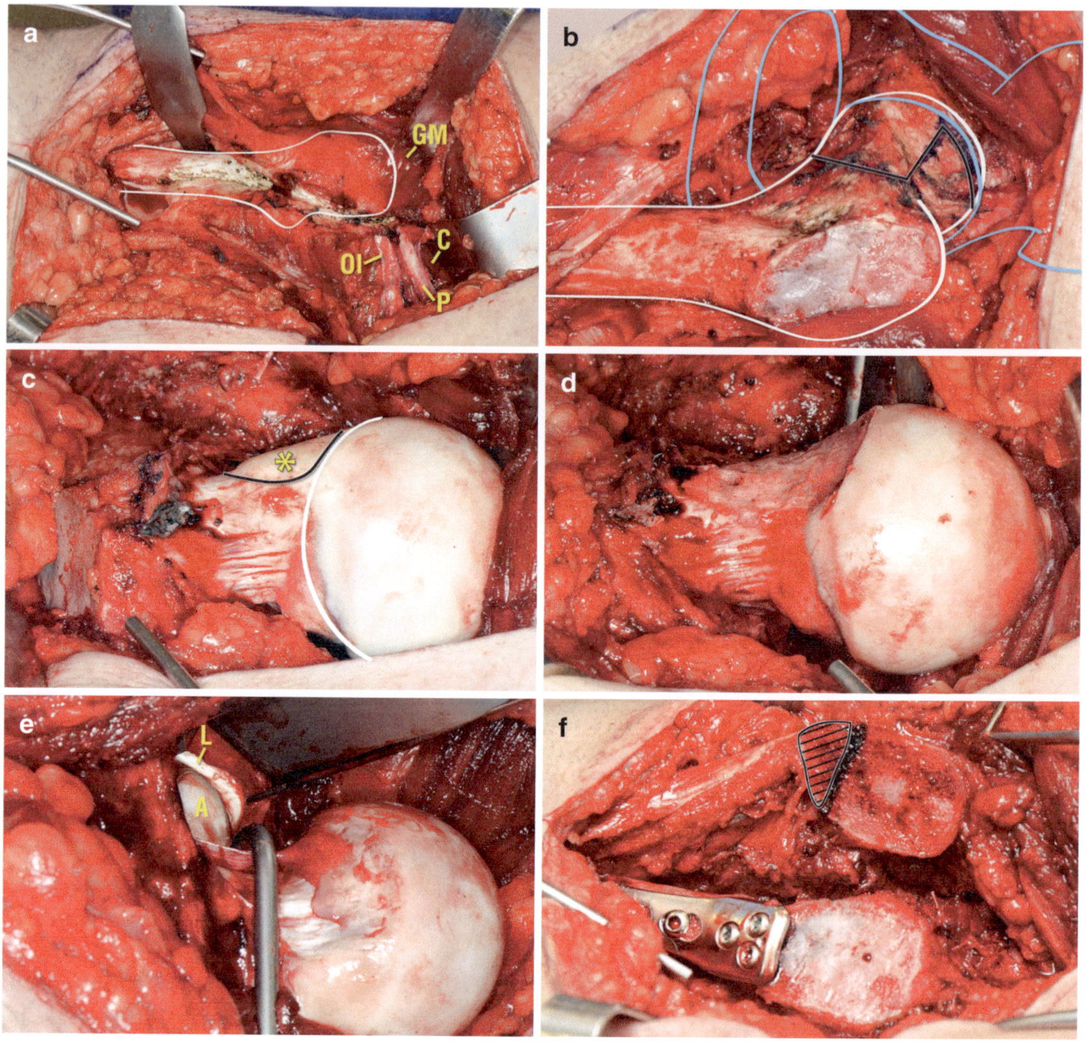

Fig. 24.3 (**a**) Once the piriformis tendon (P) has been traced back toward its insertion on the greater trochanter, the gluteus minimus has been lifted off the hip capsule (C), and the vastus lateralis has been subperiosteally elevated, the trochanter is ready to be osteotomized (*OI* obturator internus, *GM* gluteus maximus). (**b**) The abductor-vastus sling along with the trochanter has been dissected off the hip capsule, and the Z-shaped capsulotomy is planned. The vertical limb is made first avoiding injury to the labrum. This is followed by the inferior limb leaving a cuff for reattachment. The posterior limb is performed last and is made just distal to the labrum leaving a small cuff of capsule for later reattachment. (*White lines represent femoral outline. Blue lines represent pelvic outline including the acetabulum.*) (**c**) The femoral head-neck junction osteoplasty of the cam lesion (asterisk) is marked (*black line*). (**d**) Spherical contouring of the head-neck junction is established. (**e**) The acetabular cartilage (A) can be assessed, and the labrum (L) can be assessed for tears or detachment. The labrum can be reinserted onto the acetabular rim if necessary. (**f**) In this case, the plate was encroaching onto the stable trochanter, and the distal 1 cm of the trochanter had to be resected prior to reattachment

the vertical limb along the anterosuperior aspect of the femoral neck. The inferior limb of the Z-capsulotomy is then incised leaving a 5–10 mm cuff of capsule along the intertrochanteric ridge to the depth of the lesser trochanter. The vertical limb is then completed ensuring that the labrum is not accidentally incised. The posterosuperior limb is incised leaving a 5 mm cuff following the labrum posteriorly to the level of the piriformis tendon. The hip is distracted by placing a bone hook around the neck and applying traction on the leg. Large curved scissors are placed into the anterior acetabulum and used to palpate the ligamentum teres which is incised. Sometimes, the hip needs to be placed in flexion and external rotation in order to enable incision of the ligamentum teres. This can be very difficult in cases of severe slips.

The hip is then dislocated anteriorly (flexion, external rotation), and the leg is placed in a pouch. The ligamentum teres is excised as it may impede reduction of the femoral head into the acetabulum.

Osteoplasty The osteoplasty is performed by resecting the anterolateral cam leaving a spherical femoral head (Fig. 24.3c, d). Femoral head templates can be used to ensure that the cam is resected fully although are not absolutely necessary. The resection must be limited to <30% of the femoral neck width to decrease the risk of femoral neck fracture. The labrum and acetabulum are then inspected to assess for labral and chondral damage (Fig. 24.3e). If the labrum is fully detached, a repair can be performed. The acetabulum is irrigated to remove and debris, and the hip is reduced. The hip is then put through a range of motion assessing for cam impingement. Additional osteoplasty can be performed if necessary.

Flexion and internal rotation at 90° of hip flexion are then measured with the hip in neutral adduction. If flexion is <100° and internal rotation is <20°, a femoral osteotomy is performed. The hip capsule is then repaired with multiple interrupted sutures using a 0-0 Vicryl suture. The hip range of motion is then verified, and the decision to proceed with the femoral osteotomy is made. If there is adequate range of motion, the stable trochanter is roughened up to disrupt the bone wax applied, and the flipped trochanter is reduced and fixed with two 4.5 mm cortical screws.

Femoral Osteotomy

If required, the skin incision is extended distally by ~5 cm, the iliotibial band is split, and the vastus is reflected anteriorly. The goal is to add a minimal amount of flexion to enable 100–110° of flexion and to derotate the femur to achieve 20–40° of internal rotation. Valgusization can be built in to normalize the articulotrochanteric distance if abduction is limited preoperatively. Care must be taken to ensure that the piriformis fossa and femoral diaphysis relationship remains similar. As such, templating is strongly recommended. Furthermore, templating will allow for a decision of whether or not the implant will be placed through the trochanter or distal to it. If the implant will be placed through the trochanter, the trochanter should be temporarily stabilized with thread K-wires. If not, it will be fixed after the femoral osteotomy has been completed with two 4.5 mm cortical screws. The flexion should be limited to 30–40°. Additional flexion will result in excessive translation at the osteotomy site and minimal bone contact for healing. Furthermore, a large amount of flexion and/or valgus may complicate future total hip arthroplasty. The amount of derotation to be performed is based on the amount of internal rotation a patient has at 90° of flexion and neutral adduction after the cam resection has been performed. While neutral anteversion (~symmetric internal and external rotation) is desired, a minimum of 20° of internal rotation is required once the osteotomy is complete. In order to facilitate precise derotation, two large (3.2 mm) K-wires are inserted into the femur (one into the proximal femur and one into the distal femur at the level of the knee). The entry point for the blade plate or locking plate guidewire must be located at the midsagittal aspect of the femur. Cheating anteriorly will result in a larger amount of translation. Cheating posteriorly will create a piriformis fossa-diaphysis mismatch. In the case that the implant is placed at the distal edge of the trochanteric osteotomy, the distal portion of the trochanter may need to be resected prior to fixation (Fig. 24.3f).

Postoperative Imaging (Fig. 24.4)

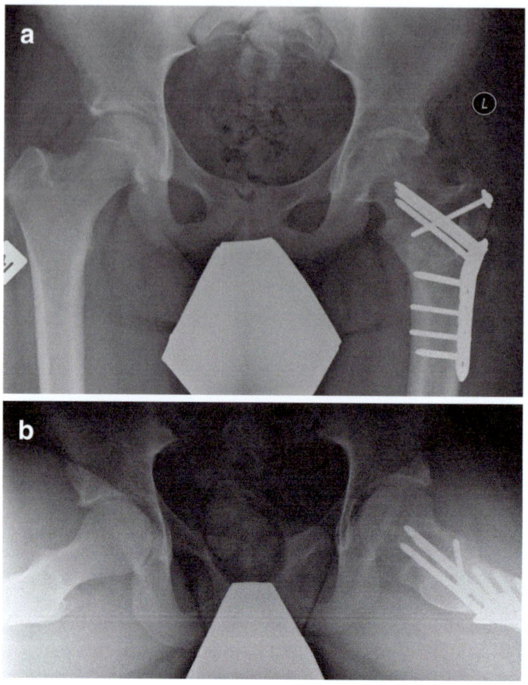

Fig. 24.4 (**a**) 12 months after an osteoplasty using the surgical hip dislocation technique and a 20° flexion, 35° internal rotation, and 25° valgus proximal femoral osteotomy, the anteroposterior pelvis radiograph show restoration of the neck shaft angle and articulotrochanteric distance. (**b**) Frog-lateral pelvis radiograph showing restoration of the femoral head version and elimination of the cam lesion at the femoral head-neck junction. The patient returned to sports with no further episodes of pain. At his 2-year follow-up, he remains asymptomatic and has 110° of hip flexion, 30° of hip abduction, 25° of internal rotation, and 50° of external rotation

Pearls and Pitfalls

- A major pitfall in treating SCFE is to attempt to correct the Southwick or posterior sloping angle completely through a flexion osteotomy. Flexion must be limited to less than 40° in order to minimize translation and maintain at least 50% bone contact at the osteotomy site.
- Ideally, the smallest amount of flexion needed should be performed, as a flexion osteotomy will deform the proximal femur resulting in a more challenging total hip arthroplasty in the future. Often, rotational correction can decrease the amount of flexion required. Also, be aware of how derotation will affect flexion and valgus. Flexion planned prior to the derotation can result in a combination of flexion and valgus. Similarly valgusization planned prior to the derotation can actually result in a combination of valgus and extension. As such, if a large amount of derotation is planned, any valgus should be limited if flexion is added to the correction.
- Valgus correction must be performed such that the mechanical axis of the lower limb is not affected. As such, careful lateralization should be planned to not disturb the relationship between the piriformis fossa and the femoral diaphysis.

Indications and Contraindications (Table 24.1)

Table 24.1 Combined osteotomy and osteoplasty for healed slipped capital femoral epiphysis deformity: surgical indications and contraindications

Indications
Moderate and severe healed slips with clinical signs of impingement
Relative contraindications
Slip angles >70°
Hip flexion >100° hip flexion and internal rotation >20° (may suffice with cam resection ± labral repair without osteotomy)
Contraindications
Tönnis 2 or greater changes to hip joint

Reference

1. Ganz R, Gill TJ, Gautier E, Ganz K, Krügel N, Berlemann U. Surgical dislocation of the adult hip a technique with full access to the femoral head and acetabulum without the risk of avascular necrosis. J Bone Joint Surg Br. 2001;83(8):1119–24.

25 Modified Dunn Procedure for Unstable Slipped Capital Femoral Epiphysis

Eduardo N. Novais and Young-Jo Kim

Introduction

The goals of unstable slipped capital femoral epiphysis (SCFE) treatment include preventing further slippage of the epiphysis, avoiding the occurrence of osteonecrosis, and restoring hip function. Although the etiology of osteonecrosis after unstable SCFE remains unsolved, injury to the retinacular nutrient vessels, increased intracapsular pressure secondary to hematoma, and kinking of the vessels have been described. The method of surgical treatment including the time to reduction has also been reported to influence the outcomes of unstable SCFE treatment. The modified Dunn subcapital realignment using the surgical dislocation approach and dissection of the retinacular flap supplying the femoral head is one alternative to the treatment of unstable SCFE. The dissection of the extended retinacular flap allows assessment and protection of the vessels that supply the femoral head.

E. N. Novais (✉) · Y.-J. Kim
Department of Orthopedic Surgery,
Boston Children's Hospital, Boston, MA, USA
e-mail: eduardo.novais@childrens.harvard.edu; young-jo.kim@childrens.harvard.edu

Brief Clinical History

This 12-year-old female presented to the emergency department with a history of fall while playing in school. She had been having some hip discomfort for the previous month without limping. Immediately after falling, she was found to have severe pain, and she was unable to stand to walk. Physical examination revealed the left lower extremity positioned in extension and external rotation with excruciating pain with any attempt to mobilize the left hip. Radiographs revealed a completely displaced SCFE.

Preoperative Imaging (Fig. 25.1)

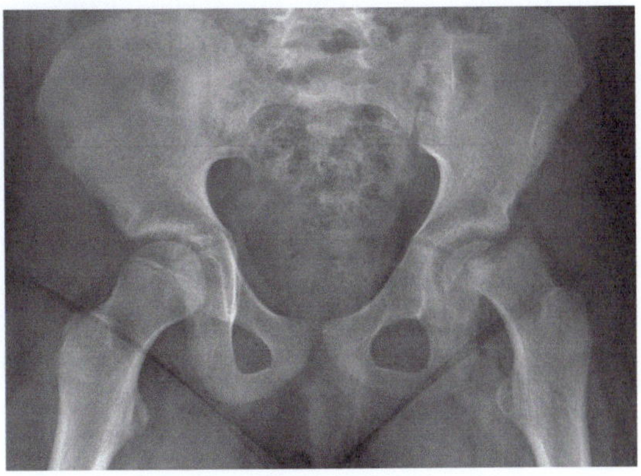

Fig. 25.1 Preoperative anteroposterior pelvic radiograph showing completely displaced slipped capital femoral epiphysis of the left hip. A lateral radiograph was not obtained due to excessive pain

R. C. Hamdy, N. Saran (eds.), *Pediatric Pelvic and Proximal Femoral Osteotomies*,
https://doi.org/10.1007/978-3-319-78033-7_25

Goals of Treatment

1. Realignment of the femoral epiphysis
2. Dissection of the retinacular flap containing the nutrient vessels and intraoperative assessment of femoral head perfusion
3. Resection of the posterior callus and anatomic fixation of the epiphysis

The treatment strategy consists of realigning the completely displaced epiphysis using the surgical hip dislocation approach [1] with dissection of the retinacular flap containing the nutrient vessels to the femoral head [2]. The modified Dunn procedure has been well described previously [3, 4]; however, other options for treatment include in situ fixation with or without a capsulotomy and open reduction through an anterolateral approach.

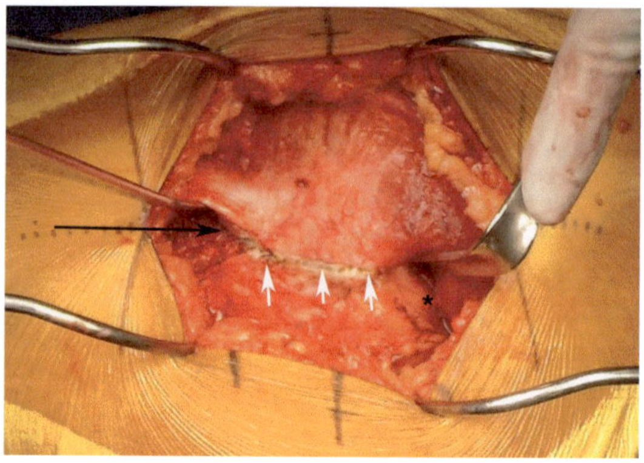

Fig. 25.2 A Hohmann retractor is placed under the vastus lateralis to facilitate the trochanteric osteotomy (*black arrow*). A line between the posterior edge of the vastus lateralis and the insertion of the gluteus medius in the greater trochanter is marked with a cautery (*white arrows*). A Langenbeck retractor is placed under the gluteus minimus exposing the piriformis tendon (*)

Surgical Details

Surgical Hip Dislocation

The patient is positioned in a lateral decubitus on a radiolucent pegboard table with all bony prominences protected with gel pads. An axillary roll should be placed under the contralateral axilla.

A lateral incision is performed longitudinally in the top of the greater trochanter, measuring approximately 15–20 cm. The subcutaneous tissue is dissected and the fascia lata identified and split longitudinally in line with the skin incision. The interval between the gluteus maximus and tensor is developed, and the fibers of the gluteus maximus are retracted posteriorly.

The piriformis tendon is identified, and the interval between the piriformis and the minimus is opened to expose the hip capsule proximally. Distally the vastus lateralis fascia is opened, and the muscle belly is dissected from the femur extraperiosteally in a posterior to anterior fashion.

A Hohmann retractor is placed under the vastus lateralis to facilitate the trochanteric osteotomy. A line between the posterior edge of the vastus lateralis and the insertion of the gluteus medius in the greater trochanter is marked with a cautery (Fig. 25.2). A trochanteric osteotomy is performed with an oscillating saw leaving a free trochanter piece that is at least approximately 1.5 cm wide. The piriformis tendon is preserved intact in the stable segment of the trochanter. The segment of the trochanter is flipped anteriorly, and the entire hip capsule is exposed.

A capsulotomy is performed using an inside out technique. The capsulotomy starts at the anterolateral corner of the stable trochanter along the femoral neck axis moving proximally until the labrum is identified. There is typically bleeding that represents the hematoma being evacuated from the capsule. The capsulotomy is extended by cutting the capsule anteriorly and distally toward the anterior-inferior aspect of the acetabulum. Finally, a posterior limb of the capsulotomy is added from the acetabular rim aiming toward the piriformis tendon. The final capsulotomy has a Z shape for the right hip and an inverted Z shape for the left hip (Fig. 25.3).

The femoral neck metaphysis is identified and instability of the capital epiphysis typically noticed. In unstable SCFE the anterior periosteum is torn and the neck displaced anteriorly. We note whether the retinacular insertion in the femoral head is preserved. The epiphysis is fixed temporarily in situ with two (2.4 mm) threaded Kirschner wires to prevent further displacement.

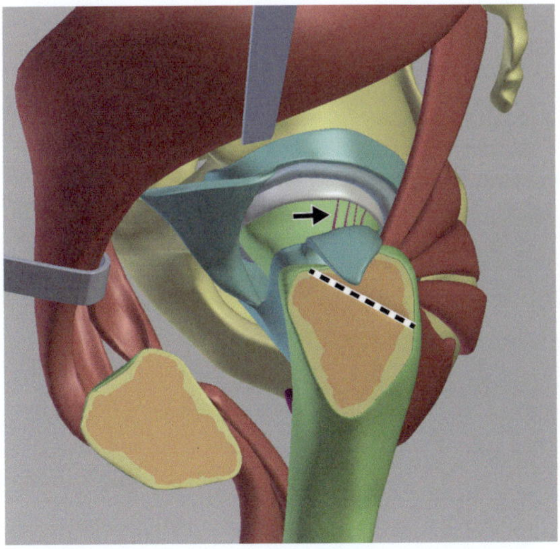

Fig. 25.3 The femoral head and neck are exposed after performing the Z-shaped capsulotomy. The vasculature to the femoral epiphysis is depicted (*black arrow*) traveling in the periosteum (*green*) of the femoral neck. Note that these are not clinically visible

The femur is partially dislocated from the acetabulum anteriorly by flexing the hip in external rotation. The ligamentum teres is resected to allow for a complete dislocation, and the acetabulum is inspected for assessment of chondral or labral injury.

Extended Retinacular Flap

A small smooth Kirschner wire (1.6 mm) is used to create a hole in the femoral head. Femoral head perfusion is monitored by observation of direct bleeding and by insertion of an intracranial pressure (ICP) probe that is connected to an ICP monitor (Fig. 25.4).

The hip is reduced, and we start to develop a periosteal sleeve around the stable trochanter and femoral neck (Fig. 25.5). We first dissect the periosteum from the anterior aspect of the femoral neck moving proximally around the greater trochanter and distally in the lateral aspect of the femoral shaft. The periosteum is opened with a knife and by a delicate periosteum elevator. In younger patients with thick periosteum, it is possible to remove the proximal aspect of the stable trochanter in one piece (see Fig. 25.5b, c). However, in adolescents we prefer to remove the proximal piece of the trochanter using a rongeur and a piecemeal technique. The posteromedial periosteum is released to the level of the lesser trochanter—approximately 4 cm distal from the greater trochanter. The femoral head is again dislocated, and the entire femoral neck is exposed after the periosteal sleeve is carefully developed anteromedially (Fig. 25.5d).

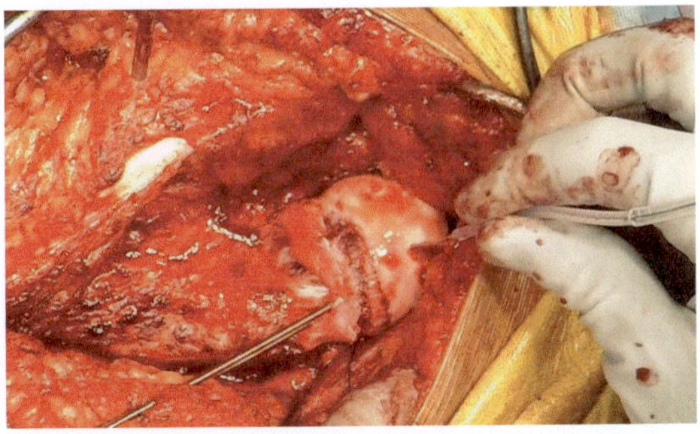

Fig. 25.4 Once the femoral head has been dislocated, the perfusion is checked by observation of active bleeding and by insertion of an intracranial pressure monitor probe

Subcapital Realignment

The two Kirschner wires are removed, and the femoral head can be displaced from the neck. A sponge is placed in the acetabulum to avoid inadvertent reduction of the femoral head into the acetabulum. A retractor is placed under the femoral neck to protect the retinacular flap (Fig. 25.6), and the posterior new bone formation (callus) is removed with a rongeur and a high-speed burr or osteotome. Identifying the native cortex of the femoral neck will help you determine the extent of callus resection. The anteromedial new bone formation is also removed to the level of the original neck. Although shortening of the femoral neck may theoretically reduce the tension on the retinaculum, the femoral neck should not be shortened more than 2–3 mm to avoid reducing the lever arm of the abductor musculature and potential instability postoperatively.

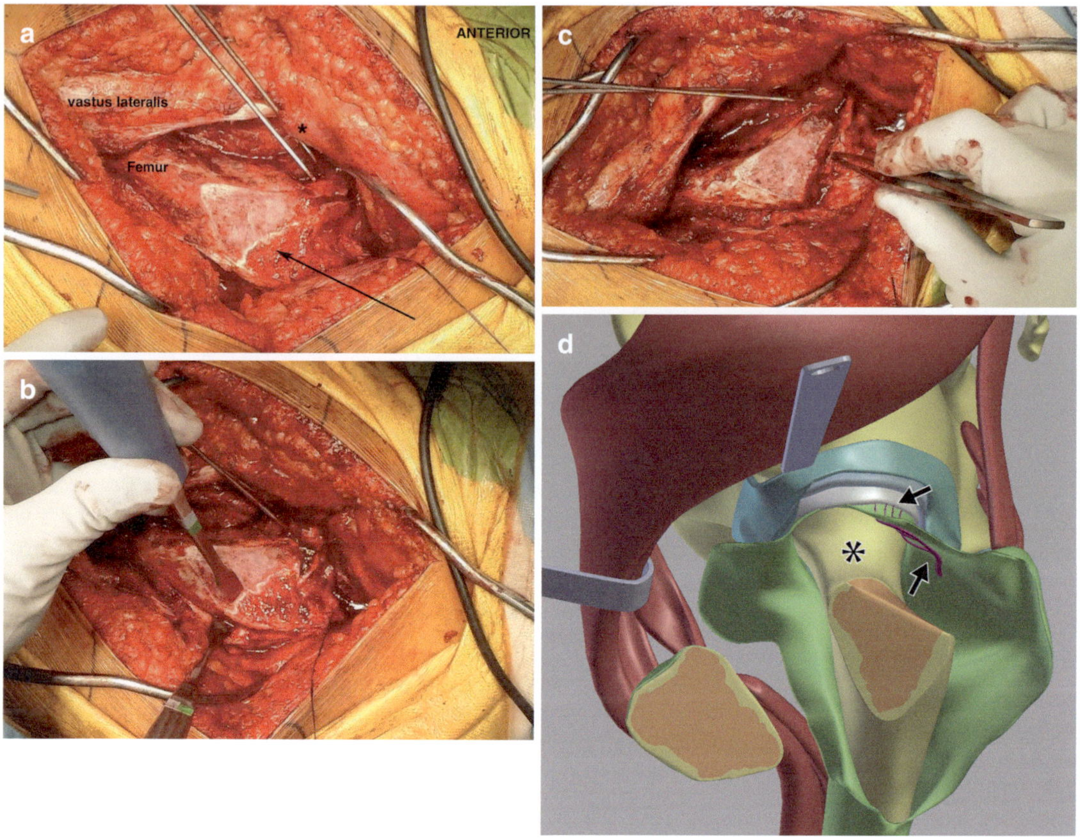

Fig. 25.5 (**a**) The trochanteric osteotomy has been performed. The remaining portion of the greater trochanter is well exposed. The *black arrow* identifies the stable trochanter proximal to the growth plate. There are two pins provisionally fixing the epiphysis (*). (**b**) An osteotomy is created at the level of the greater trochanter growth plate to allow for resection of the proximal portion of the stable trochanter. Note that a Cobb elevator is placed under the periosteum to avoid penetration of the posterior retinacular flap. (**c**) The proximal portion of the stable trochanter has been completely resected subperiosteally, leaving the retinacular flap intact as shown by the tip of the surgeon's forceps. (**d**) The femoral neck (*) is seen with circumferential subperiosteal exposure with a retinacular flap that maintains perfusion to the femoral epiphysis (*black arrows*). Note that the vasculature is traveling in the periosteum at this level and is not clinically seen

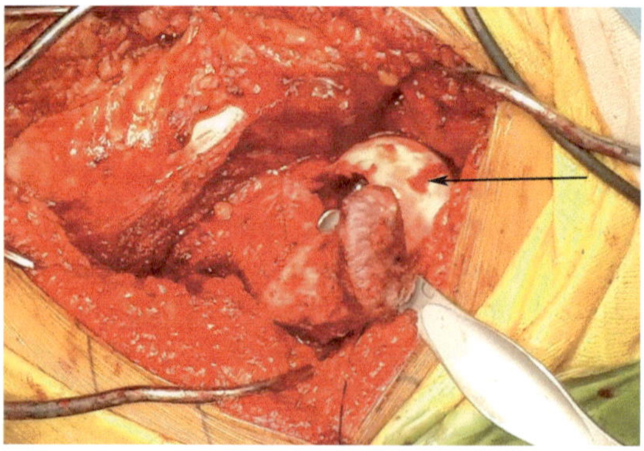

Fig. 25.6 Once the posterior and anterior periosteum has been dissected, the femoral neck is fully exposed. A retractor protects the posterior aspect of the neck to allow for resection of the new bone formation (callus). The femoral head is actively bleeding (*black arrow*)

The femoral head physis is scraped down with a curette to remove the growth plate, and the femoral head is gently reduced to the neck.

During reduction the femoral epiphysis is gently held and reduced on top of the femoral neck with constant attention to the retinacular flap to avoid excessive tension, kinking, and a potential damage (Fig. 25.7). The epiphysis is then fixed to the neck with a retrograde 3.0 mm fully threaded wire introduced through the fovea, aiming just distal to the distal end of the trochanteric osteotomy. One or two additional threaded wires are then introduced in a regular

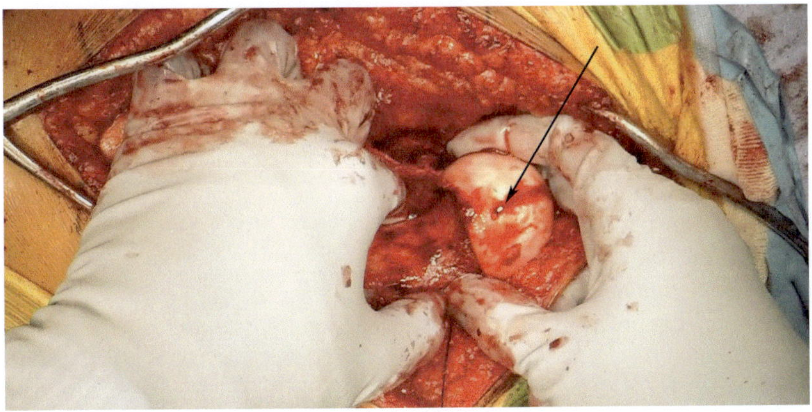

Fig. 25.7 Once the callus formation has been resected from the callus and the cartilage curetted from the epiphysis, the femoral head is carefully manipulated and reduced on top of the femoral neck. The reduction should take into consideration the varus-valgus alignment as well as the version. The femoral head is actively bleeding (*black arrow*)

fashion from the lateral aspect of the femur, aiming toward the center or inferior portion of the femoral head. We avoid placing the wires on the superior and posterior region of the femoral head. The fixation is checked under C-arm guidance to allow adequate spread of the pins in the femoral head.

The hip is then finally reduced, and the ICP monitor is again used to check the femoral head blood flow. If no blood flow is present and the retinaculum is intact, we free the retinaculum further distally, and, if needed, we shorten the neck 1–2 mm further. The periosteal sleeve should be approximated loosely. The hip capsule should also be loosely closed. The trochanteric piece is fixed with two 3.5 mm screws.

Postoperative Management

Postoperatively, patients are protected with an abduction foam pillow for the first 2 weeks and kept in a restricted non-weight-bearing protocol for about 6–8 weeks. Typically, there will be radiographic evidence of healing at 6–8 weeks after surgery, and partial weight bearing is initiated. Patients are released to full weight bearing at 10–12 weeks after surgery.

Postoperative Imaging (Fig. 25.8)

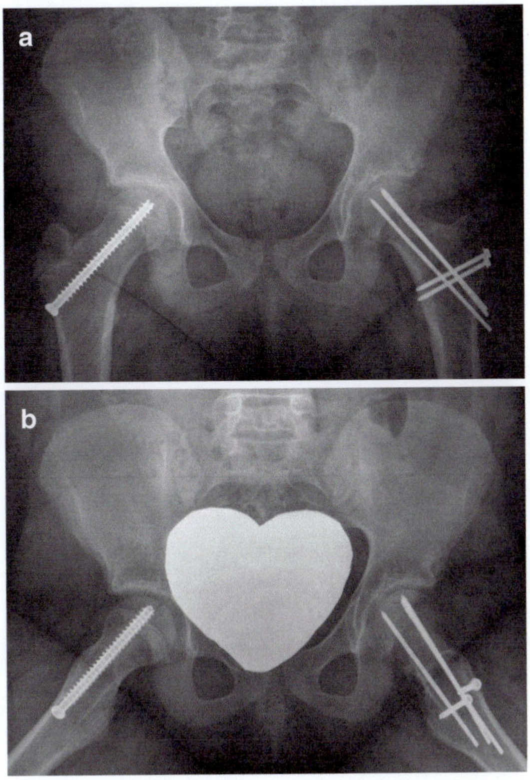

Fig. 25.8 (**a**) Anteroposterior and (**b**) lateral radiographs 2 years after modified Dunn procedure for the treatment of unstable slipped capital femoral epiphysis of the left hip showing restored anatomy of the proximal femur with normal femoral head-neck morphology

Pearls and Pitfalls

- A major pitfall in performing the modified Dunn occurs when performing the release of the stable portion of the greater trochanter and freeing the periosteal flap posteriorly. Careful dissection should be performed especially around the piriformis fossa. Although the trochanter can be resected in one piece, when the periosteum is thick, it is probably safer to use a piecemeal technique.
- Another important point is to avoid excessive tension of the periosteum during and after reduction of the epiphysis. If there is tension, the posterior aspect of the greater trochanter may need to be resected down to the level of the posterior neck.
- Shortening of the neck is not recommended, but if inadvertently performed, then the greater trochanter should be fixed with slight advancement. Shortening of the femoral neck may reduce the lever arm of the abductor musculature and lead to hip instability after surgery. An additional 1–2 mm of shortening is reasonable, however, if there is excessive tension in the retinaculum after reduction of the epiphysis. In these cases, the trochanter should be fixed with slight advancement.
- To ensure adequate bone apposition, it is important to remove the remaining physis cartilage from the epiphysis with a curette.

Indications and Contraindications (Table 25.1)

Table 25.1 Modified Dunn procedure for unstable slipped capital femoral epiphysis (SCFE): Surgical indications and contraindications

The modified Dunn using a surgical dislocation approach is an option for treatment for displaced unstable SCFE that has historically been associated with high rates of osteonecrosis. However, it is unclear at this time whether this technique is able to reduce the proportion of osteonecrosis of unstable SCFE
There is a steep learning curve associated with the procedure, and caution is recommended for the novice surgeon. This procedure should not be indicated in mild cases of stable SCFE

References

1. Ganz R, Gill TJ, Gautier E, Ganz K, Krügel N, Berlemann U. Surgical dislocation of the adult hip a technique with full access to the femoral head and acetabulum without the risk of avascular necrosis. J Bone Joint Surg Br. 2001;83(8):1119–24.
2. Ganz R, Huff TW, Leunig M. Extended retinacular soft-tissue flap for intra-articular hip surgery: surgical technique, indications, and results of application. Instr Course Lect. 2009;58:241–55.
3. Leunig M, Slongo T, Kleinschmidt M, Ganz R. Subcapital correction osteotomy in slipped capital femoral epiphysis by means of surgical hip dislocation. Oper Orthop Traumatol. 2007;19(4):389–410. (Article in English, German).
4. Ziebarth K, Zilkens C, Spencer S, Leunig M, Ganz R, Kim YJ. Capital realignment for moderate and severe SCFE using a modified Dunn procedure. Clin Orthop Relat Res. 2009;467(3):704–16.

Morscher Osteotomy

26

Étienne L. Belzile

Introduction

At this point in this book, the reader shall begin to grasp the key points that may help in the preparation and execution of osteotomies around the hip. Let us now focus the attention on proximal femoral growth disturbances affecting the lateral femoral offset, the femoral neck length, and the overall limb growth. First, a clear definition of femoral growth disturbance will be offered, followed by the description of typical indications for performing a Morscher osteotomy in the context of an open surgical dislocation. A surgical technique will be suggested. The ultimate goal of the surgical treatment must be individualized to address the level and the extent of the proximal femoral growth deformity.

Brief Clinical History

A 16-year-old boy treated for Legg-Calve-Perthes at age 10 with adductor tenotomy and a varus intertrochanteric osteotomy presents with left hip pain and limping. The patient evolved well after implant removal 1 year following his initial surgery. He participated in regular daily activities and in running sports over the preceding few years. He recalls starting to have pain after long periods of standing. He later developed associated lower back pain after running and long days of standing still. He can walk without pain, but his mother notes that he tends to walk with his left leg in external rotation. The patient is comfortable in the sitting position but reports having sharp pains in his left buttock in abduction or external rotation position.

On physical exam, the patient displays a left-sided prolonged weight-bearing limp with a Trendelenburg pelvic tilt. Clinically measured leg length is 2 cm short on the left side. Hip muscle strength is within normal except for a slight abductor weakness. Range of motion of the left hip shows pain free and fluid motion from 0° to 110° of flexion. In the 90° flexed position, internal rotation is limited to 10°, while the external rotation is close to 45°. In full extension, internal rotation is 30°, while the external rotation is accompanied by pain in the 40° position. Pure left hip abduction is less than 30° with a bony end-feel. The anterior hip impingement test is positive and the FABER (flexion, abduction, external rotation) position recreates buttock pain and is limited to a 30 cm knee to table distance.

É. L. Belzile
Department of Orthopaedic Surgery, CHU de Québec-Université Laval, Quebec City, QC, Canada
e-mail: etienne.belzile@mail.chudequebec.ca

R. C. Hamdy, N. Saran (eds.), *Pediatric Pelvic and Proximal Femoral Osteotomies*,
https://doi.org/10.1007/978-3-319-78033-7_26

Preoperative Imaging

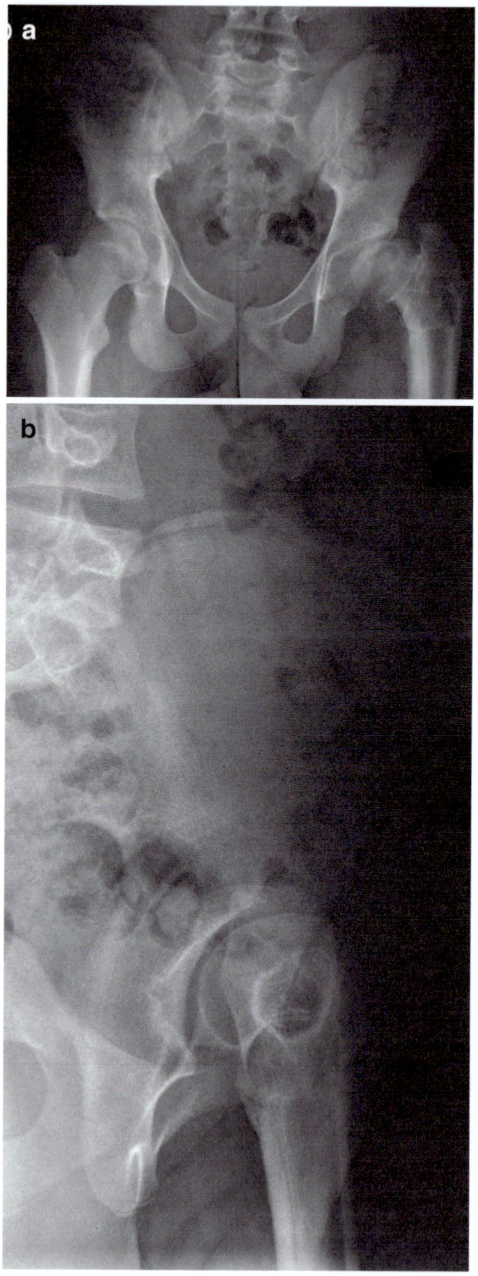

Fig. 26.1 Preoperative radiographs. (**a**) Anteroposterior pelvic standing view. (**b**) Standing false-profile view of the left hip

Radiographic imaging (Fig. 26.1) confirms a growth sequela from the adolescent femoral head osteonecrosis with a typical coxa magna and coxa breva deformity. The hip joint presents a round on flat congruence, with an acetabular index of 24°, a lateral coverage edge angle of 6.5°, an anterior coverage edge angle of −10°, and a head-neck angle of 103°. The greater trochanter is resting in-line and overhanging with respect to the femoral canal of the proximal femur. The joint space remains intact with no signs of hinging on functional views. Measured radiological leg length difference is 1.2 cm short on the left with well-aligned limbs on standing long films (Fig. 26.2).

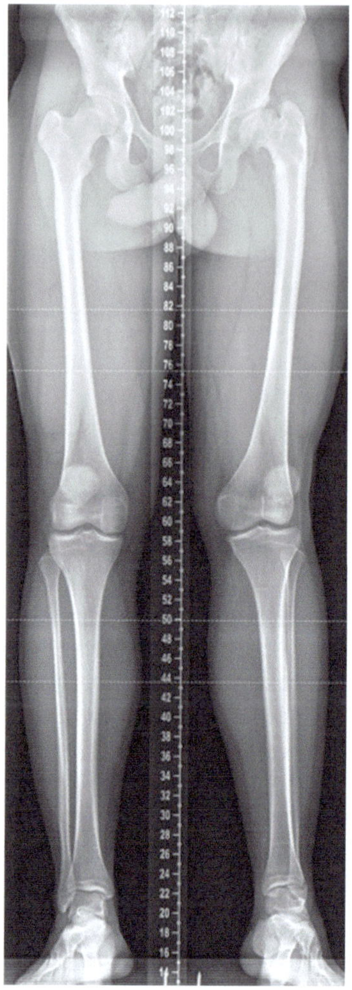

Fig. 26.2 Standing long film. Measured radiological leg length difference is 1.2 cm short on the left with well-aligned limbs

Goals of Treatment

The principles of treatment include:

- Reposition and distalize the greater trochanter.
- Lateralize the femoral shaft.
- Maximize leg length.
- Optimize joint congruence.

Treatment Strategy

The strategy offered by the Morscher osteotomy [1], also known as the true femoral neck lengthening osteotomy, aims at improving the abductor lever arm while increasing leg length. This femoral osteotomy is possible when hip joint congruence, functional hip range of motion, and adequate abductor muscle strength are present simultaneously. Its goals are threefold: (1) Distalize the greater trochanter to diminish pelvi-trochanteric impingement and optimize the abductors' lever arm; (2) lateralize the femoral shaft and truly lengthen the femoral neck to normalize the articulo-trochanteric distance; and (3) lengthen the operated leg. Surgical decision-making is challenging in patients with complex hip morphologic abnormalities. The patient should undergo proper activity modification and/or physical therapy aimed at improving core stability and movement control, with strengthening of hip muscles before considering such a surgical intervention. Maximal muscular recovery may take up to 2 years postoperatively.

Surgical Details

Surgical Hip Dislocation [2]

The patient is positioned in lateral decubitus with the affected leg free, disinfected from the 12th rib to the toes, and draped accordingly. A 20 cm skin incision is made in line with the femoral longitudinal axis, centered on the greater trochanter (GT). The proximal fascia lata is approached longitudinally along the anterior border of the gluteus maximus muscle and distally centered on the femur, for the length required for plate fixation.

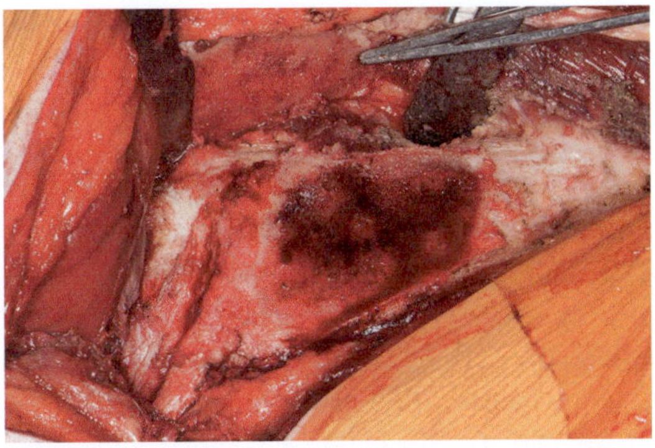

Fig. 26.3 Intraoperative photograph. Flat and trigastric trochanteric osteotomy is elevated anteriorly (with gluteus medius, gluteus minimus, and vastus lateralis attached) to expose the proximal 15 cm of lateral right femur

Gluteus maximus is retracted posteriorly; the approach is developed through the gluteus medius superficial fascial sheath to then expose gluteus medius posterior border and allow proper identification of piriformis and short external rotators. A proximal femoral subvastus approach is developed over a segment of 10–15 cm. Careful and precise dissection will assure protection of the inferior gluteal artery that runs along the piriformis muscle and tendon. The GT slide osteotomy is performed with a trochanteric fragment depth no greater than 1.5 cm and the osteotomy plane parallel to the lower leg (tibia) when the knee is flexed at 90° and the hip is in 20° of internal rotation. The resulting flat and trigastric trochanteric osteotomy is elevated anteriorly (with gluteus medius, gluteus minimus, and vastus lateralis attached) to expose anterior capsule (Fig. 26.3). A Z-shaped capsulotomy can be performed to allow for further intra-articular surgery or femoral head dislocation. Complete dislocation requires sectioning of the ligamentum teres with long curved scissors and the use of a bone hook while mobilizing the femur in external rotation and flexion. Acetabular rim, labrum, and acetabular cartilage are, at this point, fully accessible for treatment.

Relative Neck Lengthening Procedure [3]

A retinacular soft-tissue flap is developed from the superior and posterior corner of the remaining base of the GT in order to peel away the femoral head blood supply. Unlike the typical retinacular flap, this is developed without piecemeal excision of the stable trochanter. The subperiosteal peeling is performed from lateral to medial and from anterior to posterior. The femoral neck lengthening bone graft is then harvested from the excess bone that represents parts of the overgrown GT. The osteotomy must be aligned parallel to the planned intertrochanteric (IT) osteotomy, going from the lateral cortex of the femur, and aimed at the superior head-neck junction but not reaching it. Templating is strongly recommended before this procedure. Since the retinacular flap has been peeled away, the superior neck osteotomy can be safely performed so that a block of bone of at least 1 cm thick can be extracted. This graft will be required to supplement the femoral neck laterally. Before proceeding to the next step, care must be taken to make sure the GT fragment can be freely mobilized away from the iliotibial and gluteus maximus complex, or the anterior hip capsule, as well as distally before fixation (Fig. 26.4).

Morscher Femoral Osteotomy [2]

The first step toward achieving adequate fixation is the optimized positioning of the cephalic fixation (blade plate or locking plate). The initial technique proposed fixation using a 130° blade plate with a long blade of 60–75 mm, allowing medial and proximal sliding of the femoral neck fragment while offering good blade-to-neck contact. Modern-day fixation devices can offer fixed-angle locking screws using a proximal femoral plate. Such locking plates offer the choice of a few angles between 110° and 140°, depending on the manufacturer. Some fixation plates may have weight limitations but may also offer better match for smaller stature proximal femora in the adolescent. Classical technique would dictate aiming for center-to-center pin placement into the neck, but in cases of femoral head growth arrest, the morphology of the head can be aspherical, rendering the target placement more difficult to obtain. Lateral radiographs are taken as the pin placement advances into the neck to avoid intra-articular perforation or pin malposition. Once

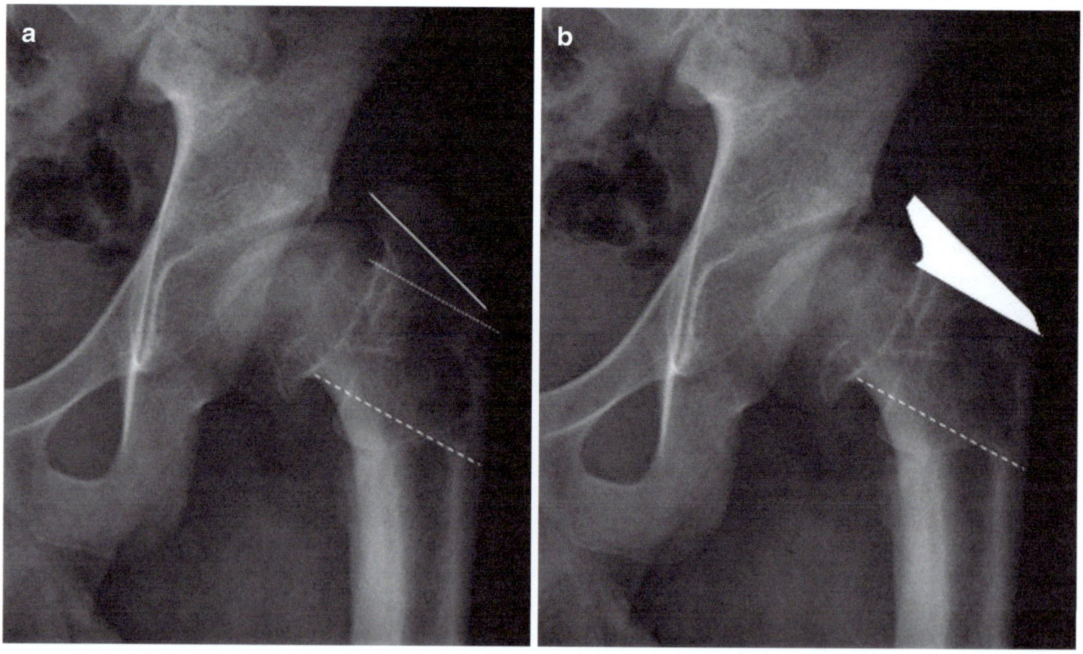

Fig. 26.4 (**a**) Anteroposterior pelvic standing radiograph focused of left hip. The *continuous line* represents the greater trochanter osteotomy; the *dotted line* is the planned neck lengthening; the *dashed line* is the planned IT osteotomy line. (**b**) The highlighted area represents the superior stable trochanteric/femoral neck bone block to be osteotomized after development of the retinacular flap

the optimal pin placement is obtained, the pin is measured for length. To that measurement, one has to add the femoral mediolateral lengthening and the thickness of the GT fragment.

When positioning the chisel, the angle of the flat portion of the blade must remain perpendicular to the long axis of the distal femur to avoid inducing extension or flexion malposition of the distal fragment upon plate reduction to the femoral shaft. Before hammering in the chisel, care must be taken to leave enough of a bony bridge between the blade entry point in the femoral neck and the future site of the IT osteotomy. Certain authors have proposed 1.5 cm, but as few as 1 cm has been used by others (Fig. 26.5). Infra-blade femoral neck fracture rarely leads to catastrophic complication but may render completion of the up-sloping medial translation lengthening procedure more challenging.

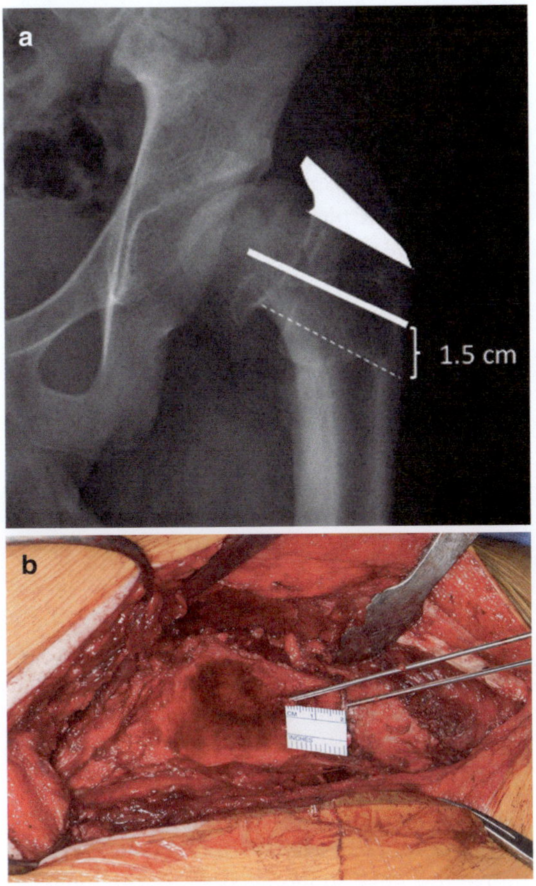

Fig. 26.5 (**a**) Anteroposterior pelvic standing radiograph focused on the left hip. A graphic representation of the blade position is represented by the plain white line. (**b**) Intraoperative photograph of a right hip; parallel K-wires may help defining the ultimate osteotomy position intraoperatively

Finally, the IT osteotomy is designed to be parallel to the cephalic fixation, up-sloping from the lateral femoral cortex to the junction between lower femoral neck and lesser trochanter. This up-sloping is designed to increase leg length as the femoral neck fragment is medialized and the femoral shaft is lateralized. The extent to which the lengthening is possible depends on the up-sloping pitch of the IT osteotomy and the femoral shaft diameter at the level of the lesser trochanter. Before performing the IT osteotomy, placement of K-wires can be useful to predict the osteotomy site and orientation (Fig. 26.6). Longitudinal markings along the anterior femur are recommended to correct for rotational malposition.

After completion of the osteotomy with an oscillating saw using subperiosteal protection anteriorly and posteriorly, calcar periosteum may require further freeing to allow for femoral neck

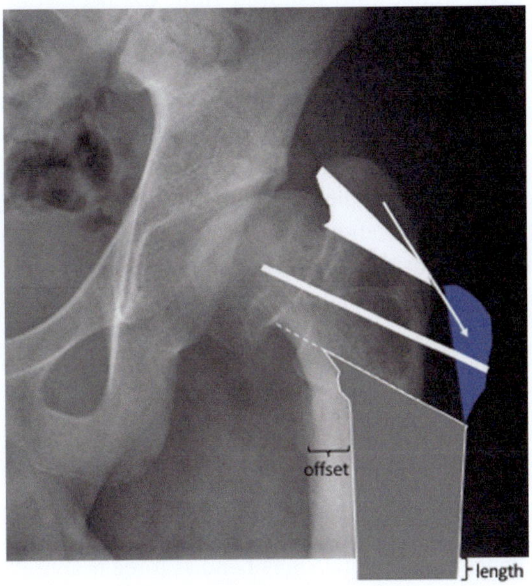

Fig. 26.6 Before performing the IT osteotomy, planning can be useful to predict the osteotomy site and orientation, as well as final distal femoral fragment (*in gray*) and GT (*in blue*) position relative to the implant and IT osteotomy. Increases in lateral offset and leg length can predicted

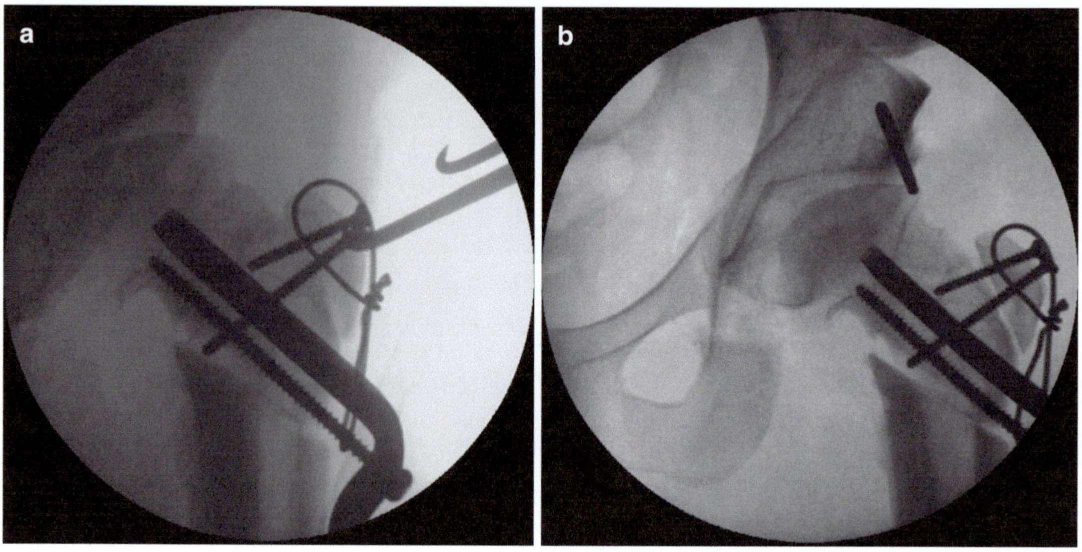

Fig. 26.7 (**a**) Final fixation of the proximal femur. (**b**) Improved hip joint coverage after periacetabular osteotomy

mobilization. The report [2] suggests performing the IT osteotomy from anterior to posterior. The femoral fragment and shaft can be held via a bone reduction clamp or an anteriorly positioned femoral distractor, using Schanz pins in the AP projection. For maximal lengthening effect, no bony wedges are removed from the neck fragment. Upon insertion of the blade plate, the vastus lateralis attachment onto the lateral edge of the GT fragment is partially released for the optional blade plate entry into the GT, followed by perforation through the bone graft before entering into the femoral neck. Once fully reduced and aligned onto the blade, final side plate apposition and fixation to the lateral cortex of the femoral shaft with preferably four bicortical screws is performed. Proper care must be taken to avoid inducing a malrotation of the distal femoral fragment as the side plate is being fixed. Some surgeons may be tempted to use the proximal femoral locking plate as a "joystick" to obtain lateral cortical apposition to the shaft, but some have encountered difficulty in bulkier patients, as the plate may bend as force is applied onto it. Additional proximal to distal compression may be applied to the osteotomy site before final fixation. Autologous bone chips are then inserted deep to the GT fragment or at the IT osteotomy site before vastus closure. The GT is further stabilized with two 4.0 or 4.5 mm cortical screws oriented parallel to each other, on each side of the blade plate, or cephalic locking screws, toward the lesser trochanter. Some may consider additional GT fixation using an Auban-style metal wire looped under the blade plate or proximal locking screws and wrapped through and under the gluteus medium tendon as an anti-proximal migration tension wire during bone healing (Fig. 26.7a).

The surgeon may consider the occasional adductor tendon release or a pie crusting of the fascia lata to release soft-tissue tension before skin closure. Hip joint coverage and congruity need to be assessed after final fixation of the proximal femur, as periacetabular osteotomy or acetabular shelf procedures may be required to improve femoral head coverage. Such complementary procedure could be performed in the same setting or in a staged fashion (Fig. 26.7b). The final position of the GT should not be in line with the femoral shaft to avoid compromising proper eventual femoral stem positioning. At closure, the posterior aponeurosis of the vastus lateralis is closed. The fascia lata and subcutaneous tissue are meticulously closed with running or single sutures, followed by skin.

Postoperative Imaging (Fig. 26.8)

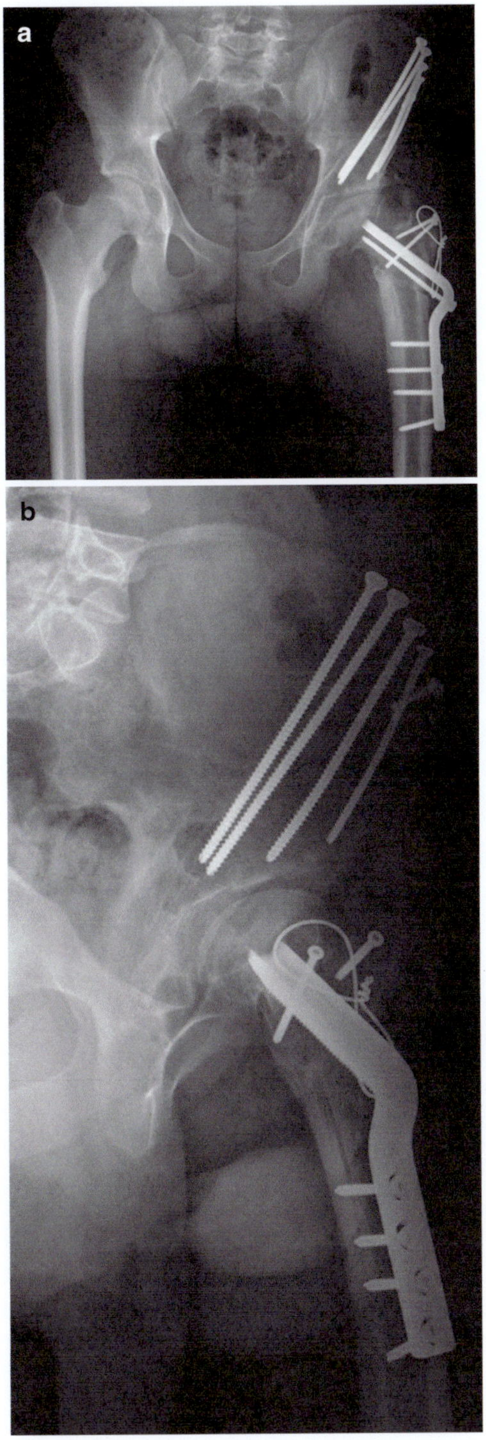

Fig. 26.8 One-year postoperative radiographs. (**a**) Anteroposterior pelvic standing view. (**b**) Standing false-profile view of the left hip

Pearls and Pitfalls (Fig. 26.9)

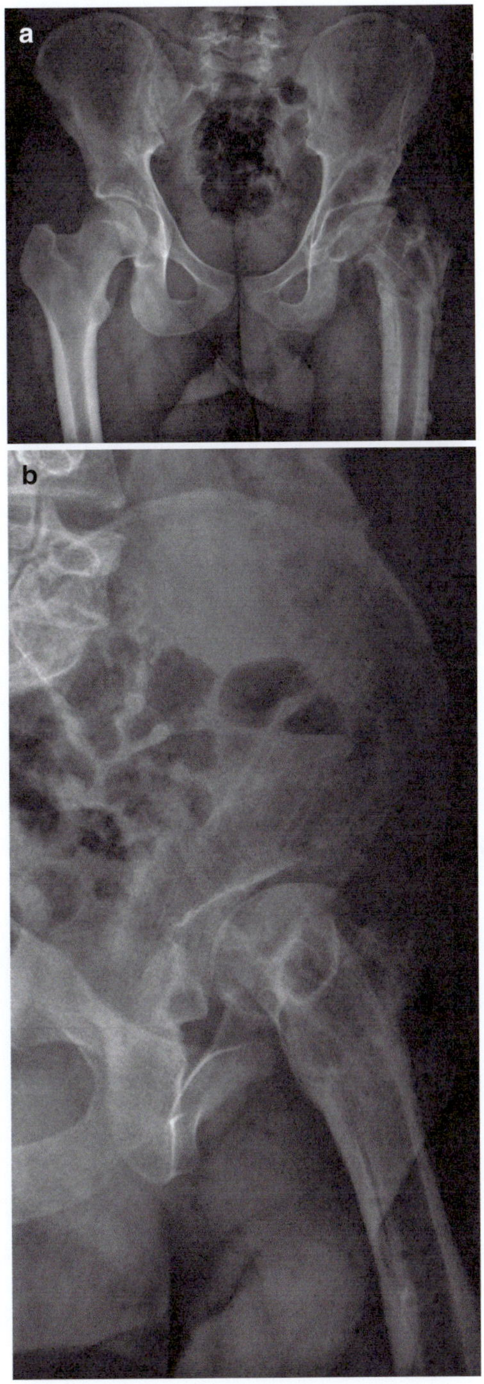

Fig. 26.9 Two-year follow-up radiographs. (**a**) Anteroposterior pelvic standing view. (**b**) Standing false-profile view of the left hip

- Postoperative mobilization is allowed with touchdown weight bearing, while hip flexion >80° and active abduction are avoided. No drains are necessary.
- Continuous passive motion of the hip from 0° to 70° has been recommended to avoid intra-articular adhesions for at least 48 hrs.
- Thromboprophylaxis should also be considered in the adult patients.
- Weight bearing on the operated leg is progressed when GT shows signs of healing at 6–8 weeks.
- A variety of pathologies can be addressed with this biomechanically powerful technique. Some surgeons would consider subsequent periacetabular osteotomy or adding a slight valgus to the described technique by adding the removal of a laterally based bone wedge on the distal femoral shaft before side plate fixation to the femoral shaft.
- The distalization of the GT risks transient abductor muscle weakness, GT fibrous union, fracture, or proximal migration.
- Minimal bony apposition at the IT osteotomy site increases risk of non-union or implant failure.
- Sliding hip screw device could also be used with the advantage of using the reaming by-products as autologous bone graft but risking a decreased bone stock of the GT fragment and less rotational control on the neck fragment.

Indications and Contraindications (Table 26.1)

Table 26.1 Morscher osteotomy: Surgical indications and contraindications

Indications
Short femoral neck due to growth disturbance
Greater trochanter overgrowth
Leg length inequality of more than 1.5 cm
Contraindications
Degenerative changes of the hip
Incongruent hip joint
Ongoing femoral head osteonecrosis

References

1. Hefti F, Morscher E. The femoral neck lengthening osteotomy. Orthop Traumatol. 1993;2(3):144–51.
2. Ganz R, Gill TJ, Gautier E, Ganz K, Krügel N, Berlemann U. Surgical dislocation of the adult hip a technique with full access to the femoral head and acetabulum without the risk of avascular necrosis. J Bone Joint Surg Br. 2001;83(8):1119–24.
3. Ganz R, Huff TW, Leunig M. Extended retinacular soft-tissue flap for intra-articular hip surgery: surgical technique, indications, and results of application. Instr Course Lect. 2009;58:241–55.

Shepherd's Crook Deformity

27

Nicole I. Montgomery, Lee S. Haruno, and John P. Dormans

Introduction

Shepherd's crook deformity is a term used to describe a pronounced coxa vara angulation (femoral neck-shaft angle <120°) and lateral bowing of the proximal femur. This deformity may be found as a sequela of fibrous dysplasia (most severely in the setting of McCune-Albright syndrome), osteogenesis imperfecta, and Paget disease. A compromise in structural integrity of the femoral neck and trochanteric region leads to progressive loss of the neck-shaft angle and bowing. This may result in pain, restricted range of motion, limb shortening, leg length discrepancy, gait alteration, and a dramatically increased risk of pathologic proximal femur fractures. Shepherd's crook deformity can be difficult to treat due to its rarity, large spectrum of severity, progressive nature, and potential for recurrence. Intralesional curettage and bone graft, once thought to halt the progression of deformity in fibrous dysplasia, has been shown to be of limited use, as the graft is resorbed over time and the bone reverts to its dysplastic state. Similarly, intertrochanteric osteotomy with a hip plate and screw has proven to be prone to failure via cutout of the cervical screw, diaphyseal screw loosening and pullout, periprosthetic fracture, and deformity below the level of the plate. Recent literature has shown promising results using proximal femoral osteotomy with intramedullary rod fixation and femoral neck stabilization to correct the neck-shaft angle and prevent progression and recurrence of deformity secondary to fibrous dysplasia.

Brief Clinical History

A 17-year-old female with history of fibrous dysplasia in the setting of McCune-Albright syndrome presented with right thigh pain and a right shorter than left leg length discrepancy. She had a remote history of thyroidectomy. The patient reported pain with ambulation and required the occasional use of crutches to limit weight bearing and improve her stability. She was observed to have restricted range of motion, a leg length discrepancy (left greater than right) of 3 cm, and an antalgic gait sparing the right lower extremity. In addition, the patient was noted to have multiple jagged-edged *café au lait* spots. Radiographs upon presentation revealed a well-defined expansile lesion in the right proximal femur with

N. I. Montgomery
Division of Orthopedic Surgery, Texas Childrens Hospital, Houston, TX, USA
e-mail: nimontgo@texaschildrens.org

L. S. Haruno · J. P. Dormans (✉)
Division of Orthopedic Surgery, Baylor College of Medicine, Texas Children's Hospital, Houston, TX, USA
e-mail: haruno@bcm.edu

R. C. Hamdy, N. Saran (eds.), *Pediatric Pelvic and Proximal Femoral Osteotomies*,
https://doi.org/10.1007/978-3-319-78033-7_27

a ground-glass appearance, coxa vara (neck-shaft angle of approximately 112°), and a shepherd's crook deformity.

Preoperative Imaging

Anteroposterior (AP) (Fig. 27.1a) and lateral (Fig. 27.1b) radiographs of the patient's right proximal femur. The neck-shaft angle is approximately 112°. Characteristic radiographic findings of fibrous dysplasia include an expansile, well-defined, sharply marginated, metaphyseal or diaphyseal ground glass or lytic lesion.

Goals of Treatment

1. Correction of coxa vara (shepherd's crook deformity) to a neck-shaft angle between 120° and 135°
2. Restoration of proper femoral alignment, including correction of rotational deformity
3. Adequate intramedullary "load-sharing" stabilization of the femoral neck following osteotomy to reduce the risk of fracture and prevent recurrence of the deformity
4. Improvement of gait, discomfort, range of motion, and pre-existing leg length discrepancy

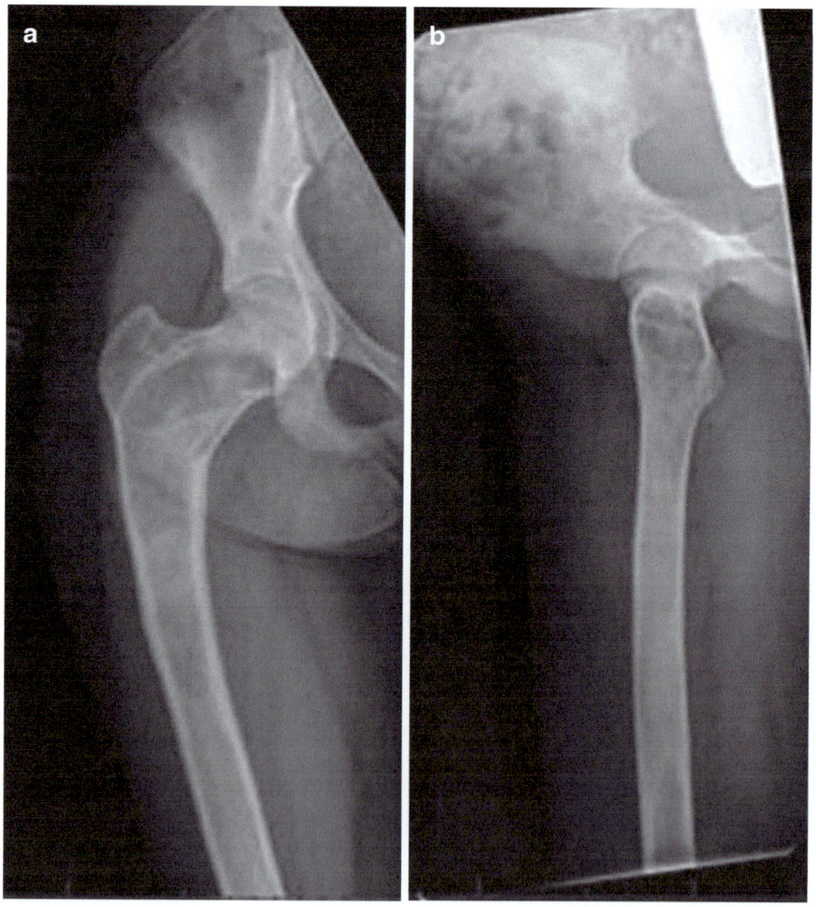

Fig. 27.1 Preoperative anteroposterior (**a**) and lateral X-rays (**b**) of the right proximal femur in a 17-year-old patient with McCune-Albright Syndrome. A shepherd's crook deformity is evident. (From Kushare et al. 2014, with permission)

Introduction

In fibrous dysplasia, there is a somatic activating mutation of the $G_s\alpha$ protein encoded by the GNAS gene resulting in an impaired ability to differentiate into mature osteoblasts. The cells instead retain a fibroblast-like phenotype, and the area is filled with undermineralized and structurally incompetent fibro-osseous tissue instead of normal bone and marrow. As a result, affected individuals are prone to deformation (i.e., lateral bowing) of weight-bearing regions in the proximal femur, eventually resulting in a shepherd's crook deformity. Patients with multiple fibrous lesions or involvement of more than one bone (polyostotic form) are considered to have more severe disease and are at higher risk of developing deformity.

Children may clinically present with pain, gait alterations, recurrent stress fractures, and shortening of the affected limb (with subsequent leg length discrepancy). Early surgical intervention should be favored in instances where the deformity is progressive or predicted to dramatically worsen. A recent study by Ippolito et al. [1] has successfully correlated progression with a proprietary classification scheme based on plain film radiographs. Fibrous dysplasia affecting the intertrochanteric region of the femoral neck may be considered high risk for progression.

Treatment Strategy

Most cases of shepherd's crook deformity are observed in childhood and early adolescence. The deformity is commonly associated with polyostotic fibrous dysplasia (either isolated or in the setting of endocrinopathies such as McCune-Albright syndrome) and to a lesser extent with other conditions that impair the structural integrity of the bone, including osteogenesis imperfecta or Paget disease.

Femoral osteotomy has been the favored approach to managing shepherd's crook deformity. However, due to its rarity and the spectrum of deformities, there is less consensus regarding the specific surgical techniques to create the best long-term outcomes for patients. Intralesional curettage and bone graft, once thought to halt the progression of deformity in fibrous dysplasia, has been shown in recent studies to be of limited use, as the graft is resorbed over time and the bone reverts to its dysplastic state. Similarly, intertrochanteric osteotomy with a hip plate and screw has proven to be prone to failure via cutout of the cervical screw, diaphyseal screw loosening and pullout, periprosthetic fracture, and deformity below the level of the plate. Fixation methods following osteotomy that do not address stabilization of the femoral neck, such as flexible intramedullary nails and telescoping intramedullary rods (Fassier-Duval), have also been shown to be inadequate.

Therefore, the current preferred treatment method is intertrochanteric or subtrochanteric osteotomy followed by stabilization with a cervicodiaphyseal (cephalomedullary) intramedullary nail. Ideally, a correction of the varus deformity to a femoral neck-shaft angle of >120° should be obtained. In cases of very severe deformity (neck-shaft angle of less than 100°), a two-staged procedure involving initial stabilization with a hip plate followed by removal of the plate once the osteotomy has healed (to avoid long-term plate associated pitfalls), and subsequently stabilization of the entire femur with an intramedullary nail has been proposed. Challenges associated with intramedullary nailing include correction of rotational deformity and difficult reaming due to sclerotic borders. In patients with coxa vara and significant lateral bowing of the femoral shaft, multiple osteotomies may be undertaken for correction and placement of the intramedullary nail. It has been suggested in the literature that patients presenting with an acute pathological femoral neck fracture in the setting of shepherd's crook deformity may have both the fracture and deformity corrected concurrently.

Surgical Details

Preoperative radiographs should include the pelvis and the entire length of the femur (see Fig. 27.1). Osteotomies should be templated based on the individual's deformity and mapped in advance of the procedure. In addition, the osteotomy should be planned to match the neck-shaft angle of the selected intramedullary implant (usually 125° or 130°). A single, subtrochanteric valgus producing osteotomy and placement of intramedullary nail will be described in this section; however, sometimes multiple complex osteotomies may be necessary.

The procedure is done in a supine (or occasionally a lateral decubitus position) on a radiolucent table. The supine position allows for better assessment of rotation and femoral version after fixation, as both legs can be prepped free to compare the rotational profiles.

For ease, the starting point for a standard trochanteric entry nail should be obtained prior to destabilizing the femur and undertaking the osteotomy. After creation of the entry point with the entry reamer, the guidewire can be introduced into the proximal femur, stopping just proximal to the planned osteotomy site. Following this, an approximately 10 cm longitudinal incision is made laterally along the proximal femur from the greater trochanter distally along the lateral midpoint of the femur. This incision is taken down to the iliotibial band, which is then incised in line with the incision and lateral midpoint of the femur.

Retractors are placed to expose the vastus lateralis and vastus ridge. The vastus lateralis fascia is incised posteriorly and in an "L" shape along the vastus ridge, and the muscle is reflected anteriorly until the proximal femur is visualized. Subperiosteal dissection is carried around the femur circumferentially at the planned osteotomy site. Retractors are placed around the femur, and the planned osteotomy (either straight or lateral closing wedge) is performed with an oscillating saw. A clamp can be placed to reduce the osteotomy site and check the correction with fluoroscopic images.

Once the correction and reduction is deemed adequate, the intramedullary nail guidewire is then advanced distally to the level of the superior pole of the patella. The nail is then reamed, placed, and cephalomedullary screw(s) are then drilled and placed in the standard fashion. Prior to placing the distal interlocking screws, the femur may be "set" to the desired rotation. Once the interlocking screws are placed, the rotational profile can be assessed and compared to the contralateral leg. Final AP and lateral fluoroscopic images should be obtained of the entire length of the femur prior to closing the wounds and leaving the operating room.

Postoperative Imaging

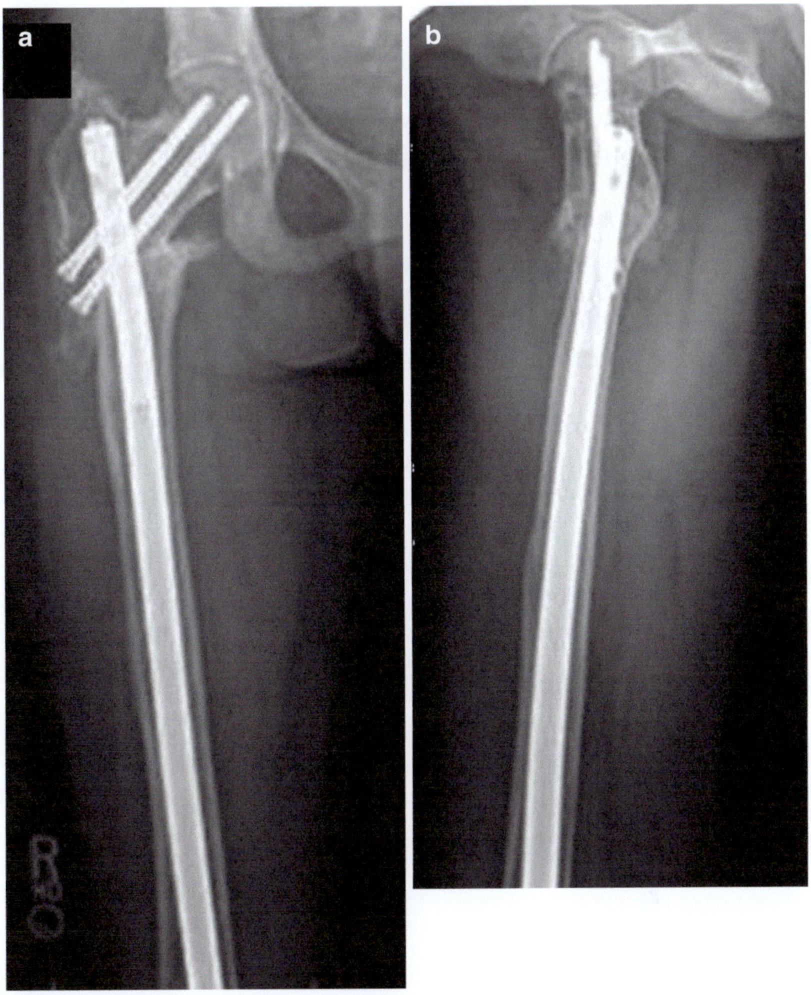

Fig. 27.2 Anteroposterior (**a**) and lateral (**b**) X-rays of the patient in Fig. 27.1 following subtrochanteric osteotomy and intramedullary nail fixation. (From Kushare et al. 2014, with permission)

AP (Fig. 27.2a) and lateral (Fig. 27.2b) radiographs of the patient's right femur following a valgus medial displacing osteotomy, intramedullary nailing, and screw fixation of the femoral neck. Following osteotomy, the neck-shaft angle has been corrected to approximately 127° from 112° initially.

Indication (Table 27.1)

Table 27.1 Shepherd's crook deformity: indication

Progressive shepherd's crook deformity of the proximal femur

Pearls and Pitfalls

- Curettage and bone graft alone is not recommended and may be associated with bleeding, recurrence of the disease, and progression of deformity. Biopsy with intra-operative frozen sections sometimes needed for confirmation of diagnosis.
- The deformity (including any rotational abnormality) is corrected with an osteotomy and appropriate stabilization of the femoral neck, and entire femur with intramedullary fixation ("recon nail") should be considered to prevent progression of the deformity (i.e., a loss of the neck-shaft angle).
- Treatment should be customized to each individual, and preoperative planning and templating is essential. A staged approach may be used for severe deformity. Multiple osteotomies may be needed to correct diaphyseal deformity as well.
- Close follow-up is necessary to monitor for bone fragment necrosis, loss of fixation, pathologic micro/macro fractures, and worsening of the neck-shaft angle.

Reference

1. Ippolito E, Farsetti P, Boyce AM, Corsi A, De Maio F, Collins MT. Radiographic classification of coronal plane femoral deformities in polyostotic fibrous dysplasia. Clin Orthop Relat Res. 2014;472(5):1558–67.

Suggested Reading

Guille JT, Kumar SJ, MacEwen GF. Fibrous dysplasia of the proximal part of the femur: long-term results of curettage and bone-grafting and mechanical realignment. J Bone Joint Surg Am. 1998;80(5):648–58.

Ippolito E, Farsetti P, Valentini MB, Potenza V. Two-stage surgical treatment of complex femoral deformities with severe coxa vara in polyostotic fibrous dysplasia. J Bone Joint Surg Am. 2015;97(2):119–25.

Ippolito E, Valentini M, Lala R, De Maio F, Sorge R, Farsetti P. Changing pattern of femoral deformity during growth in polyostotic fibrous dysplasia of the bone: an analysis of 46 cases. J Pediatr Orthop. 2016;36(5):488–93.

Kushare IV, Colo D, Bakhshi H, Dormans JP. Fibrous dysplasia of the proximal femur: surgical management options and outcomes. J Child Orthop. 2014;8(6):505–11.

Leet AI, Boyce AM, Ibrahim KA, Weintroub S, Kushner H, Collins M. Bone-grafting in polyostotic fibrous dysplasia. J Bone Joint Surg Am. 2016;98(3):211–9.

28 Coxa Vara in Osteogenesis Imperfecta

Reggie C. Hamdy

Introduction

Osteogenesis imperfecta (OI) is a heterogenous genetic disorder of connective tissue that causes low bone mass, bone fragility, multiple fractures, and reduced mobility and function. The type and severity of OI are variable. The Sillence classification has designated four types: Type I is a mild form, Type II is lethal at birth, Type III is very severe with multiple fractures often at birth, and Type IV is of mixed severity. Several other types were added later. Long bone deformities, including coxa vara, are typical findings in patients with OI, specifically in the more severely affected.

Definition Coxa vara is *defined* as any decrease in the neck-shaft angle (NSA) below 110° (Fig. 28.1). The normal development of the NSA is shown in Fig. 28.2. This deformity may be observed in numerous *congenital and acquired conditions* such as proximal focal femoral deficiency (PFFD) (Fig. 28.3a), congenital short femur (Fig. 28.3b), developmental coxa vara (Fig. 28.3c), and some types of skeletal dysplasias (Fig. 28.3d), secondary to any pathology that may lead to damage to the capital femoral epiphysis growth plate such as Perthes disease, slipped capital femoral epiphysis, and developmental dysplasia of the hip (DDH), and specifically in children with bone fragility such as OI and fibrous dysplasia (FD). In a large series of 283 patients with OI [1], coxa vara was present in 10% of patients, most commonly in patients with Type III OI (almost 50% of all, patients) and was almost absent in the mildest form of Type I showing that coxa vara is clearly associated with the extent of bone fragility.

Pathogenesis The exact *pathogenesis* of coxa vara in children with OI is not very clear; however, it is largely believed that one of the main causes is repeated minor fractures of the femoral neck. As the majority of patients with coxa vara have undergone femoral rodding procedures, it is possible that the biomechanical effects of femoral rods and the trauma caused by insertion of the rods contribute to the development of coxa vara.

Clinical presentation of coxa vara includes pain around the hip region partially caused by weak hip abductors due to the decreased abductor lever arm (Fig. 28.4) and decreased abduction due to trochanteric impingement. Genu valgum may develop in some cases in an attempt to compensate for the decreased abduction of the hip (Fig. 28.5).

R. C. Hamdy
Division of Orthopaedic Surgery, McGill University Health Centre, Montreal, QC, Canada

The Montreal Children's Hospital, Montreal, QC, Canada

Shriners Hospital for Children – Canada
Montreal, QC, Canada
e-mail: rhamdy@shriners.mcgill.ca

R. C. Hamdy, N. Saran (eds.), *Pediatric Pelvic and Proximal Femoral Osteotomies*,
https://doi.org/10.1007/978-3-319-78033-7_28

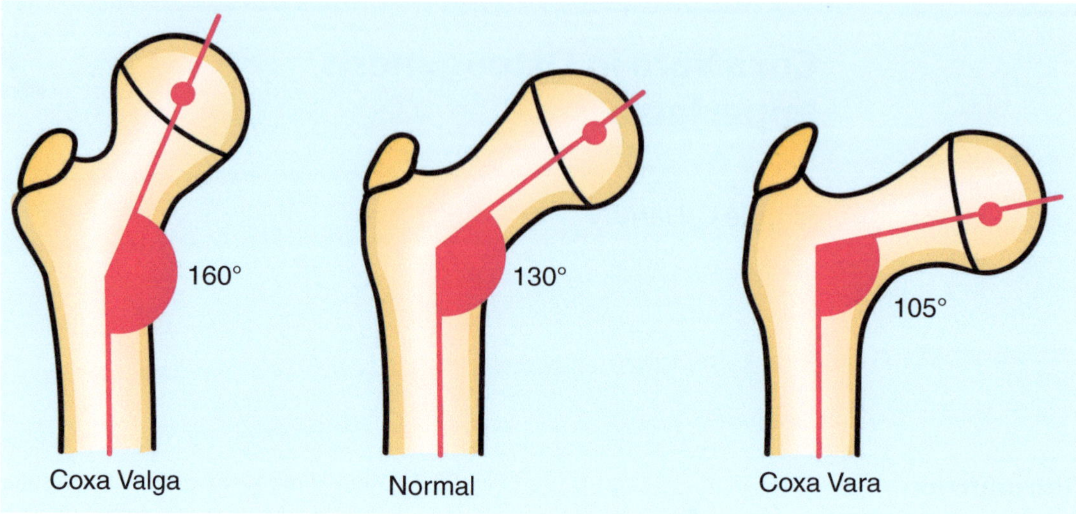

Fig. 28.1 Neck-shaft angle

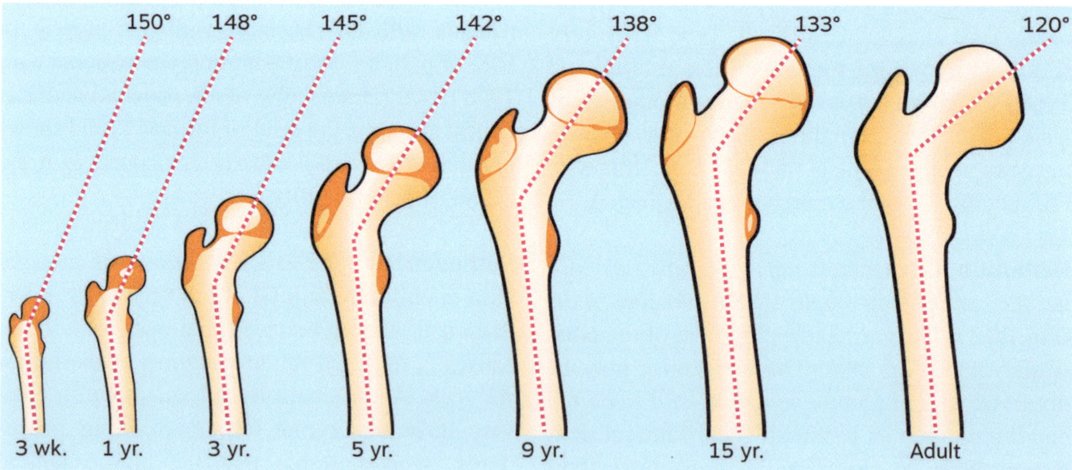

Fig. 28.2 Normal development of the neck-shaft angle

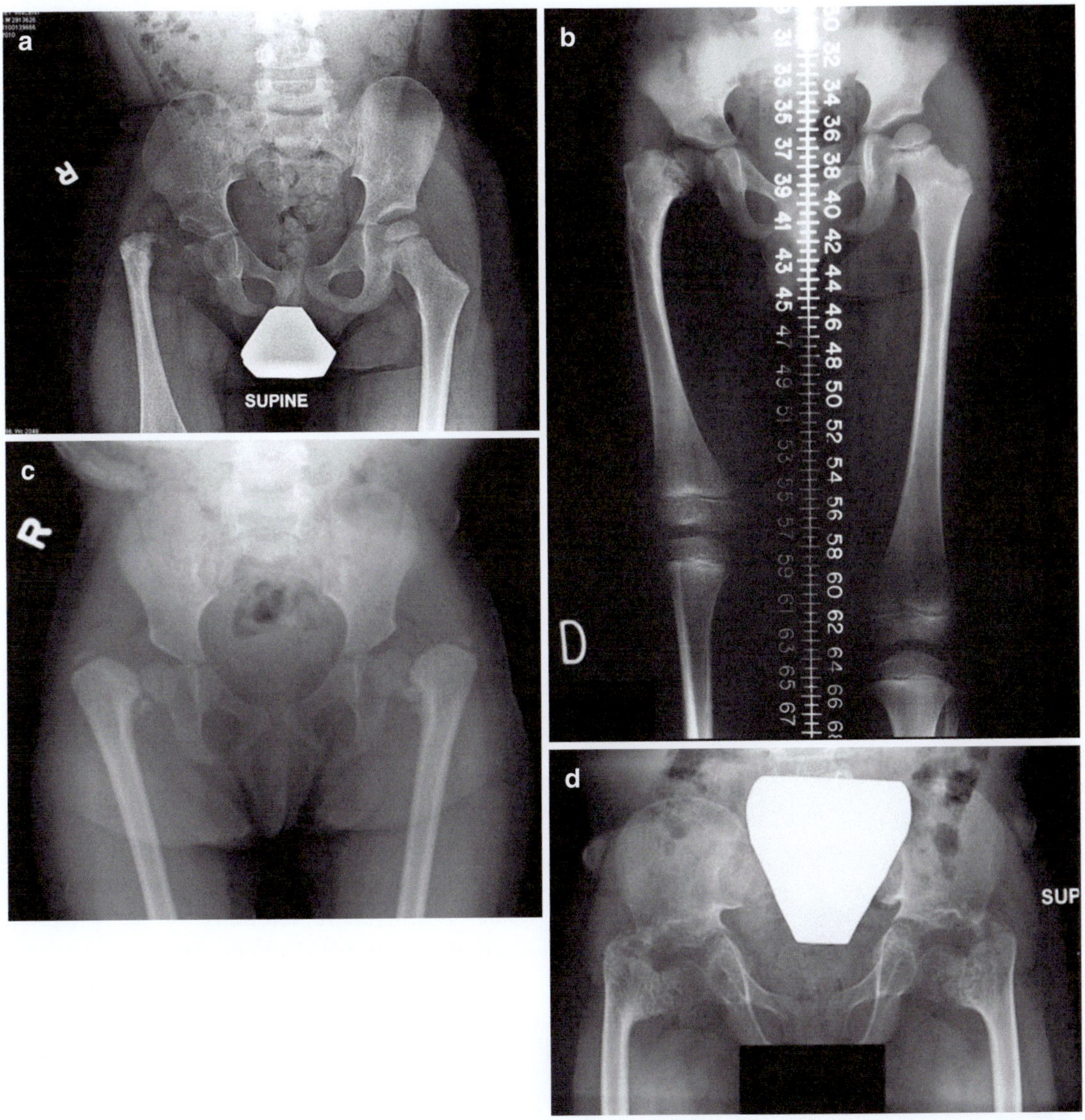

Fig. 28.3 Various causes of coxa vara. (**a**) Coxa vara in proximal focal femoral deficiency. (**b**) Coxa vara in congenital short femur. (**c**) Developmental coxa vara. (**d**) Skeletal dysplasia

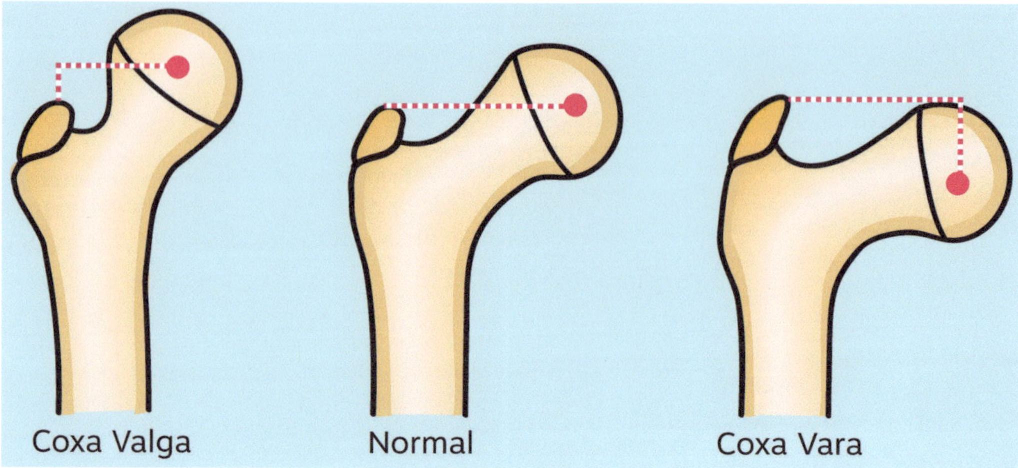

Fig. 28.4 Relation between the tip of the greater trochanter and the center of the femoral head

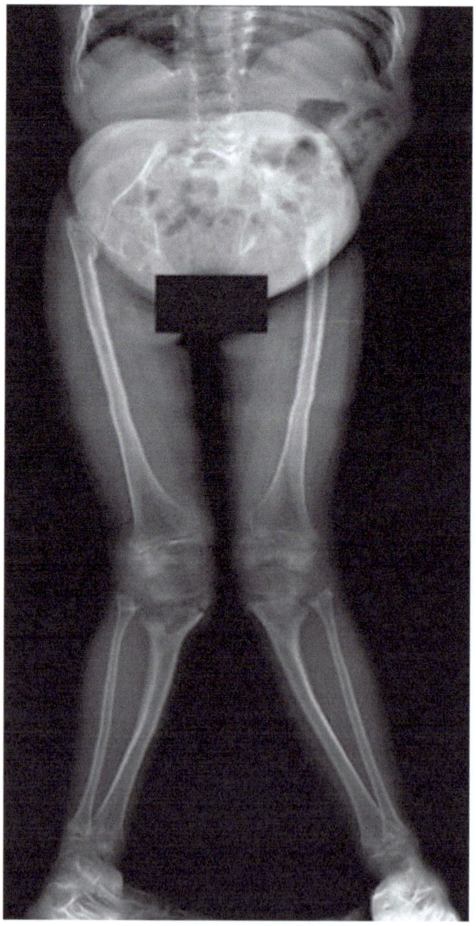

Fig. 28.5 Genu valgum associated with coxa vara

Gait abnormalities are common. In unilateral cases, a Trendelenburg gait develops, caused by the limb length discrepancy and weak abductors. In bilateral cases, a waddling gait develops.

Radiological examination of coxa vara includes the neck-shaft angle (Fig. 28.6a), head-shaft angle (Fig. 28.6b), and the Hilgenreiner epiphyseal angle (Fig. 28.6c).

It is important to exclude radiologically false coxa vara, especially in children with OI. Sagittal plane procurvatum deformity of the proximal third of the femoral shaft can give the appearance of a false coxa vara on anteroposterior (AP) radiograph in the presence of a normal neck-shaft angle. Hence, a lateral radiograph is extremely important to evaluate whether procurvatum is present. A proper AP radiograph taken with the hip in hyper extension will give a better projection of the true neck-shaft angle in these cases. An example of false coxa vara is shown in Fig. 28.7.

Brief Clinical History

This is a 4-year-old girl with OI Type III. Since the age of 8 months, she has been receiving bisphosphonate treatment (zolendrate intravenously). At the age of 2 years, she had bilateral femoral rodding with Fassier-Duval (FD) rods.

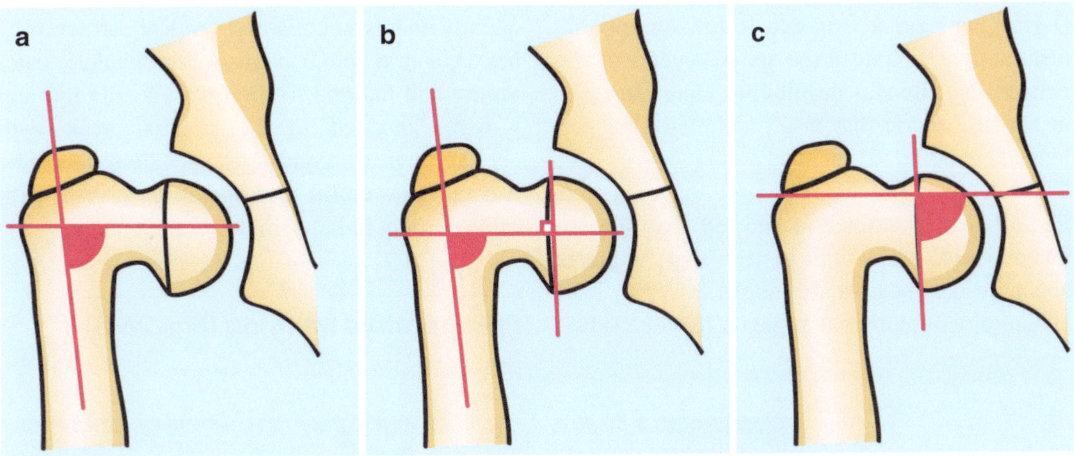

Fig. 28.6 Radiological examination of coxa vara include (**a**) the neck-shaft angle, (**b**) head-shaft angle, and (**c**) the Hilgenreiner epiphyseal angle

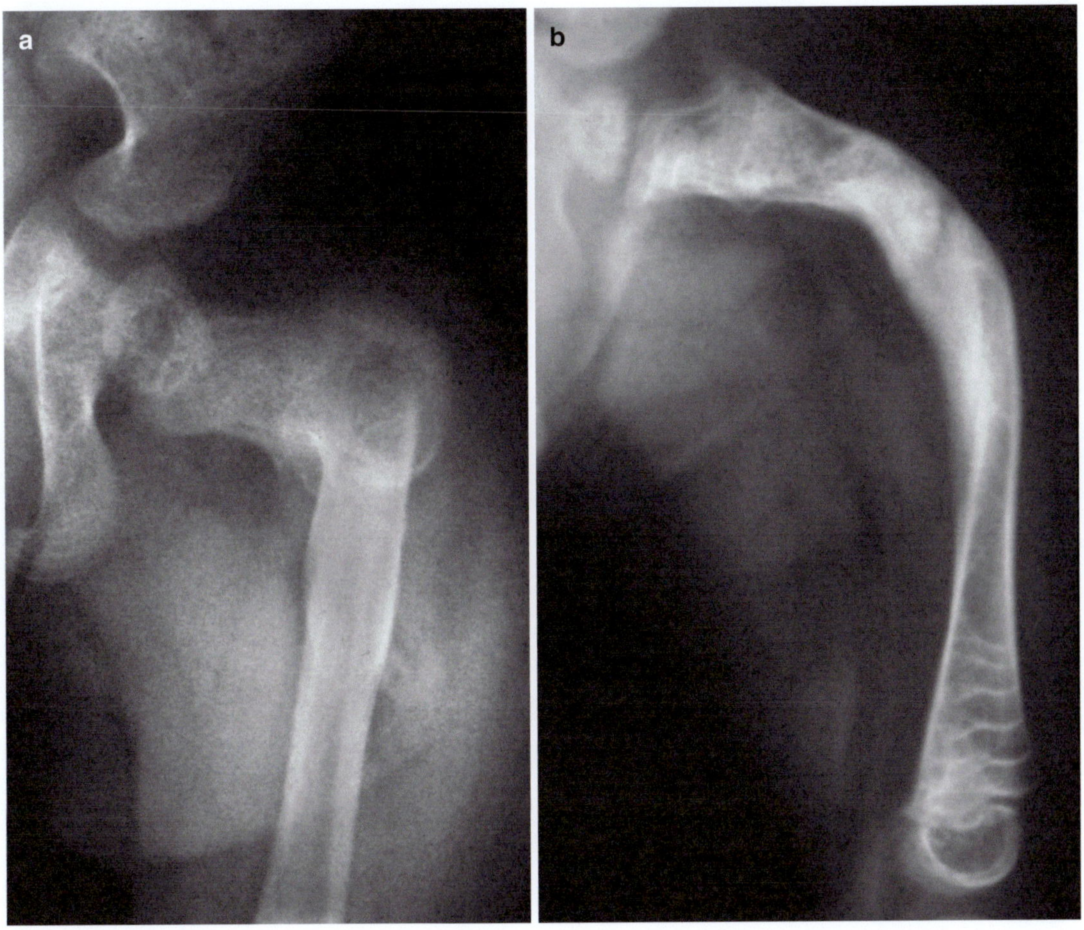

Fig. 28.7 An example of false coxa vara

During her regular 6 month follow-up appointment at the OI clinic at the age of 4 years, it was noticed that she was developing increasing pain in her hip region that was precipitated by prolonged walking. Clinical examination revealed Trendelenburg gait and decreased hip abduction. Radiological examination showed that she has bilateral coxa vara with a neck-shaft angle of about 100°, head-shaft angle of 90°, and Hilgenreiner epiphyseal angle of 70°. She subsequently underwent bilateral surgical correction of her coxa vara with a valgus subtrochanteric osteotomy and internal fixation with an FD rod and K-wires inserted in the femoral neck with cerclage wires around the upper diaphysis. She had an uneventful postoperative course with improvement in her symptoms and gait.

Preoperative Imaging (Fig. 28.8)

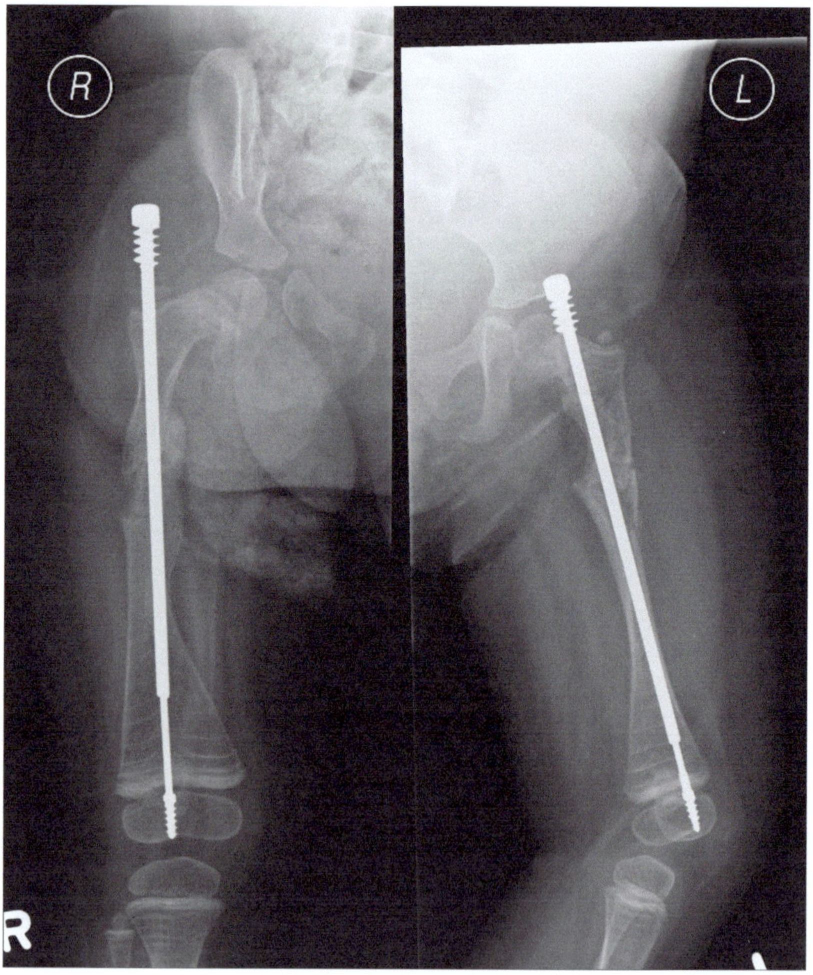

Fig. 28.8 Preoperative X-rays

Goals of Treatment

- Irrespective of the cause of OI, the goal of treatment is to prevent progression of the deformity and restore the normal anatomy of the proximal femur by performing a subtrochanteric valgus osteotomy that will increase the neck-shaft angle to at least 120°.
- In this case with weak bone, stabilization of the osteotomy by cephalo-medullary internal fixation to protect both the femoral neck and the diaphysis is required.
- The valgus osteotomy will eliminate the Trendelenburg gait by restoring normal articulo-trochanteric distance and normal abductor lever arm.
- Recurrence of the deformity has been reported to be directly related to the direction of the physis and the mechanical forces that the physis is subjected to. The goal is to obtain a Hilgenreiner epiphyseal angle of less than 35°. This will convert the shear forces acting on the physis to compressive forces.

Treatment Strategy

Surgical treatment of coxa vara is indicated when the patient becomes symptomatic or if there is progression of the deformity radiologically. To attain the goals mentioned above, a valgus subtrochanteric osteotomy is performed. Stabilization of the osteotomy largely depends on the underlying bone pathology. In cases with normal bone, such as developmental coxa vara, a plate construct such as a blade plate, locking plate, or dynamic hip screw is usually all that is required. However, in cases of weak, osteopenic bone, as in the present case (and cases with fibrous dysplasia—discussed in detail in another chapter), cephalo-medullary fixation is indicated. This technique will allow the desired correction to be obtained along with lateral translation of the femoral shaft. It will also provide protection to the femoral neck and eliminate the stress riser effect that may be caused by a plate construct. This technique allows stable fixation and does not require immobilization in a hip spica.

Surgical Details

- Under general anesthesia, the patient is placed supine on the operating table.
- An appropriate saline bag is placed under the operative hemi-pelvis to position the patient into a semi-lateral position (Fig. 28.9).
- Ensure that intraoperative fluoroscopy view scan be obtained (Fig. 28.10).
- The whole lower limb is prepped free.
- A direct lateral approach starting at the greater trochanter is used (or the previous scar is used if and FD rod has already been inserted).
- Subcutaneous tissue is dissected, tensor fascia lata incised, and the proximal femur exposed.
- The first K-wire is inserted in the middle of the femoral neck on the AP view (see Fig. 28.10c) and from anterior to posterior in the lateral view (see Fig. 28.10d).
- The second K-wire is inserted parallel to the first wire on the AP view (see Fig. 28.10e) and from posterior to anterior (see Fig. 28.10f).
- A subtrochanteric osteotomy is performed with a power saw, leaving at least 2 cm distal to the insertion of the K-wires (see Fig. 28.10g).
- The two K-wires are used as a joystick to position the proximal fragment into the desired amount of valgus (see Fig. 28.10h).
- Retrograde drilling for the insertion of the FD rod is performed from the lateral cortex of the proximal fragment (see Fig. 28.10i).
- The male and then female FD rod is inserted in an antegrade fashion (see Fig. 28.10j).

The two K-wires are bent over the proximal fragment (see Fig. 28.10k), and cerclage wires are applied with tension of about 30 kg. The K-wires are crossing in the femoral neck as seen on the lateral view to allow space for insertion of the FD rod (see Fig. 28.10l).

- The wound is irrigated and closed in layers.
- If fixation is not very stable, the patient is immobilized in a half spica for 6 weeks. The patient is kept non-weight bearing until evidence of union.

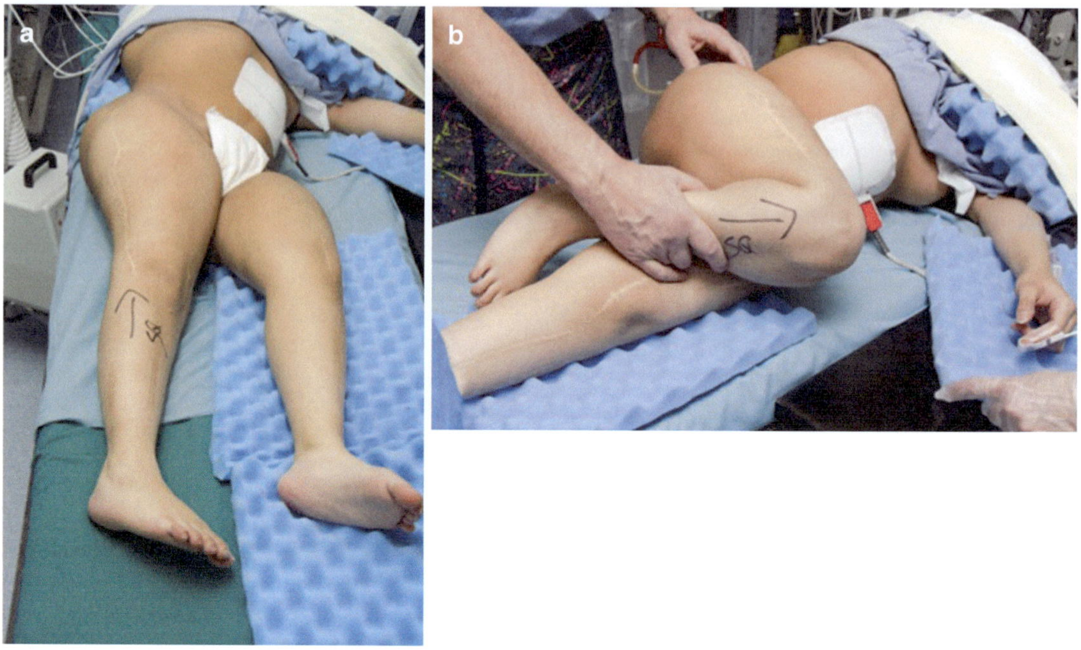

Fig. 28.9 Positioning of the patient on translucent operating table

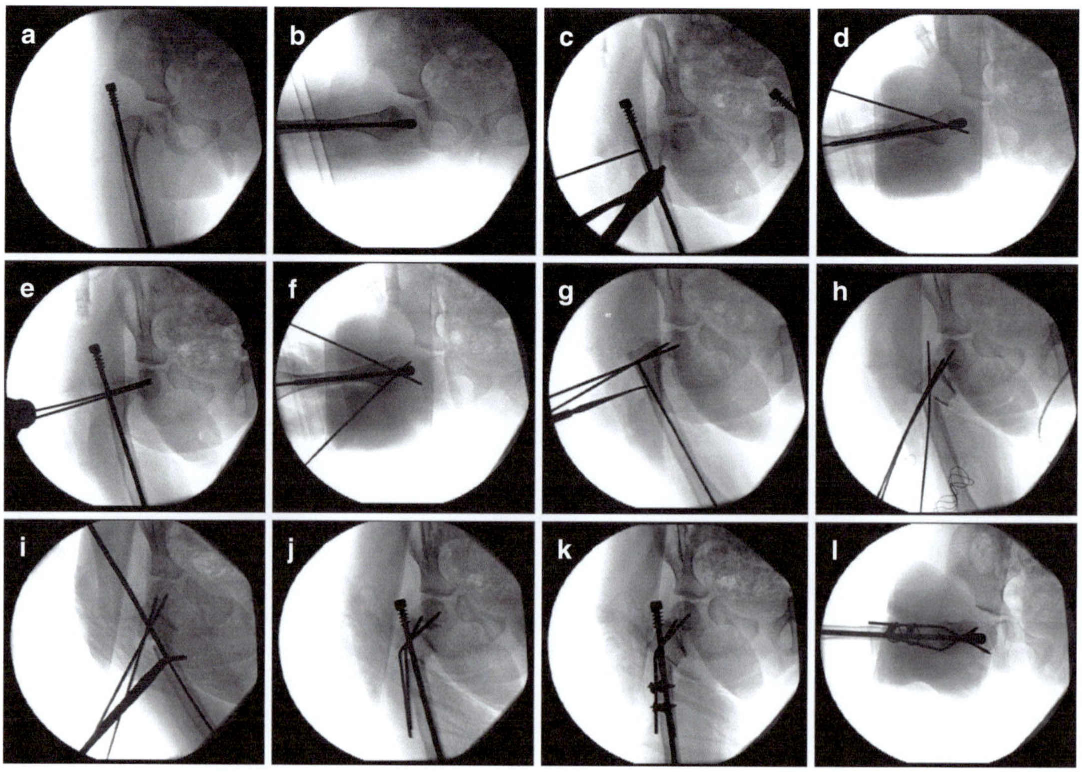

- The key steps of the surgery are shown in Fig. 28.11:
  a. Insertion of the two K-wires in the femoral neck
  b. Site of the subtrochanteric osteotomy
  c. Preparation of the distal fragment
  d. Retrograde drilling of the lateral cortex
  e. Removal of triangular fragment of the medial distal diaphysis
  f. Insertion of the FD rod
  g. Cerclage wires after bending the K-wires

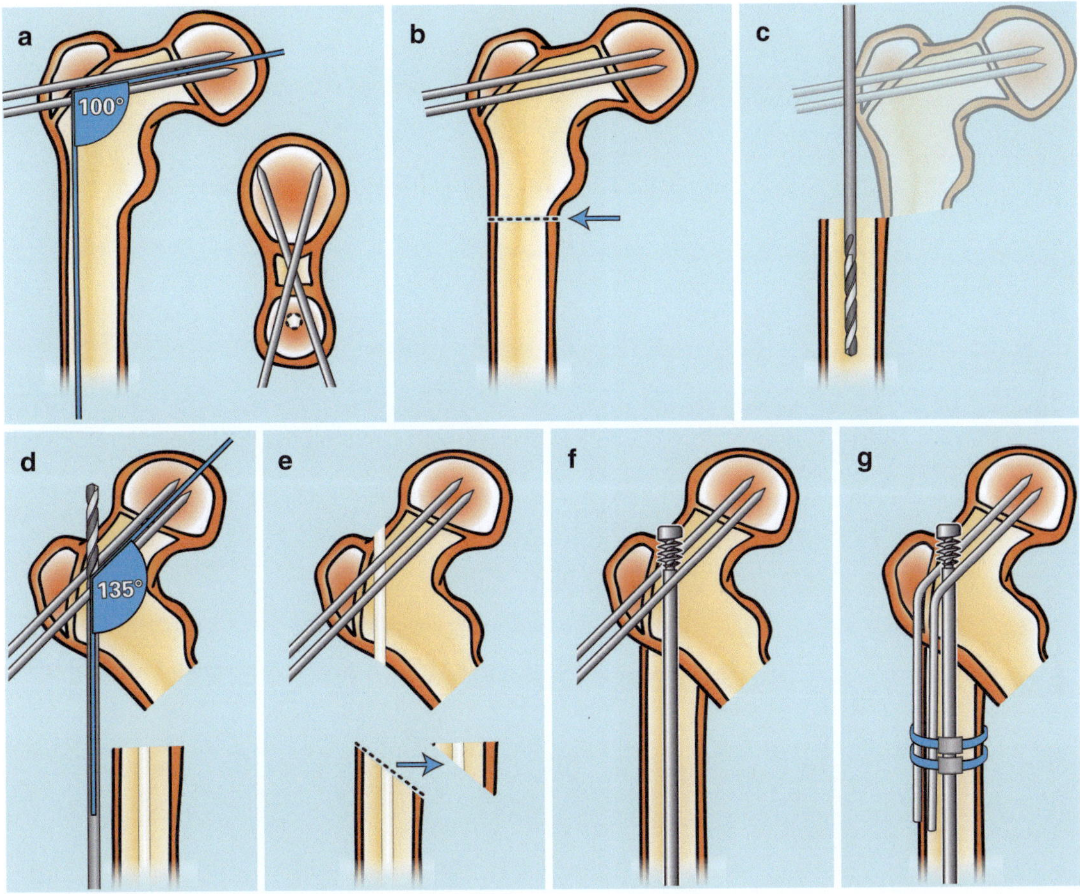

Fig. 28.11 Key steps of the surgical correction (see text)

Fig. 28.10 Fluoroscopic pictures showing surgical details. (**a**) Anteroposterior view showing coxa vara and FD rod. (**b**) Lateral view showing the FD rod slightly posterior in the femoral neck. (**c**) AP view showing entry point of the first K-wire in the middle of the femoral neck. (**d**) First K-wire inserted from anterior to posterior. (**e**) Second K-wire inserted parallel to first wire on the AP view. (**f**) Second K-wire inserted from posterior to anterior direction. (**g**) Site of subtrochanteric osteotomy (female component of FD rod removed). (**h**) Subtrochanteric osteotomy completed. Two K-wires used as a joystick to obtain correct and planned valgus correction. Drill inserted retrograde through lateral part of the femoral neck into the proximal fragment. (**i**) Antegrade insertion of the FD drill bit followed by insertion of the male and then female component. (**j**) K-wires are bent over the diaphysis—after insertion of the FD rod. (**k**) Cerclage wires applied at two points. (**l**) Lateral view showing crossing of K-wires in the femoral neck to allow space for the insertion of the FD rod

Postoperative Imaging

Four years postsurgery, imaging shows that the correction is maintained (Fig. 28.12).

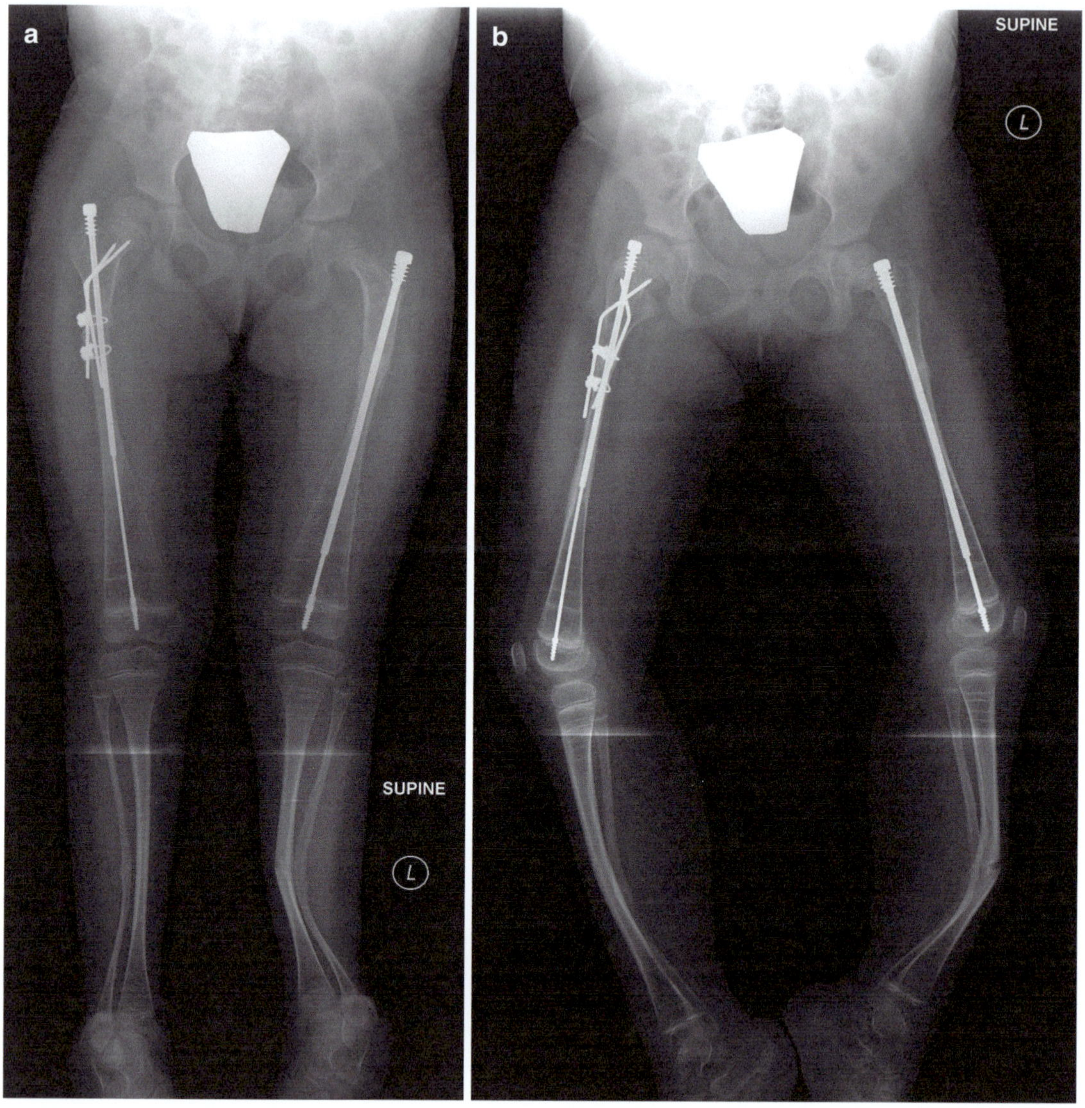

Fig. 28.12 Postoperative X-rays

Pearls and Pitfalls

- Before the surgery, ensure that there is enough adduction to accommodate for the optimal amount of valgus correction. If necessary, soft tissue releases adductors, psoas at the pelvic brim, and even abductor slide at the iliac crest may be necessary.
- Verify that the deformity to be corrected is a true and not a false coxa vara.
- The use of two K-wires has a dual purpose: first, to allow manipulation of the proximal fragment to obtain adequate valgus correction without the fear of fracturing the femoral neck and, second, to obtain cephalo-medullary fixation as is usually indicated in fragile osteope-

nic bone. Furthermore, in cases of OI, there are multiple deformities in the shaft of the femur that may need correction.

- Antegrade insertion of the guide wire of the FD rod in the proximal fragment is very difficult due to the presence of the coxa vara deformity. Therefore, retrograde insertion through the lateral part of the femoral neck is indicated. This also allows lateral translation of the femur during insertion of the FD nail. The entry point on the lateral cortex and the angulation of the drill will determine the amount of valgus obtained and the position of the FD rod.
- Do not use the largest FD rod, as this may lead to absorption of the bone.
- Resection of a triangular part of the medial distal diaphysis will allow some bone-to-bone contact and provide some stability to the osteotomy.

Indication (Table 28.1)

Table 28.1 Coxa vara in osteogenesis imperfecta: surgical indication

A Hilgenreiner epiphyseal angle of more than 60° or documented progression of varus deformity is the standard criteria for surgical correction, particularly when clinical symptoms such as limping are present

Complications (Table 28.2)

Table 28.2 Coxa vara in osteogenesis imperfecta: surgical complications

Recurrence of the deformity always remains a concern. The patient and family should be made aware of this possibility. Correction of the Hilgenreiner epiphyseal angle to less than 35° may decrease the incidence of recurrence
Hardware failure secondary to proximal migration of the intramedullary rod has been reported with this technique, requiring exchange rodding

Reference

1. Aarabi M, Rauch F, Hamdy RC, Fassier F. High prevalence of coxa vara in patients with severe osteogenesis imperfecta. J Pediatr Orthop. 2006;26(1):24–8.

Suggested Reading

Fassier F, Ashby E, Hamdy RC. Case 86: Coxa vara in a nine-year-old boy with osteogenesis imperfecta. In: Rozbruch SR, Hamdy R, editors. Limb lengthening and reconstruction surgery atlas: pediatric deformities. Cham: Springer; 2015. p. 619–22.

Fassier F, Glorieux FH. Osteogenesis imperfecta. In: DuParc J, editor. Surgical techniques in orthopaedics and traumatology 55-050-D-30. New York: Elsevier; 2003. p. 1–8.

Fassier F, Sardar Z, Aarabi M, Odent T, Haque T, Hamdy R. Results and complications of a surgical technique for correction of coxa vara in children with osteopenic bones. J Pediatr Orthop. 2008;28(8):799–805.

Fassier FR. Osteogenesis imperfecta. In: Sanjeev S, editor. Pediatric lower limb deformities: principles and techniques of management. Cham: Springer; 2016. p. 255–65.

Trejo P, Rauch F. Osteogenesis imperfecta in children and adolescents—new developments in diagnosis and treatment. Osteoporos Int. 2016;27(12):3427–37.

Proximal Femoral Reorientational Osteotomies for the Hip Deformities in Children with Arthrogryposis Multiplex Congenita

29

Harold J. P. van Bosse

Introduction

Children with arthrogryposis and severe hip contractures face great difficulties with ambulation and often even with comfortable positioning for seating. These multiplanar joint deformities are a challenge for treatment. The surgical goal is to align the lower extremity in a functional position relative to the body, exploiting the most optimal range of hip motion available. While flexion or flexion-abduction contractures can be improved with a percutaneous anterior soft tissue release of the hip, the more severe contractures can reliably be corrected with a reorientational osteotomy of the proximal femur. This procedure leaves the actual "ball in socket" hip joint undisturbed but aligns the lower extremity with the body axis.

Brief Clinical History

A 17-month-old girl presented with arthrogryposis multiplex congenita (AMC), most likely amyoplasia, with severe hip contractures. She began sitting at 7 months, but she was not yet rolling over because of her hip contractures. Similarly, she was unable to crawl or stand due to the lower limb positioning. Her examination revealed bilateral hip flexion to 170° but with a 70° hip flexion contracture on the right and 65° on the left. Frogleg abduction was 90° bilaterally, and regular abduction was 140° bilaterally; adduction was limited to 50° short of neutral on the right and 40° short of neutral on the left. With the hips flexed, hip external rotation on the right was 70°, left was 60°, and internal rotation was −30° on the right, −20° on the left. With the hips extended, external rotation is 90° bilaterally, whereas internal rotation was −30° on the right and −40° on the left.

Radiographs revealed that both hips were well contained within their acetabuli, with mild acetabular dysplasia. The hips were in a widely abducted position, reflecting their natural resting position due to the contracture.

H. J. P. van Bosse
Shriners Hospital for Children,
Philadelphia, PA, USA
e-mail: HvanBosse@Shrinenet.org

R. C. Hamdy, N. Saran (eds.), *Pediatric Pelvic and Proximal Femoral Osteotomies*,
https://doi.org/10.1007/978-3-319-78033-7_29

Preoperative Imaging (Fig. 29.1)

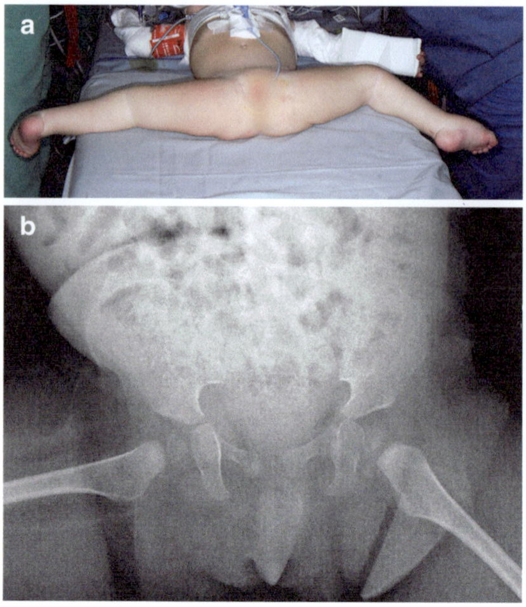

Fig. 29.1 Preoperative findings. (**a**) Clinical photograph of the patient featured, demonstrating her hip/lower extremity positioning at rest. (**b**) Anteroposterior supine pelvis radiograph in the same at rest position. In both images, the patients extreme hip abduction contracture is apparent

Goals of Treatment

The principles of treatment include:

- Initially reducing the soft tissue contracture if possible and thereby increase the total arc of motion of the hip joint, so that a lesser correction needs to occur through the bony procedure.
- Realign the lower extremity with the body axis, to place the available hip motion into the best motion domain possible. Essentially, the hip joint will be left unaltered, but the knee will be brought directly forward, positioning the available hip flexion-extension total arc of motion where it is most functional.

Treatment Strategy

The first step is assessing if there are any soft tissue contractures that can be readily released at the beginning of the operative procedure. These would include the conjoint tendon of the Sartorius and tensor fascia lata (flexion-abduction contracture), the adductor longus (hip adduction contracture), or occasional the hamstrings (hip extension-adduction contractures). Then it is necessary to assess which pre-operative position of the hip, in terms of abduction and internal-external rotation, will allow the greatest flexion-extension total arc of motion, as the goal of the procedure is to maintain this position of the upper femur when bringing the rest of the lower extremity in line with the body axis.

Surgical Details

Patient Positioning

The patient is positioned supine, with a transverse bump under the sacrum, to allow good access to the lateral hip region and maximal hip extension. In most cases, bilateral hips need to be addressed in the same surgical setting, so a "diaper drape" is used, with the Foley catheter brought directly superiorly up over the abdomen and chest, and the perineum and Foley initially prepped into the field prior to draping them out (Fig. 29.2a). The anterior superior iliac spines (ASIS) are included in the surgical field, which also extends posteriorly as far possible to provide maximally hip exposure (Fig. 29.2b). If the contralateral hip is dislocated, requiring an open reduction, the reorientation osteotomy is performed first, so that there is minimal time between completing the open reduction and application of a hip spica cast. Otherwise, a Petrie cast is used, both for unilateral and bilateral reorientational osteotomies.

Percutaneous Anterior Hip Release

The hip is first examined to see if a percutaneous anterior hip release will be appropriate and possible. The contralateral hip is fully flexed, to stabilize the pelvis. By flexing the hip, the pelvis will be oblique, with flexed hip side high. The ipsilateral hip is adducted in a flexed position, so as to align it straight down from the oblique pelvis, then the hip is extended to demonstrate the flexion contracture (Fig. 29.3a). If a tight cord can be felt directly infe-

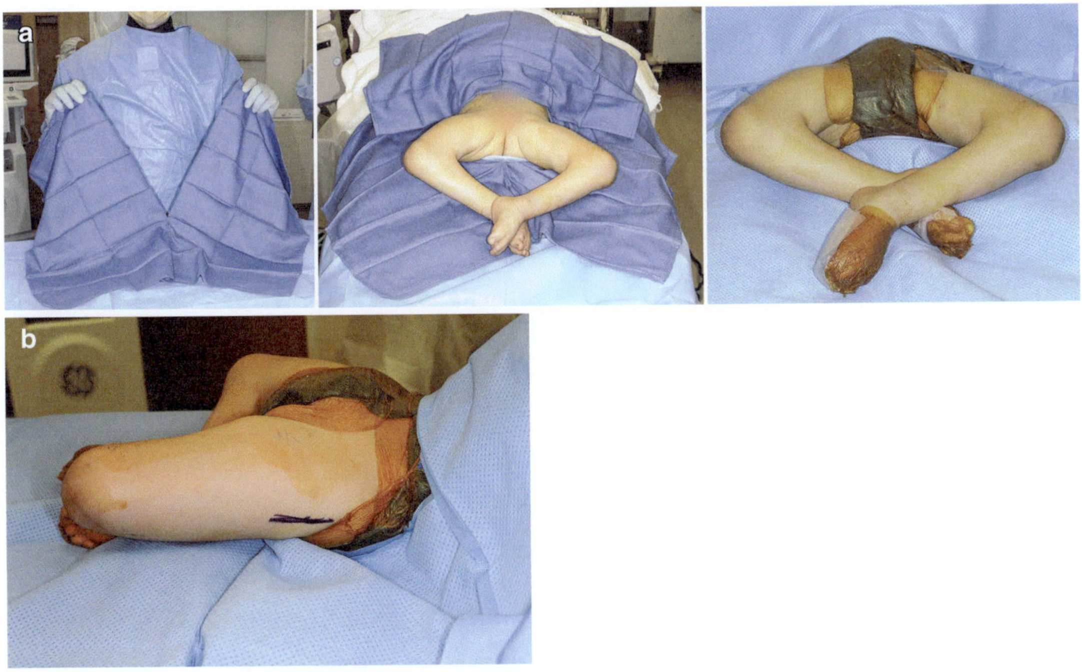

Fig. 29.2 Draping. (**a**) Left: the "diaper drape," two surgical towels stapled together along their inferior quarter length. Middle: placement of the diaper drape from inferiorly, and coming proximally on either side of the pelvis, as posteriorly as possible. The genitals have been blurred, as has the Foley catheter extending directly superiorly. Right: completed draping, with a surgical towel placed vertically to cover the foley and genitalia. All edges are then sealed with an adhesive draping material. (**b**) Side view of the left hip demonstrating full exposure to the lateral hip and pelvis region

rior to the ASIS, then the percutaneous anterior hip release will be helpful to address the flexion-abduction contracture (Fig. 29.3b). The tight cord is the conjoin tendon of the sartorius and the tensor fascia lata. A 15-blade scalpel is brought just medial to the conjoined tendon, 10–20 mm distal to the ASIS. The conjoined tendon is transected from medial to lateral, with continued incision of the fascia lata laterally and posteriorly down to the tip of the greater trochanter (Fig. 29.3c, d). If a significant contracture remains, a contracted rectus femoris tendon may be palpated deep in the incision; it can similarly be transected with the scalpel. Lastly, if the lateral fibers of the fascia overlying the iliacus muscle can be palpated, this fascia too can very carefully be incised to improve hip extension.

Proximal Femoral Reorientational Osteotomy

Prior to incision, a guidewire is placed on the skin, overlaying the pelvis from ASIS to ASIS, and held in place with an adhesive drape; this will be called the pelvis axis wire (Fig. 29.4a). A standard incision for proximal femoral osteotomies is made, starting just distal to the level of the palpable tip of the greater trochanter and extending longitudinally distally. The incision is positioned directly lateral, regardless of how posterior the greater trochanter is. In cases of severe external rotation contractures, the incision initially will appear very anteriorly on the anatomic thigh, since this region of the skin will become the lateral thigh after the reorientation (see Fig. 29.2b).

The fascia lata is split in line with the surgical incision. A 1 cm incision is made in the vastus lateralis fascia as posteriorly possible, and a Hohmann retractor is placed subperiosteally over the anterior aspect of the femur, thereby elevating the vastus lateralis anteriorly. The fascial incision is continued proximally and distally to accommodate the length of the blade plate. Proximally at the vastus ridge, the incision is brought directly anteriorly, releasing the vastus lateralis and allowing it to be subperiosteally elevated anteri-

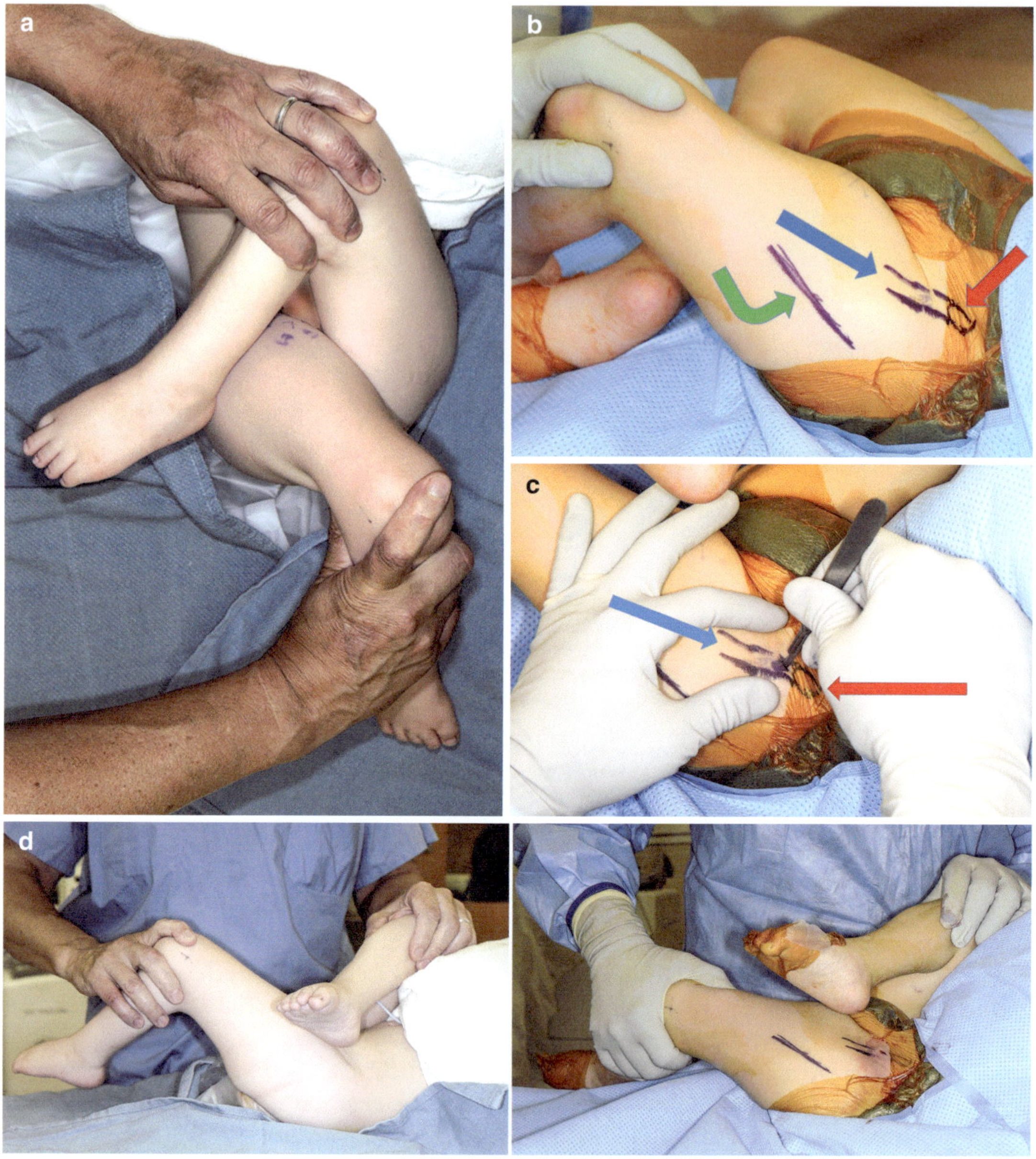

Fig. 29.3 Anterior hip release. (**a**) In order to best appreciate the typical arthrogrypotic hip flexion-abduction contracture, the contralateral hip is fully flexed; the ipsilateral hip is held flexed, then adducted, prior to extending. The adduction actually brings the limb in alignment with the pelvis, which has obliqued with the flexion of the contralateral hip. (**b**) A view of the left hip, with the red arrow indicating the anterior superior iliac spine and the blue arrow aligning with the conjoin tendon of the contracted sartorius and the tensor fascia lata. The curved green arrow indicates the planned incision for the proximal femoral reorientational osteotomy to follow. (**c**) Performing the percutaneous anterior hip release, with palpation through the skin of the fascia being incised. (**d**) Comparison of pre-procedure left hip flexion contracture (left, 35°) to post-procedure (right, 15°)

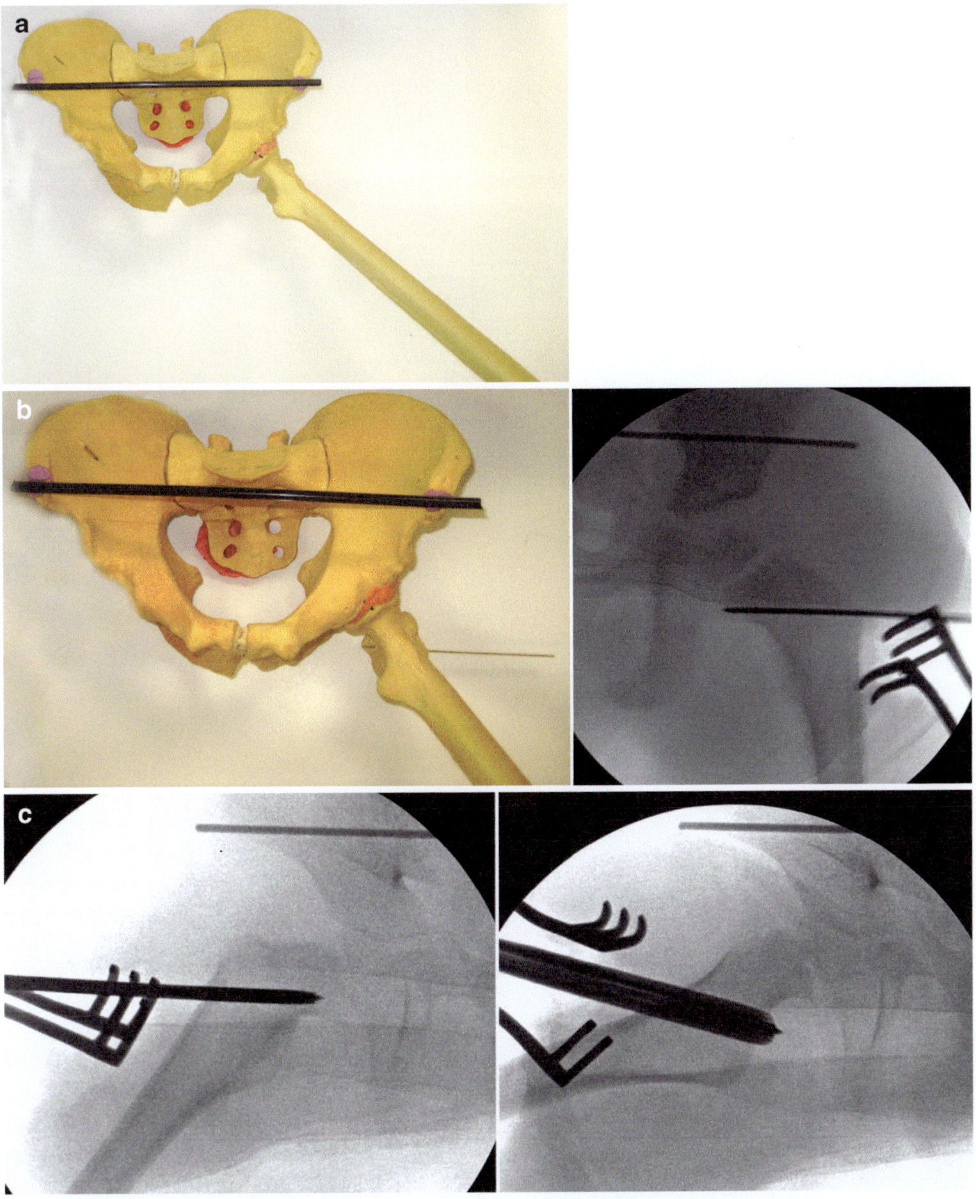

Fig. 29.4 Reorientational osteotomy. (**a**) Pelvis model with the hip/lower extremity in the characteristic position of an arthrogrypotic hip contracture: flexion, abduction, and external rotation. The pelvis axis wire is shown traversing from one anterior superior iliac spine to the other. (**b**) Pelvis model and fluoroscopic surgical view, demonstrating the path of the guide wire for the cannulated proximal femoral blade plate, parallel to the pelvis axis wire. (From van Bosse and Saldana 2017, with permission). (**c**) Fluoroscopic views of the right proximal femur, showing the trajectory of the guide wire and seating chisel with the hip in its natural resting position (left) and on maximally externally rotated view (right), in order to demonstrate the oblique positioning and bicortical purchase of the seating chisel. (**d**) Pelvis model showing an anterior and a lateral view of the seating chisel. Note that the blade of the seating chisel is in the transverse plane of the pelvis and is parallel to the pelvis axis wire in all planes (From van Bosse and Saldana 2017, with permission). (**e**) Lateral view of the pelvis and femur, indicating the two osteotomy lines. The red line is the first cut, parallel to the blade of the seating chisel. The blue line is the second cut, squaring off the end of the distal fragment. The resulting bone fragment removed is a wedge (From van Bosse and Saldana 2017, with permission). (**f**) Anterior view of the pelvis and femur, after the osteotomized ends have been approximated, acutely correcting the rotation, to bring the knee directly anterior. The 90° angulated blade plate is used for fixation (From van Bosse and Saldana 2017, with permission). (**g**) Postoperative anteroposterior (AP) and frogleg lateral views of pelvis. On comparing the AP view to the pre-operative AP pelvis (Fig. 29.1b), the positioning of the proximal femoral metaphyses can be seen to be very similar, with the greater trochanter directly posterior on both the pre-operative and post-operative views

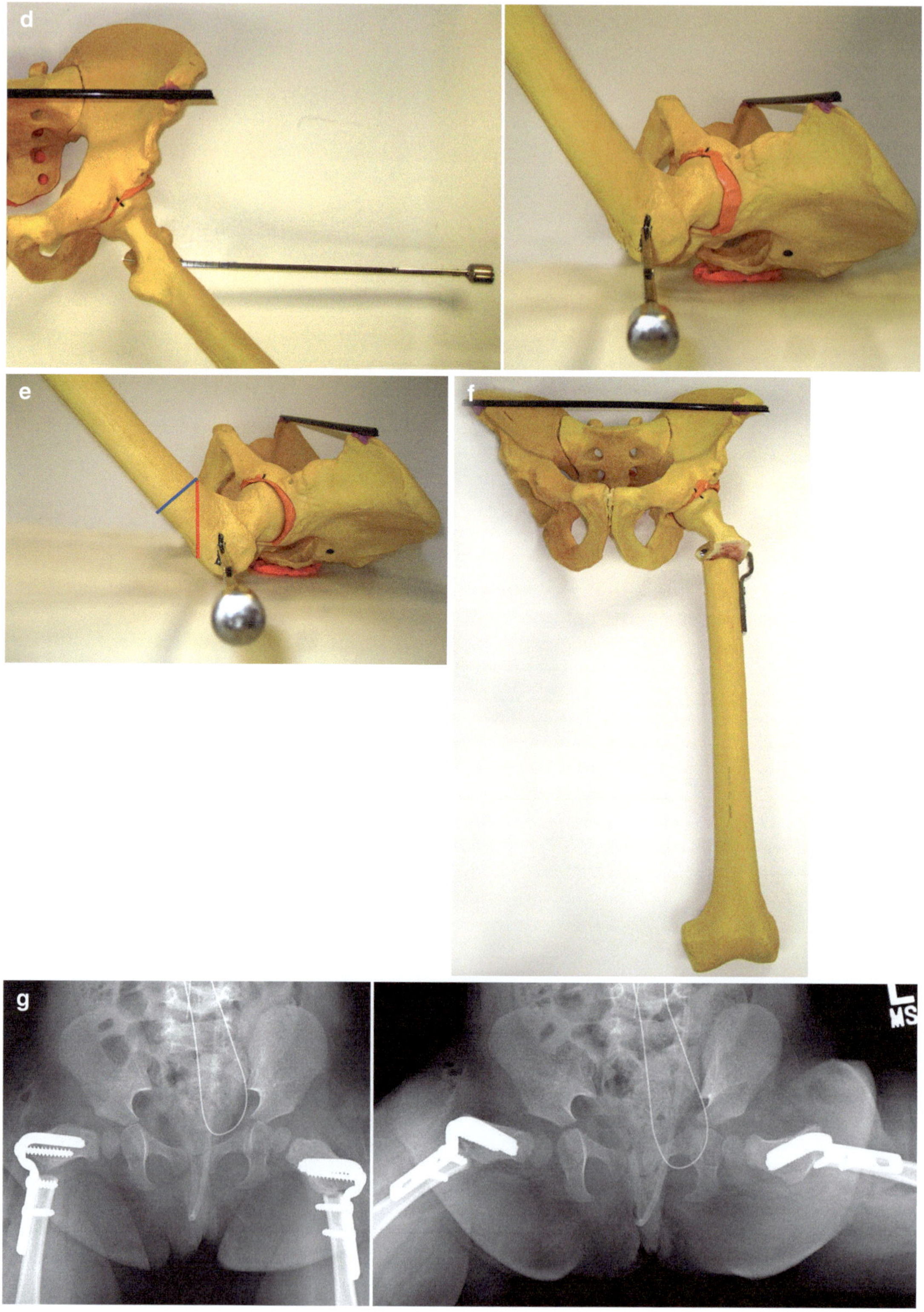

Fig. 29.4 (continued)

orly. In many cases of AMC, the vastus lateralis muscle has essentially been replaced by fibroadipose tissue, in which case a midline longitudinal split of the fascia is done instead.

The hip and lower extremity are held in their natural resting position, usually a combination of flexion, abduction, and external rotation. Under fluoroscopic guidance, a guidewire for a cannulated 90° proximal femoral blade plate system is advanced into the proximal femur, parallel to the pelvic axis wire in all planes (Fig. 29.4b). The wire is placed at a level on the femur where it will traverse the greatest length of femoral neck. Due to the external rotation of the hip, the wire will often exit the posterior femoral neck, in essence providing bicortical support for fixation (Fig. 29.4c).

The seating chisel from the cannulated blade plate set is advanced over the guidewire, with the hip still in its resting position, and the chisel held parallel to the transverse plane of the pelvis (Fig. 29.4d). Once a satisfactory depth is attained, the chisel is backed out slightly for ease of extraction later.

Two osteotomy cuts are made, the first is approximately 5–8 mm distal and parallel to the flat surface of the seating chisel. The second osteotomy squares the end of the distal fragment with a resulting wedge of bone removed (Fig. 29.4e). By marrying the two osteotomy surfaces together and acutely derotating the limb to bring the knee directly anterior, the deformity of the lower limb is corrected. A 90° proximal femoral blade with offset is impacted over the guidewire. The femoral shaft is reduced to the plate while correcting for rotation. We have used a three-hole plate, only filling the proximal two holes, which allows for easier plate removal later. A metaphyseal screw is added, if it can be accommodated within the proximal fragment (Fig. 29.4f, g).

Only skin and subcutaneous tissue are closed, in three layers, with a running stitch of absorbable suture in the subcutaneous fascial layer then interrupted buried suture stitches in the subcutaneous layer followed by a running subcuticular stitch. A Petrie cast (bilateral long leg casts with a bar spanning the ankles) is applied, unless a contralateral open hip reduction was performed, then a bilateral hip spica cast is placed. If radiographs at 3 weeks show adequate healing, standing is allowed in the Petrie cast. The cast is removed at 6 weeks, and an aggressive standing/gait training program is started, usually with knee-ankle-foot orthoses (KAFO).

Clinical Case Follow-Up

A.D. is now 8 years old and 6 and one-half years past her bilateral reorientational osteotomies. She began walking independently at 3 and one-half years of age and now keeps up with her peers in regular activities using only AFOs. Her current hip examination shows flexion of 145°on the right, 135° on the left, with 10° flexion contractures. Frogleg abduction is 65° on the right, 60° on the left, with regular abduction of 65° bilaterally; adduction is 20° on the right and 15° on the left.

Postoperative Imaging (Fig. 29.5)

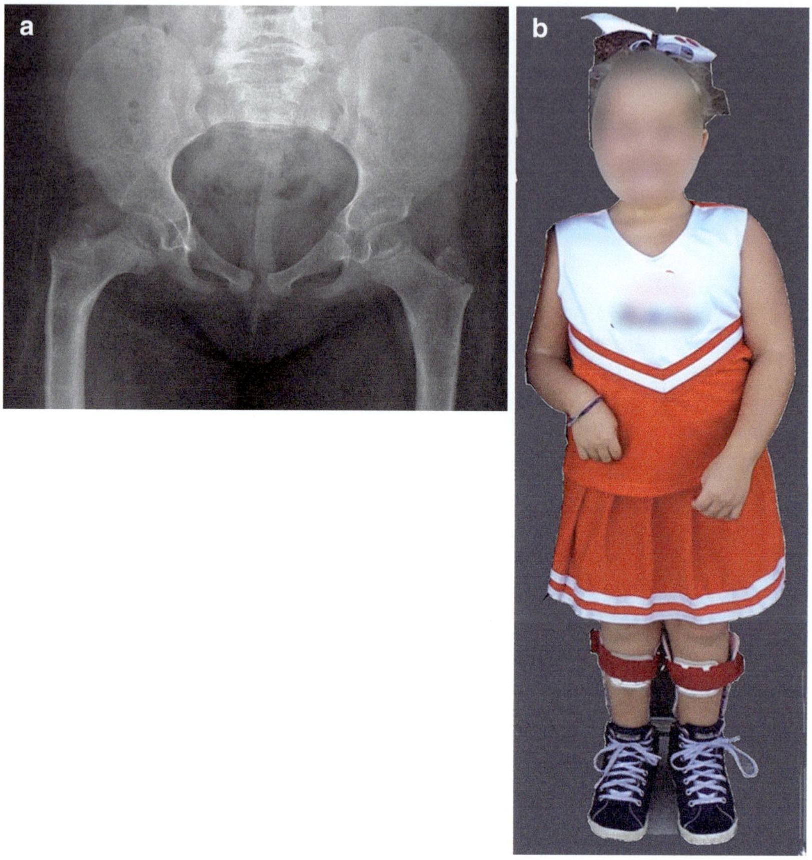

Fig. 29.5 Follow-up. (**a**) Anteroposterior pelvis view 4 years postoperatively; the fixation plates were removed 12 months after the procedure. Note the proximal femoral remodeling, with the greater trochanters having a nearly normal position. (**b**) Photograph of the patient standing at 8 years of age, 6 and one-half years after the procedure. She is able to keep up with her peers in regular activities

Pearls and Pitfalls

- When correcting moderate to severe hip flexion contractures, the osteotomy cuts will result in an anterior spike emanating distally from the proximal fragment. This needs to be trimmed to prevent mechanical impingement or encroachment on the neurovascular structures in full flexion.
- Hips lacking flexion are difficult to treat. Our best strategy at this time is to strip the gluteus maximus and abductors off the linea aspera (posterior hip release). Then, when placing the seating chisel, the hip is flexed as best possible, and the seating chisel is rotated parallel to the coronal plane of the pelvis. This will allow the hip to flex to 90° after the osteotomy; it may be necessary to shorten the femur to allow safe correction without stretching the sciatic nerve. This flexion may be difficult to maintain, since it is uncomfortable initially for the patients, and they tend to fight it; the gluteus maximus is a very strong muscle. I impose strict rules on sitting upright with a lap belt to force hip flexion.
- There is no upper age limit to when the procedure can be done, even in the skeletally mature. In general, as part of our treatment protocol, we try to perform the reorientational osteotomies between 12 and 18 months, so that weight-bearing therapies can be started directly thereafter.
- Our philosophy is that hip deformities in children with AMC should be corrected,

regardless of perceived ability to ambulate. Even if the children do not walk functionally, they still benefit from the improved sitting position and the ability to be positioned comfortably in a stander. By and large, though, we have found that children with AMC more often surprise us by what they can achieve, rather than disappoint us by what they cannot.

- Our treatment algorithm is to cast AMC foot deformities (clubfoot or congenital vertical talus) as a neonate/infant, address hip contractures and/or congenital dislocations between 12 and 18 months, and then correct knee flexion contractures after the fourth birthday.

Indications and Contraindications (Table 29.1)

Table 29.1 Proximal femoral reorientational osteotomies for the hip deformities in children with arthrogryposis multiplex congenita: surgical indication and contraindication

Indication
Congenital (arthrogrypotic) multiaxial hip contractures that preclude stable seating and/or efficient walking or crawling, regardless of the perceived potential for sitting or ambulating
Contraindication
Uniplanar hip contractures that can be treated with soft tissue releases (anterior hip release or adductor tenotomy) or simple derotational osteotomy

Suggested Reading

van Bosse HJ, Saldana RE. Reorientational proximal femoral osteotomies for arthrogrypotic hip contractures. J Bone Joint Surg Am. 2017;99(2):55–64. https://doi.org/10.2106/JBJS.16.00304.

Part III

Combined/Miscellaneous Osteotomies and Procedures Around the Hip Joint

Combined Pinning and Arthroscopic Osteoplasty for Stable Slipped Capital Femoral Epiphysis

30

Benjamin F. Ricciardi, Hannes M. Manner, and Michael Leunig

Introduction

In the past, the natural history of mild slipped capital femoral epiphysis (SCFE) was thought to be benign, and in situ pinning was considered the standard of care. Recently, open and arthroscopic studies have found high rates of intra-articular damage to the acetabular cartilage and labrum even in mild SCFE. Additionally, more recent clinical studies have found hip pain in one-third of patients with a mild SCFE and reduced Tegner and Lysholm scores at intermediate follow-up relative to age-matched controls. Femoroacetabular impingement (FAI), caused by the anterior metaphyseal prominence of the femoral neck entering the acetabulum, appears to be a source of this intra-articular injury. It is believed that by removing the prominent metaphyseal bone and reestablishing an appropriate head-neck offset, femoral osteoplasty will eliminate impingement and reduce subsequent intra-articular damage. Based on the increasing evidence of early articular damage after mild SCFE, the senior author (ML) began treating all mild slips with in situ pinning and immediate arthroscopic head-neck osteoplasty in 2008.

B. F. Ricciardi
Orthopedic Surgery, University of Rochester Medical Center, Rochester, NY, USA

Department of Pediatric Orthopedics, Schulthess Clinic, Zurich, Switzerland

H. M. Manner
Department of Orthopedic Surgery, Schulthess Clinic, Zurich, Switzerland
e-mail: hannes.manner@kws.ch

M. Leunig (✉)
Orthopedic Surgery, University of Rochester Medical Center, Rochester, NY, USA
e-mail: michael.leunig@kws.ch

Brief Clinical History

This 11-year-1-month-old female presented with a 2-month history of right groin pain with ambulation. On examination, the patient was able to ambulate without assistance but had been provided crutches by their referring physician. On the right side, she had 100° hip flexion, 10° internal rotation at 90° of hip flexion, 80° external rotation at 90° of hip flexion, and 40° of abduction. On the left side, she had 110° of hip flexion, 35° internal rotation at 90° of hip flexion, 60° of external rotation at 90° of hip flexion, and 45° of abduction. Impingement testing consisting of hip flexion, adduction, and internal rotation produced groin pain on the right side. Frog-leg lateral radiographs of the hip showed a deformity consistent with a mild slipped capital femoral epiphysis including posterior tilt and translation of the epiphysis with a slip angle of 26°. Based on increasing evidence of early articular damage after mild SCFE due to femoroacetabular impingement from the prominent anterior metaphysis, our preference is to treat all mild slips with in situ pinning and concurrent hip arthroscopy with removal of prominent metaphyseal bone to reestablish a normal contour to the head-neck junction.

R. C. Hamdy, N. Saran (eds.), *Pediatric Pelvic and Proximal Femoral Osteotomies*,
https://doi.org/10.1007/978-3-319-78033-7_30

Preoperative Imaging (Fig. 30.1)

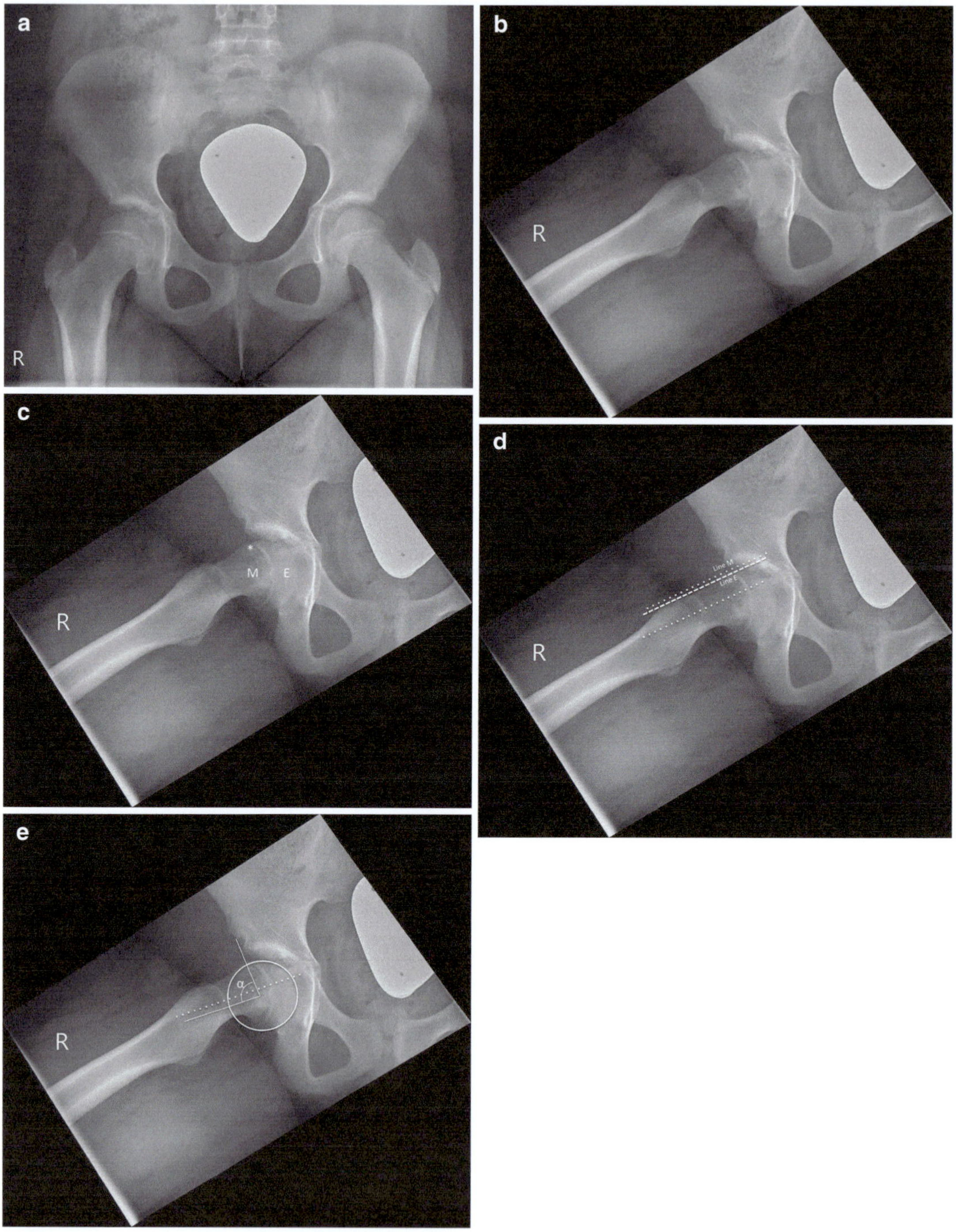

Fig. 30.1 Anteroposterior pelvis (**a**) and frog-leg lateral (**b**, **c**) radiographs show a mild right slipped capital femoral epiphysis deformity with posterior translation of the epiphysis (*E*) and anterior prominence (*) of the metaphyseal (*M*) region of the femoral neck. (**d**) Epiphyseal-metaphyseal offset of the right hip. (**e**) Alpha angle of the right hip

Goals of Treatment

The principles of treatment include:

Stable in situ fixation of the epiphysis
Debridement of prominent anterior metaphyseal bone to reestablish head-neck contour (goal: internal rotation of at least 20° with no visualized impingement between the acetabular rim and anterior femoral neck)

Treatment Strategy

The treatment strategy consists of addressing the stable SCFE and reducing the risk of intra-articular injury due to subsequent FAI. The mild stable SCFE is addressed by percutaneous pinning with a partially threaded screw in the center of the epiphysis and perpendicular to the physis. Arthroscopic femoral osteoplasty of prominent anterior metaphyseal bone is then performed at the time of percutaneous pinning (see Leunig et al. 2010) in order to restore the head-neck contour and reduce subsequent FAI.

Surgical Details

Percutaneous Pinning

The patient is positioned supine on a standard fracture table with both feet placed in well-padded boots and a well-padded perineal post. No traction is placed at this stage, and no attempt at reduction of the deformity is made. The operative hip rests in 0°of extension and is allowed to lie in a comfortable rotational position based on their deformity. Ensure that appropriate anteroposterior and lateral views can be obtained fluoroscopically prior to prepping and draping. After sterile prepping and draping, a guide wire is placed percutaneously onto the anterior femoral neck and directed into the center of the epiphysis, perpendicular to the physis under fluoroscopic guidance. Appropriate depth of the guide wire is assessed on the lateral view taking care to avoid joint penetration. A 6.5 mm partially threaded screw is then placed over the guide wire. Anteroposterior, lateral, and oblique views are used to ensure that the screw is central within the epiphysis and no joint penetration took place.

Hip Arthroscopy

After in situ fixation, the legs were positioned in 40° of abduction, 0–20° of flexion, and maximal internal rotation. Gentle traction is applied to the abducted operative hip with slight countertraction on the nonoperative hip. Joint distraction is achieved by adducting the operative hip and verified fluoroscopically. Standard anterolateral and midanterior portals are established. An interportal capsulotomy is performed, and a standard diagnostic arthroscopy of the central compartment is undertaken with a particular focus on assessing existing labral and chondral pathology. Attention is then turned to the peripheral compartment. With the camera in the midanterior portal, the retinacular branches of the medial femoral circumflex artery are directly visualized, and completion of the T-capsulotomy down to the intertrochanteric line is performed with hip extended. The head-neck junction is now well-visualized, and periosteum is removed from the anterior femoral neck to identify the metaphyseal prominence. Fluoroscopy is used to identify the physis and identify a starting point for the femoral osteoplasty. A 5.5 mm burr from the anterolateral portal is used to remove the metaphyseal prominence up to the level of the physis until the head-neck junction is restored to a more natural contour on fluoroscopy. Traction is released, and the hip is flexed to 45° and 30° of abduction. This allows visualization of the anteroinferior aspect of the deformity. In order to reach the level of the physis, relative extension of the hip will become necessary. The inferior retinacula of Weitbrecht define the anteroinferior limit of the resection. A 5.5 mm burr is used to carry the resection to the level of the physis with fluoroscopic confirmation of appropriate resection. The goal is to achieve internal rotation of at least 20° with no visualized impingement between the acetabular rim and anterior femoral neck.

Intraoperative and Postoperative Imaging (Figs. 30.2 and 30.3)

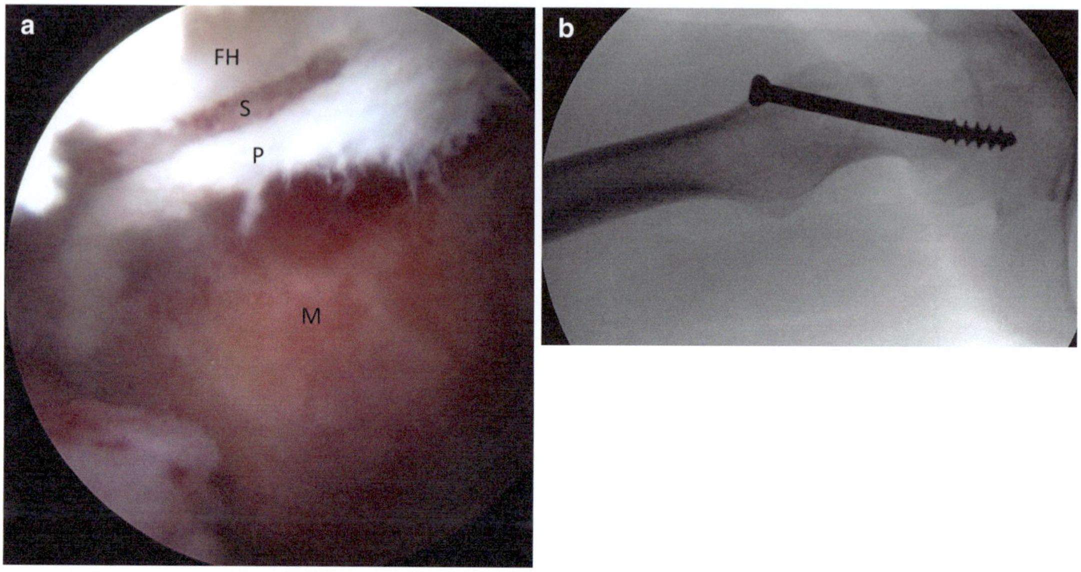

Fig. 30.2 (**a**) Intraoperative arthroscopic view of the right hip shows resection of the proximal anterior metaphysis (*M*) carried up to the level of the physis (*P*). The anterior separation (*S*) between the metaphysis and femoral head (*FH*) can be seen. (**b**) Fluoroscopy is used to confirm appropriate debridement with restoration of appropriate head-neck offset

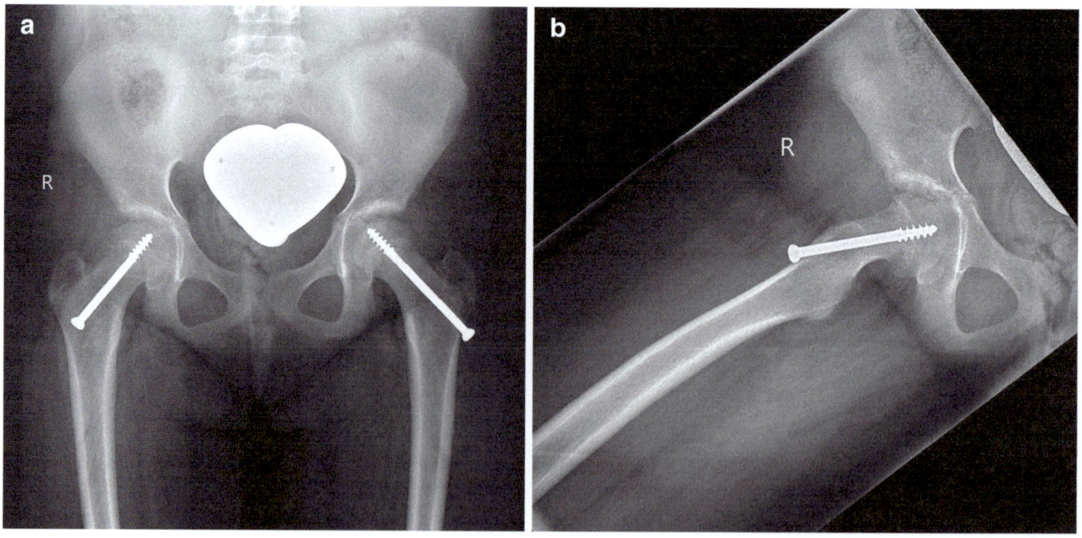

Fig. 30.3 Postoperative anteroposterior (**a**) and frog-leg lateral (**b**) images show stable positioning of the right mild slipped capital femoral epiphysis deformity with restoration of a normal contour of the head-neck junction. Prophylactic pinning of the left side was performed in conjunction with the right side

Pearls and Pitfalls

Pearls

- Always ensure that multiple oblique fluoroscopic views are obtained for (1) percutaneous pinning to avoid joint penetration and (2) assess the completeness of femoral osteoplasty.
- Relative extension of the hip during femoral osteoplasty will become necessary to complete resection of the metaphyseal prominence to the level of the physis.

Pitfalls

- Osteoplasty does not realign the epiphysis with the femoral shaft or increase the articular weight-bearing area. In slip angles higher than 30°, the epiphysis insufficiently corresponds with the anterosuperior acetabulum under axial loading. This may result in higher intra-articular contact stresses and intra-articular injury. In moderate to severe slips, even substantial osteoplasty would not eliminate impingement and might critically decrease the neck's structural integrity. We prefer subcapital realignment for all stable SCFE with slip angles greater than 30°.
- It is important to pay attention to hips with anterior overcoverage of the acetabulum due to acetabular retroversion, a morphological finding that is not rare in SCFE hips. Under such circumstances, even a decent osteoplasty may not be sufficient, and the level of impingement may just shift distally on the femoral neck; therefore, such hips may require additional rim trimming or, in the experience of the senior author, be even better treated with subcapital realignment. In cases of substantial acetabular retroversion, reverse PAO may also be an option in combination with pinning and osteoplasty.
- It is important to note that in situ pinning does not restore leg length like subcapital realignment due to persistent malposition of the epiphysis, and patients (and parents) should be informed about persistent mild shortening after the procedure.

Indications and Contraindications (Table 30.1)

Table 30.1 Combined pinning and arthroscopic osteoplasty for stable slipped capital femoral epiphysis: surgical indications and contraindications

Indications
Stable SCFE
Mild deformity (<30° slip angle)
Acute-on-chronic or chronic
Contraindications
Unstable SCFE
Moderate to severe deformity (>30° slip angle)
Acute

SCFE slipped capital femoral epiphysis

Suggested Reading

Dodds MK, McCormack D, Mulhall KJ. Femoroacetabular impingement after slipped capital femoral epiphysis: does slip severity predict clinical symptoms? J Pediatr Orthop. 2009;29(6):535–9.

Fraitzl CR, Kafer W, Nelitz M, Reichel H. Radiological evidence of femoroacetabular impingement in mild slipped capital femoral epiphysis: a mean follow-up of 14.4 years after pinning in situ. J Bone Joint Surg Br. 2007;89(12):1592–6.

Leunig M, Horowitz K, Manner H, Ganz R. In situ pinning with arthroscopic osteoplasty for mild SCFE: a preliminary technical report. Clin Orthop Relat Res. 2010;468(12):3160–7.

Leunig M, Casillas MM, Hamlet M, Hersche O, Notzli H, Slongo T, Ganz R. Slipped capital femoral epiphysis: early mechanical damage to the acetabular cartilage by a prominent femoral metaphysis. Acta Orthop Scand. 2000;71(4):370–5.

31 Osteochondroplasty and Acetabular Rim Trimming by Surgical Hip Dislocation for Femoroacetabular Impingement

Benjamin D. Martin and Matthew E. Oetgen

Introduction

Femoroacetabular impingement is typically a combination of cam- and pincer-type impingement. The surgical hip dislocation approach described by Ganz allows for 360° access to the femoral head and acetabulum for osteochondroplasty, acetabular rim trimming, and labral repair. The cam lesion is removed to restore sphericity and offset of the head-neck junction. The edge of the acetabulum can be resected, or trimmed, to address acetabular over-coverage, and areas of cartilage and labral damage due to the cam lesion can be repaired, resected, or treated with microfracture, as needed. To accomplish this, the labrum must be detached from the acetabular rim and later repaired back to reconstruct this anatomic structure. Intraoperative assessment is essential to confirm that all aspects of the impingement are addressed by observing the femoral head and the labrum as the hip is taken through a range of motion.

B. D. Martin
Division of Orthopaedic Surgery and Sports Medicine, Children's National Health System, Washington, DC, USA
e-mail: bdmartin@childrensnational.org

M. E. Oetgen (✉)
Division of Orthopaedic Surgery and Sports Medicine, Children's National Health System, Washington, DC, USA

The George Washington University School of Medicine and Health Sciences, Washington, DC, USA
e-mail: moetgen@childrensnational.org

Brief Clinical History

Case 1

A 12 + 4-year-old female presented with a 2-year history of progressive left hip and groin pain. She had been treated 3 years prior for a left-sided slipped capital femoral epiphysis (SCFE) with bilateral in situ hip pinning. The right hip was treated at that time prophylactically due to her relative skeletal immaturity and risk of subsequent slip of that side. While she had initially been asymptomatic following this procedure, the patient complained of progressive left-sided hip and groin pain over the past 2 years. Initially the hip was painful only with activities that required hip flexion past 90°, but the symptoms progressed to more constant groin pain with any hip motion over the past 6 months. The patient walked with an antalgic gait on the left side with a 40° external foot progression angle on the left and a 10°external foot progression angle on the right. She had a slightly shorter left leg, resulting in pelvic obliquity that was corrected with a 1.5 cm block under the left foot. The left hip range of motion (ROM) was limited by pain at 90° hip flexion and 5° of hip internal rotation. The right

R. C. Hamdy, N. Saran (eds.), *Pediatric Pelvic and Proximal Femoral Osteotomies*,
https://doi.org/10.1007/978-3-319-78033-7_31

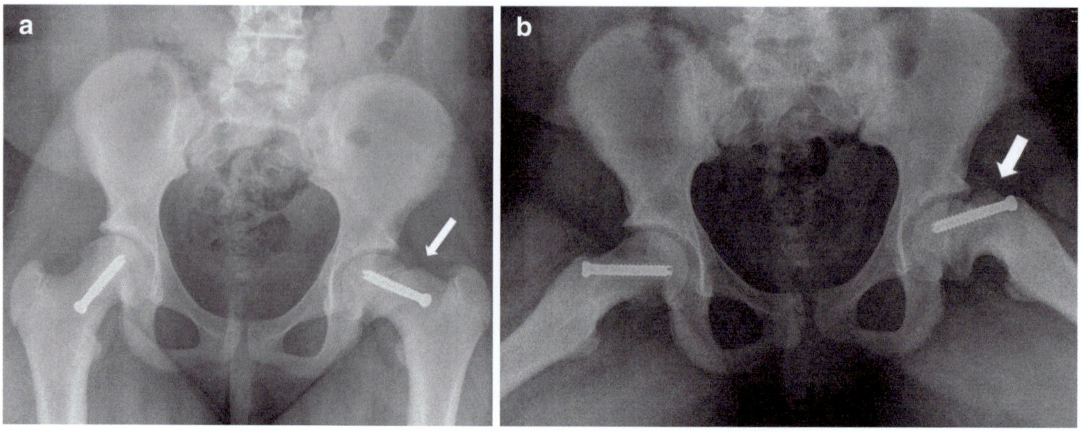

Fig. 31.1 Case 1. (**a**) Anteroposterior radiograph of the pelvis showing a healed SCFE deformity of the left hip with previously placed cannulated screw and residual varus angulation of the hip and a large cam lesion on the femoral neck (*arrow*). (**b**) Frog lateral radiograph showing significant retroversion of the left hip and the cam lesion extending to the anterior aspect of the femoral neck (*arrow*)

hip had an asymptomatic ROM of 120° of hip flexion and 30° of internal rotation. Radiographs demonstrated a healed severe SCFE on the left with the femoral hardware to be intact. The lateral center-edge angle on the left was measured to be 35°. Frog lateral radiograph demonstrated a large anterior femoral neck cam lesion. Magnetic resonance imaging (MRI) was not obtained preoperatively due to concern of inadequate visualization caused by scatter from the femoral hardware.

Preoperative Imaging for Case 1 (Fig. 31.1, anteroposterior and frog lateral of the pelvis)

Case 2

A 15-year-old male who was an active soccer player presented with 3 months of increasing left hip pain. The pain had been progressively worse over the previous 3 months, progressing from pain with maximal hip flexion to pain with hip flexion past 90° and with any hip internal rotation past neutral. Despite an initial trial of nonsteroidal anti-inflammatory medication, rest, and physical therapy, the patient's symptoms persisted. Radiographs demonstrated a broad left-sided anterior cam lesion. An MRI scan was obtained, which demonstrated an anterior labral tear.

Preoperative Imaging for Case 2 (Fig. 31.2a, b, anteroposterior and frog lateral of the pelvis; Fig. 31.2c, shoot through lateral of the left hip; Fig. 31.2d magnetic resonance image scan showing anterior labral tear and reduced femoral neck offset due to cam lesion)

Goals of Treatment

The ultimate goal is to remove the pathologic structure(s) leading to the abnormal contact between the femoral neck and the acetabulum. Cam lesions are removed via osteochondroplasty to restore sphericity of the femoral head and offset at the head-neck junction. If the acetabular rim is involved as a part of pincer impingement, or there is cartilage delamination from the cam lesion, this area can be addressed and labral pathology, such as fraying or frank labral tears can be repaired as well.

Treatment Strategy

Satisfactory femoral head osteochondroplasty and acetabular rim trimming are dependent on 360° visualization of the femoral head and acetabulum, which is best accomplished through a

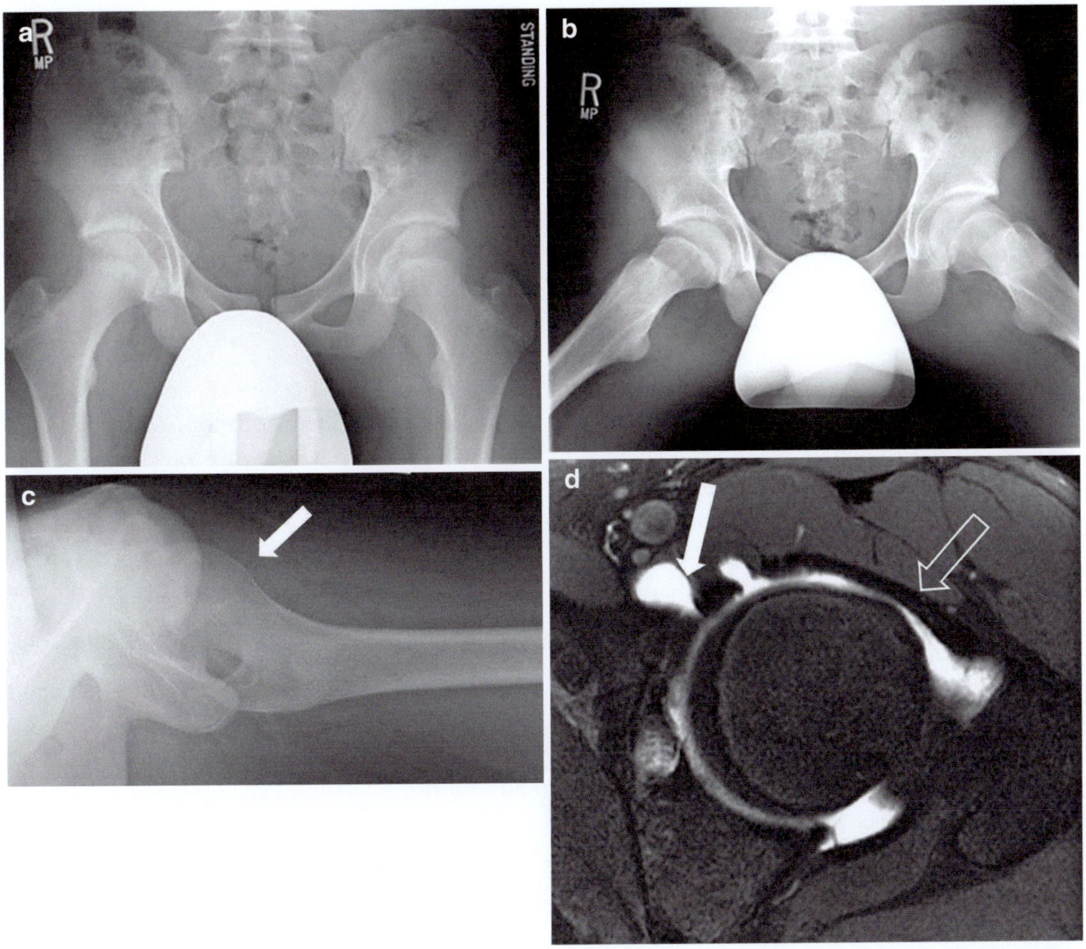

Fig. 31.2 Case 2. (**a**) Anteroposterior radiograph of the pelvis. (**b**) Frog lateral radiograph of the pelvis. (**c**) Shoot through lateral of the left hip demonstrating anterior cam lesion of the femoral neck (*arrow*). (**d**) Axial MRI cut of the left hip demonstrating anterior labral tear (solid arrow) with paralabral cyst and anterior femoral neck cam lesions (*open arrow*)

surgical hip dislocation approach as described by Ganz et al. (2001). With this exposure, cam and pincer impingement, along with the associated intra-articular pathology and joint damage, can be readily addressed.

Surgical Details

Surgical Hip Dislocation

The procedure is performed in the lateral decubitus position using a beanbag for patient positioning on a radiolucent flattop table. An epidural catheter is offered to patients to provide pain control until the second postoperative day. Effort is made to have the operative leg in a neutral position (without having to hold it during the procedure) by placing blankets over the well-padded down leg. A straight lateral incision is centered over the greater trochanter approximately 15 cm in length. Cerebellar retractors assist in adequate visualization, especially in patients with significant adipose depth. The iliotibial (IT) band is opened distal to the greater trochanter in the center of the femoral shaft using electrocautery or curved Mayo scissors. While holding the anterior leaf of the IT band with Kocher clamps, the dissection is carried proximally until the anterior edge of the gluteus maximus is identified. The gluteus maximus is teased off of the undersurface of the anterior fascial leaf, allowing it to fall posteriorly without splitting the muscle.

The insertion of the piriformis tendon and the most medial aspect of the greater trochanter are identified. A mark is made 5–8 mm lateral to this as well as at the posterior edge of the vastus lateralis. The greater trochanter is osteotomized using an oscillating saw along that line, leaving the vastus lateralis and abductor complex attached to the trochanteric fragment, which is typically between 10 and 15 mm in thickness. A small cuff of gluteus medius is left behind. A smooth Hohmann retractor is placed onto the anterior aspect of the stable trochanter, and bone wax is placed on the stable trochanter to decrease bleeding for the remainder of the case. The vastus lateralis is dissected off the femur distally. Superiorly, the interval between the piriformis tendon and the gluteus minimus is developed down to the capsule. It is important to remain proximal to the piriformis tendon to protect the blood supply to the femoral head. The gluteus medius and gluteus minimus are dissected off the joint capsule while abducting the leg and holding the muscle on tension with 90° retractors. Placing free standing retractors, such as a sharp Holman retractor or Kirschner wires, into the pelvis superior to the acetabulum provides good visualization without requiring an additional assistant for soft tissue retraction. As the dissection proceeds anteriorly, flexing and externally rotating the hip relaxes the anterior aspects of the gluteus medius muscle to allow exposure of the anterior capsule medially until the direct head of the rectus tendon is identified.

A "Z"-shaped capsulotomy is performed, starting in the middle of the neck to avoid injury to the femoral head cartilage. The inferomedial limb is opened down to the iliopsoas tendon, and the superoposterior limb is released to the piriformis tendon. A superior cuff of capsule is left behind to allow for repair during closure. The labrum should be visualized while cutting the capsule by elevating the edges with Kocher clamps to ensure that iatrogenic labral damage is not introduced. At this point, visualization into the hip joint is possible, and, with good retraction of the soft tissues and hip capsule, impingement of the femoral neck cam lesion and anterolateral acetabular rim can be observed while taking the hip through a range of motion. This impingement typically occurs with flexion and internal rotation, and this visualization is important to begin to estimate the extent of osteochondroplasty that will be required.

A bone hook around the base of the femoral neck is used to break the suction effect of the joint and to provide distraction so that the ligamentum teres can be cut with long curved Mayo scissors. The hip is then safely dislocated with traction, flexion, and external rotation. The leg is placed into a sterile bag positioned between the legs of the assistant. The femoral head can now be completely visualized and inspected for areas that are not spherical. A 360° view of the acetabulum is achieved by placing Hohmann retractors about the acetabulum and providing axial pressure along the femoral shaft to push the head posteriorly.

Acetabular Rim Trimming and Labral Repair

The labrum is examined for obvious tears, and the cartilage of the acetabulum is inspected with a nerve hook to feel for areas of cartilage damage or delamination. The junction of the labrum and acetabular edge is also probed for small, less obvious tears. If there is cartilage delamination or acetabular over-coverage leading to pincer impingement that requires intervention, the labrum is taken down from this area. This is performed by developing a bucket handle-type release of the labrum at the chrondrolabral junction with a knife, thus allowing this section of the labrum to be retracted away from the acetabular rim (Fig. 31.3a). The area of acetabular over-coverage and/or areas of cartilage delamination are resected using a combination of a rongeur and a high-speed burr. Assessment of the preoperative center-edge angle will assist in planning the amount of rim resection to be performed;

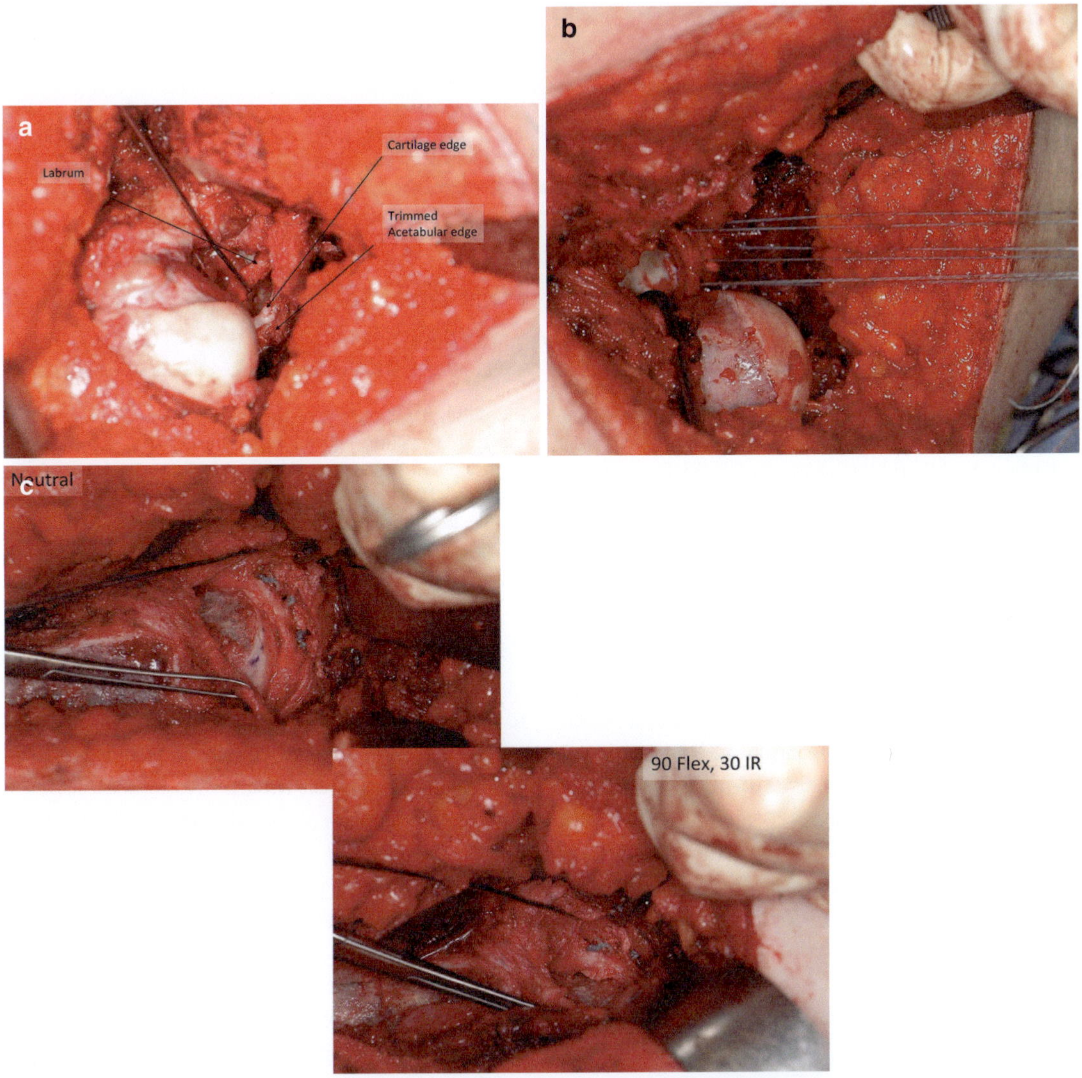

Fig. 31.3 Intraoperative photos of rim trimming and labral repair. (**a**) Intraoperative photo showing the labrum after release from the chondrolabral junction of the hip and trimming of the over covered acetabular rim. (**b**) Suture anchors have been placed in the bed of the acetabular rim in an extra-articular fashion. The sutures are shown having been placed through the labrum, prior to being tied down. (**c**) Intraoperative photo demonstrating the final labrum repair. The hip has been relocated in the acetabulum and the suture anchor knots tied on the outside of the joint, securing the labrum back in place (*top*). No impingement is noted with the hip flexed to 90° (*bottom*)

however, judicious resection should be undertaken as over-resection of the anterior, or lateral acetabulum may lead to postoperative instability. The center-edge angle can be measured on intraoperative fluoroscopy to quantify the amount of acetabular resection. After completing this rim resection, the bed of the acetabular edge is prepared with a burr to ensure a bed of bleeding bone. The labrum is then repaired back to that acetabular bed using suture anchors. Anchors are carefully placed to ensure that they are extra-articular, and all knots are tied on the outside edge of the labrum (Fig. 31.3b, c). The anchors are spaced approximately 1 cm apart to ensure a stable labral reconstruction (Fig. 31.4). If there is no evidence of acetabular over-coverage on preoperative or intraoperative assessment, however, a labral tear is noted on inspection; labral repair

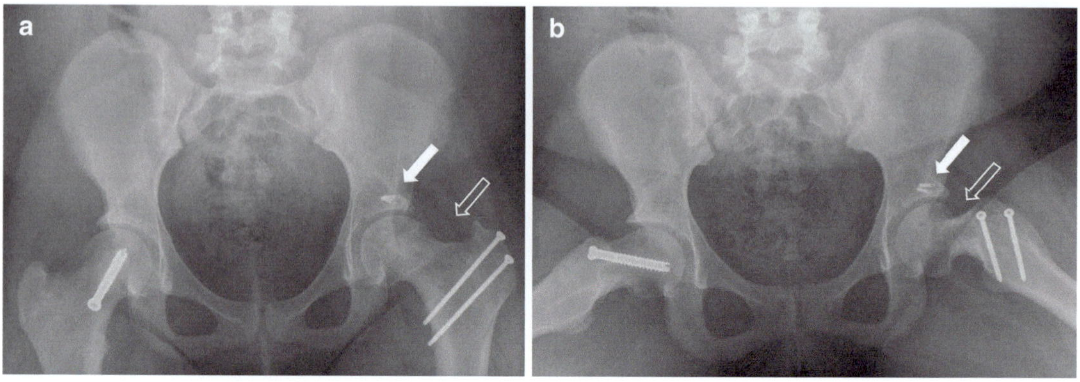

Fig. 31.4 Case 1. (**a**) Anteroposterior radiograph of the pelvis 1 year after a surgical hip dislocation, acetabular rim trimming, labral repair, and cam debridement. Suture anchors have been placed in the superior acetabulum for labral repair (*solid arrow*), and femoral neck offset has been restored (*open arrow*). (**b**) Frog lateral radiograph of the pelvis 1 year after a surgical hip dislocation, acetabular rim trimming, labral repair, and cam debridement. Suture anchors have been placed in the superior acetabulum for labral repair (*solid arrow*), and femoral neck offset has been restored (*open arrow*)

via suture anchors is performed in a similar fashion as described above.

If there is no evidence of acetabular overcoverage on the preoperative radiographs, no evidence of clinical pincer deformity on intraoperative acetabular inspection, and no labral tear identified with inspection, the focus of intervention is then moved to the femoral neck cam lesion.

Femoral Neck Osteochondroplasty (Fig. 31.5)

The sphericity of the femoral head is then evaluated. The cam lesion is typically in the anterior and anterolateral aspect of the femoral head-neck junction. Cartilage surrounding the lesion is often reddish in color, indicating that it should be resected (see Fig. 31.5a). Resection is best done with multiple passes of osteotomes, starting at the area of head-neck junction and directed distally to avoid iatrogenic damage to the femoral head (see Fig. 31.5b, c). Consistent visual and radiographic reevaluation of femoral head sphericity and head-neck offset should be performed to avoid excessive resection of the femoral neck. It is important to avoid deviation onto the lateral aspect of the femoral head and neck to avoid injury to the ascending cervical arteries supplying blood flow to the femoral head. Resection should be limited to less than 30% of the femoral neck. Bone wax is spread onto the resected area to stop bleeding and prevent bony re-overgrowth.

The hip is then reduced into the acetabulum and taken through a range of motion while observing the head-neck junction looking for persistent area of impingement. Ideally the femoral head should tuck under the labrum without significant deformation of the labrum. If there is an area that still impinges, the femoral head is dislocated again and the area resected. Maximal hip range of motion without impingement is the goal.

After confirming that both the femoral and acetabular components of the impingement have been addressed, the joint is thoroughly irrigated to remove debris and excess bone wax before the final reduction of the head into the acetabulum. In most cases the ligamentum teres is completely resected from its insertion on the femoral head prior to final relocation of the hip. Once the hip is reduced into the acetabulum, the capsule is repaired with heavy sutures in an interrupted fashion. After removing the bone wax from the stable trochanter, two or three bicortical 3.5 mm screws are used for fixation of the trochanteric fragment. The fascia and skin are closed in routine fashion.

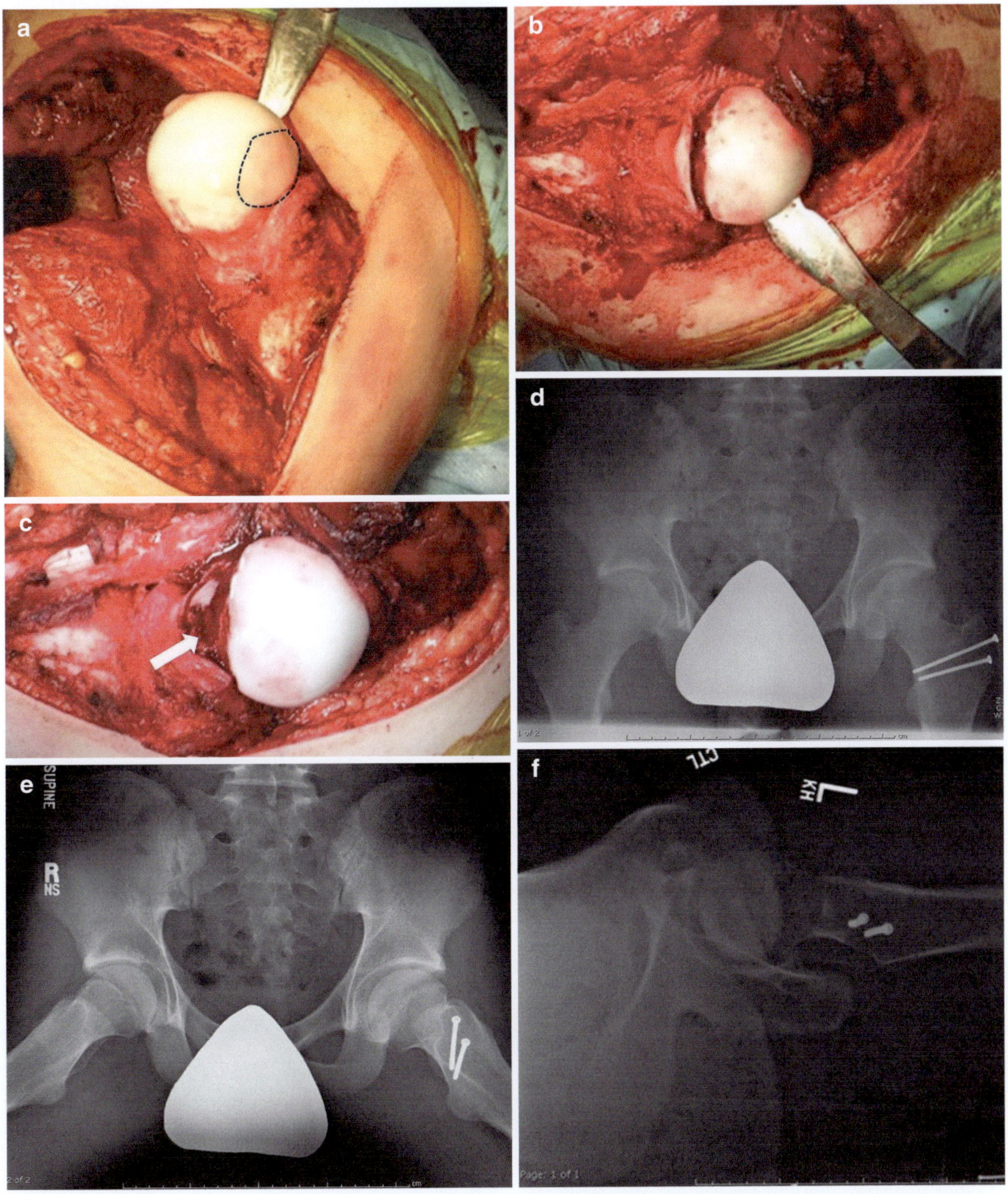

Fig. 31.5 Case 2. (**a**) Intraoperative photo of the left hip after surgical dislocation. Notice area of cam lesion that is to be resected (*outlined in dotted line*). (**b**) Intraoperative photo showing beginning of the femoral neck osteoplasty. Notice osteotomy was started at the head-neck junction and proceeds distally. (**c**) Image of femoral head after osteochondroplasty is completed. Notice resected area indicated by bleeding bone (*arrow*). (**d**) Anteroposterior radiograph of the pelvis after surgical hip dislocation and osteochondroplasty. (**e**) Frog lateral radiograph of the pelvis after surgical hip dislocation and osteochondroplasty. (**f**) Shoot through lateral of the left hip after surgical hip dislocation and osteochondroplasty demonstrating resection of femoral neck cam lesion showing improvement of head-neck offset

Postoperative Imaging for Case 1 (See Fig. 31.4)

The patient underwent a surgical hip dislocation, acetabular rim trimming, labral repair (notice suture anchors in superior acetabulum used for labral repair), and femoral neck osteochondroplasty to resect the femoral neck cam lesion.

Postoperative Imaging for Case 2 (Fig. 31.5d–f)

The patient underwent a surgical hip dislocation. Visual inspection of the labral revealed a frayed anterior labral (as opposed to a frank tear as suggested by the MRI) that was not amenable to repair, thus was judiciously debrided. A femoral neck osteochondroplasty was performed to resect the femoral neck cam lesion and to improve the femoral neck offset to eliminate the femoroacetabular impingement.

Pearls and Pitfalls

- Following the technique described by Ganz is necessary to avoid avascular necrosis of the femoral head by inadvertent injury to the ascending branches of the medial circumflex artery. Care should be taken when resecting the far posterolateral aspect of the cam lesion on the femoral neck. While there is no specific anatomic landmark for this, protection of the vascular supply to the femoral neck through the ascending cervical arteries should be constantly assessed during resection.
- Adequate visualization is essential. It is important to ensure that the capsule is open wide and retractors are strategically placed to see the acetabulum. This is accomplished with two or three Hohmann retractors. These are inserted in the space between the capsule and the labrum. A Hohmann retractor carefully placed around the transverse acetabular ligament in the inferior aspect of the acetabulum is helpful. With the hip dislocated, axial pressure along the femoral shaft pushes the femoral head posteriorly and allows for a better view of the acetabulum.
- Reducing the femoral head and ranging the hip to evaluate for deformation of the labrum aid in assessing if further resection is necessary. This can be done a few times if necessary. Flexion and internal rotation is the typical position of impingement.
- All components of the impingement, both femoral and acetabular, should be addressed. Time should be spent inspecting the acetabular cartilage, labrum, and femoral head-neck junction intraoperatively for potential areas that require resection.

Indications and Contraindications (Table 31.1)

Table 31.1 Osteochondroplasty and acetabular rim trimming by surgical hip dislocation for femoroacetabular impingement: Surgical indications and contraindications

Indications
Isolated cam lesion
Isolated pincer over-coverage
Mixed impingement
Contraindication
Advanced arthritis (Tönnis $\geq$2 or greater)

Acknowledgment The authors would like to thank Daniel J. Sucato MD, MS, and Neil Saran MD for their help in supplying images for this chapter.

Suggested Reading

Anwander H, Siebenrock KA, Tannast M, Steppacher SD. Labral reattachment in femoroacetabular impingement surgery results in increased 10-year survivorship compared with resection. Clin Orthop Relat Res. 2017;475(4):1178–88.

Espinosa N, Beck M, Rothenfluh DA, Ganz R, Leunig M. Treatment of femoro-acetabular impingement: preliminary results of labral refixation. Surgical technique. J Bone Joint Surg Am. 2007;89(Suppl 2, Pt 1):36–53.

Espinosa N, Rothenfluh DA, Beck M, Ganz R, Leunig M. Treatment of femoro-acetabular impingement: preliminary results of labral refixation. J Bone Joint Surg Am. 2006;88(5):925–35.

Ganz R, Gill TJ, Gautier E, Ganz K, Krugel N, Berlemann U. Surgical dislocation of the adult hip a technique with full access to the femoral head and acetabulum without the risk of avascular necrosis. J Bone Joint Surg Br. 2001;83(8):1119–24.

Unstable Hip in a Child with Down Syndrome

32

Claire E. Shannon and Simon P. Kelley

Introduction

Hip instability in Down syndrome (trisomy 21) is a spectrum of disease that presents with characteristic features at specific ages. Well-defined treatment options exist for each manifestation of hip instability. The final common pathway for the untreated unstable hip is painful degenerative hip disease with significant functional limitations. Traditionally, the results of treatment of hip instability were poor in this population; however, an improved understanding of the pathoanatomy and the development of contemporary algorithms for hip reconstruction have led to improved outcomes. Habitual dislocation of the hip presenting before age 8 years of age is treated with proximal femoral varus derotational osteotomy (VDRO). Older children who have developed secondary acetabular dysplasia are managed with an acetabular reorientation osteotomy with or without a femoral osteotomy. Individuals with evidence of degenerative arthritis, with or without fixed hip dislocation, are not suitable for hip preservation surgery but have been shown to be good candidates for total hip arthroplasty.

Brief Clinical History

A 4-year-old female with trisomy 21 and known hip instability since infancy presents for follow-up. She was treated with a Pavlik harness for an extended period of time as an infant for clinical hip instability and was felt to have achieved acceptable stability around 8 months of age. She was subsequently followed annually and noted to have developed habitual dislocation of both hips at the age of 3 years. The left hip was reduced but dislocatable, whereas the right hip was dislocated at rest but easily reducible. At the age of 4 years, she underwent bilateral varus derotational osteotomies of the proximal femurs in order to achieve concentrically reduced, stable hips.

C. E. Shannon
Division of Orthopaedics, Department of Orthopaedic Surgery, The Hospital for Sick Children, Toronto, ON, Canada

S. P. Kelley (✉)
Department of Surgery, University of Toronto, Toronto, ON, Canada

The Hospital for Sick Children, Toronto, ON, Canada
e-mail: simon.kelley@sickkids.ca

R. C. Hamdy, N. Saran (eds.), *Pediatric Pelvic and Proximal Femoral Osteotomies*,
https://doi.org/10.1007/978-3-319-78033-7_32

Preoperative Imaging (Fig. 32.1)

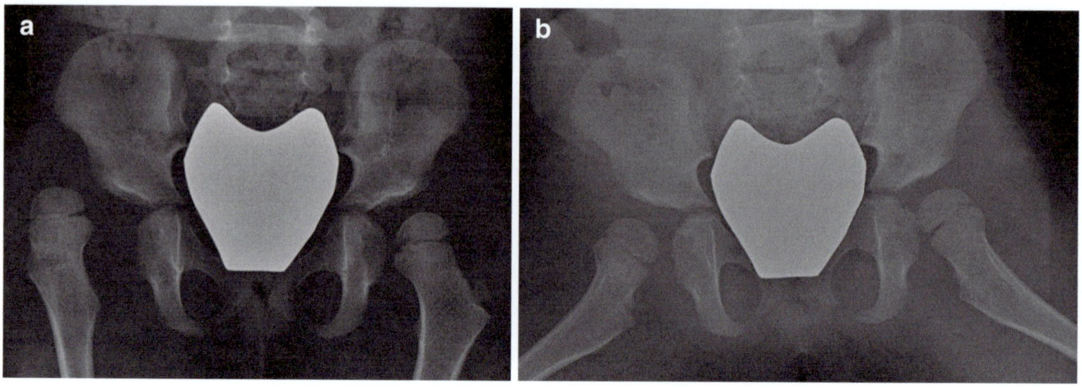

Fig. 32.1 (**a**) Anteroposterior radiograph at age 3 years with right hip dislocation and left hip subluxation. Acetabulae show dysplasia and widened (*V-shaped*) teardrop. (**b**) Frog-leg lateral radiograph at age 3 years showing positional reduction of right hip

Goals of Treatment

Goals of treatment depend on the severity of the disease and age of presentation but include:

- Reduction of the hip
- Maintain hip stability
- Prevent resubluxation
- Correct acetabular dysplasia
- Prevent secondary acetabular changes

Treatment Strategy

Instability of the hip in patients with trisomy 21 is notoriously difficult to manage. Historical efforts at treatment were met with frequent redislocations and high rates of complications. This was compounded by the low life expectancy for patients with trisomy 21 in that era, predominantly due to cardiac disease. At present, due to advances in the recognition and treatment of the medical comorbidities seen in these patients, life expectancy has almost doubled; however, this makes management of hip instability even more important for quality of life measures. Current approaches to hip instability in trisomy 21 are based on an improved understanding of the pathoanatomy, which includes a combination of soft tissue laxity, proximal femoral dysplasia, and acetabular retroversion.

Infants with trisomy 21 may present with reducible hip dislocations. These may respond well to conservative management with the harness/bracing techniques as used in developmental dysplasia of the hip but may require significantly prolonged treatment periods to achieve stability due to the tissue hyperlaxity. Due to the underlying pathoanatomy, many of these hips will progress to habitual dislocation when the child becomes ambulatory. Expectant management is the mainstay in this phase.

In the habitual dislocation phase, the treatment strategy seeks to contain the hip and to prevent further progression of changes, using a stepwise menu of procedures. Varying theories exist in the literature regarding the source of the primary structural abnormality and, therefore, the initial management. Some authors propose proximal femoral dysplasia in the setting of tissue hyperlaxity as the primary deficiency. This is managed with proximal femoral varus osteotomy with the aim of achieving a neck-shaft angle (NSA) of 105–110° and restoration of Shenton's line. Obtaining a lesser varus correction than this risks continued hip subluxation and/or dislocation. Excessive femoral anteversion may be present and addressed at this time, but care must be taken to avoid creating instability due to the relative retroversion of the acetabulum. When assessing femoral anteversion, plain radiographs may be misleading because the soft tissue laxity allows a wide variety of hip positions to be present upon imaging. It can therefore be particularly difficult to discern what is a true and excessive valgus NSA vs. a purely rotational abnormality. Thorough clinical assessment, along with an examination under fluoroscopic imaging at the time of corrective surgery, will help determine the true components of the proximal femoral dysplasia. Femoral anteversion should not be corrected to less than 20° for fear of creating functional (or true, in the case of overcorrection) retroversion on the background of a retroverted acetabulum. Other authors have shown acetabular retroversion and believe this to be a primary issue (along with soft tissue laxity) contributing to hip instability. Our experience in treating young children with trisomy 21 and hip instability has demonstrated success in correcting proximal femoral morphology alone (without acetabular reorientation) to deal with instability in the younger age group. Treatment of acetabular retroversion, should it be desired, is with a redirectional osteotomy, such as a triple osteotomy in the skeletally immature, or by Bernese periacetabular osteotomy in the skeletally mature, with or without proximal femoral osteotomy. These procedures are discussed in other chapters of this book. Soft tissue procedures alone have no role in these patients with pathologic tissue hyperlaxity. Attempts at soft tissue reconstruction will invariably "stretch out" over time, leading to recurrence of instability.

Patients in the subluxation phase are typically older than 8 years and have begun to develop secondary acetabular changes over and above the underlying retroversion, often demonstrating a reduced center-edge angle of Wiberg, increased Tonnis angle, and a widened or dysmorphic teardrop. The treatment of choice in this stage of disease is acetabular reorientation to provide increased anteversion, as well as lateral and anterior coverage, with or without proximal femoral osteotomy. Proximal femoral osteotomy alone is unlikely to be successful due to the more significant secondary acetabular dysplasia present in the adolescent. Skeletally immature patients should undergo a triradiate sparing procedure such as a triple osteotomy. Patients who have closed triradiate cartilages should be managed with a Bernese periacetabular osteotomy. Osteotomies that do not provide increased anteversion (Salter, Pemberton) are contraindicated and will exacerbate the posterior undercoverage, thus increasing the instability.

Fixed dislocations in the setting of degenerative joint disease typically preclude the use of hip preservation procedures described above. These patients should be managed with total hip arthroplasty to improve pain and mobility. This topic is discussed in a number of published case series and is outside the scope of this text.

Surgical Details

Proximal Femoral Varus Osteotomy for Habitual Dislocation

Positioning Position the patient supine on a radiolucent table with a small bump under the flank of the surgical side. Prepare and drape the entire hindquarter, from the base of the ribcage to the midline both dorsal and ventral. If performing bilateral procedures, isolate the groin from the surgical field with an impermeable dressing.

Approach A standard direct lateral approach to the proximal femur is used. A 10–15 cm longitudinal incision is made, centered over the lateral aspect of the femur, with the greater trochanter as the most proximal extent. The fascial layer is exposed and split in line with the skin incision. The vastus lateralis is released sharply from its origin with an L-shaped incision, transecting the tendinous portion at the vastus ridge and elevating the muscle longitudinally along the posterolateral aspect of the femur. Care should be taken to avoid disruption of the gluteus maximus tendon at the distal aspect of the vastus lateralis dissection. The vastus lateralis is elevated subperiosteally from posterolateral to superomedial, using a Hohmann retractor to aid exposure. A periosteal elevator is then carefully used to carry the subperiosteal dissection around the posterior aspect of the proximal femur from the level of the lesser trochanter to the distal extent of the incision.

Varus Derotational Osteotomy

A 90° blade plate is the implant of choice for most patients due to the typically narrow femoral neck morphology in trisomy 21 (particularly in the anterior to posterior dimension); however, a 100° or 110° proximal femoral locking plate may be considered if adequate bony real estate is available. The blade plate typically offers a broader shoulder than the locking plate and thus the opportunity for more significant medialization of the femoral shaft, which may be of benefit to restoring a neutral mechanical axis of the entire limb.

Guide Wire Insertion A guide wire is inserted under fluoroscopic guidance into the femoral neck from the proximal lateral femur as a directional aid. The guide wire should be centered in the neck on the lateral view and in the superior aspect of the femoral neck on the anteroposterior (AP) view to allow insertion of the seating chisel in the midportion of the femoral neck. The angle of the wire on the AP view will help determine the varus correction (acting as a guide for the seating chisel). To aid accurate insertion of the guide wire in the AP plane, a metallic triangle of a known geometry is used. For example, in a hip with a native 140° NSA, a correction of 30° of varus is required to achieve a NSA of 110° (140°–110° = 30°). Thus, a 60° metallic triangle is aligned with the straight lateral border of the proximal femur. This ensures the guide wire is inserted at an angle 30° from perpendicular to the femoral shaft (Fig. 32.2a).

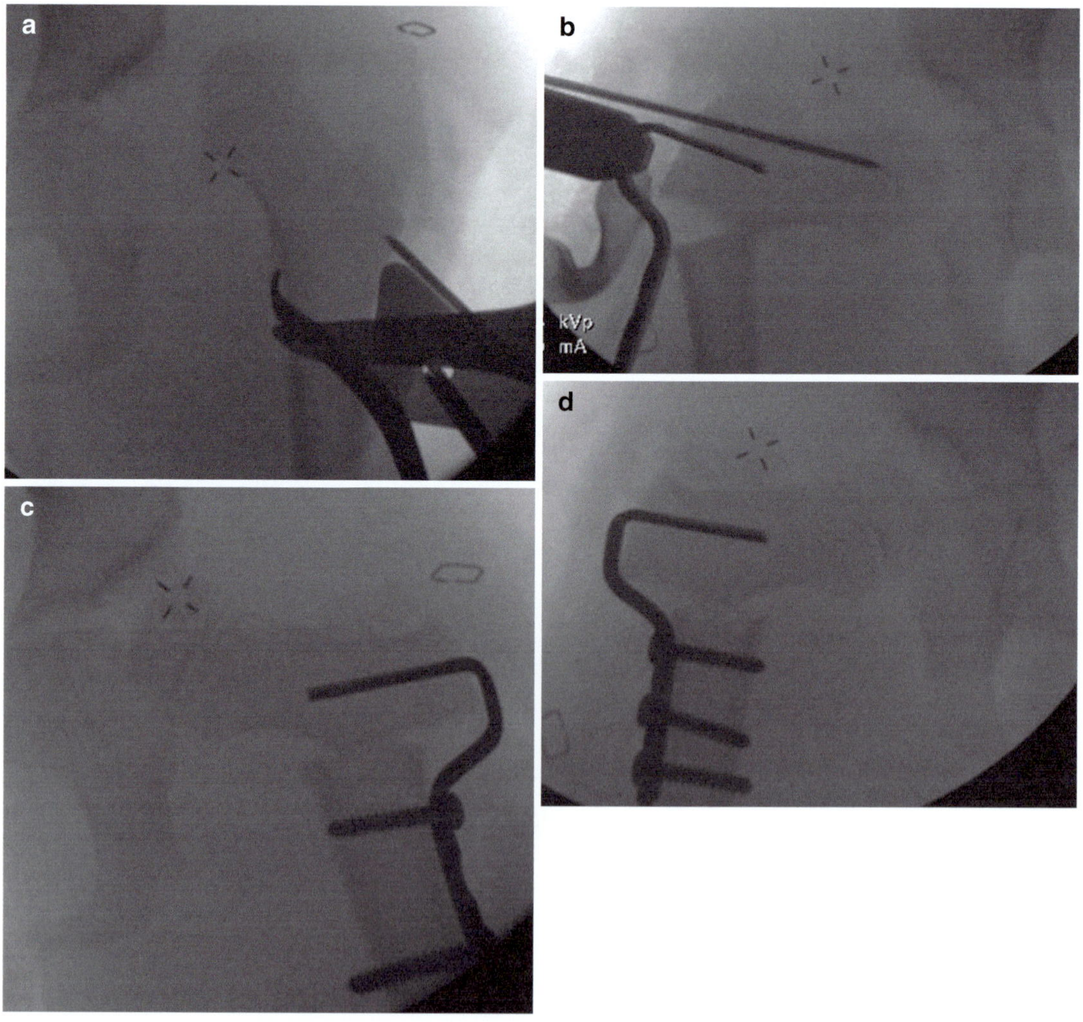

Fig. 32.2 Intraoperative radiographs of bilateral varus derotational osteotomies. (**a**) Guide wire placement using a metallic triangle to create a varus correction with the preselected 90° blade plate that results in a 105–110° neck-shaft angle. (**b**) Osteotomy cuts—proximal cut is parallel to blade, and distal cut is perpendicular to femoral shaft. (**c**) Initial plate fixation showing obligatory medialization of the femoral shaft to restore overall mechanical axis of limb. (**d**) Final fixation demonstrating the desired 105–110° neck-shaft angle

Further detail concerning geometric planning of VDRO can be found in Chap. 19 of this book.

Chisel Insertion An appropriately sized 90° blade plate is then selected based on a blade width that will fit comfortably within the width of the femoral neck. To help with sizing, the corresponding seating chisel can be held over the femoral neck under a lateral fluoroscopic view. The seating chisel should be projected to lie completely within the width of the femoral neck. The seating chisel is then carefully inserted into the femoral neck, parallel but inferior to the pre-inserted guide wire. The chisel should be advanced into the femoral neck, stopping short of the subcapital physis. Frequent fluoroscopic checks should be made to ensure accurate trajectory of the seating chisel. A more proximal start point will allow for insertion of a longer blade due to the cylindrical shape of the femoral neck.

Osteotomy Once the chisel is seated in the appropriate position, a varus wedge osteotomy is performed. The level of the osteotomy is marked on the bone and must occur within the shoulder region of the plate, approximately 10 mm distal to the chisel. Two parallel K-wires are inserted into the anterior surface of the femur above and below the osteotomy site to monitor rotation. Hohmann retractors are placed circumferentially around the femur at the level of the osteotomy. The first cut is made with an oscillating saw parallel to the chisel blade, taking care not to extend into the femoral neck. The second cut is made perpendicular to the femoral shaft either at the same start point as the first cut or more distal if femoral shortening is required (Fig. 32.2b). The wedge of the bone is removed and kept as potential bone graft. The seating chisel is then carefully removed, and the preselected plate is inserted by hand into the blade track. A mallet may be used to provisionally seat the blade. A Verbrugge clamp is then used to reduce the femoral shaft to the distal aspect of the plate.

Derotation and Distal Fixation If derotation of the femur is desired, this is performed now. Femoral anteversion is assessed prior to the osteotomy by examination under fluoroscopy. In full extension, the lower limb is internally rotated until a true AP of the femoral neck is seen (this corresponds to the smallest measurable neck-shaft angle). The amount of internal rotation required from the patella forward position of the leg corresponds to the amount of femoral anteversion. Care is taken not to overcorrect the femur rotation. A minimum of 20° residual anteversion is required. The plate is then fixed to the shaft of the femur with a screw, using compression technique followed by a second positional screw (Fig. 32.2c). A narrow tamp is then used to complete insertion of the blade portion of the plate, resulting in the desired medialization of the femoral shaft, and the final screw fixation is performed (Fig. 32.2d). Figure 32.3 shows intraoperative radiographs of a varus derotational osteotomy performed with a proximal femoral locking plate as an alternative to the blade plate.

Closure and Postoperative Care

The vastus lateralis tendon is repaired, followed by closure of the wound in standard layered fashion. Postoperative immobilization with Petrie casting is recommended for 6–8 weeks. This allows for stabilization of the soft tissues and protected weight bearing, which is difficult to ensure in this patient population without casting.

Complications

Three particular postsurgical complications do appear to have an increased incidence in this patient population. Redislocation or resubluxation was traditionally a common reason for failure of treatment; however, improved understanding of the pathoanatomy of hip instability in trisomy 21, specifically, abolishment of soft tissue reconstruction alone and the need to reduce the NSA to 105–110° using proximal femoral osteotomies, has significantly reduced this complication. Postoperative infection rates of up to 20% have been reported for this patient population. This is thought to be secondary to immunodeficiency associated with trisomy 21, although supportive literature on this finding is sparse. Appropriate perioperative precautions should be taken, as with any procedure in a child with inherent risks of infection. Although no evidence exists in the literature regarding increased risk of fracture in patients with trisomy 21, the authors have noted an increased incidence of peri-implant fracture in this group. Patients with trisomy 21 may have a lower bone mineral density by area due to smaller bone size and lower actual density. Furthermore, they are also subject to external factors, such as hypotonia, low activity levels, and endocrine abnormalities that put them at risk of falls and skeletal insufficiency. The authors recommend removing proximal femoral hardware after bony union on this basis. Figure 32.4a shows a radiograph of a peri-implant fracture around a blade plate in a patient with trisomy 21 after bony union of a VDRO. Figure 32.4b shows a radiograph of a fracture fixation using a proximal femoral locking plate.

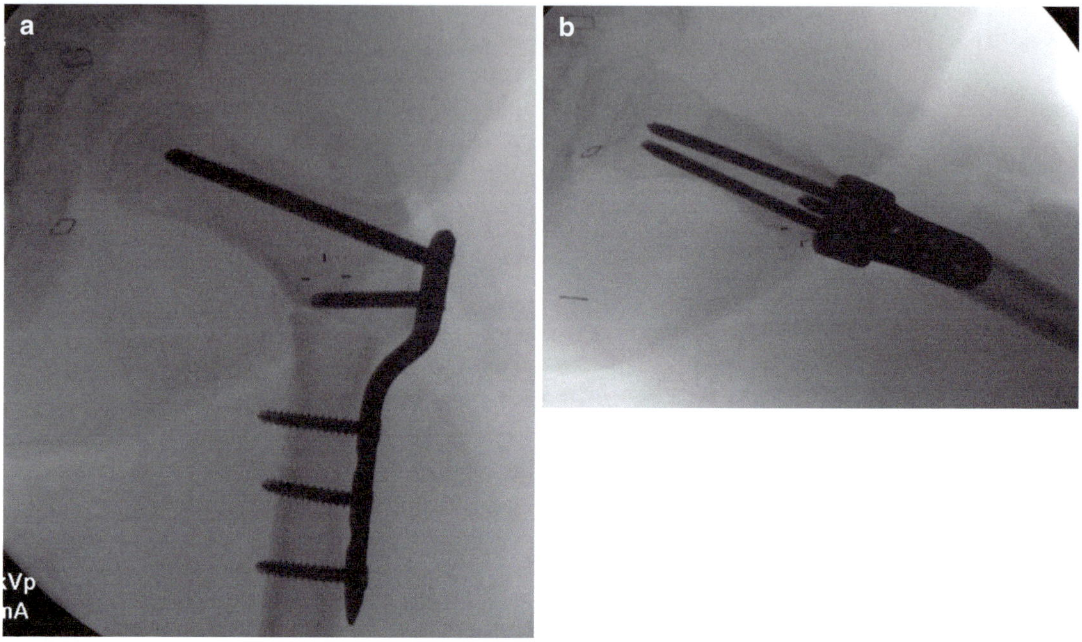

Fig. 32.3 Intraoperative radiographs of a varus derotational osteotomy performed with a proximal femoral locking plate

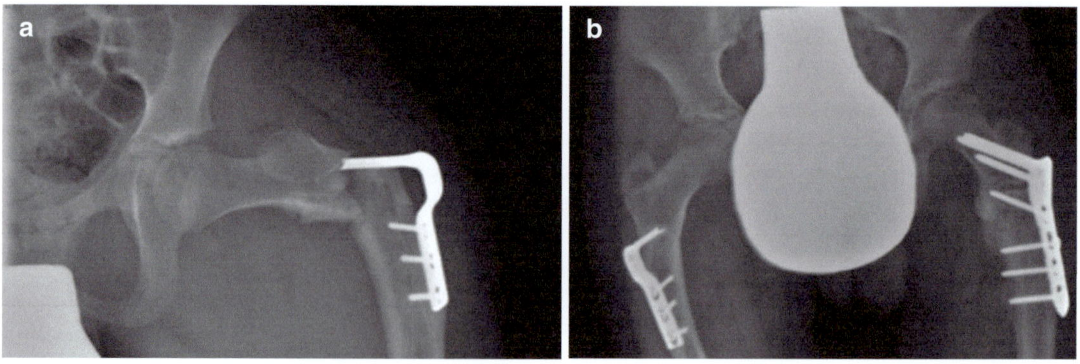

Fig. 32.4 (**a**) Radiographs of a peri-implant fracture of the left hip around a blade plate in a patient with trisomy 21 a number of years after bony union of a varus derotational osteotomy. Also note that despite excellent initial position and fixation, over many years, the right proximal femur has grown away from, and off, the blade plate. This increases the risk of peri-implant fracture and is a further indication for implant removal (**b**) Fracture fixation using a proximal femoral locking plate

Postoperative Imaging (Figs. 32.5 and 32.6)

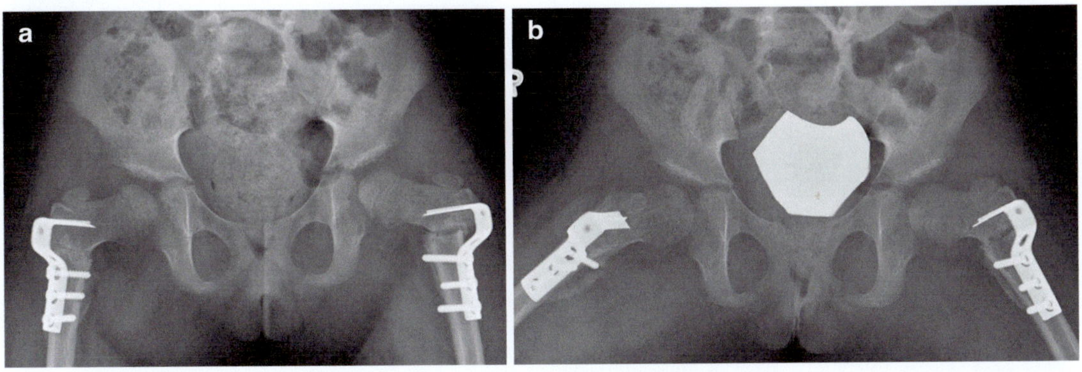

Fig. 32.5 Early postoperative (**a**) anteroposterior and (**b**) frog lateral radiographs of the hips showing varus correction of bilateral proximal femora, with resulting neck-shaft angles of 110°. Both hips are now enlocated, Shenton's arc is restored, and the hips remain stable bilaterally. Note that the femoral necks are directed toward the triradiate cartilage

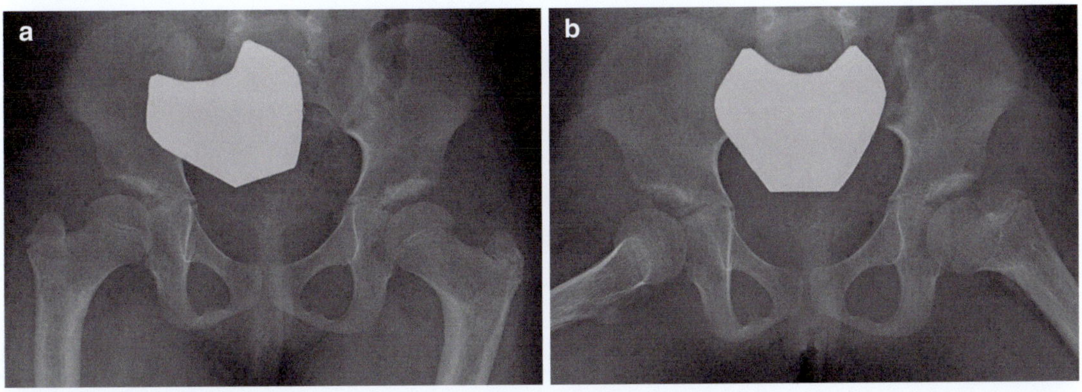

Fig. 32.6 (**a**) Anteroposterior and (**b**) frog lateral radiographs 2 years postoperatively, after undergoing removal of implants. Some remodeling of the femoral necks has occurred. The hips remain concentrically reduced and clinically stable. Note the improved acetabular coverage and development compared to preoperative radiographs in Fig. 32.1

Pearls and Pitfalls

- Soft tissue procedures alone are inadequate to treat to hip instability in hyperlaxity conditions.
- Avoid undercorrection of proximal femoral varus. Goal NSA is 105–110°.
- Avoid overcorrection of femoral rotation. A minimum of 20° residual anteversion is required to maintain stability due to relative acetabular retroversion.
- Postoperative cast immobilization is necessary to protect weight bearing and to stabilize soft tissues.
- Implant removal after bony union should be highly considered to avoid peri-implant fracture.

Indications and Contraindications (Tables 32.1 and 32.2)

Table 32.1 Proximal femoral osteotomy: surgical indications and contraindications

Indications
Hip instability with lack of degenerative change
Increased proximal femoral anteversion
Concentrically reducible hip
Contraindications
Degenerative changes of the hip joint
Secondary acetabular changes (femur alone)

Table 32.2 Pelvic osteotomy: surgical indications and contraindication

Indications
Hip instability with lack of degenerative change
Secondary acetabular changes
Concentrically reducible hip
Acetabular retroversion
Contraindication
Degenerative changes of the hip joint

Suggested Reading

Katz DA, Kim YJ, Millis MB. Periacetabular osteotomy in patients with Down's syndrome. J Bone Joint Surg Br. 2005;87(4):544–7.

Kelley SP, Wedge JH. Management of hip instability in trisomy 21. J Pediatr Orthop. 2013;33(Suppl 1):S33–88.

Knight D, Alves C, Wedge JH. Femoral varus derotation osteotomy for the treatment of habitual subluxation and dislocation of the pediatric hip in trisomy 21: a 10 year experience. J Pediatr Orthop. 2011;31(6):638–43.

Sales de Gauzy J. Pelvic reorientation osteotomies and acetabuloplasties in children. Surgical technique. Orthop Traumatol. 2010;96(7):793–9.

Sankar WN, Millis MB, Kim YJ. Instability of the hip in patients with down syndrome: improved results with complete redirectional acetabular osteotomy. J Bone Joint Surg Am. 2011;93(2):1924–33.

Steel H. Triple osteotomy of the innominate bone 1973. J Bone Joint Surg Am. 2004;86(3):644.

Taylor D, Macdonald MP, Koshavili Y, Gross AE. Total hip arthroplasty to treat congenital musculoskeletal abnormalities in the juvenile down syndrome hip: review of literature with case. J Pediatr Orthop B. 2012;21(3):235–9.

Weber M, Ganz R. The Bernese periacetabular osteotomy. Orthop Traumatol. 2002;10(2):93–112.

33 Proximal Femoral Head Resection and Interpositional Arthroplasty

Elizabeth Ashby and Deborah M. Eastwood

Introduction

Despite preventative screening programmes in some countries, hip dislocation is still a common problem in many severely affected, non-ambulant patients with cerebral palsy. There are two scenarios where pain and stiffness affect all aspects of patient comfort and care and where a proximal femoral excision with an interpositional arthroplasty (myoplasty) must be considered: (1) the enlocated hip following hip reconstruction that is associated with a poor clinical outcome and (2) the dislocated hip, which due to anatomical or clinical factors is not reconstructible. Both indications are most common in patients assessed as IV or V on the Gross Motor Function Classification Scale (GMFCS).

Where pain, difficulty sitting in a wheelchair for more than about 45–60 mins and/or perineal care are significant problems, proximal femoral excision with interposition myoplasty and aggressive management of the associated tonal abnormalities will reduce pain, ease care and improve sitting tolerance to 3 h or more. Examples of both scenarios are described.

Brief Clinical History

Case 1

A 7-year-old girl with spastic bilateral cerebral palsy, Gross Motor Function Classification Scale (GMFCS) level IV, presented with stiff hips. X-ray showed bilateral hip subluxation with migration percentages of 35–40%. She underwent bilateral soft tissue releases and proximal femoral varus osteotomies. At the age of 16 years, the right hip became painful. X-ray showed re-subluxation of the hip joint. She underwent open hip reduction, revision soft tissue releases and revision proximal femoral osteotomy. Her hip pain subsided. At the age of 18 years, she underwent spinal fusion to the pelvis for deformity correction. She developed increasing right hip pain, stiffness and difficulty with perineal care with the groin crease scar from her previous adductor release splitting regularly. By age 22 years, she was unable to sit comfortably for more than an hour in her customised chair. Her hip was in 10° of fixed adduction and had a flexion range of 30–60°. Total hip arthroplasty was considered but rejected on clinical grounds because of her spasticity.

E. Ashby
Department of Orthopaedics, Evelina Children's Hospital, London, UK
e-mail: elizabethashby@doctors.org.uk

D. M. Eastwood (✉)
Department of Orthopaedic Surgery, Great Ormond Street Hospital for Children, London, UK
e-mail: Deborah.Eastwood@gosh.nhs.uk

R. C. Hamdy, N. Saran (eds.), *Pediatric Pelvic and Proximal Femoral Osteotomies*,
https://doi.org/10.1007/978-3-319-78033-7_33

Right proximal femoral resection with interposition myoplasty was performed. Her hip pain resolved completely, her limb was mobile, and she was able to sit comfortably for 4–6 h.

Case 2

A 14-year-old boy with dystonic, total body cerebral palsy, GMFCS level V, presented with a painful, chronically dislocated, right hip. The hip was very stiff and irritable, and he could not sit comfortably for more than 20 mins. Despite the obvious erosion of the femoral head, a hip reconstruction was attempted, but the femoral head could not be mobilised sufficiently. Therefore, a proximal femoral resection with interposition myoplasty was performed. This provided good pain relief and allowed the boy to sit comfortably in his chair. Subsequently he has undergone a spinal fusion, but despite the persisting pelvic obliquity, his 'hip' is mobile, and perineal care and dressing remain easy to achieve and comfortable.

Preoperative Imaging

Case 1: Fig. 33.1a
Case 2: Fig. 33.1b

Goals of Treatment

1. Pain relief
2. Allow comfortable sitting in a customised wheelchair
3. Improve 'joint'/lower limb mobility to facilitate perineal hygiene, washing and dressing, and ease of hoisted transfers

Treatment Strategy

1. Maximise nonoperative treatment measures with medications such as baclofen, trihexyphenidyl and analgesics [including, if appropriate, intra-articular injections of local anaesthetic and/or ITB (intrathecal baclofen)] to reduce pain and spasm (determine whether the spasm is due to spasticity or dystonia or both).
2. Identify/confirm the hip as the principal site of pain.
3. In the dislocated hip, assess whether reconstruction is feasible: a deformed or eroded femoral head is not necessarily a contraindication to reconstruction with symptomatic relief.
4. If reconstruction not technically possible, proceed to proximal femoral excision with interposition myoplasty.

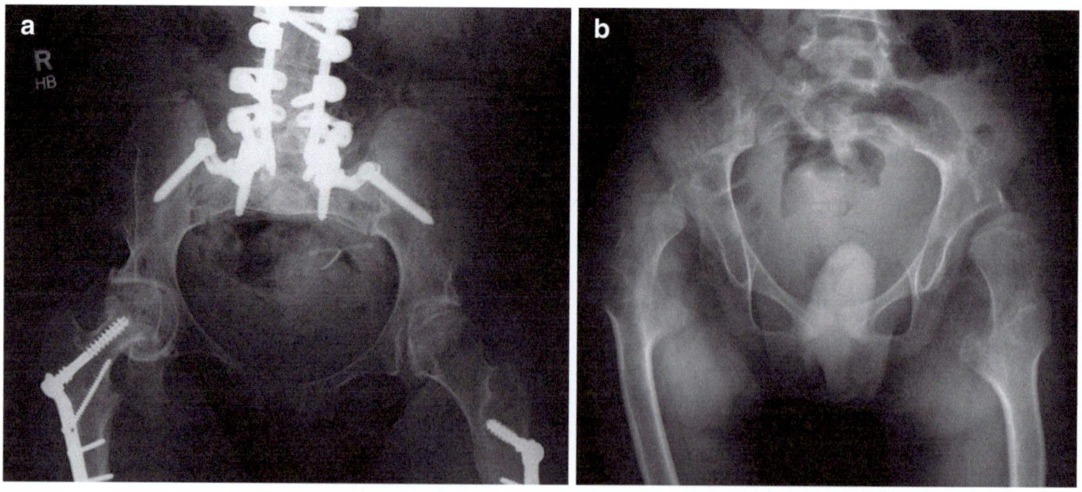

Fig. 33.1 *Case 1*. (**a**) Anteroposterior radiograph of both hips. The lower lumbar spine is fused to the pelvis. Both hips are in joint with severe loss of joint space on the right side. Note the chronic constipation which can also be a cause of pain and difficulty sitting comfortably as can her IUCD (intrauterine contraceptive device). *Case 2*. (**b**) Anteroposterior radiograph of both hips. The right hip is dislocated, and there is a significant erosion of the superior aspect of the right femoral head. The left hip is subluxated

5. If a reconstructed hip remains or becomes painful, consider proximal femoral excision with interposition myoplasty.

Surgical Details (Figs. 33.2 and 33.3)

Preoperative Planning

1. Liaise with community team of paediatricians, physiotherapists, occupational therapists and wheelchair services to ensure postoperative care plans are in place.
2. Ensure that tone management has been maximised, anticipate perioperative increase in spasm and ensure appropriate collaboration with anaesthetic team for postoperative period.
3. Consider increasing medications for the perioperative period.
4. Ensure that general health and nutritional status has been optimised.

Surgical Procedure

1. Prophylactic intravenous cephalosporin (or institutional preferred antibiotic) given at induction.
2. Intraoperative calf pumps, thromboembolic deterrent stockings and low-molecular-weight heparin should be considered for venous thromboprophylaxis in all patients age 16 years and older.
3. Anterior approach to the hip (*depending on position of femoral head and siting of previous scars*).
4. Extraperiosteal release of the glutei and vasti from the proximal femur and release of iliopsoas (*if it has not been divided previously*).

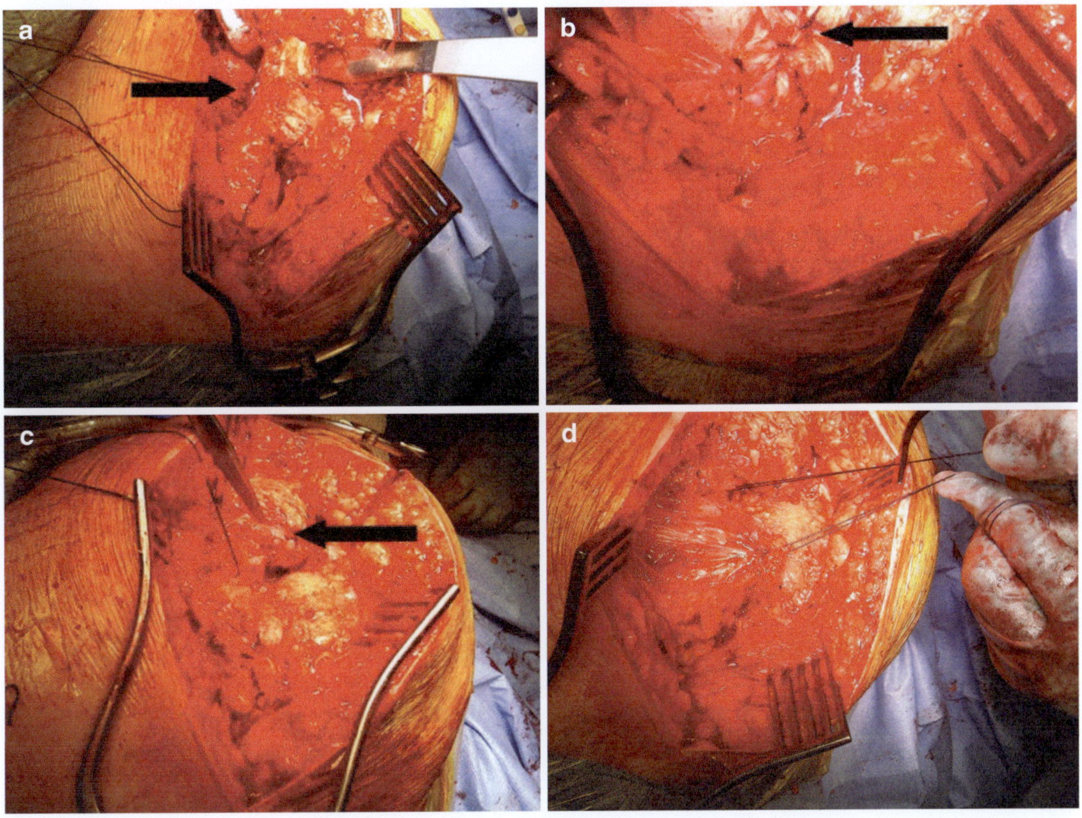

Fig. 33.2 (**a**) Proximal femur exposed and excised below the level of the lesser trochanter (*black arrow*) (patient's head to the left of the photograph; hip is flexed). (**b**) Closure of the capsule over the acetabulum with the psoas sutured to the gluteus medius and minimus (*black arrow*). (**c**) Closure of the vastus medialis and lateralis over the proximal femoral stump (*black arrow*). (**d**) Final result of interposition myoplasty (From Patel et al. 2015, with permission)

5. Capsulotomy to expose the femoral head and to release it from its capsular attachments.
6. Resection of the proximal femur 3–4 cm below the lesser trochanter.

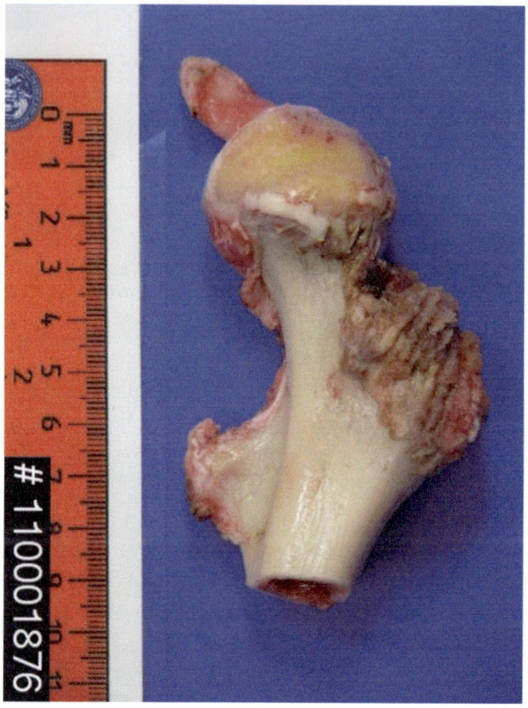

Fig. 33.3 Resected femoral head specimen showing the extent of the erosion of the articular cartilage: note that the femoral cut is only 1 cm below the base of the lesser trochanter; a further 2 cm was excised subsequently

7. Acetabulum covered with a double-breasted capsular repair.
8. Iliopsoas, gluteus medius and minimus tenodesed and sutured to the capsule.
9. Vastus medialis and lateralis closed over the femoral stump using transosseous sutures: before tying the sutures, ensure that the cut end of the femur is smoothed to reduce the risk of the bone 'cutting' through its muscle envelope.
10. Repair the fascia lata and complete the closure in layers.
11. Use an absorbable skin suture.
12. Ensure no residual adductor muscle tightness/contracture.
13. Postoperative control of pain and muscle spasm tailored to the individual patient. This could include an epidural, intravenous analgesia, botulinum toxin injections, increased doses of baclofen and additional doses of diazepam (or similar).
14. Skin traction may be useful in the first few days to help with positioning and spasm.

Postoperative Imaging

A single postoperative image is helpful to confirm immediate status, but later imaging is required on clinical grounds only (Figs. 33.4).

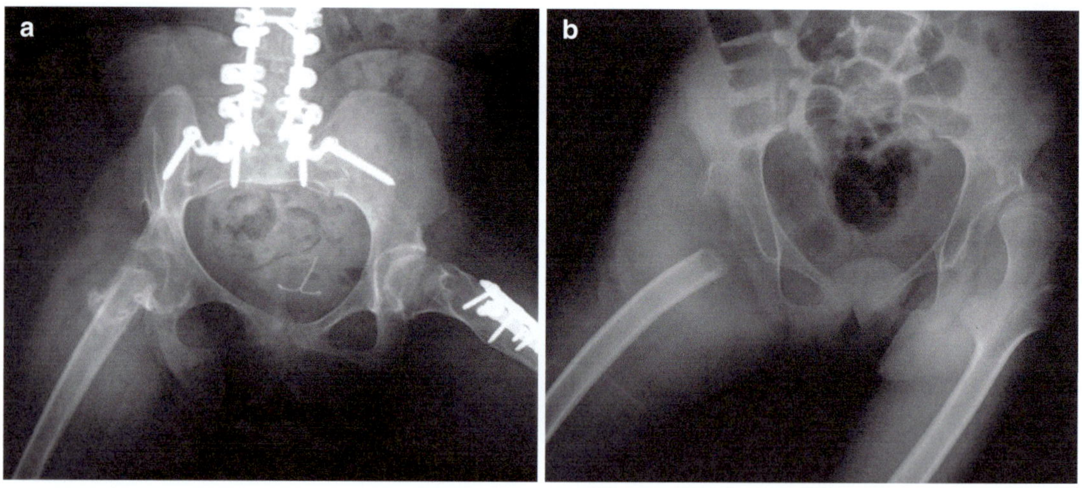

Fig. 33.4 *Case 1*. (**a**) Anteroposterior radiograph of both hips. The right proximal femur has been excised. The left hip remains in joint. *Case 2*. (**b**) Anteroposterior radiograph of both hips. The right proximal femur has been excised. The left hip remains subluxated

Pearls and Pitfalls

- Ensure you are prepared: involve a multidisciplinary team including a neurologist, physiotherapist and occupational therapist early, and anticipate additional causes of perioperative pain.
  - Constipation
  - Gastro-oesophageal reflux
  - Urinary retention
- Consider inserting a NG feeding tube if the child is self-feeding and malnourished.
- Many patients have had previous hip surgery: determine the direction of the dislocation and the site of previous scars, and place your scar accordingly.
- Always resect at least 3 cm of femur distal to the lesser trochanter.
- Ensure adequate closure/cover of the acetabulum.
- Ensure an adequate myoplasty is performed around the femoral stump: it is the integrity of this soft tissue envelope that maintains some 'control' over the mobility of the limb and reduces the risk of troublesome proximal migration.
- Proximal femoral migration is inevitable (see Figs. 33.2a, b) and not a significant problem as long as the femoral stump remains within its muscle envelope and does not move posterolaterally to protrude through the buttock.
- Heterotopic ossification does occur but is not usually a problem in the presence of a well-covered femoral stump.
- Families are used to a stiff and painful hip: they are often disconcerted by the extreme mobility of the 'hip' after excision arthroplasty. Traction can be useful until they have become familiar and comfortable with the new clinical picture.
- The wheelchair will require temporary adaptations in the immediate postoperative period and a more formal review at 6-8w post surgery.
- A review of tone medication must take place at the 6–8 w post-surgery check.

Indications and Contraindications (Table 33.1)

Table 33.1 Proximal femoral head resection and interpositional arthroplasty: surgical indications and contraindications

Indications
A reconstructed hip that remains painful and stiff despite regular analgesia and adequate muscle spasm control
A painful, anterior or posterior hip dislocation in which reconstruction is not feasible or unlikely to allow comfortable sitting
Contraindications
Patient not medically fit to undergo a general anaesthetic
Pain not arising from the dislocated hip

Suggested Reading

Dartnell J, Gough M, Paterson JM, Norman-Taylor F. Proximal femoral resection without post-operative traction for the painful dislocated hip in young patients with cerebral palsy: a review of 79 cases. Bone Joint J. 2014;96-B(5):701–6.

Knaus A, Terjesen T. Proximal femoral resection arthroplasty for patients with cerebral palsy and dislocated hips: 20 patients followed for 1-6 years. Acta Orthop. 2009;80(1):32–6.

Leet AI, Chhor K, Launay F, Kier-York J, Sponseller PD. Femoral head resection for painful hip subluxation in cerebral palsy: is valgus osteotomy in conjunction with femoral head resection preferable to proximal femoral head resection and traction? J Pediatr Orthop. 2005;25(1):70–3.

McCarthy RE, Simon S, Douglas B, Zawacki R, Reese N. Proximal femoral resection to allow adults who have severe cerebral palsy to sit. J Bone Joint Surg Am. 1988;70(7):1011–6.

Patel NK, Sabharwal S, Gooding CR, Hashemi-Nejad A, Eastwood DM. Proximal femoral excision with interposition myoplasty for cerebral palsy patients with chronic hip dislocation. J Child Orthop. 2015;9(4):263–71.

34 Pelvic Support Osteotomy

Karl E. Rathjen, Mikhail L. Samchukov, Alexander M. Cherkashin, and John G. Birch

Introduction

Prior to the development of effective total hip arthroplasty, "pelvic support" osteotomies were described as salvage reconstructive procedures for osteoarthritic hips to reduce pain and Trendelenburg limp while preserving hip motion. In addition to modest efficacy at best, iatrogenic shortening and valgus deformity significantly restricted the role of these osteotomies in clinical practice, even before the introduction of total hip arthroplasty. Ilizarov introduced important secondary reconstructive deformity correction and lengthening strategies, using his gradual correction and adaptable circular fixator to improve clinical results over the original procedures. Occasional patients with relatively mobile hips and minimal pain but poor hip function due to septic destruction, irreducible dislocation, or neurogenic functional impairment who are not reasonable candidates for total hip arthroplasty may benefit from pelvic support osteotomy with Ilizarov's methods of external fixation, gradual deformity correction, and distal reconstruction. We describe here a patient with fixed, neurogenic hip dislocations and symptomatic Trendelenburg gait associated with trisomy 21 (Down syndrome) treated effectively by pelvic support osteotomy and distal deformity reconstruction.

K. E. Rathjen · J. G. Birch (✉)
Department of Pediatric Orthopedics, Texas Scottish Rite Hospital for Children, Dallas, TX, USA
e-mail: karl.rathjen@tsrh.org; John.Birch@tsrh.org

M. L. Samchukov
Department of Pediatric Orthopedics, Center of Excellence for Limb Lengthening and Reconstruction, Texas Scottish Rite Hospital for Children, Dallas, TX, USA
e-mail: Mikhail.samchukov@tsrh.org

A. M. Cherkashin
Department of Pediatric Orthopedics, Division of Clinical Implementation and Data Management, Center of Excellence for Limb Lengthening and Reconstruction, Texas Scottish Rite Hospital for Children, Dallas, TX, USA
e-mail: alex.cherkashin@tsrh.org

Brief Clinical History

This patient originally presented for orthopedic evaluation at the age of 9 years with a history of trisomy 21 and complaints of flatfeet, waddling gait, and right knee pain. He had generally good health previously with mild gross motor milestone delay. Clinical examination at that time revealed bilateral patellar instability in extension, flexible planovalgus feet, and a smooth arc of hip motion without pain but Trendelenburg gait bilaterally. Radiographs demonstrated bilateral previously unrecognized severe hip dysplasia (Fig. 34.1). He returned at age 11 with a complaint of deteriorating gait. At that time, he was noted to have cervical myelopathy and significant C1–2 instability (Fig. 34.2). He was treated by

R. C. Hamdy, N. Saran (eds.), *Pediatric Pelvic and Proximal Femoral Osteotomies*, https://doi.org/10.1007/978-3-319-78033-7_34

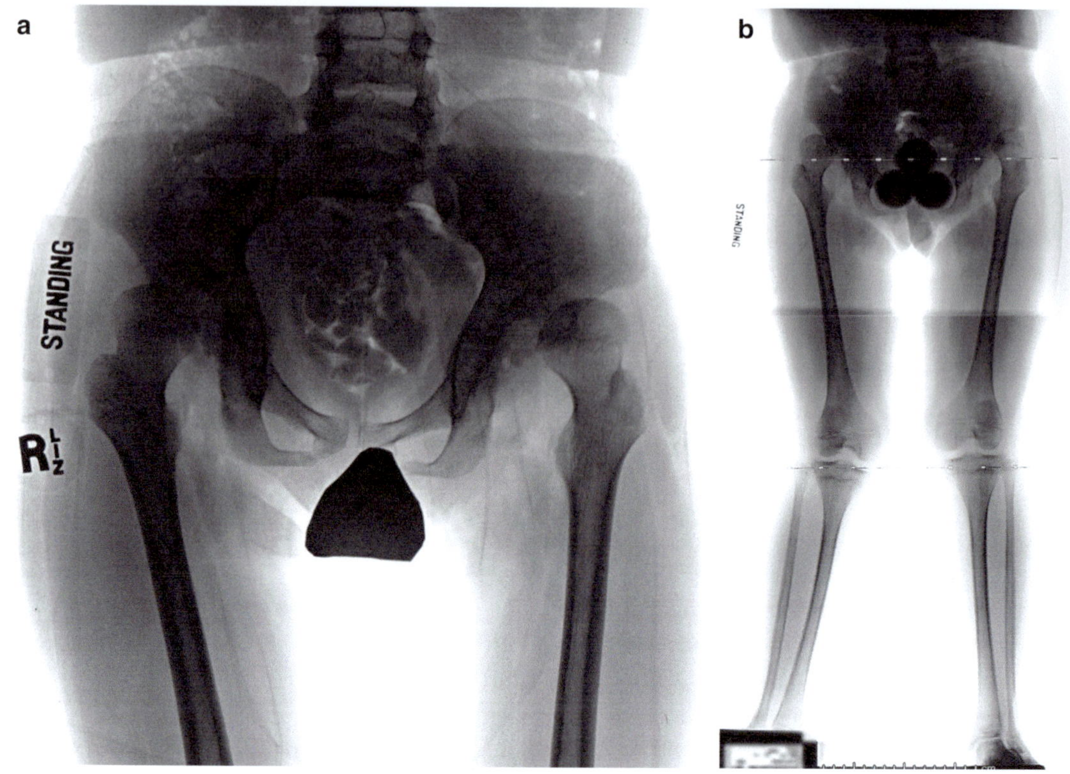

Fig. 34.1 Radiographic appearance of the patient on presentation to our institution at age 9. His complaints included waddling gait and right knee pain. (**a**) Anteroposterior (AP) radiograph of the pelvis demonstrates bilateral previously unrecognized hip dislocations with severe acetabular dysplasia. (**b**) AP radiograph of the lower extremities demonstrating bilateral distal femoral valgus deformities but no significant leg length inequality

posterior cervical decompression and instrumented occiput-C2 fusion, with resolution of the myelopathic symptoms (Fig. 34.3).

He returned at age 13 with complaints of left knee pain, decreased exercise tolerance, and decreased independent ambulation. He had some discomfort with hip motion and progressive changes of bilateral hip dysplasia (Fig. 34.4a). He was not felt to be a suitable candidate for hip reduction/acetabular osteotomy, fusion, or total hip arthroplasty. Because of the deterioration in gait and independent ambulation, he was considered for pelvic support reconstruction on the symptomatic (left) side.

Preoperative examination (Fig. 34.4b–d) demonstrated effectively no leg length discrepancy and distal femoral valgus deformity (masked by knee flexion in stance). He underwent pelvic support osteotomy with distal reconstruction consisting of application of a circular external fixator, an upper femoral valgus osteotomy, and simultaneous distal femoral osteotomy for gradual valgus deformity correction and minor lengthening (Figs. 34.5, 34.6, 34.7, 34.8, 34.9, and 34.10). The fixator was removed 4 months after application.

Five years after reconstruction, he maintained and actually increased his mobility over all preoperative abilities, remained asymptomatic in both lower extremities, and has required no further orthopedic treatment to date (Fig. 34.11).

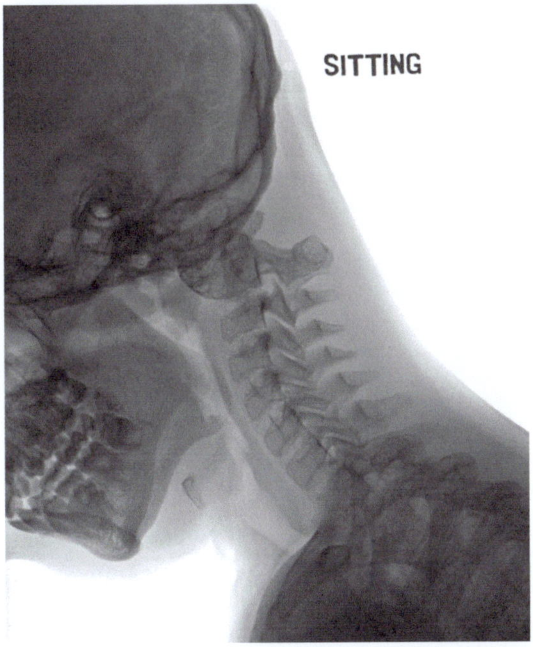

Fig. 34.2 On re-presentation at age 11, with complaints of deteriorating gait and exercise tolerance, he was noted to have signs of cervical myelopathy and significant C1–2 instability on flexion radiographs of the cervical spine

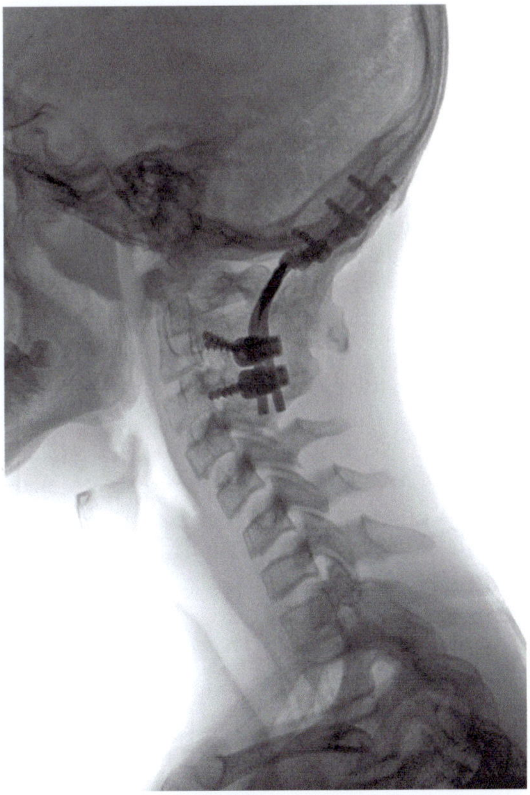

Fig. 34.3 He subsequently underwent posterior decompression and instrumented fusion from occiput to C2. He had resolution of the complaints and myelopathic signs and remained stable 5 years postoperatively (despite radiographic evidence of rod fracture)

Preoperative Imaging

Crucial radiographic images include:

1. Standing anteroposterior (AP) view of the lower extremities with a block under the affected extremity to level the pelvis, if necessary. This film will document the functional leg length discrepancy, the double limb stance relationship between the affected upper femur and pelvis, deformities in the affected extremity which need to be taken into consideration for deformity correction planning, and mechanical axis restoration planning.
2. AP views of the pelvis with the affected extremity in maximum abduction and adduction to document the coronal arc of motion and the relationship of the upper femur to the pelvis and plan the level of upper femoral osteotomy and degree of valgus production required.
3. Lateral view of the affected femur to identify and quantify sagittal plane deformities that may need to be taken into account in deformity correction planning.
4. If lengthening is anticipated, a dedicated lateral view of the knee in full extension may be valuable for radiographic assessment of any possible knee flexion deformity/subluxation during the course of treatment.

Other images may be helpful but are not always needed. These include:

1. Scanogram of the lower extremities to document the actual bony leg length discrepancy.

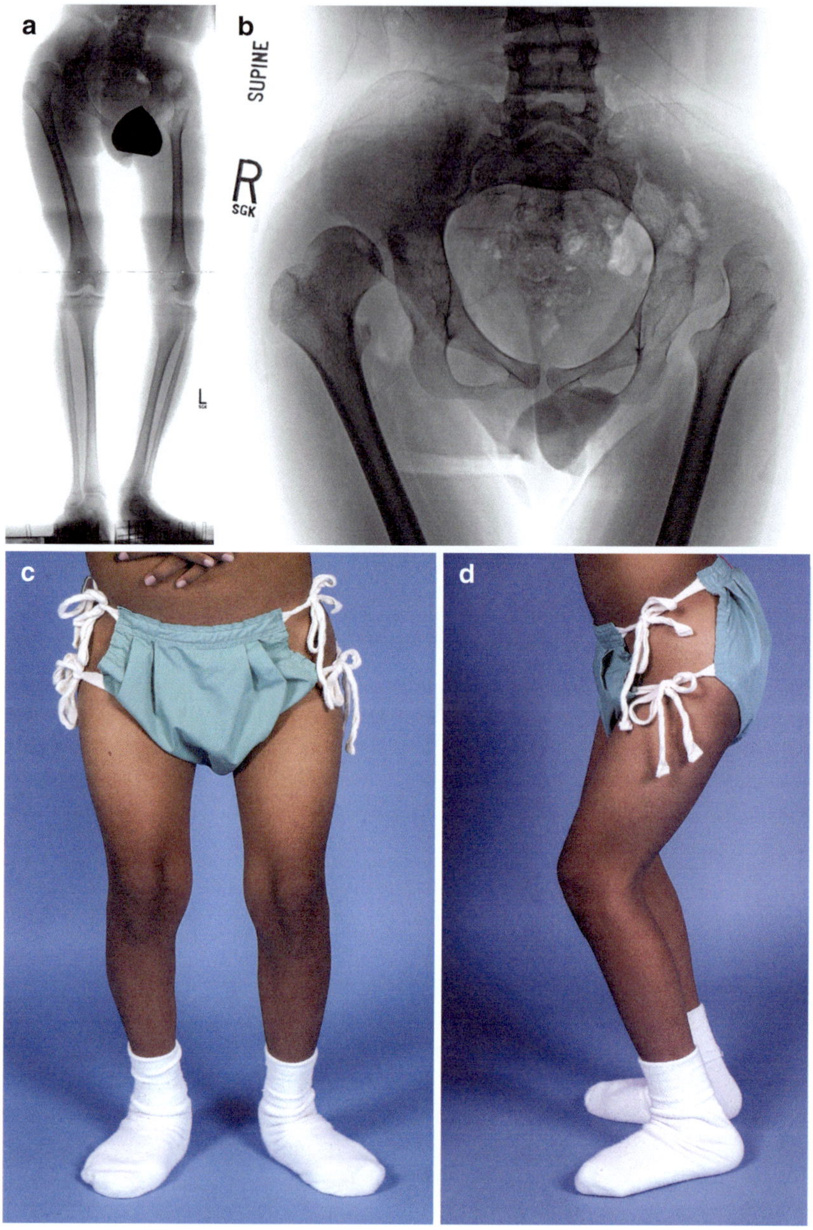

Fig. 34.4 Appearance on presentation at age 13 with new complaints of left knee pain, deteriorating exercise tolerance, and trouble walking without support. (**a**) Standing anteroposterior (AP) film demonstrates bilateral acetabular dysplasia and relatively equal leg lengths. Valgus deformity in the distal femur is masked by his tendency to stand with his knees flexed. (**b**) AP film of the pelvis demonstrates progression of bilateral hip dysplasia. (**c**) Clinical appearance viewed from the front. (**d**) Clinical appearance viewed from the left side. Note his tendency to stand with his knees flexed (masking his distal femoral valgus deformity)

2. An affected side single-leg standing AP film of the pelvis to document the relationship of the upper femur to the pelvis in this position.
3. CT of the pelvis and upper femur with 3-D reconstruction may be performed to aid in planning the best position to maximize contact between the pelvis and repositioned upper femur.

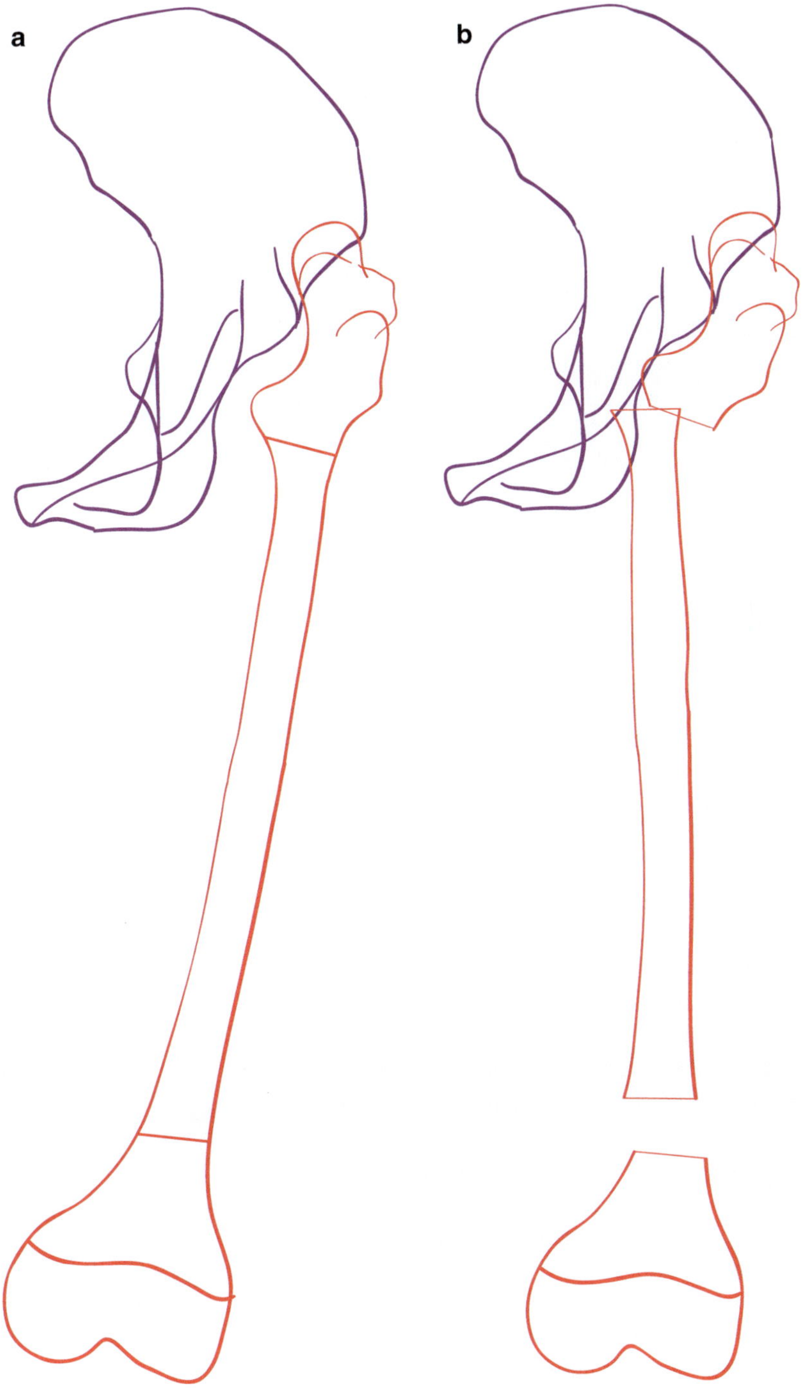

Fig. 34.5 (**a**, **b**) Outlines of the surgical plan. The plan is to adduct the proximal fragment maximally and correct distal valgus deformity and minor leg length inequality through a second distal femoral osteotomy

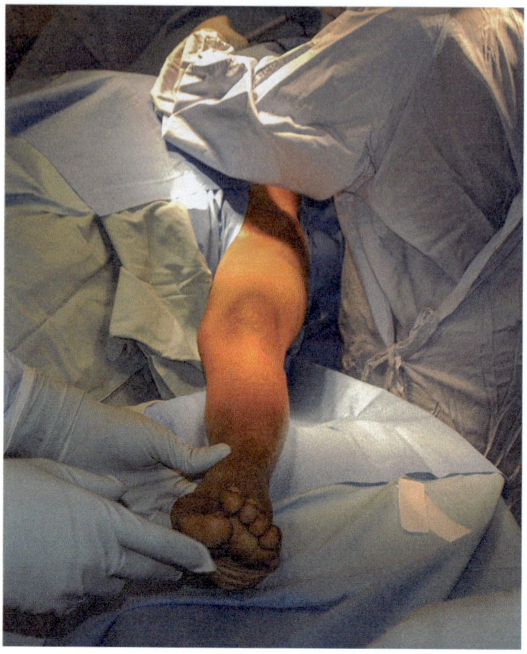

Fig. 34.6 Intraoperative positioning. The entire affected extremity is draped free from the hemipelvis distally. In this case, the articulated OR table leg support has been removed, and the leg rests on a separate table

Goals of Treatment

The primary goal of treatment is to obliterate the Trendelenburg gait (and associated abductor muscle pain, if relevant) by increasing upper femoral adduction in single limb stance so that further adduction at the (surrogate) hip is not possible while maintaining functional flexion and extension of the hip and maximizing contact between the pelvis and upper femur to increase and distribute weight bearing surfaces between them.

An associated primary goal is to restore the mechanical alignment of the limb (through the knee from the surrogate hip articulation to the ankle) by adducting the distal femur to compensate for the upper femoral valgus osteotomy. The exact location of this deformity correction will be determined by the effect of the upper femoral valgus osteotomy on the mechanical axis and pre-existing deformity in the femur.

Important secondary goals include correction of pre-existing deformities (such as distal femoral valgus deformity) and correcting leg length inequality to maximize limb function.

Treatment Strategy

Treatment strategy begins with careful selection of the patient based on the criteria outlined in "Indications and Contraindications," followed by careful analysis of the patient's radiographic deformity. Preoperative clinical assessment includes:

1. Careful documentation of the hip arc of motion, including maximum abduction and flexion, and the presence of any hip flexion contracture. The relatively painless nature of that arc of motion should be confirmed.
2. Assessment of hip flexor and abductor strength, if present. A hip with no abductor power will have the Trendelenburg gait eliminated postoperatively only if the upper femoral osteotomy results in no clinical adduction of the hip.
3. Identification and quantification of secondary deformity (such as distal femoral valgus or knee instability) and functional leg length inequality.

Next, the preoperative imaging described above should be analyzed to determine:

1. The amount of adduction of the proximal fragment desired
2. The level of the upper femoral osteotomy to maximize contact between the upper femur and the pelvis, while allowing the amount of valgus-production desired
3. The level of secondary osteotomy and varus production required to bring the limb into

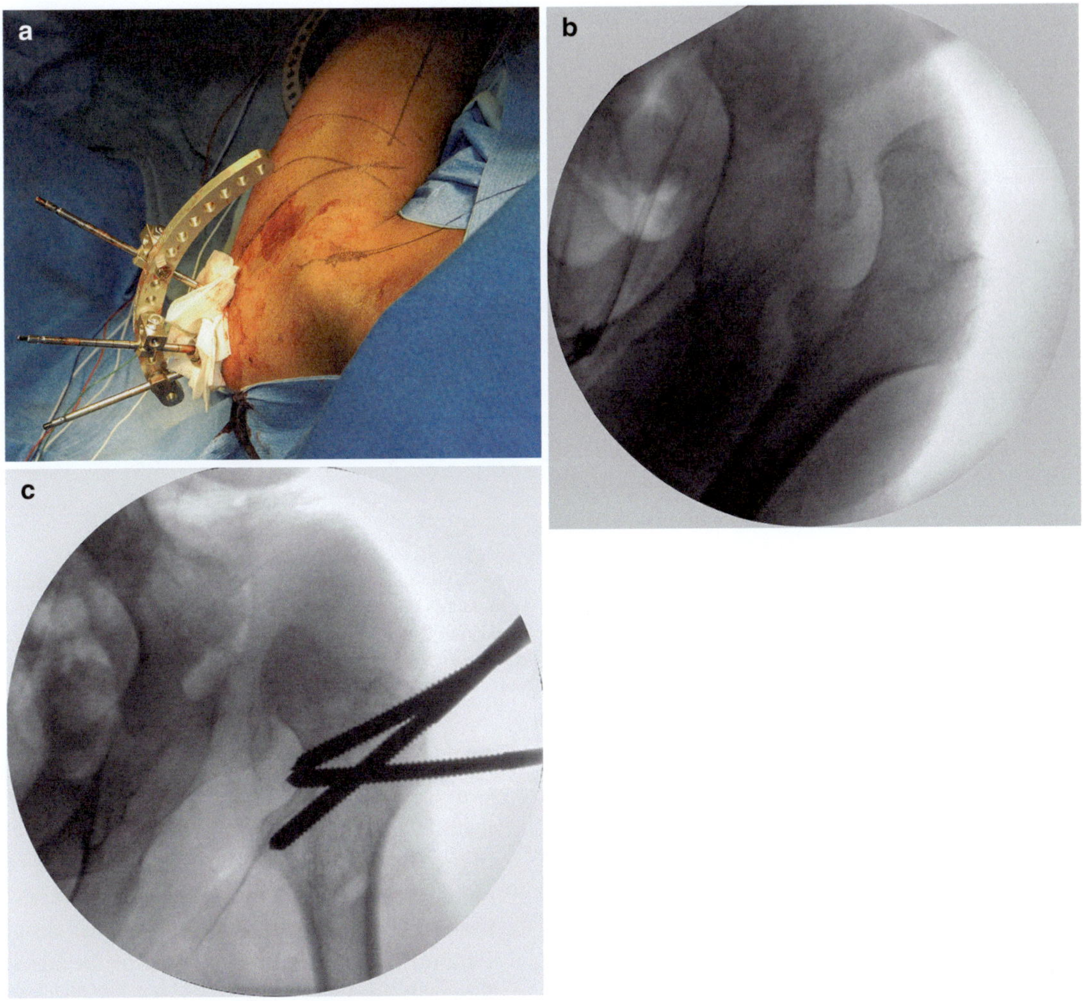

Fig. 34.7 Fixation of the upper femur with half-pins secured to a two-arch block. (**a**) The leg is placed in maximum adduction; the upper femoral fixation will be placed orthogonal to the anticipated distal femoral mechanical axis (intraoperative and/or postoperative adjustment may be required). Note that anatomic landmarks of the intercrestal line, axis of the distal femur, and osteotomy level have been marked on the skin to aid proper fixator orientation. (**b**) Radiographic appearance of the proximal femur in maximal adduction. (**c**) Radiographic appearance after proximal fragment fixation

proper mechanical alignment (such that the knee is on the mechanical axis of the limb)

4. The existence of other deformities in the femur (such as distal femoral valgus), their impact on postoperative correction goals and limb function, and thus the need to correct them by osteotomy
5. The extent of residual leg length discrepancy (if any) and development of a plan to manage it

Finally, an external fixation apparatus that will allow acute and gradual correction of deformities, sequentially during the same treatment session, should be selected and constructed for use

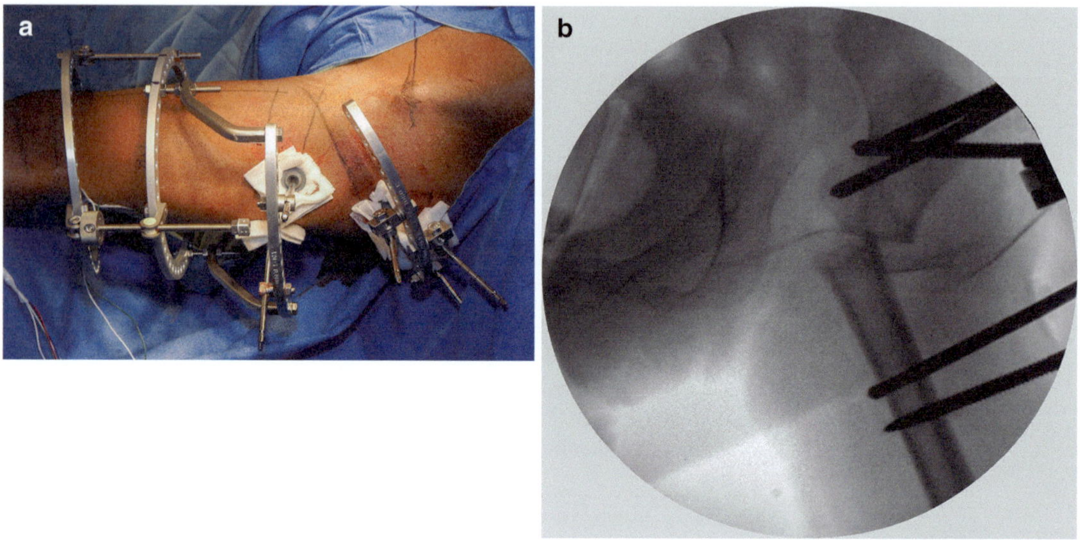

Fig. 34.8 (**a**) Clinical appearance of the fixator after fixation, prior to upper femoral osteotomy. Note the orientation of the upper and lower fixator segments, which will be brought into parallel after osteotomy. (**b**) Intraoperative radiographic appearance after proximal femoral osteotomy and displacement. Note that the intercalary fragment is in valgus and has been allowed to displace medially and proximally to maximize segment contact with the pelvis and medialize the weight-bearing axis of the limb

in the patient. In most cases, hybrid circular fixators are ideal for this purpose, but other fixators or combination of external and internal fixation strategies may be used.

Surgical Details

1. The patient is positioned supine on a radiolucent table top with the entire affected extremity and hemipelvis draped free to allow circumferential access to the entire limb. Placing the patient on a substantial lower spinal bump may suffice, but the ideal is to use a table with separate, adjustable leg extensions, abducting the contralateral extremity maximally to allow an assistant to work from the medial side of the affected extremity, removing the leg extension on the affected side, and supporting the affected lower leg on an adjustable table (see Fig. 34.6). The key is to have circumferential access to the entire affected leg and hemipelvis.
2. Fluoroscopy is used to mark on the patient's skin all appropriate landmarks, including the level and angle of proximal fixation, the level of proximal osteotomy, the mechanical axis of the intercalary fragment, the level of the knee, the intended level of the (subsequent) distal femoral osteotomy, and the axis of the distal femoral segment.
3. Preoperative fixator assembly to mimic the deformity and intended upper femoral valgus production will be helpful in most cases. In this case, an acute upper femoral valgus-producing osteotomy and distal femoral valgus osteotomy for valgus correction and minor lengthening are planned (see Fig. 34.5). The uppermost support block was secured to the upper femur with three half-pins (see Fig. 34.7). The intercalary and distal segment fixation components were assembled, slid over the patient's leg, and secured orthogonally to the patient's femur (see Fig. 34.8a). The fixator is secured to the affected limb with half-pins and wires. We use self-tapping and

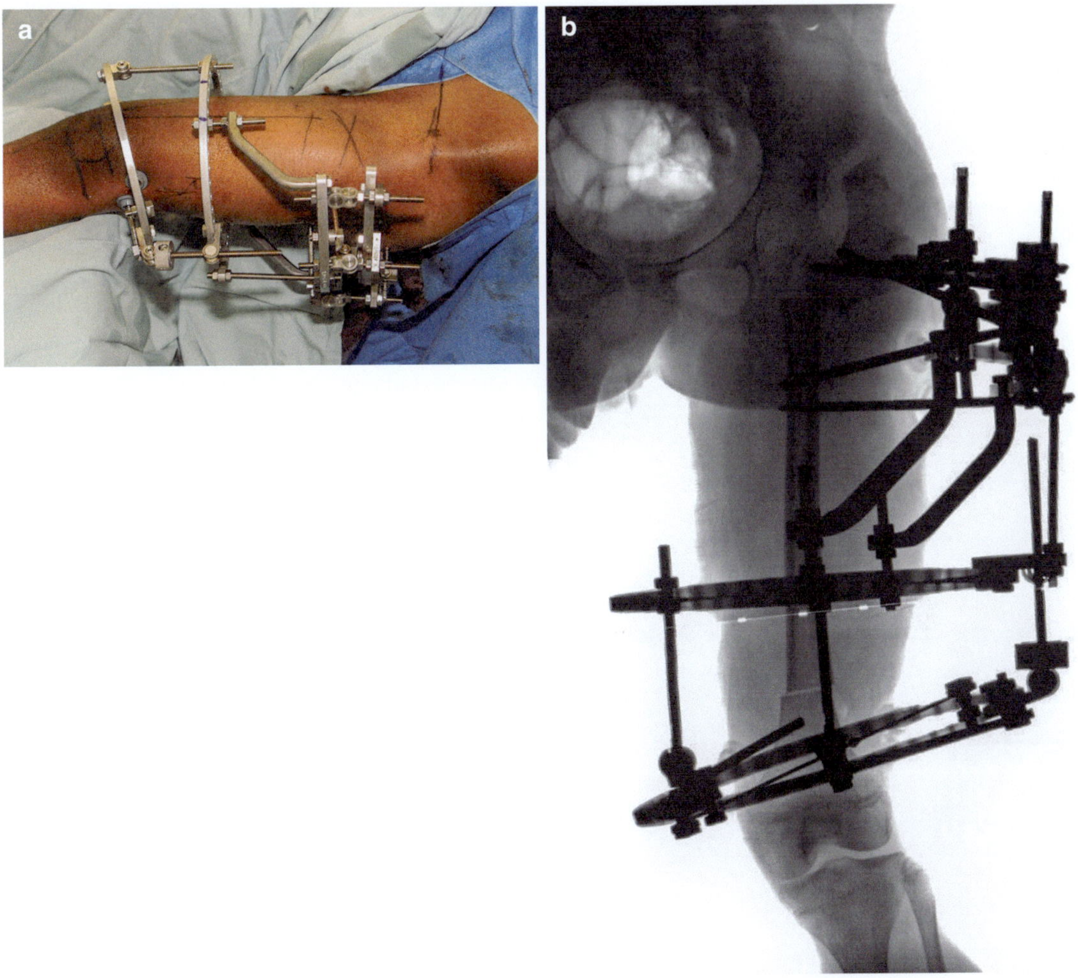

Fig. 34.9 (**a**) Clinical appearance of the apparatus at the completion of surgery. Note that the upper and lower fixator segments are now parallel (compare to Fig. 34.8a). (**b**) Radiographic appearance after proximal femoral osteotomy and displacement and distal femoral osteotomy for valgus deformity correction and mild lengthening

drilling 5 mm half-pins almost exclusively in the proximal and intercalary segments of the femur and a hybrid of half-pins and 1.8 mm olive wire in the distal segment. Fixation must be adequate for bone manipulation and stability, while minimizing soft tissue tethering.

4. Percutaneous or limited open osteotomy is performed at the intended level of the upper femur, the bone fragments displaced acutely as desired, and the fixator segments (re)connected. (see Figs. 34.8a and 34.9a)
5. In this patient, because proximal fixation was secure and full osteotomy displacement achieved and only minor angular deformity correction and lengthening planned at the distal osteotomy site, the distal osteotomy was performed at the same stage (see Fig. 34.9b).
6. After wound closure and soft tissue release around pin sites performed, a bulky compressive dressing is applied to the limb and baseline radiographs obtained.

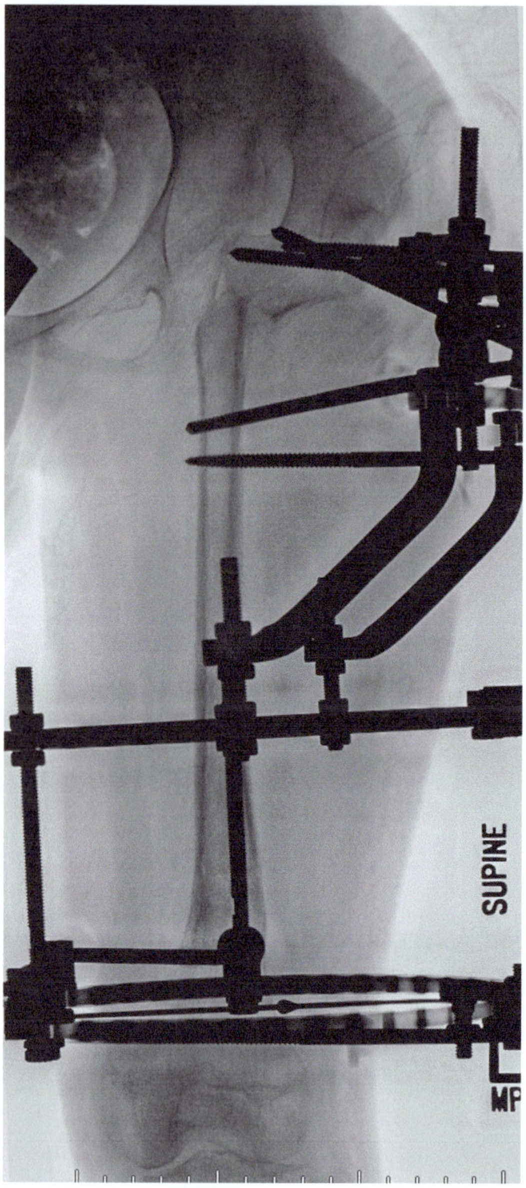

Fig. 34.10 Radiographic appearance of the femur at the end of correction

Postoperative Care and Imaging

The patient is encouraged to weight-bear as tolerated as soon as possible, with upper extremity aid as needed. In addition to general mobility, muscle strengthening, and joint range of motion exercises, the physical therapy program should emphasize active and gentle passive affected side adduction to insure that adduction range of motion is reduced to only a few degrees (documented radiographically by an AP film of the pelvis with the upper femur in maximum adduction). If adduction range obliteration is inadequate, manipulation of the distal segment into further valgus, either gradually or acutely, is required.

Once final upper segment position has been achieved, radiographs of the upper femur centered on the osteotomy site should be taken every 2 weeks to confirm maintenance of fragment position, until adequate healing of the osteotomy site is confirmed to allow proceeding with the second osteotomy, if needed. At that time, a standing AP film of the lower extremity should be taken to confirm the level of the second osteotomy and the "target" position of the distal-most fragment onto the new weight-bearing axis of the limb.

After the second osteotomy, therapy continues, and radiographs are taken as necessary to monitor regenerated formation in the distraction gap. Adequate fragment realignment is confirmed with a standing AP film of the lower extremities. At that point, once-monthly films of the osteotomy sites should be taken to confirm adequate consolidation to initiate fixator removal (see Fig. 34.10). We prefer in most cases to remove such complex fixators by gradual destabilization by judicious sequential half-pin removal and fixator "destabilization."

Pearls and Pitfalls

- Patient selection is key: the patient must have adequate range of motion of the hip worth preserving, not have articular pain as the primary or dominant complaint, and be able to comply with prolonged, staged, external fixation treatment.
- Alternative reconstructive procedures (hip fusion, total joint arthroplasty) must be

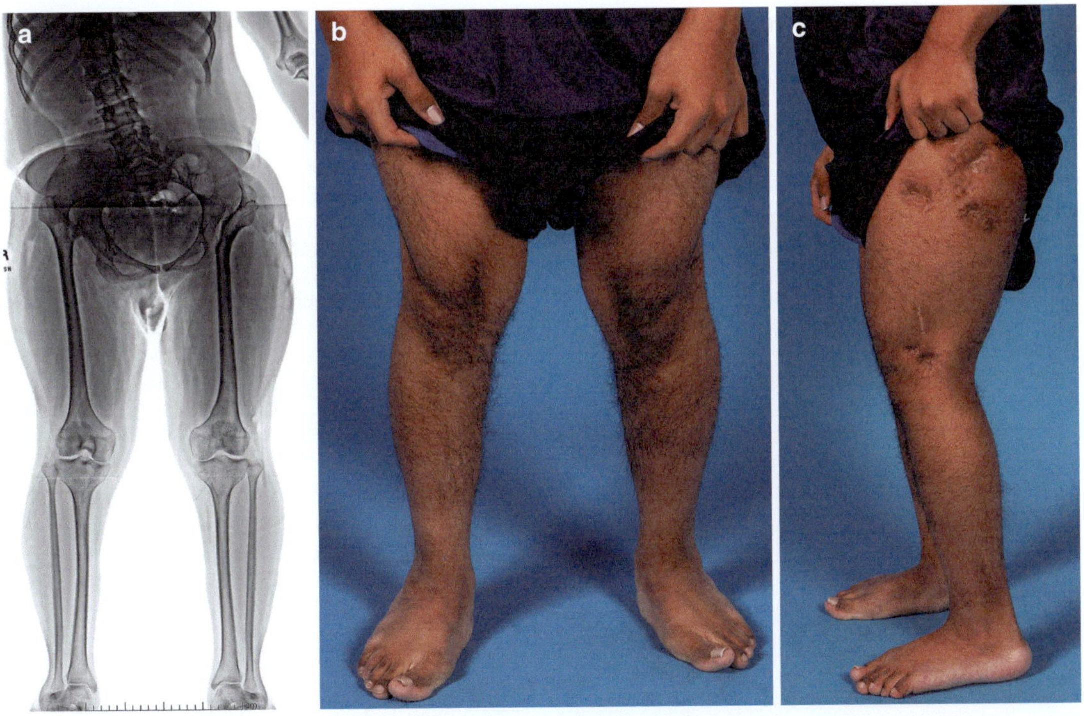

Fig. 34.11 At 5 years postoperatively, the patient has exceeded his best preoperative ambulatory abilities and is without complaint in either extremity. The right leg remains untreated. (**a**) Standing anteroposterior radiograph of the lower extremities. (**b**) Clinical appearance viewed from the front. (**c**) Clinical appearance viewed from the patient's left side

deemed inappropriate short-term options for the patient.

- The initial stage of reconstruction (upper femoral valgus osteotomy) even with distal realignment will have no positive effect on a pre-existing leg length discrepancy or even accentuate shortening of the affected extremity. Both surgeon and patient must be cognizant of this and plan subsequent leg lengthening (either as a sequential stage of the reconstruction, or a subsequent one) as indicated.
- Some patients may be equivocal as to whether they are more affected by the Trendelenburg gait or an associated significant leg length discrepancy. In such patients, asking them to wear an appropriate-size shoe lift (accommodating their associated Trendelenburg gait) so that they can decide which characteristic is their primary concern may be very helpful.
- It is extremely important to minimize soft tissue bunching around fixation sites by stretching the tissues apart as far as possible before inserting pins into the femur at the level of planned valgus correction (which will squeeze the soft tissues together) and to release any residual tethering around the pin sites prior to completing surgery.
- Even when the anticipated goal of angular correction can be accomplished acutely, the ability to adjust this correction by manipulation of an external fixator is very valuable. In our experience, internal fixation of the proximal osteotomy (and acceptance of the outcome) in the desire of avoiding upper femoral external fixation is not wise.

Indications and Contraindications (Table 34.1)

Table 34.1 Pelvic support osteotomy with distal reconstruction: surgical indications and contraindications

Indications
There should be adequate range of motion of the involved hip (or surrogate, in cases of septic destruction or dislocation) to warrant preservation, as opposed to hip fusion
Painful motion of the hip should not be a major complaint, as results of pelvic support procedures primarily for pain relief have unpredictable results. Minor activity-related or muscle fatigue pain is not a contraindication, however
The patient should not be an appropriate candidate for total hip arthroplasty in the short term. Usual (relative) contraindications to total hip arthroplasty include young age, severely distorted anatomy or bone size preventing insertion of implants, and active infection
Careful consideration should be given to the possibility that the patient would be a candidate for total hip arthroplasty in the long term, since upper femoral valgus deformity produced by pelvic support osteotomy may make such reconstruction very difficult or impossible
The patient must be able to tolerate prolonged, bulky external fixation, to comply with pin-care and therapy protocols, and to accept sequential osteotomies as indicated in the particular patient
Contraindications
Limited, nonfunctional range of motion of the affected hip, particularly with pain as a primary or significant complaint
Hip fusion or total joint arthroplasty is reasonable surgical alternatives in the short-term management of the patient
Long-term possibility of total joint arthroplasty can be a relative contraindication because the deformity produced by the upper femoral valgus osteotomy may make arthroplasty difficult or impossible without preceding corrective osteotomy
The presence of active periarticular deep infection is a contraindication and should be resolved completely medically and surgically before considering pelvic support osteotomy
A patient who is unable or unwilling to comply with prolonged, staged treatment therapy and pin-care protocols using external fixation

Suggested Reading

Dimitrios P, Nayagam S. The pelvic support osteotomy: indications and preoperative planning. Strategies Trauma Limb Reconstr. 2008;32(2):83–92.

Haas J. A subtrochanteric osteotomy for pelvic support. J Bone Joint Surg. 2592;1943:281–91.

Ilizarov GA. Transosseous osteosynthesis. Theoretical and clinical aspects of the regeneration and growth of tissue. New York: Springer; 1992. p. 701–18.

Inan M, Bowen RJ. A pelvic support osteotomy and femoral lengthening with monolateral fixator. Clin Orthop. 2005;440:192–8.

Mahran MA, El Gebeily MA, Ghaly NA, Thekab MF, Hefny HM. Pelvis support osteotomy by Ilizarov's concept: is it a valuable option in managing neglected hip problems in adolescents and young adults. Strategies Trauma Limb Reconstr. 2011;6(1):13–20.

Samchukov ML, Birch JG. Restoration of pelvic support and limb length by the Ilizarov method. Bull Hosp Jt Dis. 1992;52(1):7–11.

SUPERhip and SUPERhip2 Procedures for Congenital Femoral Deficiency

35

Dror Paley

Introduction

Congenital femoral deficiency (CFD) presents a spectrum of deficiency, deformity and dysplasia of the upper femur, hip joint and acetabulum. The Paley classification divides this spectrum into separate pathoanatomical groups that can be treated using discreetly different operative procedures specific to the pathoanatomy of each type of CFD. The SUPERhip1 procedure is used to reconstruct Paley type 1 CFD cases, while the SUPERhip2 procedure is used to reconstruct Paley type 2 CFD cases.

Brief Clinical History

Classification of Congenital Femur Deficiency [1] (Fig. 35.1)

Type 1: *intact femur* with mobile hip and knee

(a) normal ossification proximal femur
(b) delayed ossification proximal femur (neck, subtrochanteric or combined neck subtrochanteric types)

Type 2: *mobile pseudoarthrosis* (greater trochanteric apophysis present), knee usually mobile

(a) femoral head mobile in acetabulum
(b) femoral head partially fused to acetabulum
(c) femoral head and acetabulum completely fused or absent

Type 3: *diaphyseal deficiency* of femur (greater trochanteric apophysis absent)

(a) distal physis present; knee motion ≥45°
(b) distal physis present knee motion <45°
(c) complete deficiency of distal femur or fusion of distal femoral remnant to tibia (distal physis absent)

Type 4: *distal deficiency of femur* (proximal end normal).

D. Paley (✉)
Paley Orthopedic and Spine Institute, St. Mary's Medical Center, West Palm Beach, FL, USA
e-mail: dpaley@paleyinstitute.org

R. C. Hamdy, N. Saran (eds.), *Pediatric Pelvic and Proximal Femoral Osteotomies*, https://doi.org/10.1007/978-3-319-78033-7_35

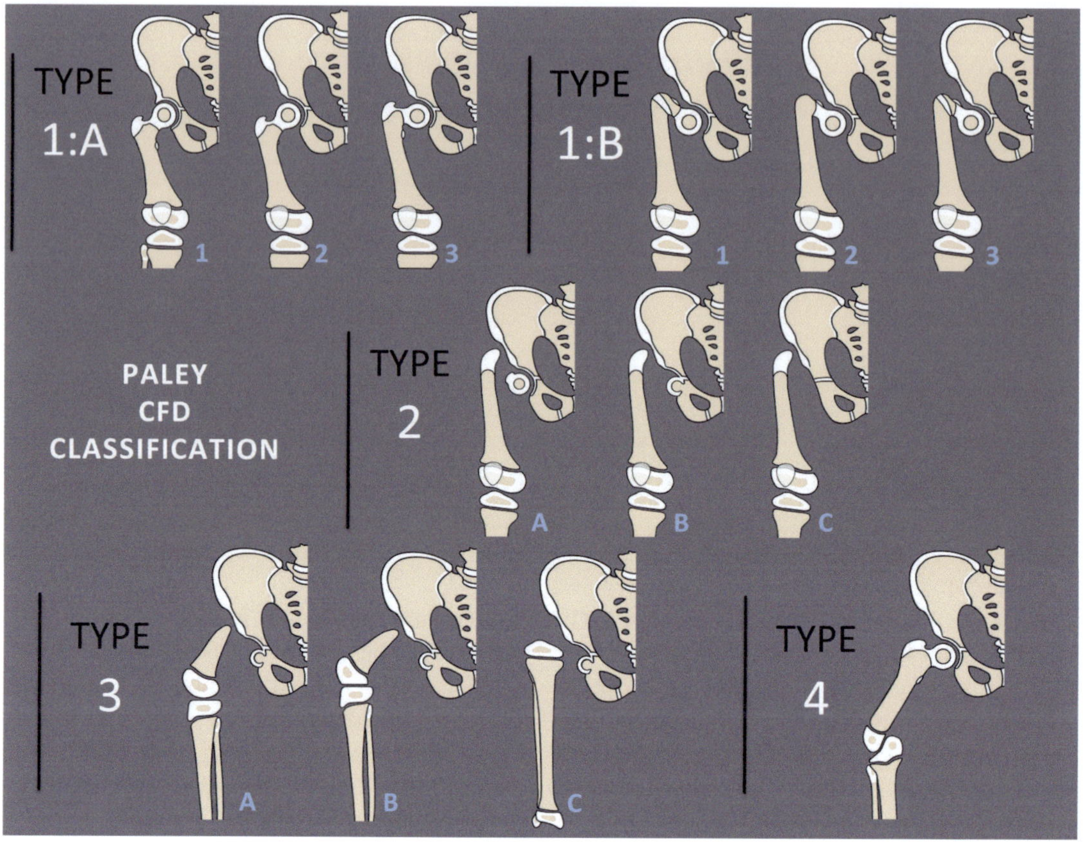

Fig. 35.1 Paley classification of congenital femoral deficiency. (© 2014 The Paley Foundation, with permission. All rights reserved)

Model Paley Type 1b Pathoanatomy [2] (Fig. 35.2)

To understand the complex deformity of the Paley type 1b deformity it is useful to create a simple model consisting of three bone segments: pelvis, proximal femur to the level of the lesser trochanter with a 130° neck shaft angle and greater trochanter at the normal level of the center of the femoral head, and distal femur from the subtrochanteric region to the knee joint. Start by placing the femoral head in the acetabulum anatomically and flexing it 90°. Then abduct the femur 45° relative to the pelvis, in the flexed position. Next, attach the distal femur to the distal end of the proximal femur with the knee rotated externally 45°. This construct is the model of the Paley 1b CFD. Note that the flexion of the upper femur makes the neck appear retroverted since the normal neck shaft angle points posteriorly. Abducting the proximal femur now makes the neck look in varus from the frontal view, despite the neck shaft angle measuring 130°. Finally, adding the distal femur in external rotation adds actual retroversion to the pseudo retroversion from the flexion and also makes the

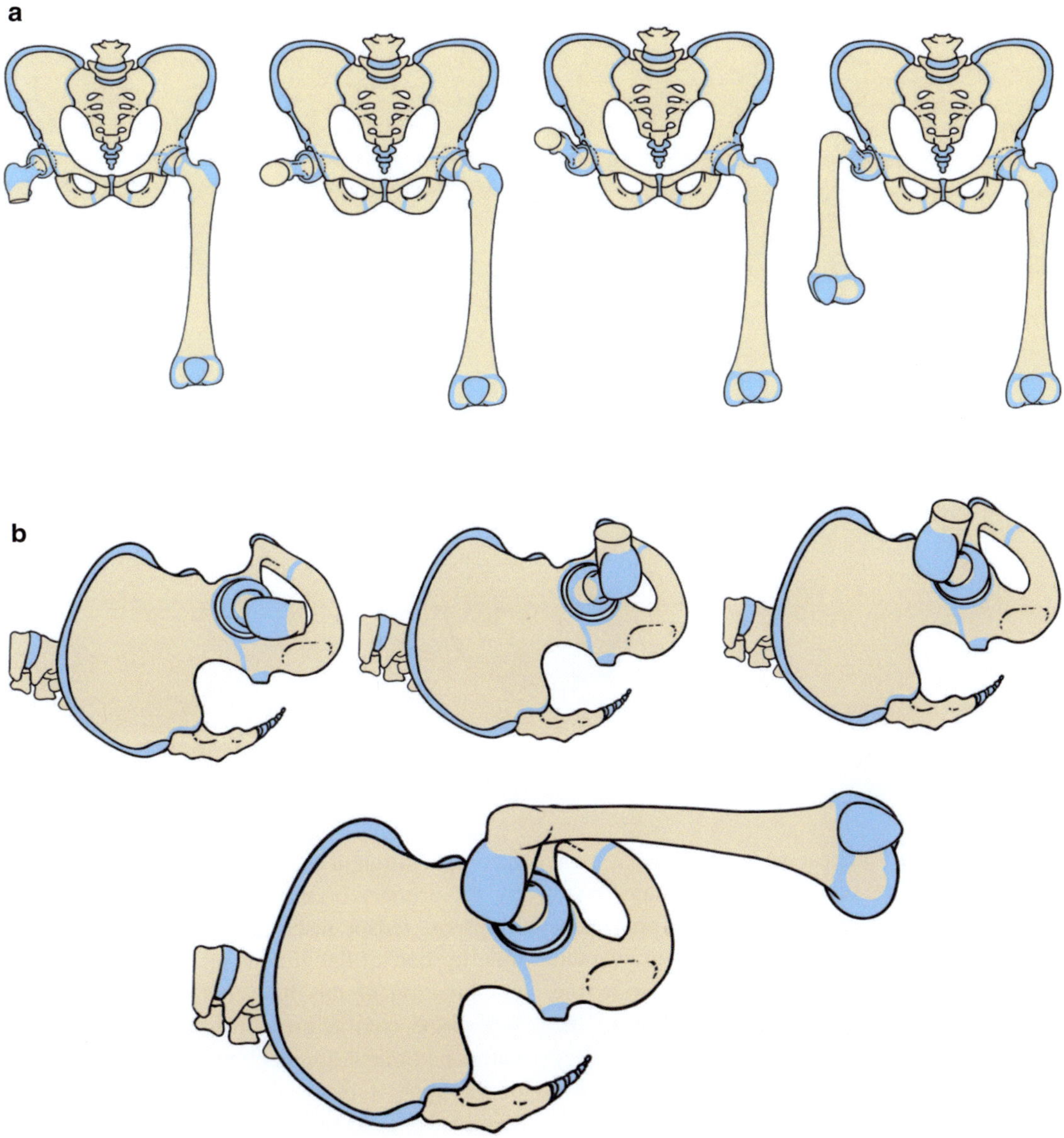

Fig. 35.2 (**a**) Model of congenital femoral deficiency (CFD) hip deformity, anteroposterior view. Hip neutral (*left*). Hip flexed 90° (*left middle*). Hip abducted in flexion (*right middle*). Distal femur externally rotated and connected to proximal hip flexion, abduction position (*right*). (**b**) Model of CFD hip deformity, lateral view. Hip neutral (*top left*). Hip flexed 90° (*top middle*). Hip abducted in flexion (*top right*). Distal femur externally rotated and connected to proximal hip flexion, abduction position (*bottom*). (**c**) Model of CFD hip deformity, inferior view. Hip neutral (*top left*). Hip flexed 90° (*top right*). Hip abducted in flexion (bottom). ()

c

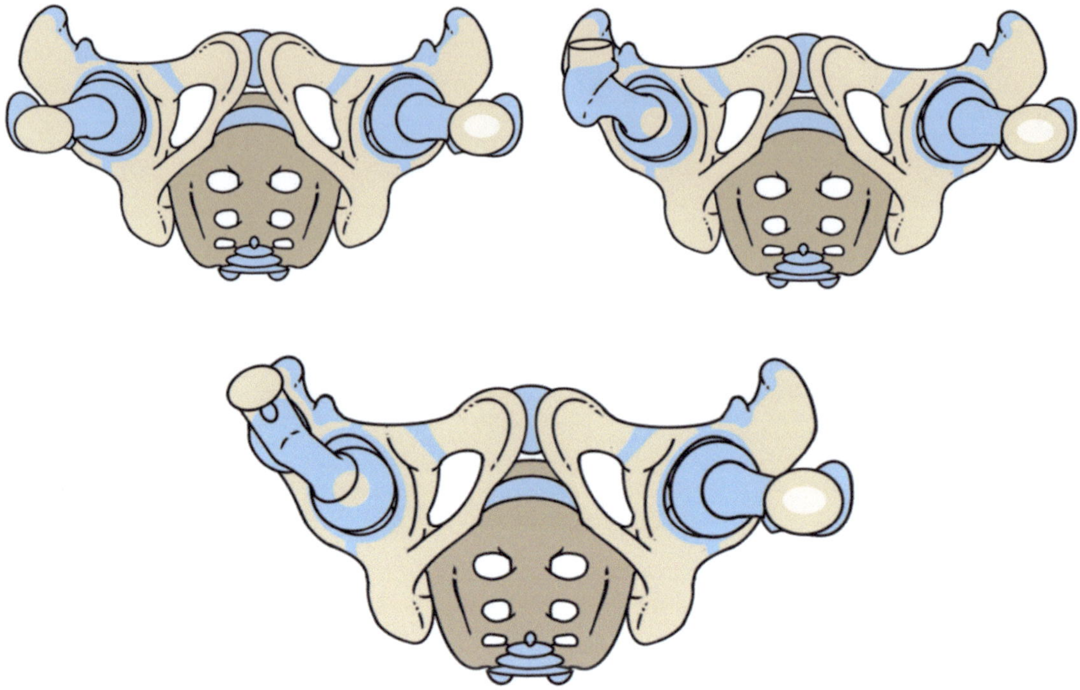

Fig. 35.2 (continued)

pseudo coxa vara appear as a severe coxa vara. The junction of the two parts of the femur form a large bend which can be palpated as a prominent bump. This bump is not the greater trochanter, which is located medial and posterior to the bump. Due to the flexion and abduction of the proximal femur, the greater trochanter lies very close to the ilium and points towards the sacrum. The muscles attaching to the tip of the greater trochanter; gluteus medius and minimus and piriformis are relatively short either primarily or secondary to this persistant position. They act as a tether preventing the proximal femur returning to its normal anatomic position. Similarly the severe flexion position of the proximal femur is tethered by the primary or secondary contracture of the iliopsoas, tensor fascia lata, rectus femoris and anterior half of the gluteus medius muscles. The combination of this bony deformity with these soft tissue contractures forms the basis for the pathoanatomical approach to surgical correction of the upper femoral deformity associated with some Paley type 1a and all Paley type 1b cases.

Case 1: Paley type 1a CFD (Fig. 35.3)

Eight-year-old girl with CFD with large LLD and failed previous attempts to correct hip deformity and lengthen femur. Fixed adduction, flexion deformity of hip. Knee stable (see Fig. 35.3a, b).

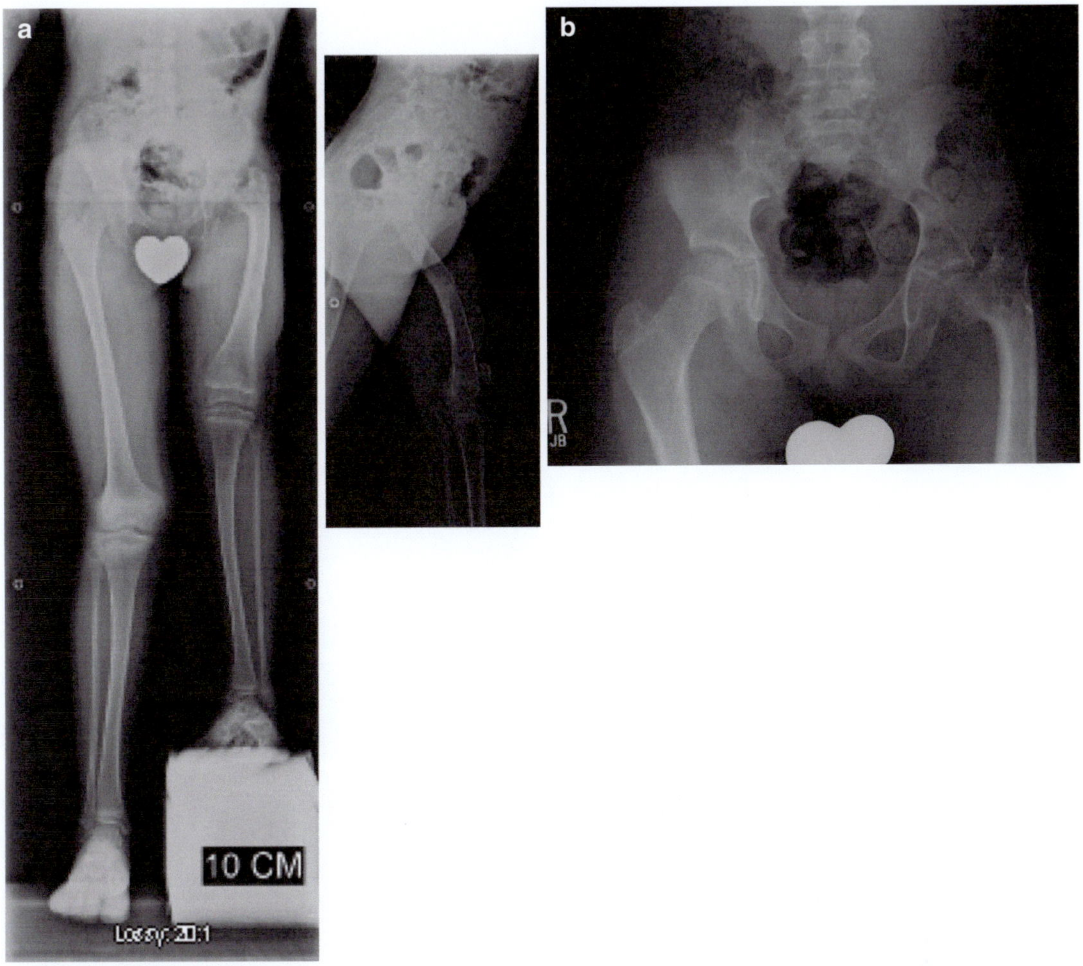

Fig. 35.3 (**a**) Radiographs of 8 year old girl with left type 1a congenital femoral deficiency and 10 cm leg length discrepancy. Erect leg radiograph (*left*) and lateral femur with knee in full extension. There is severe coxa vara and a very high greater trochanter. There is also mild fibular hemimelia. The knee comes into full extension. (**b**) Anteroposterior (AP) pelvis radiograph showing the coxa vara and dysplastic acetabulum. (**c**) Intraoperative fluoroscopic views with blade plate inserted into femoral neck. The varus angulation (angle between plate and femoral shaft) is 45° of varus (*left*) and 15° of flexion. The wires in the femur outline the planned first osteotomy. (**d**) Intraoperative fluoroscopic views after SUPERhip osteotomy showing correction of the coxa vara (*left*). The greater trochanter is now at the level of the center of the femoral head. The full extent of the acetabular dysplasia can be appreciated after the valgus osteotomy of the femur (left). A periacetabular triple osteotomy was performed to cover the femoral head (*right*). (**e**) AP pelvis radiograph after healing of the femoral and pelvic osteotomies. (**f**) Photographs taken during lengthening of the femur and tibia simultaneously with a femoral and tibial external fixator with a hinge connecting the frames at the knee. She was able to be active even with these two external fixators in place. In these pictures she is shown competing in a swim meet. (**g**) Erect leg radiograph after lengthening. The hip correction and stability are maintained. Hemiepiphysiodesis plates can be seen on the medial proximal and distal tibia to correct valgus. The long lateral radiograph shows full knee extension. (**h**) Even after two lengthening surgeries her flexibility and range of motion is excellent

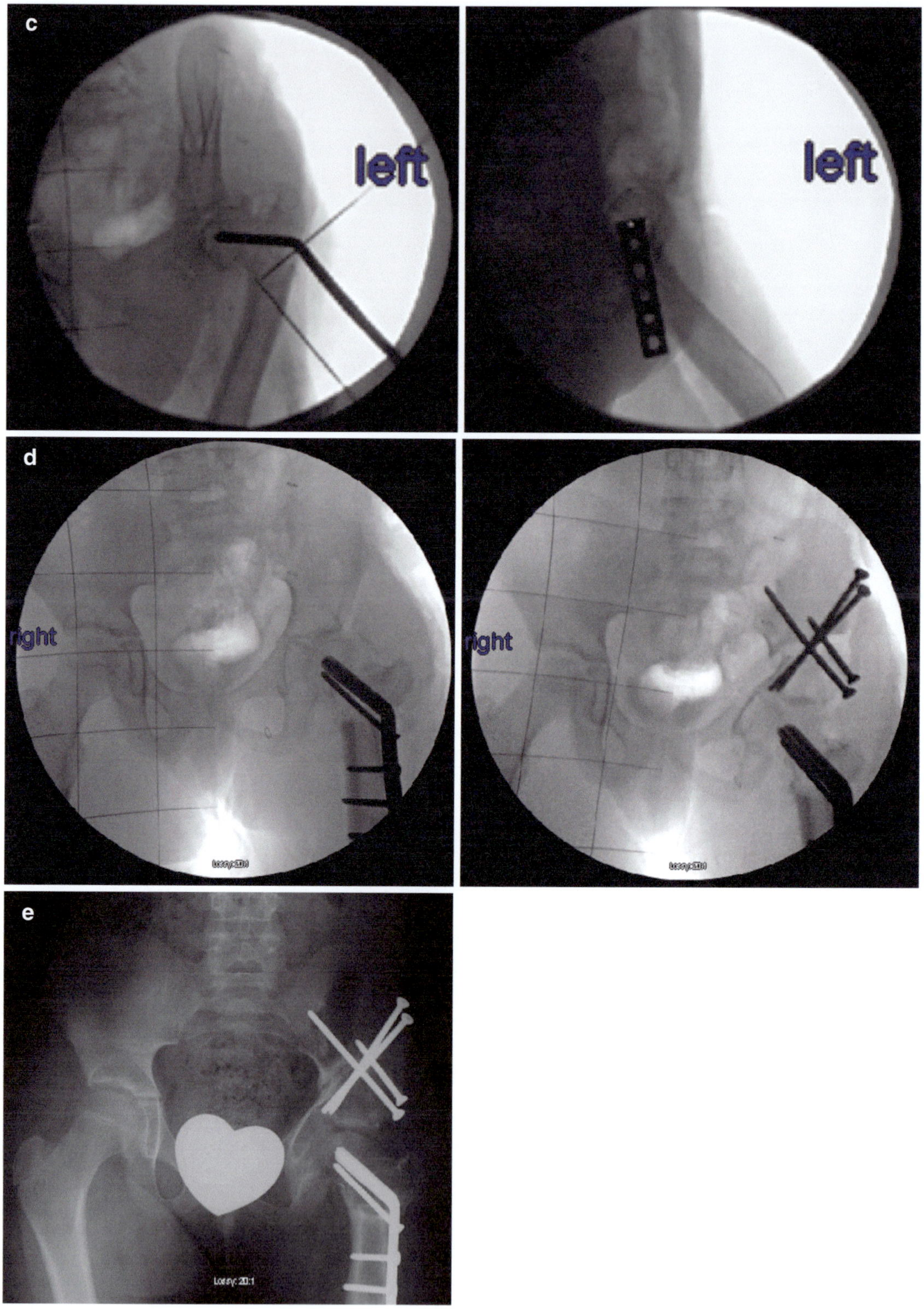

Fig. 35.3 (continued)

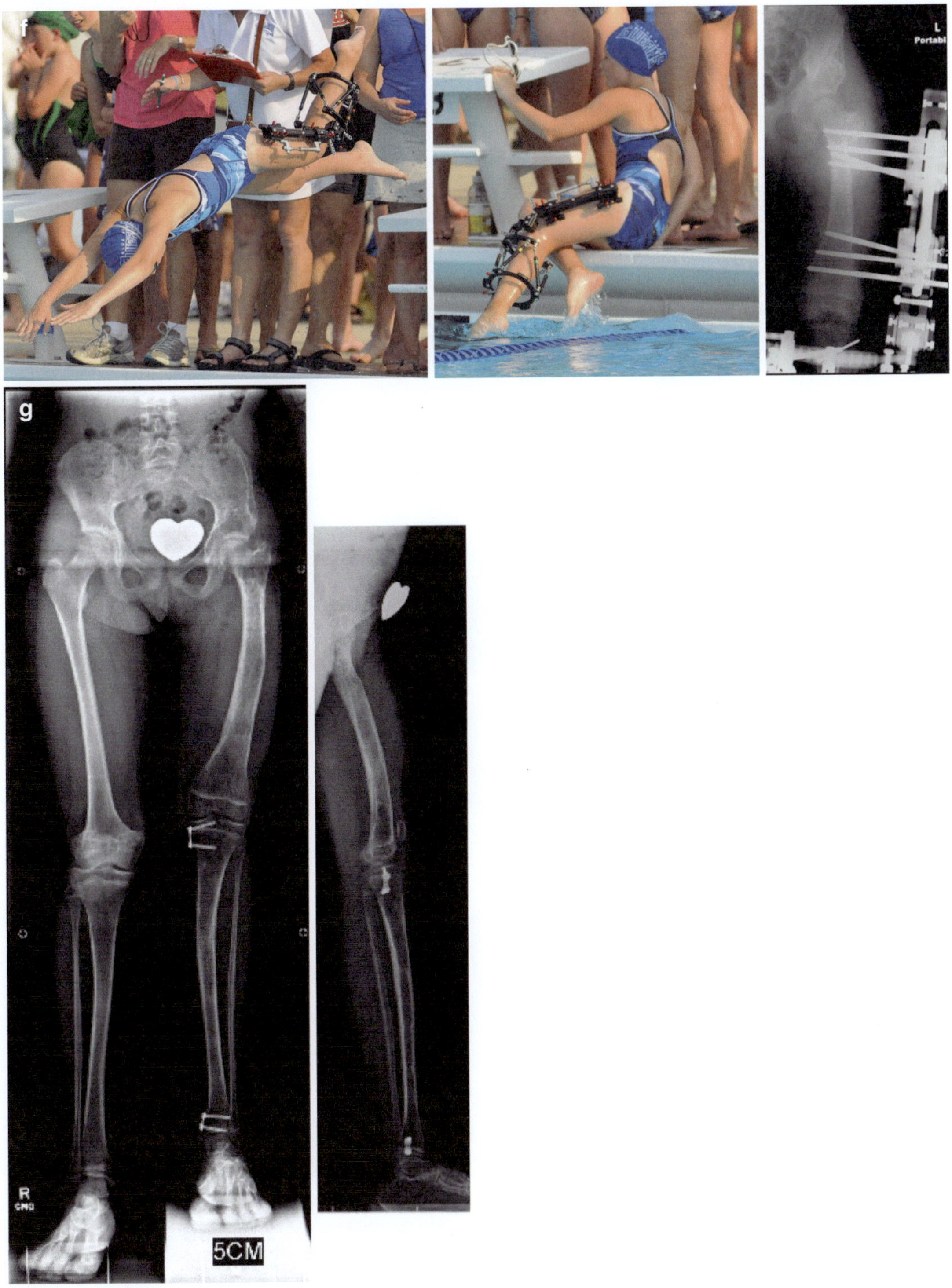

Fig. 35.3 (continued)

h

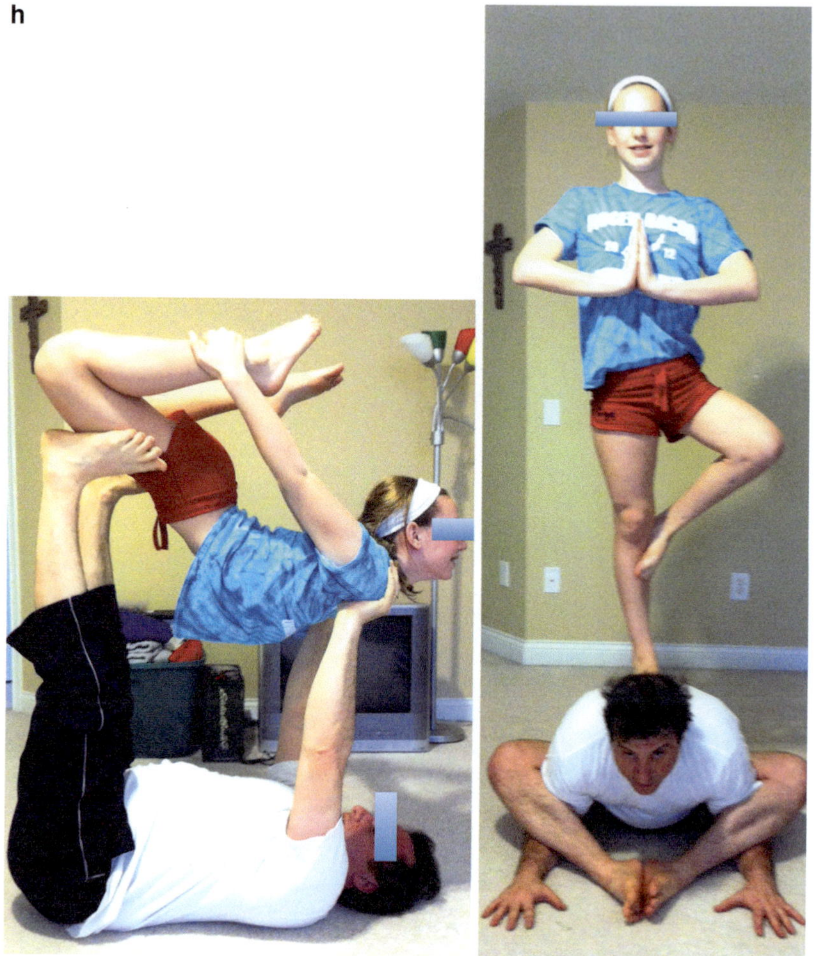

Fig. 35.3 (continued)

Case 2: Paley type 1b neck type CFD (Fig. 35.4)

Two-year-old girl with right CFD an large leg length discrepancy (LLD).

She has a fixed flexion, external rotation deformity of the hip. Her hip lacks abduction. Her knee has significant anteroposterior instability (see Fig. 35.4a, b).

Case 3: Paley type 1b subtrochanteric type CFD (Fig. 35.5)

Two-year-old girl with left CFD and a large LLD. She has a fixed flexion, adduction, external rotation deformity of the hip. She has a fixed flexion deformity of the knee (see Fig. 35.5a).

Case 4: Paley type 2a CFD (Fig. 35.6)

Six-year-old girl with right CFD and large LLD. Lacks abduction and internal rotation of hip. Knee has mild fixed flexion deformity (see Fig. 35.6a, b).

Preoperative Imaging

Radiographs of the lower limbs are taken to assess leg length discrepancy, evaluate the hip and knee deformities, femoral and acetabular dysplasia [3]. In children that can stand still, an anteroposterior (AP) radiograph is taken standing on a lift of known magnitude to approximately level the pelvis (see Fig. 35.3a). In infants the

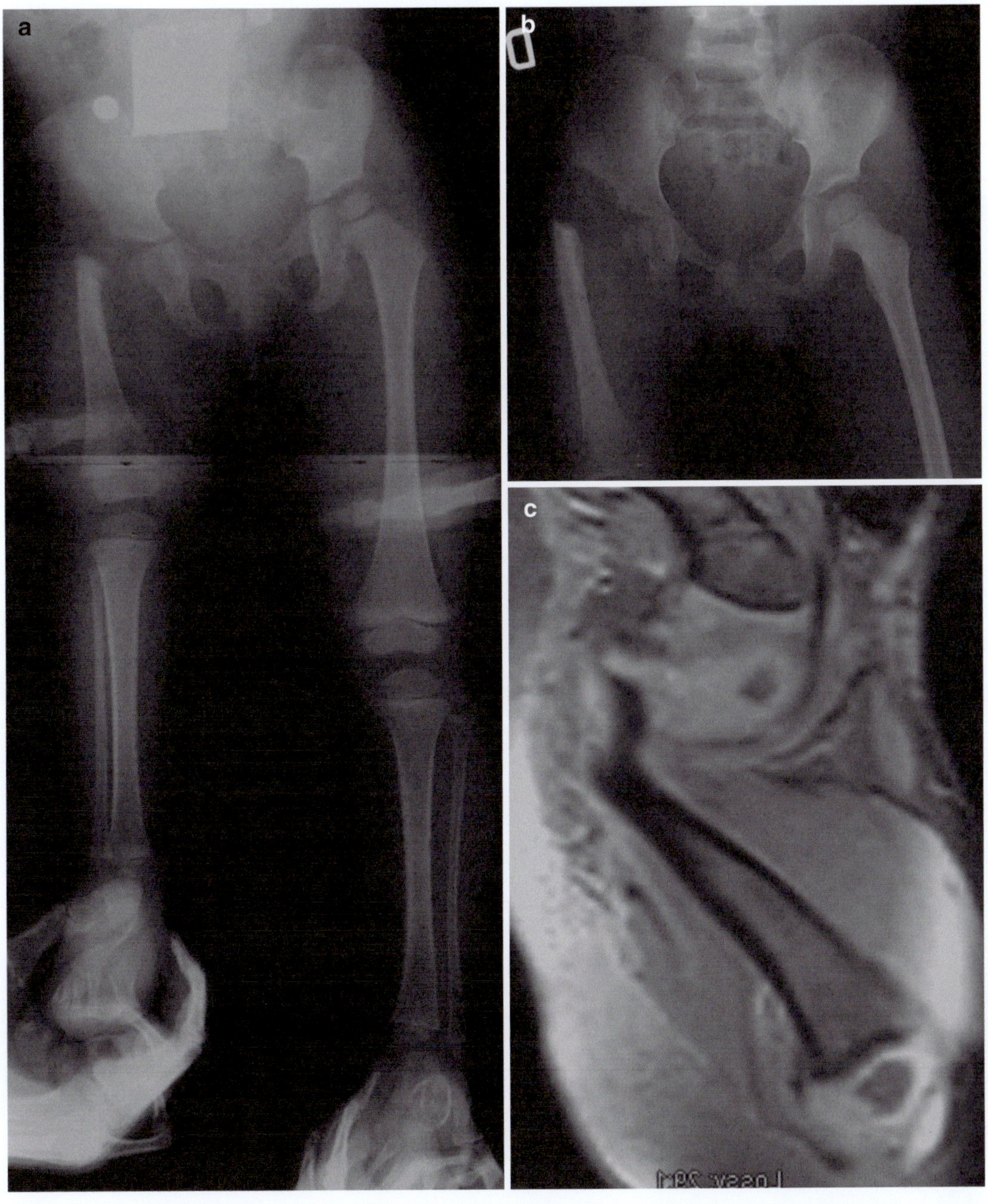

Fig. 35.4 (**a**) Long anteroposterior (AP) radiograph at age 24 months. Congenital femoral deficiency type 1b neck type. (**b**) AP pelvis showing lack of ossification of femoral neck. Note that the femur is not migrating proximally or medially indicating that there is some tissue preventing the femoral shaft from moving proximal or medial. (**c**) MRI showing cartilagenous femoral neck. This is referred to as delayed ossification of the femoral neck. (**d**) Lateral (*left*) and AP (*right*) radiographs of the femur after the SUPERhip procedure. Note the beginning of early ossification of the femoral neck in the superior neck region where the bone morphogenic protein was placed. (**e**) The femoral neck is ossified and there is obvious growth of the distal femoral physis away from the distal end of the plate. (**f**) Standing radiograph a year after the SUPERhip procedure. (**g**) external fixator in place during lengthening of 8 cm of the femur. The external fixator extends to the knee with a hinge. (**h**) After 8 cm lengthening the external fixator was removed and the femur rodded to prevent fracture. (**i**) Erect leg radiograph during the second lengthening, using Precice Lengthening Nail (Nuvasive Specialized Orthopedics, Irving CA, USA). Hemiepiphysiodesis plate in place to treat the genu valgum. (**j**) Erect leg radiograph (*right*) and long lateral radiograph (*left*) after completion of lengthening with Precice nail and after screw epiphysiodesis of left distal femur

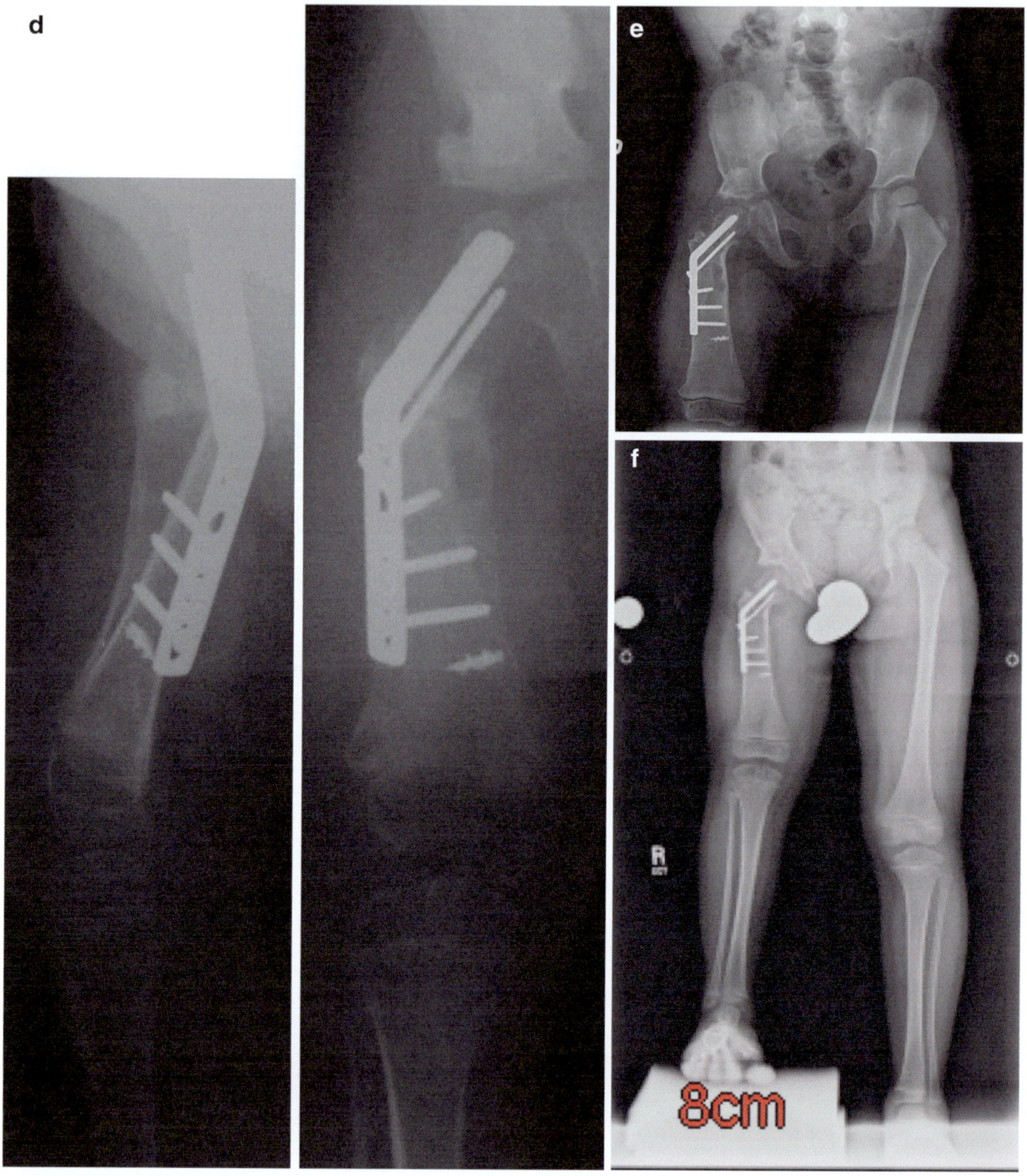

Fig. 35.4 (continued)

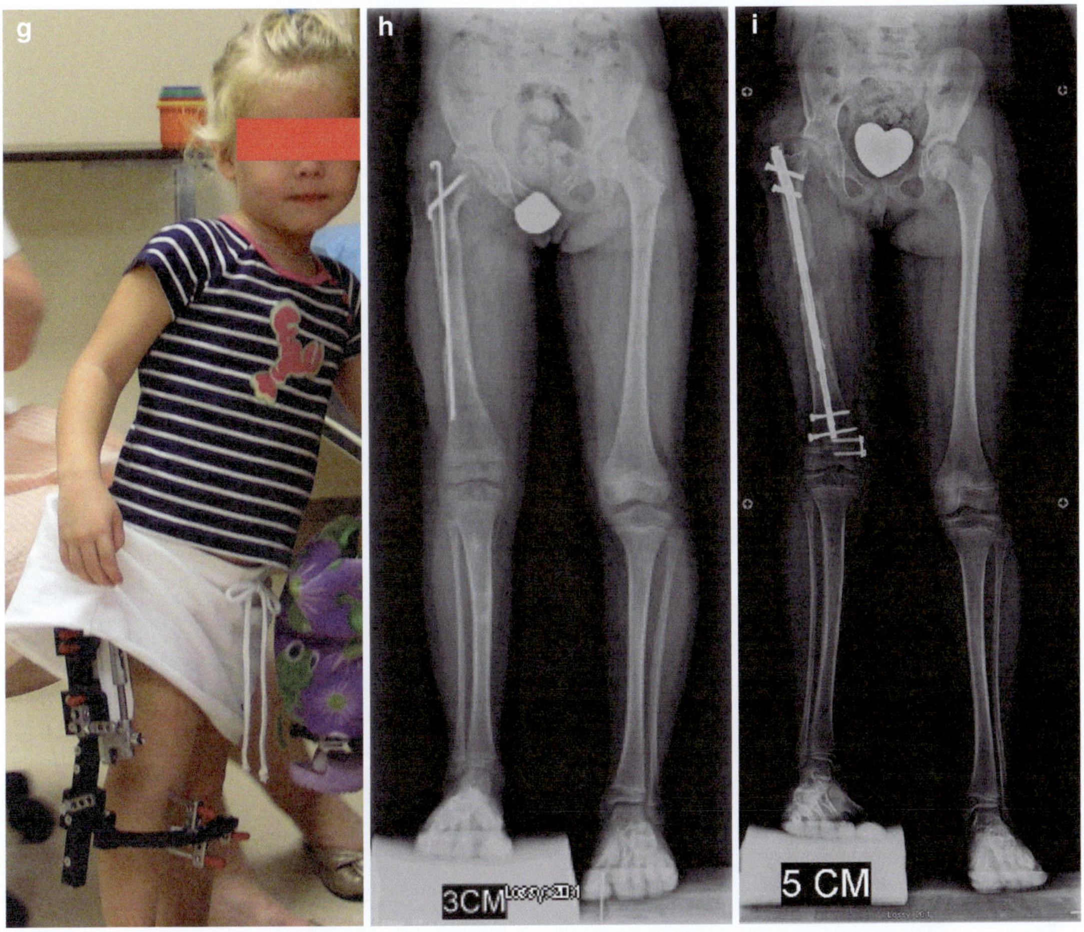

Fig. 35.4 (continued)

j

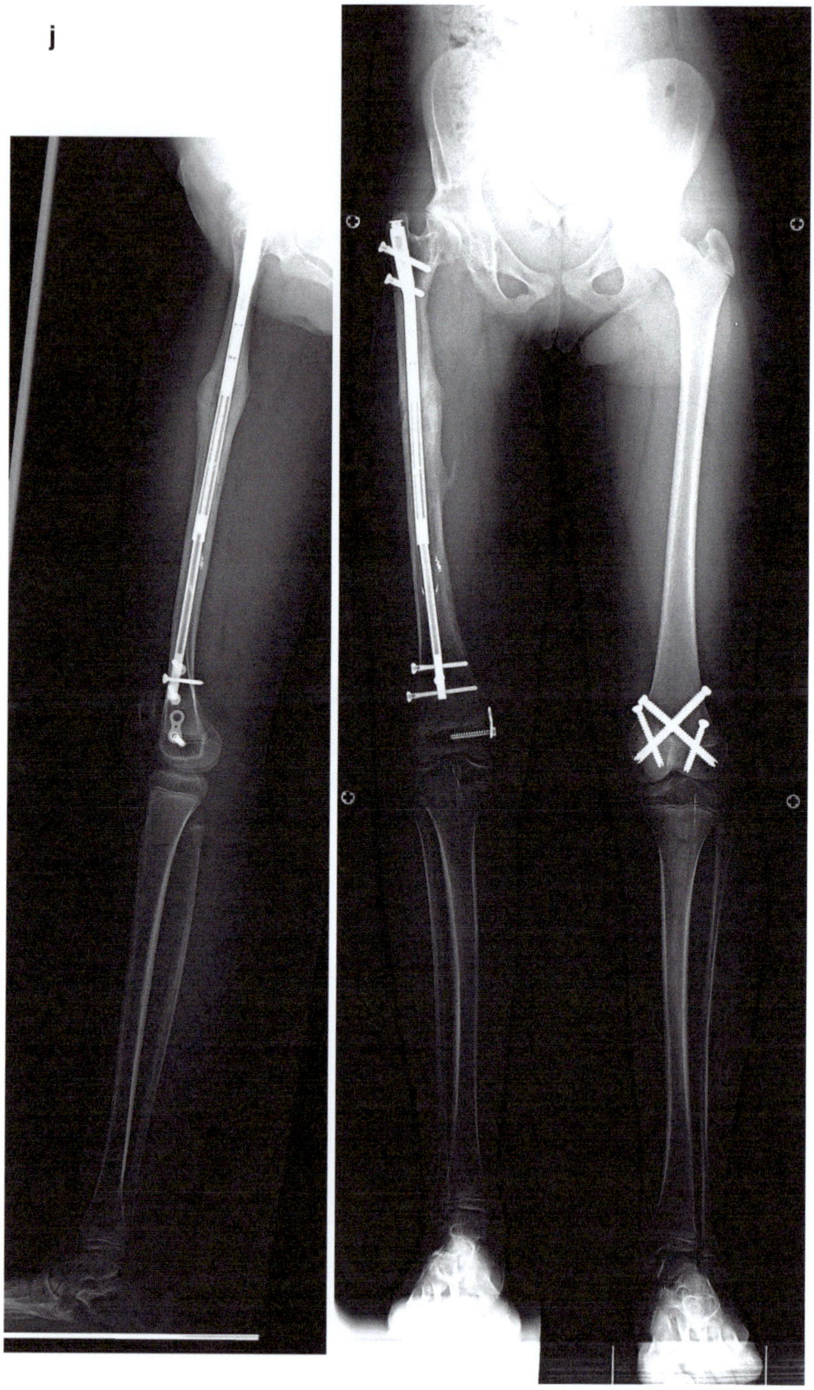

Fig. 35.4 (continued)

radiographs are taken supine with both feet pulled down by a parent to keep the hip and knee in maximum extension (see Figs. 35.4a and 35.5a). The x-ray should include the pelvis, both femurs and both tibias and feet. This x-ray is used to measure the length discrepancy between the femurs and tibias. Total leg length discrepancy including the foot can be measured from a standing x-ray by measuring from the top of the hip joints. A simulated standing lateral radiograph of both feet can also be taken to directly measure the foot height differences. The sum of femur, tibia and foot height difference gives the total LLD. A long lateral radiograph of the femur and tibia with the knee in maximum extension is also used to evaluate for knee flexion deformity (see Figs. 35.3a, 35.5a, and 35.6b). A supine AP pelvis radiograph (see Figs. 35.3b and 35.6a) is used to study acetabular dysplasia and ossification of the femoral neck.

Magnetic resonance imaging is useful if there is delayed ossification of the femoral neck (see Fig. 35.4c) or subtrochanteric region (see Fig. 35.5b). It can help determine whether a cartilagenous femoral neck is present or not distinguishing between a delayed ossification of the femoral neck (type 1b) vs a true pseudarthrosis of the femoral neck (type 2).

Goals of Treatment

1. Correct femur/hip deficiency, deformity and dysplasia
2. Make the hip stable
3. Serial lengthenings of femur to equalize limb length discrepancy.

One cannot equalize the limb length discrepancy in the presence of significant femoral deformity or hip dysplasia. Therefore surgery to correct the upper femoral deformity and to secure hip stability is preparatory to femoral lengthening and must be performed prior to beginning with a lengthening program.

Treatment Strategies

Paley type 1a:

(a) extra-articular release of contractures by lengthening the tethering soft tissues without weakening these muscles
(b) subtrochanteric corrective osteotomy with shortening to acutely correct all of the bony deformities so that the normal anatomy of the femur is restored
(c) treat acetabular dysplasia

Paley type 1b neck type hip surgery:

(a) Extra-articular release of contractures by lengthening the tethering soft tissues without weakening these muscles
(b) Subtrochanteric corrective osteotomy with shortening to acutely correct all of the bony deformities so that the normal anatomy of the femur is restored
(c) Cause the delayed ossification of the femoral neck to ossify
(d) Treat acetabular dysplasia

Paley type 1b subtrochanteric type hip surgery:

(a) Extra-articular release of contractures by lengthening the tethering soft tissues without weakening these muscles
(b) Subtrochanteric corrective osteotomy with shortening to acutely correct all of the bony deformities so that the normal anatomy of the femur is restored
(c) Resect the region of delayed ossification of the subtrochanteric femur
(d) Treat acetabular dysplasia

Paley type 2a hip surgery:

(a) Extra-articular release of contractures by lengthening the tethering soft tissues without weakening these muscles

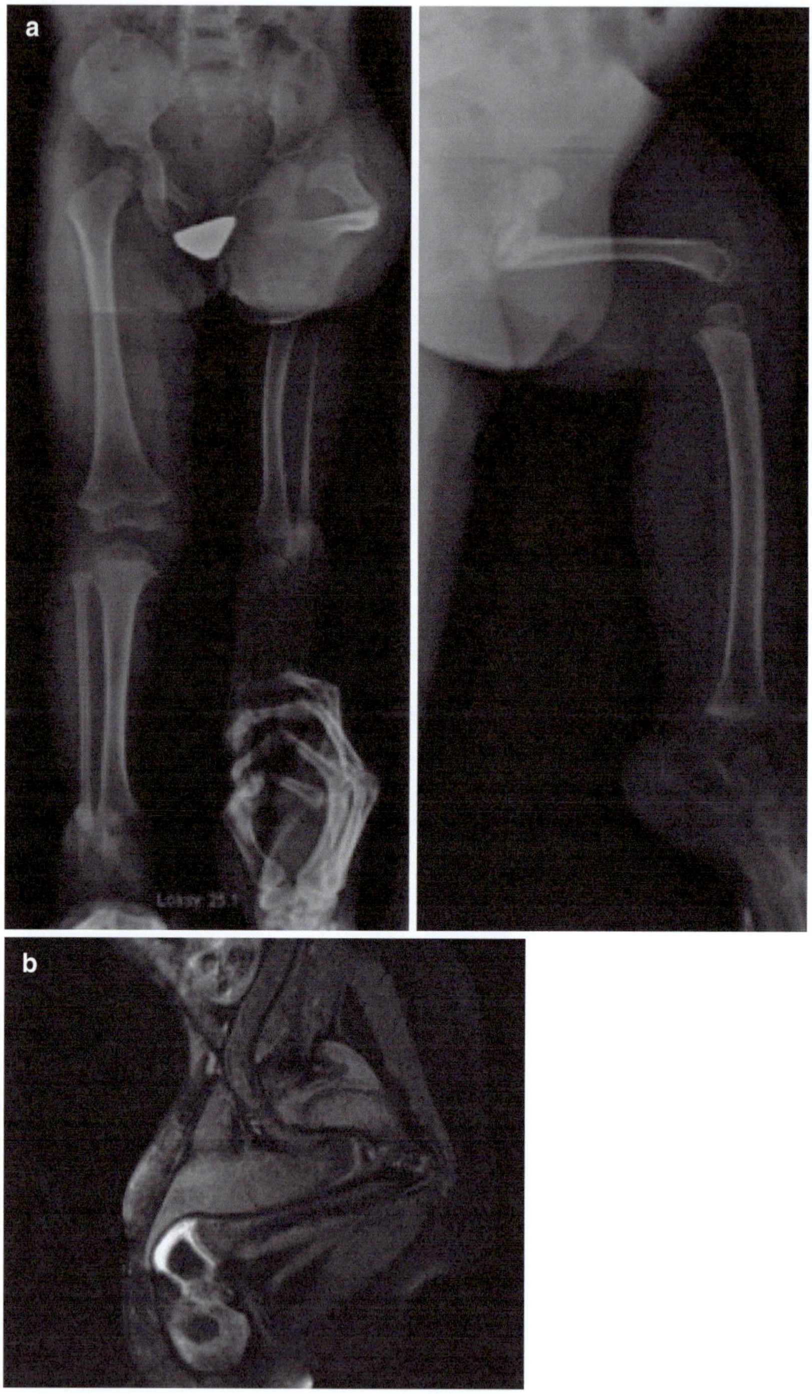

Fig. 35.5 (**a**) Long anteroposterior (AP) pull down radiograph showing severe bend in left subtrochanteric region of femur (*right*) and long lateral radiograph in maximum extension showing severe knee flexion contracture. This is a type 1b congenital femoral deficiency, subtrochanteric type. (**b**) Magentic resonance image showing the greater than 90° bend in the femur and the region of delayed ossification in the subrochanteric region. (**c**) Erect leg radiograph after SUPERhip procedure with posterior knee capsulotomy. There has been significant growth stimulation (the distal end of the femoral plate was next to the distal physis after surgery) The knee comes into full extension and flexes 90°. (**d**) AP femur radiograph during lengthening with external fixator in place. (**e**) Erect legs radiograph after lengthening. The rodding was done to prevent fracture

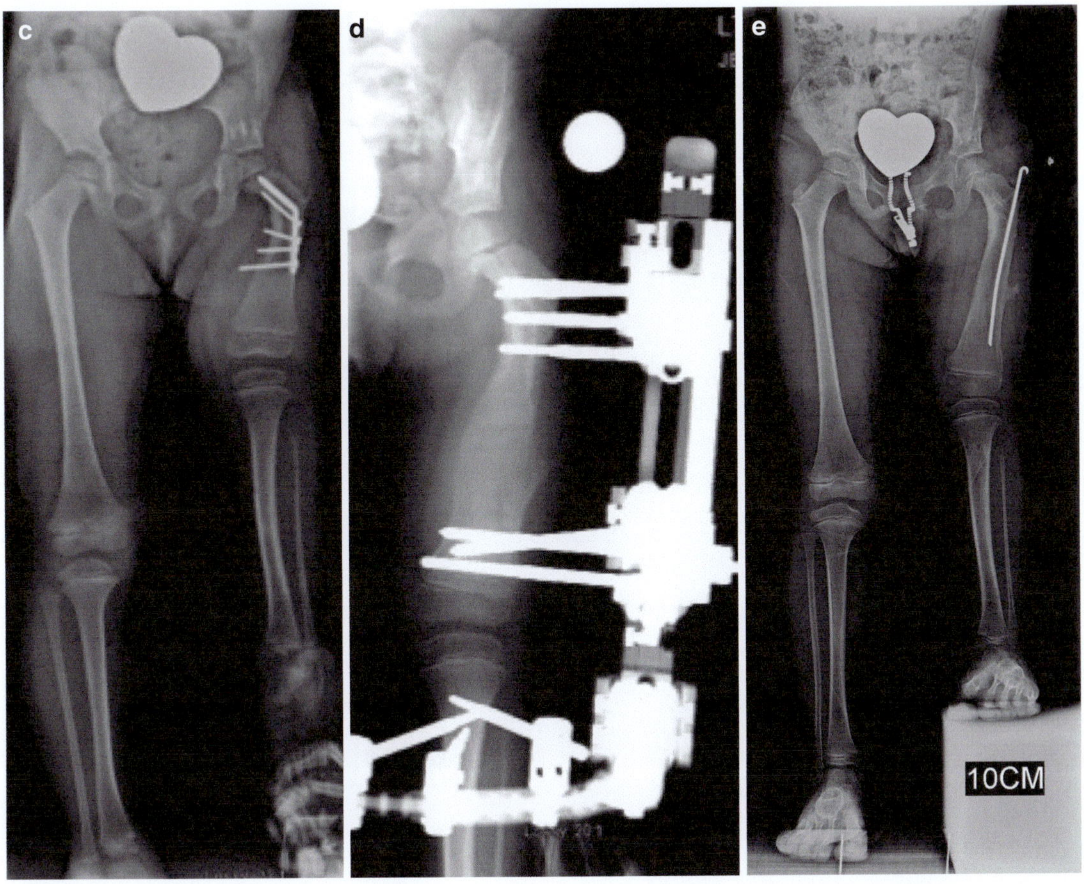

Fig. 35.5 (continued)

(b) Reconstruct femoral neck
(c) Unite new femoral neck to mobile femoral head

Paley type 2b hip surgery:

(a) Extra-articular release of contractures by lengthening the tethering soft tissues without weakening these muscles
(b) Reconstruct femoral neck
(c) Separate femoral head fusion from acetabulum and make the femoral head mobile
(d) Unite new femoral neck to mobile femoral head

Paley types 1a and 1b lengthening surgery:

(a) Lengthen through distal femoral osteotomy
(b) Apply external fixator to femur articulated to the tibia with a knee locking bar
(c) Extend the external fixator to the pelvis with a hip hinge only if hip stability or femoral neck integrity are suspect

Paley types 2 lengthening surgery:

(a) Lengthen through distal femoral osteotomy
(b) Apply external fixator to femur articulated to tibia and articulated to pelvis for knee and hip motion respectively

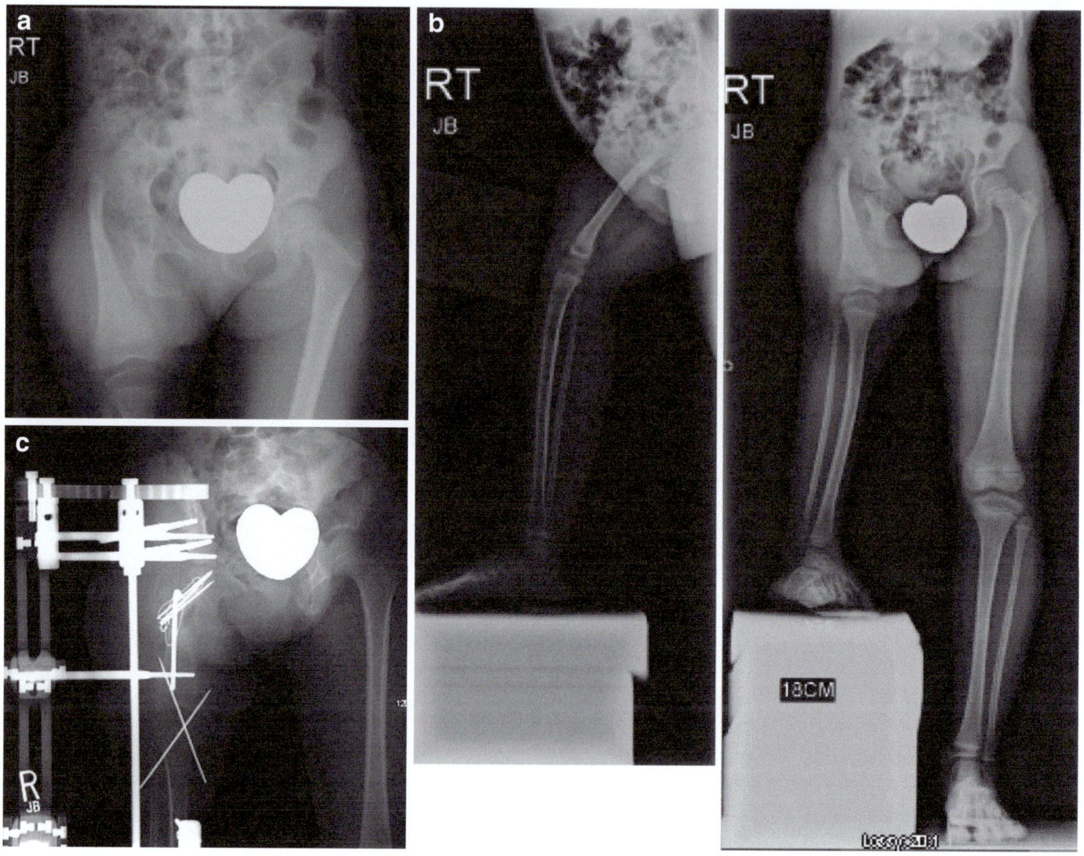

Fig. 35.6 (**a**) Anteroposterior pelvis radiograph showing high riding femur. The ossific nucleus of the femoral head is also clearly visible. (**b**) Erect leg radiograph showing the LLD *(right)*. The knee has a mild flexion deformity (*left*). (**c**) After SUPERhip2 procedure with neutralizing external fixator in place. (**d**) Final radiograph before lengthening. There has been a lot of growth stimulation. (**e**) Erect leg radiograph during 8 cm lengthening of right femur. The external fixator is seen in place. (**f**) Radiographs showing the bone is healed and a rod is in place to prevent from fracture

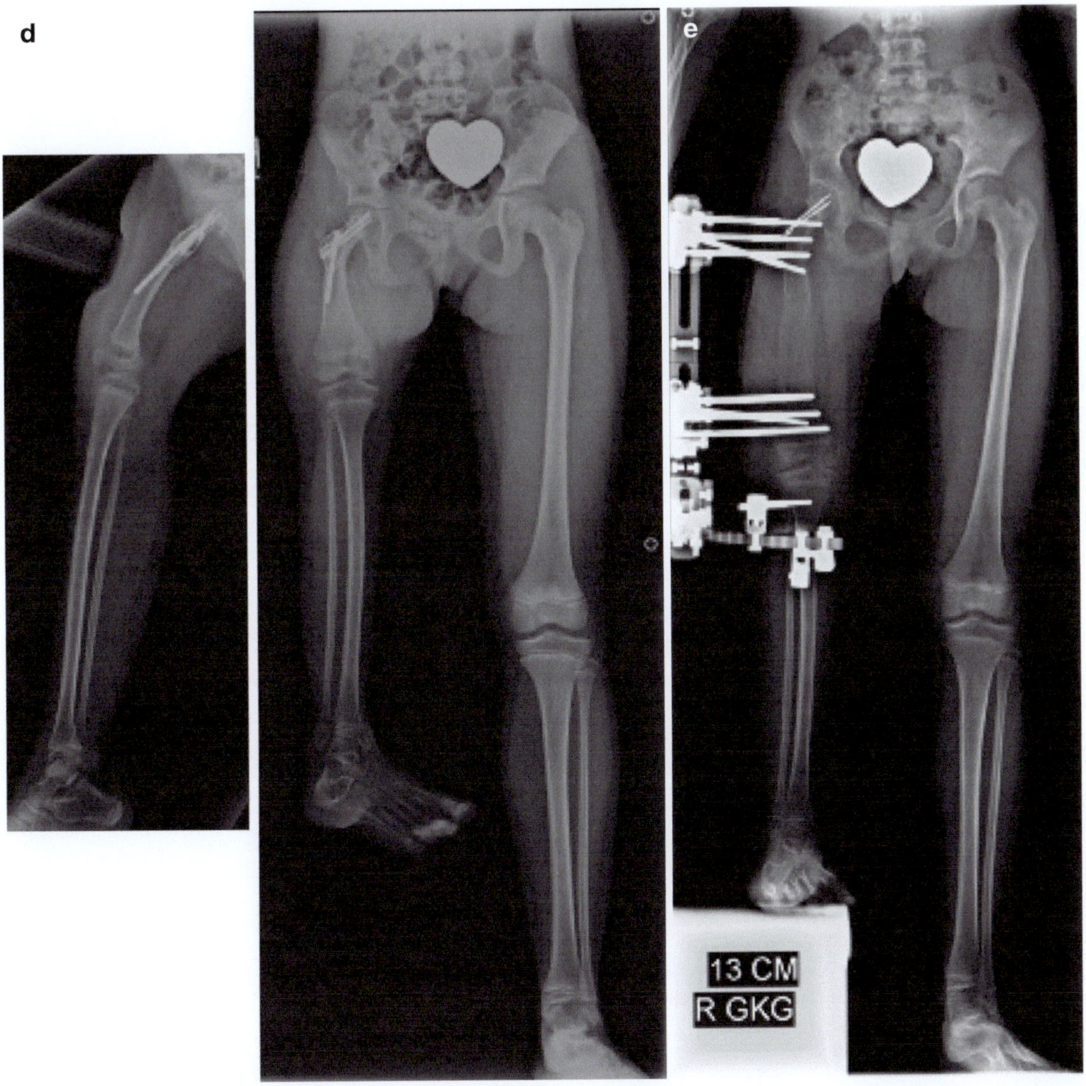

Fig. 35.6 (continued)

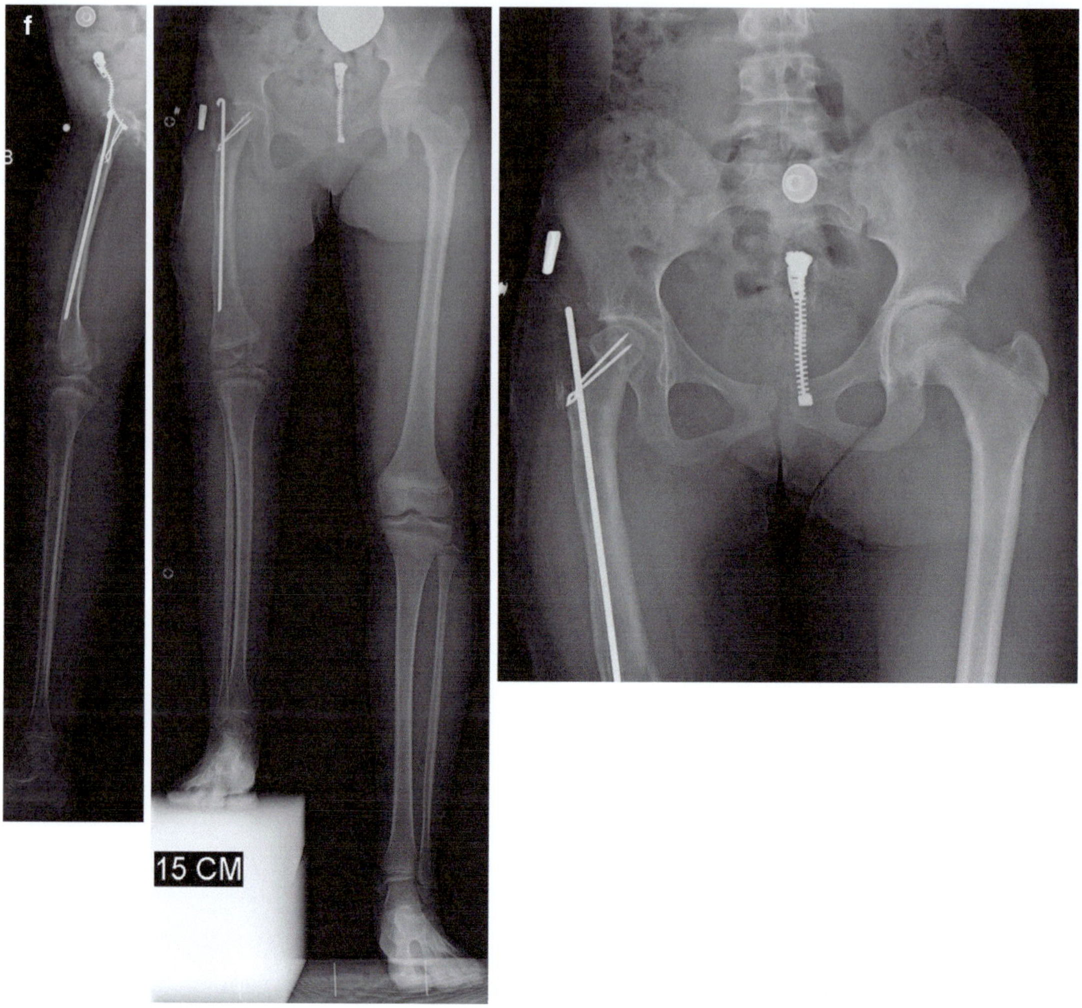

Fig. 35.6 (continued)

Surgical Details

SUPERhip Surgical Technique [2, 4–8] (Figs. 35.7, 35.8, and 35.9)

1. *Positioning, prepping and draping (see Fig. 35.7a, b)*. An epidural is placed by the anesthesia service with a catheter running up the back on the non-operative side. A Foley catheter is placed and also routed to the non-operative side. The patient should be moved to the edge and foot of the radiolucent table in a supine position. The ipsilateral arm should be appropriately padded and placed across the patient's chest. A radiolucent bump (usually a folded towel or sheet) is placed beneath the ipsilateral ischium to roll the pelvis 45° towards the opposite side. The bump should not be beneath the iliac crest or lower back. The entire side should be prepped and draped free from the nipple to the toes. The drapes should extend from the mid buttocks to the scrotal/labial-thigh fold. The lower limb should be completely free of the drapes.

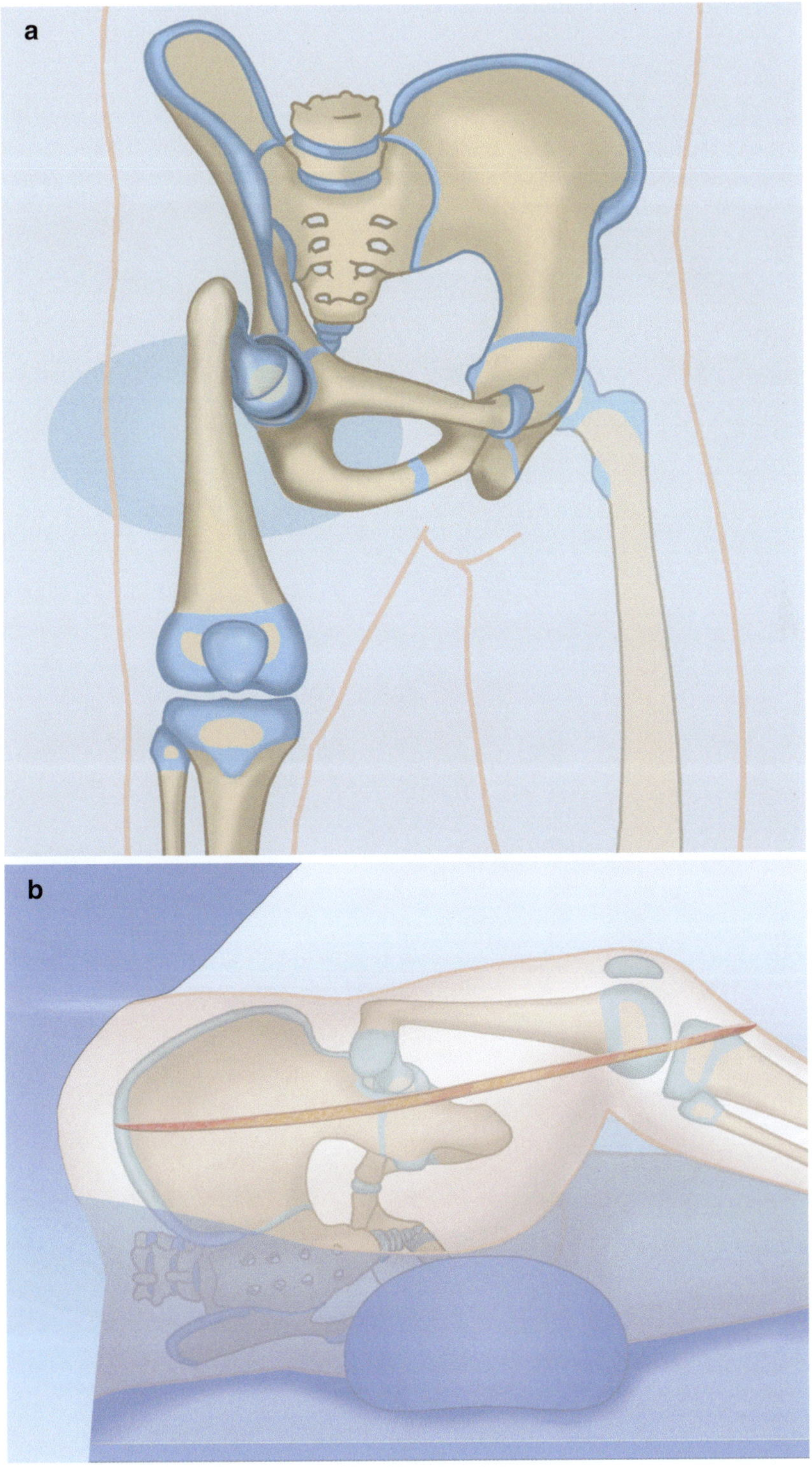

Fig. 35.7 (**a**–**j**) Illustrations of SUPERhip procedure soft tissue releases: see steps of surgery corresponding to each figure. (© 2014 The Paley Foundation, with permission. All rights reserved)

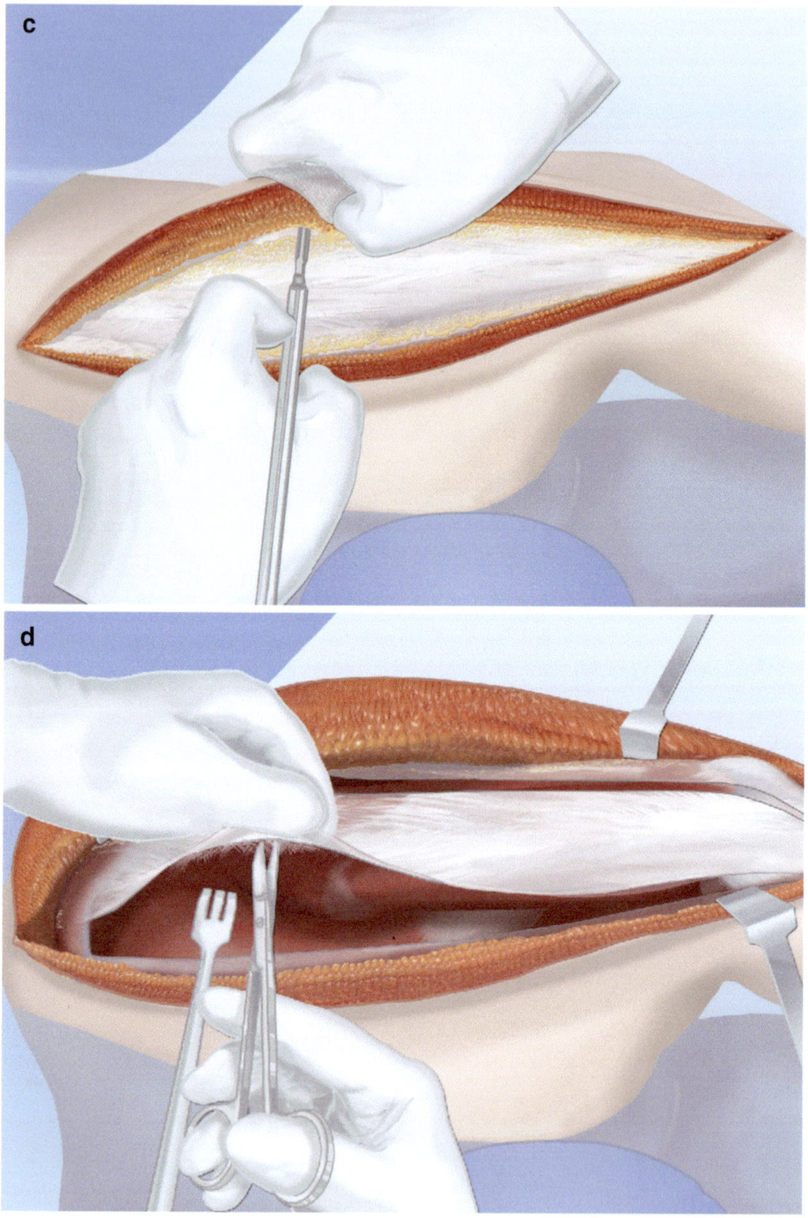

Fig. 35.7 (continued)

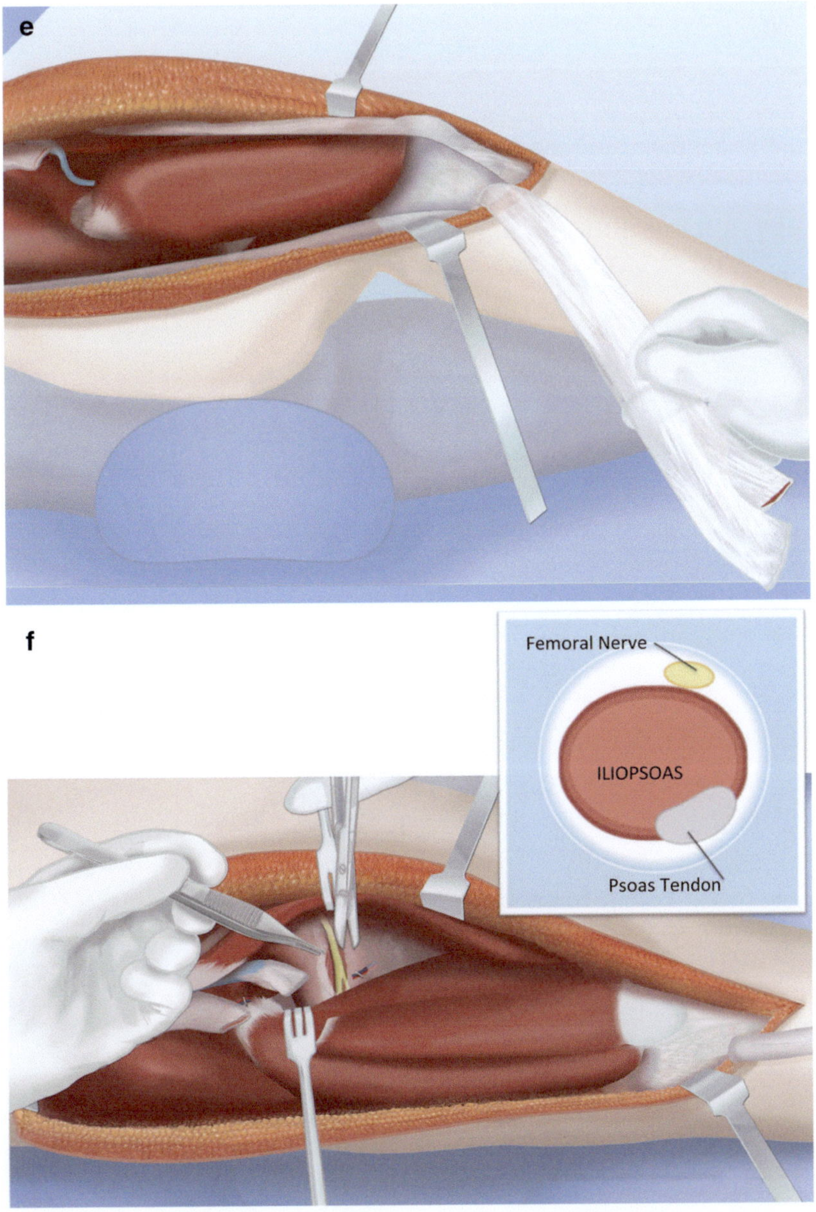

Fig. 35.7 (continued)

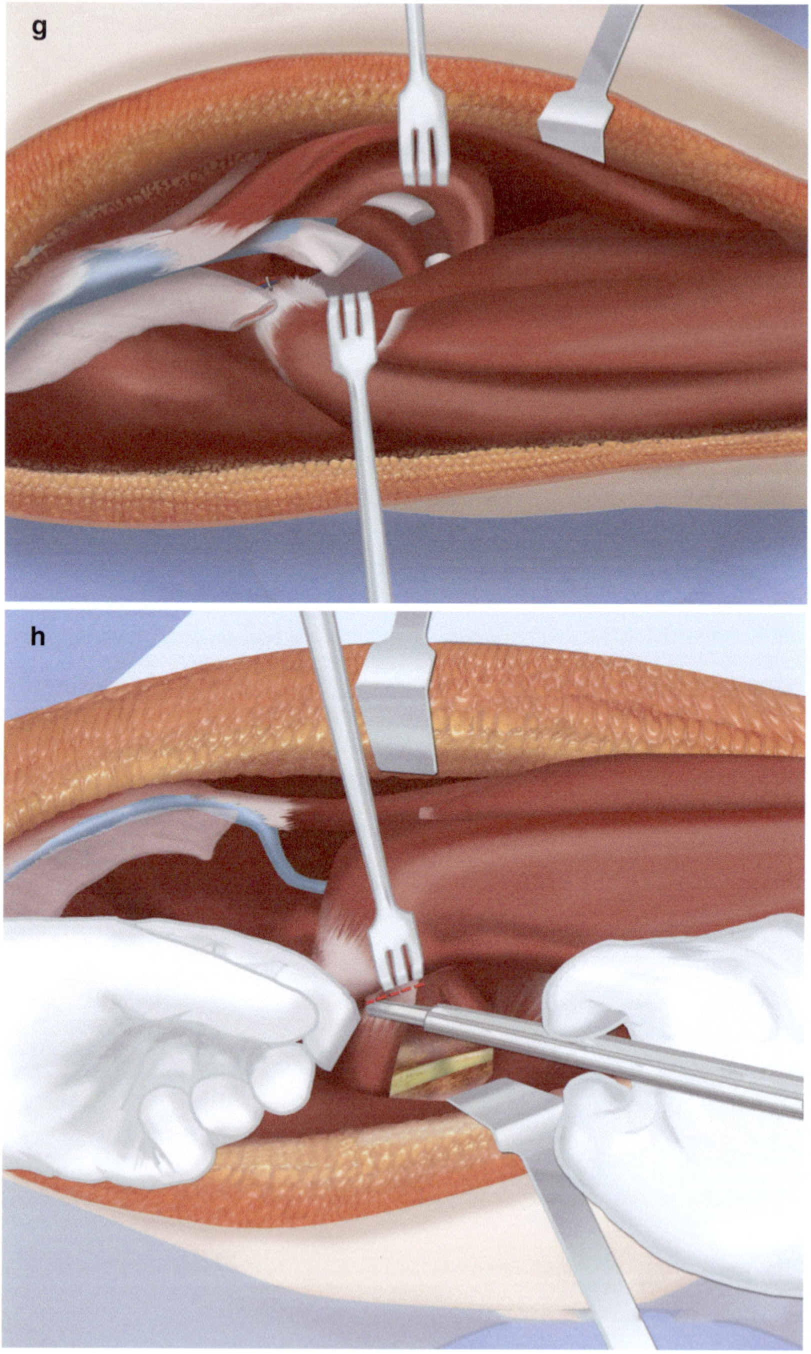

Fig. 35.7 (continued)

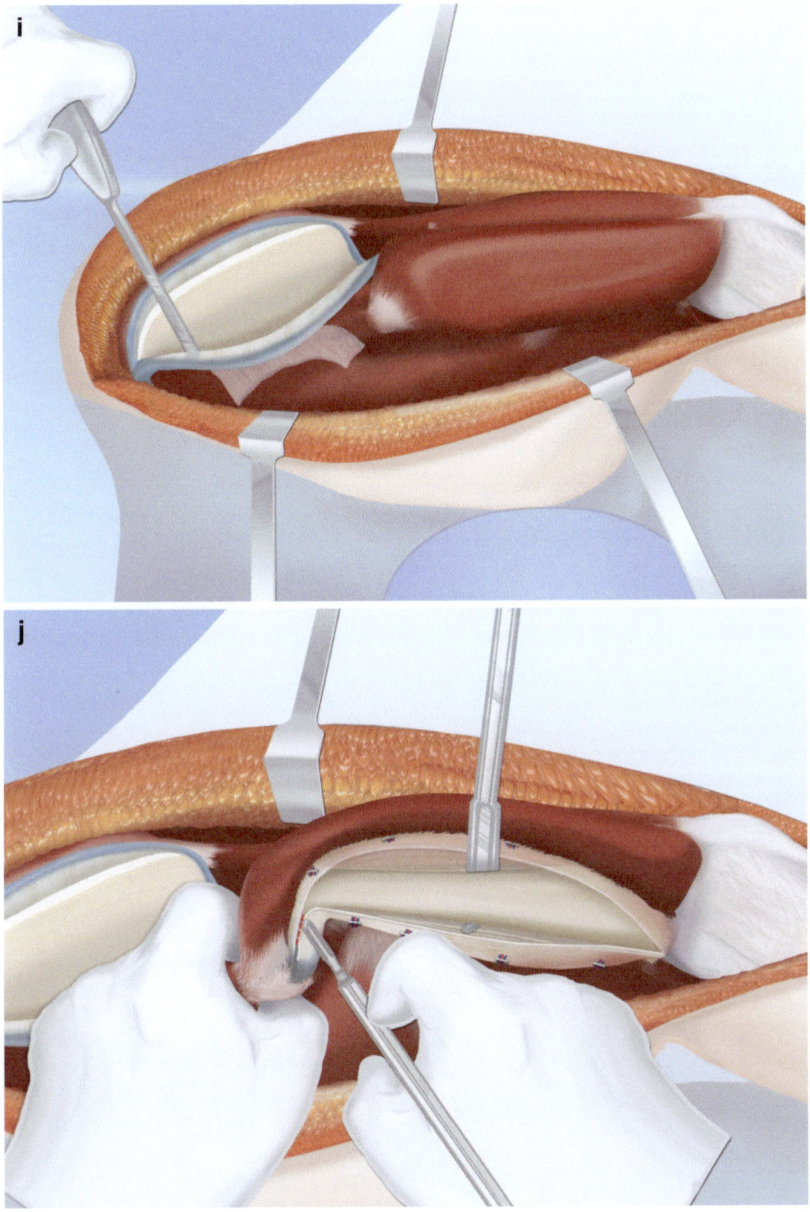

Fig. 35.7 (continued)

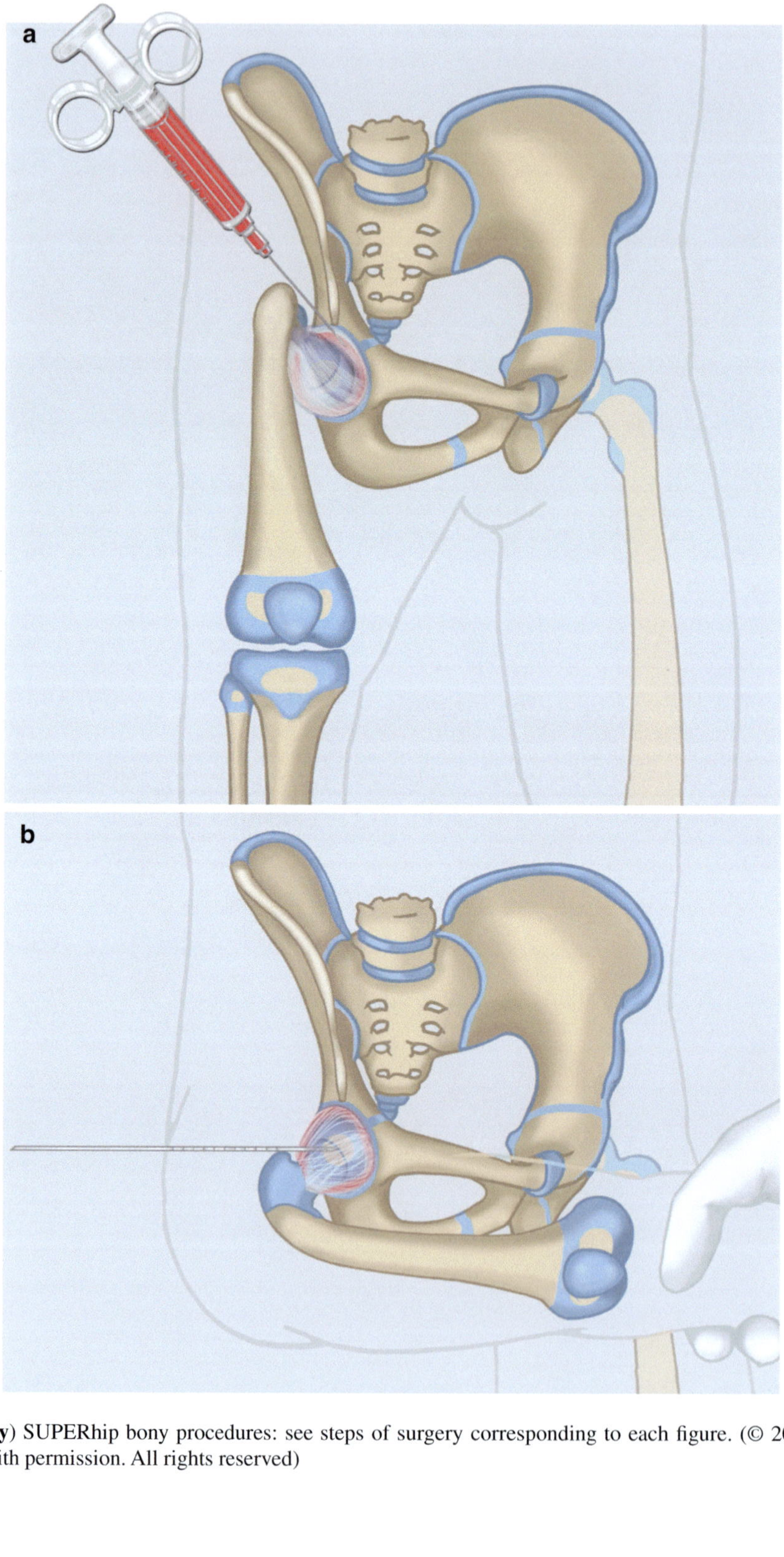

Fig. 35.8 (**a–y**) SUPERhip bony procedures: see steps of surgery corresponding to each figure. (© 2014 The Paley Foundation, with permission. All rights reserved)

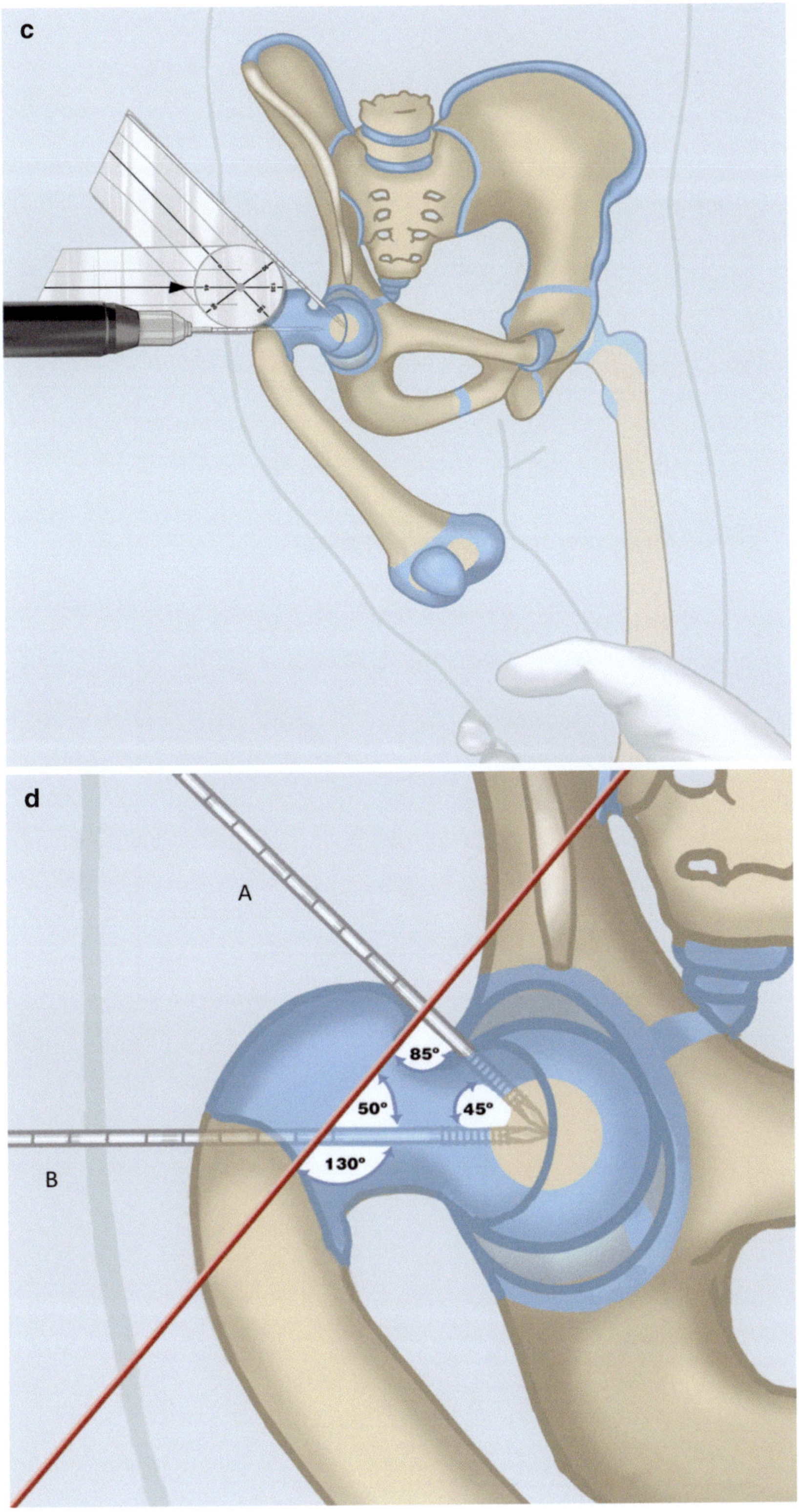

Fig. 35.8 (continued)

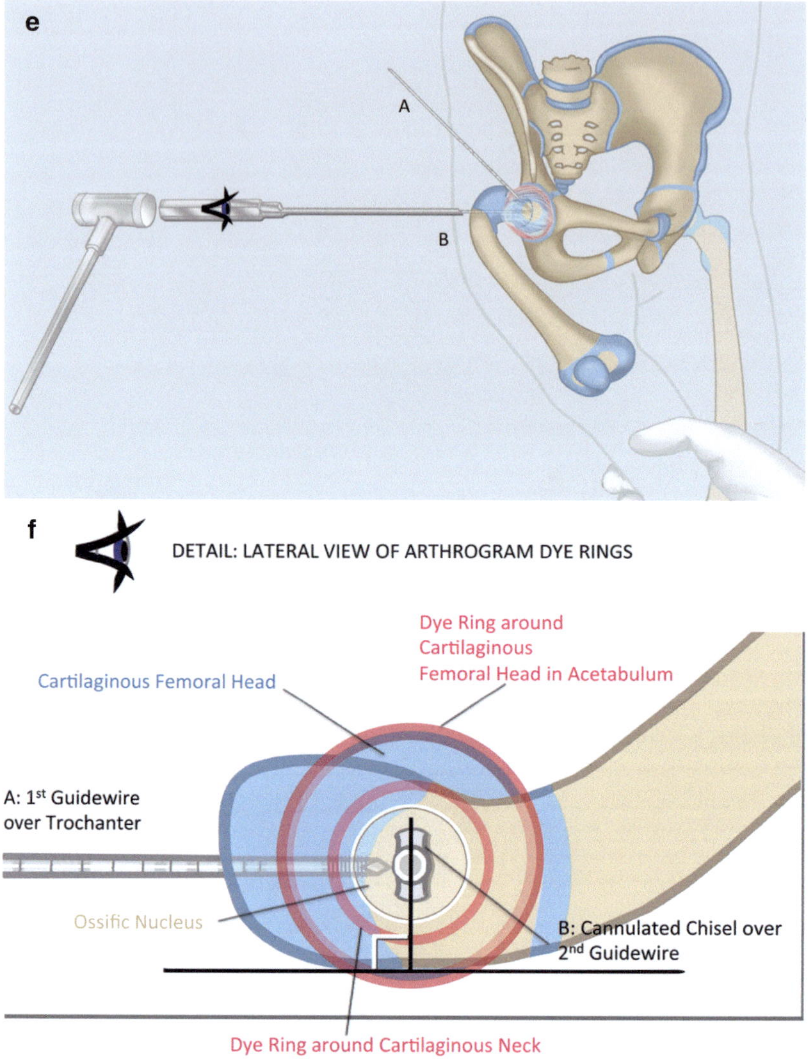

Fig. 35.8 (continued)

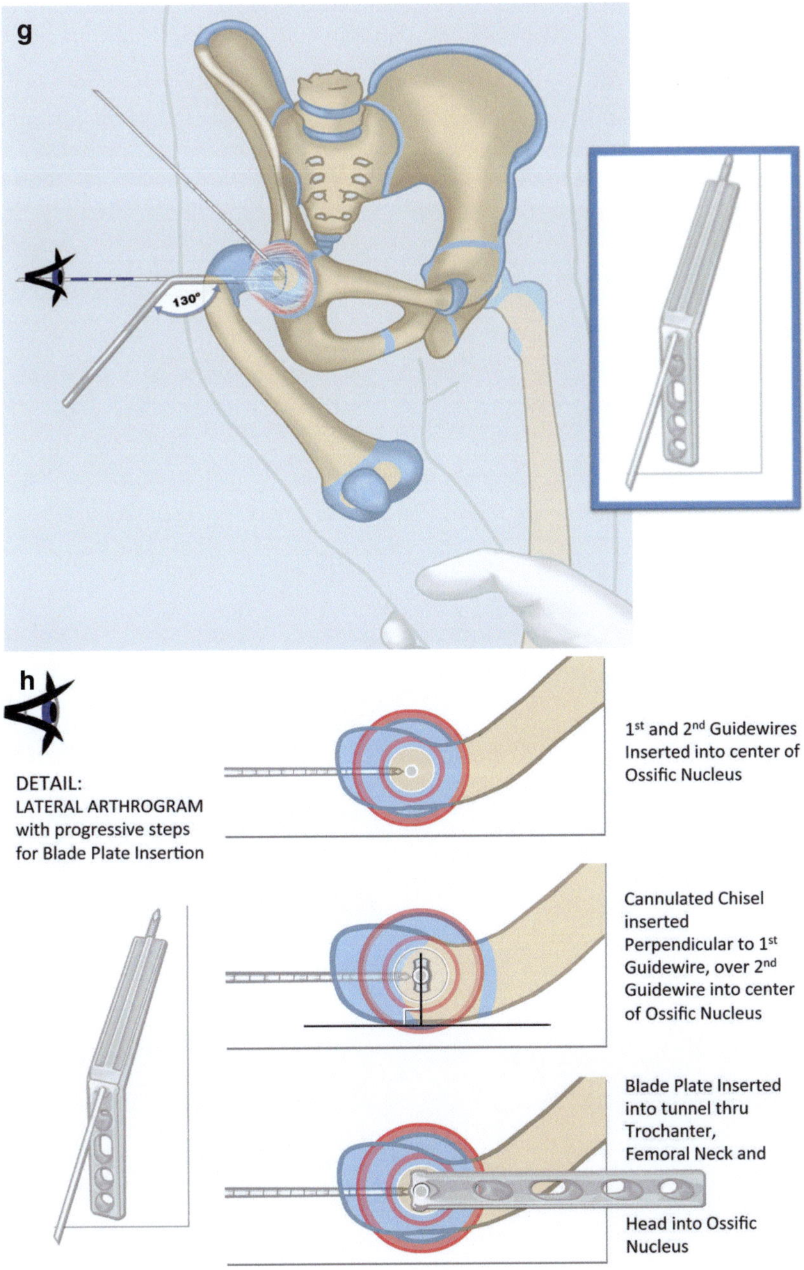

Fig. 35.8 (continued)

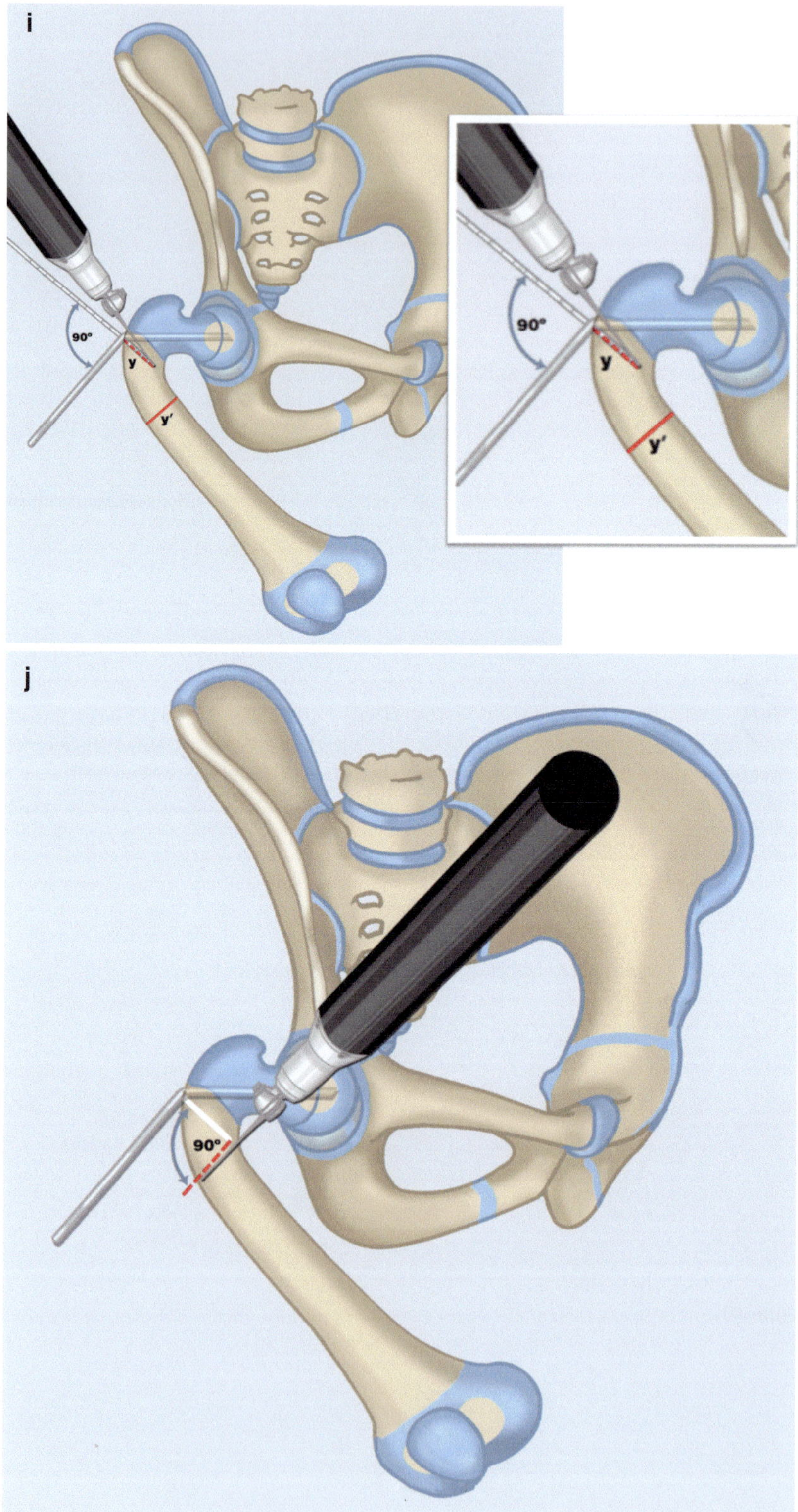

Fig. 35.8 (continued)

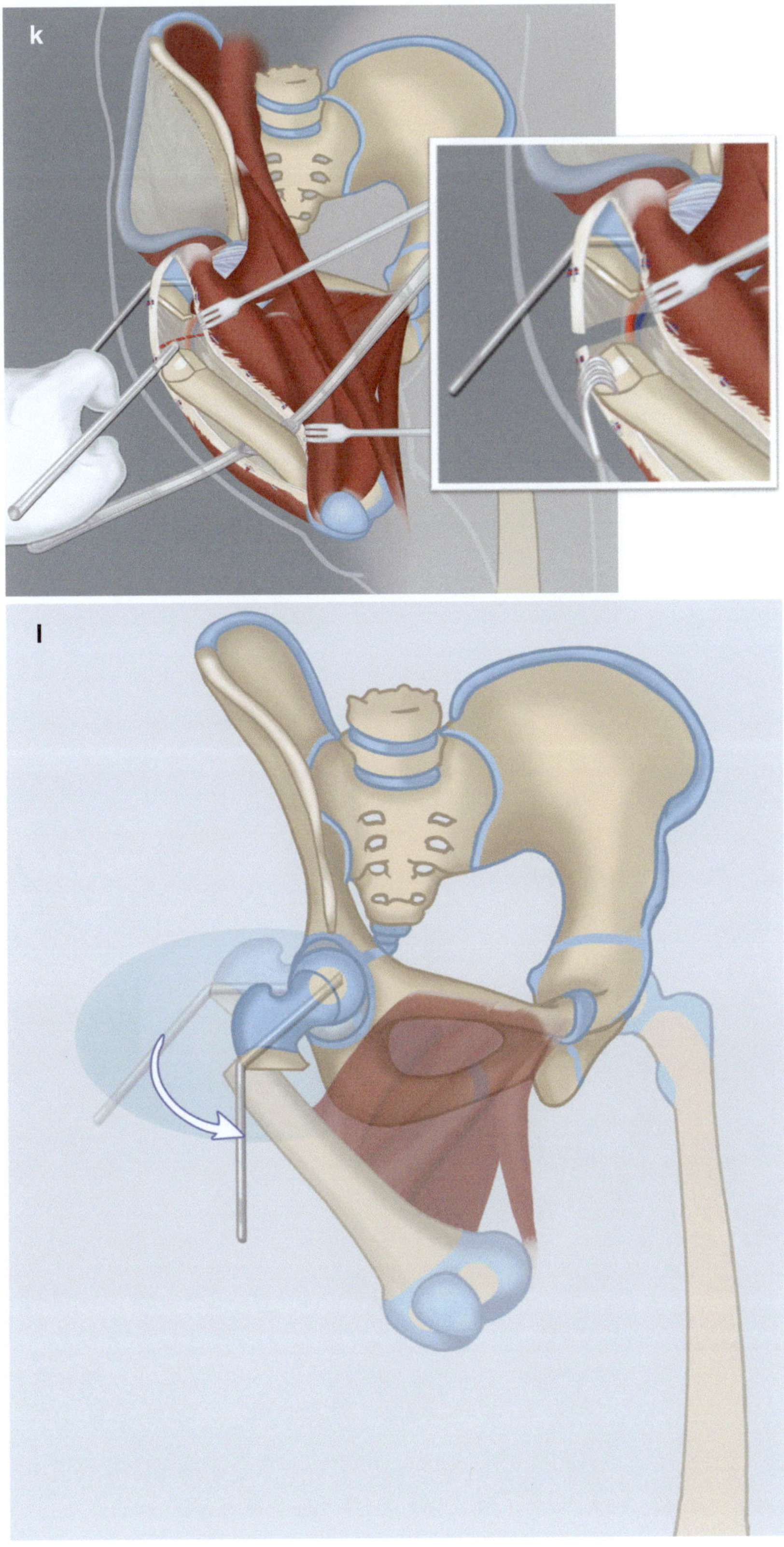

Fig. 35.8 (continued)

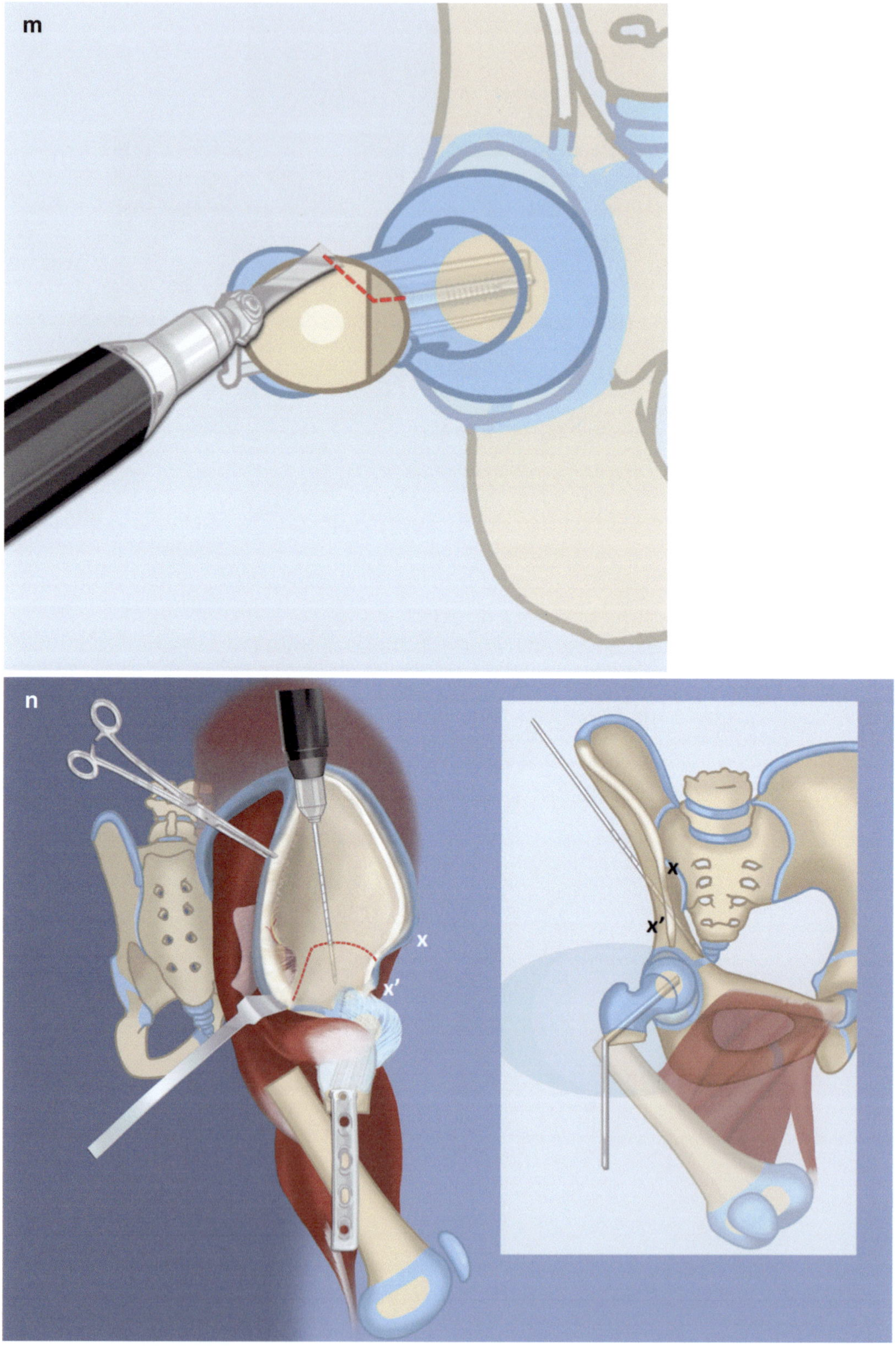

Fig. 35.8 (continued)

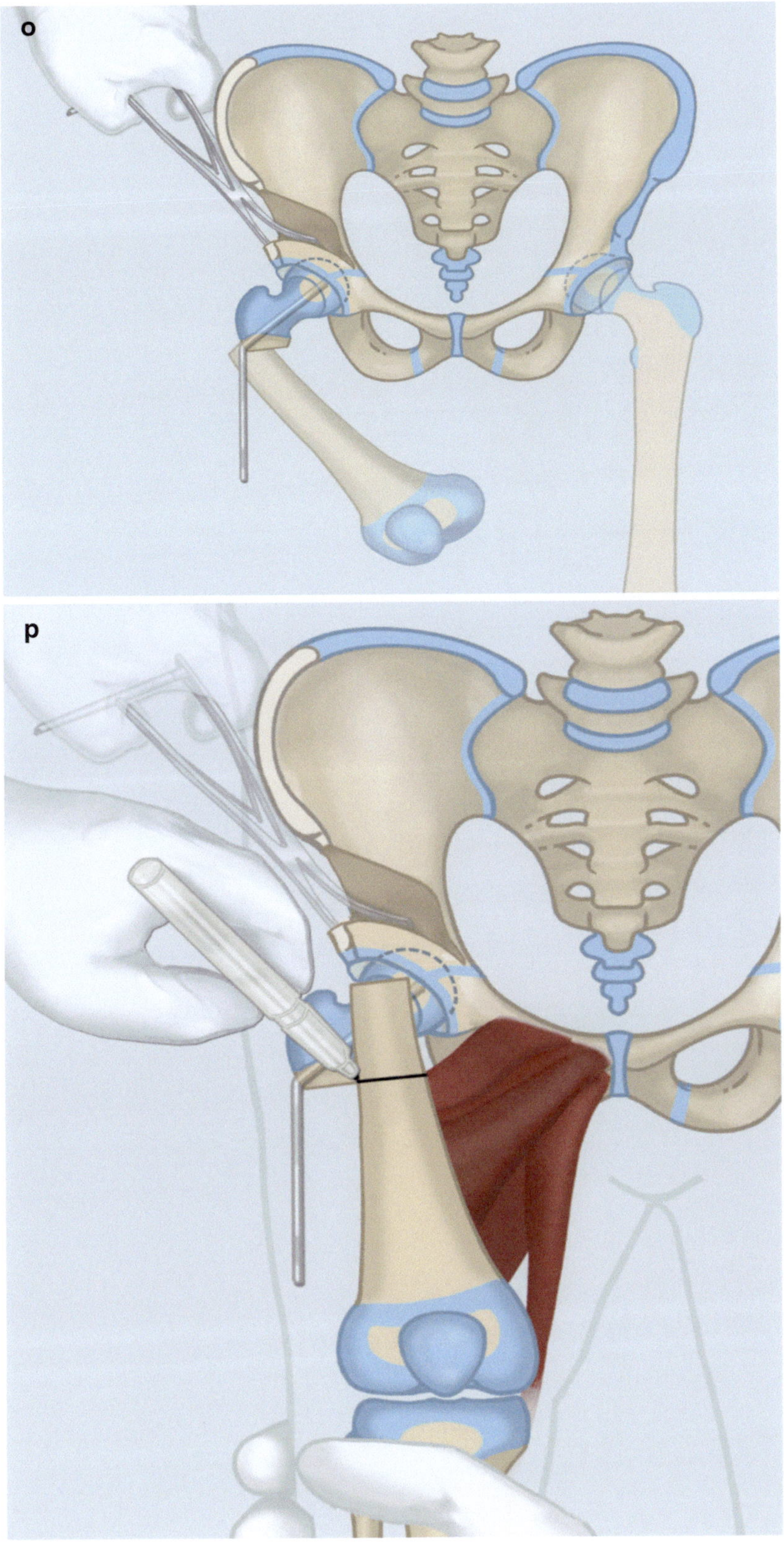

Fig. 35.8 (continued)

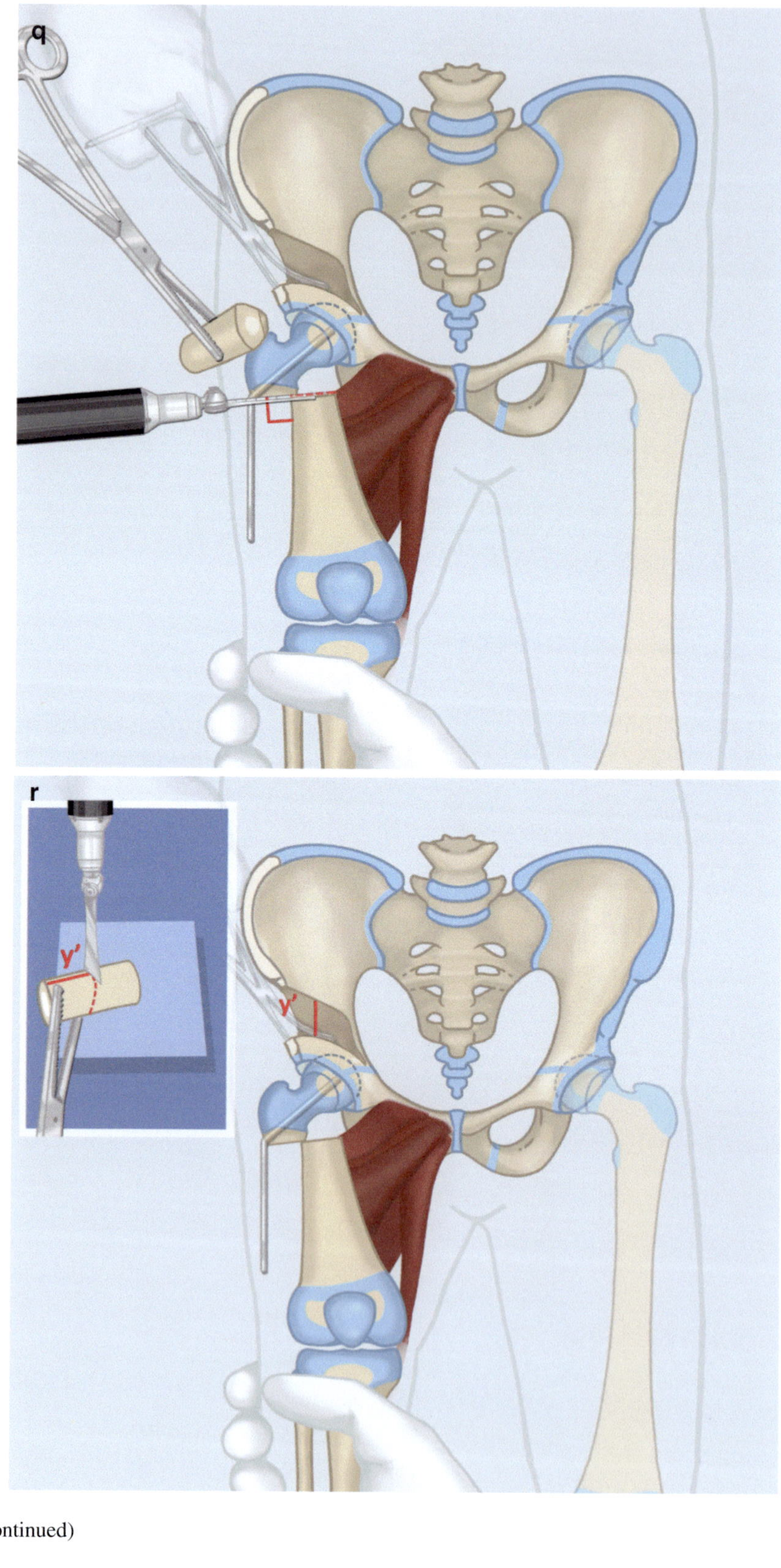

Fig. 35.8 (continued)

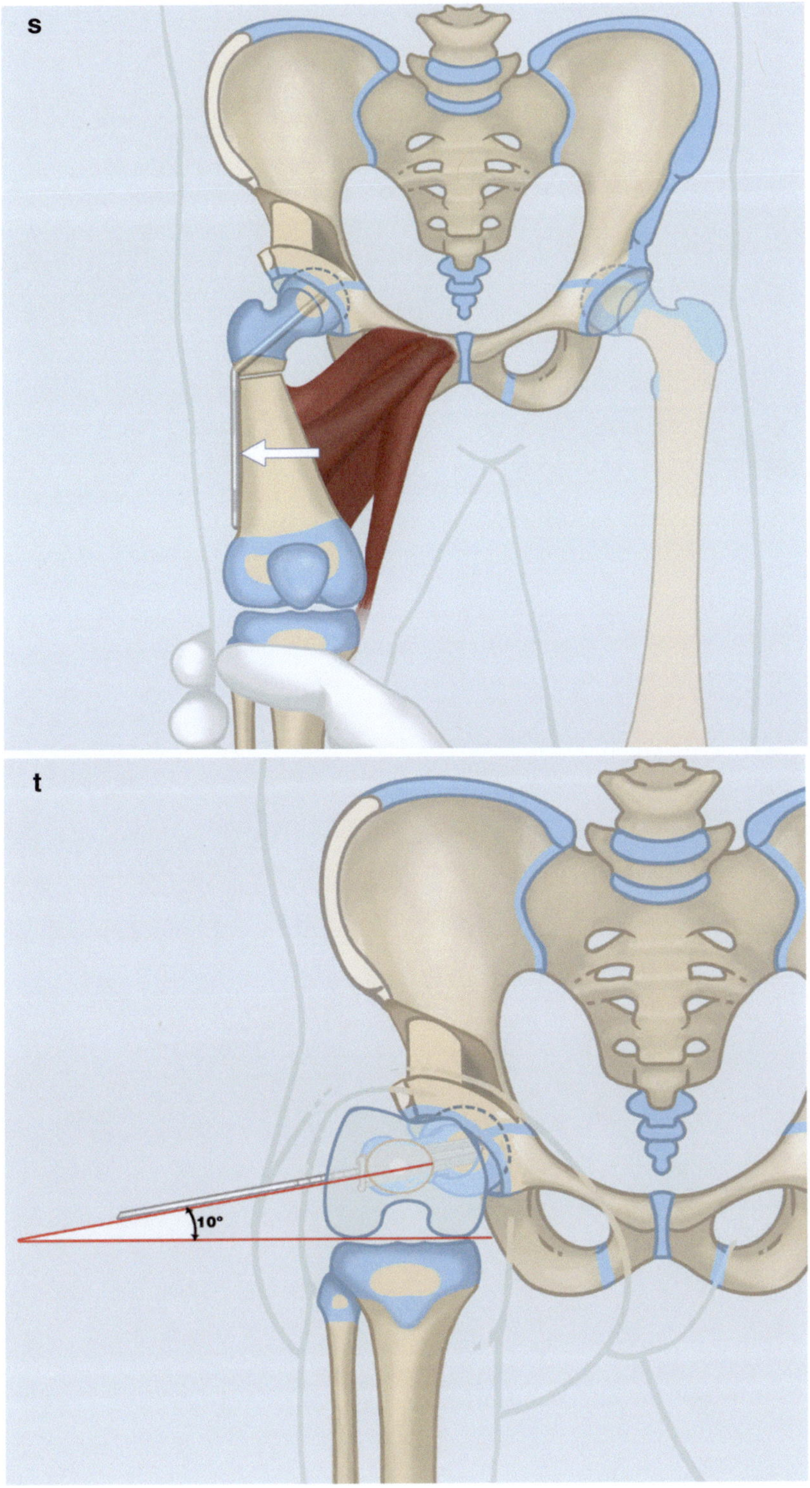

Fig. 35.8 (continued)

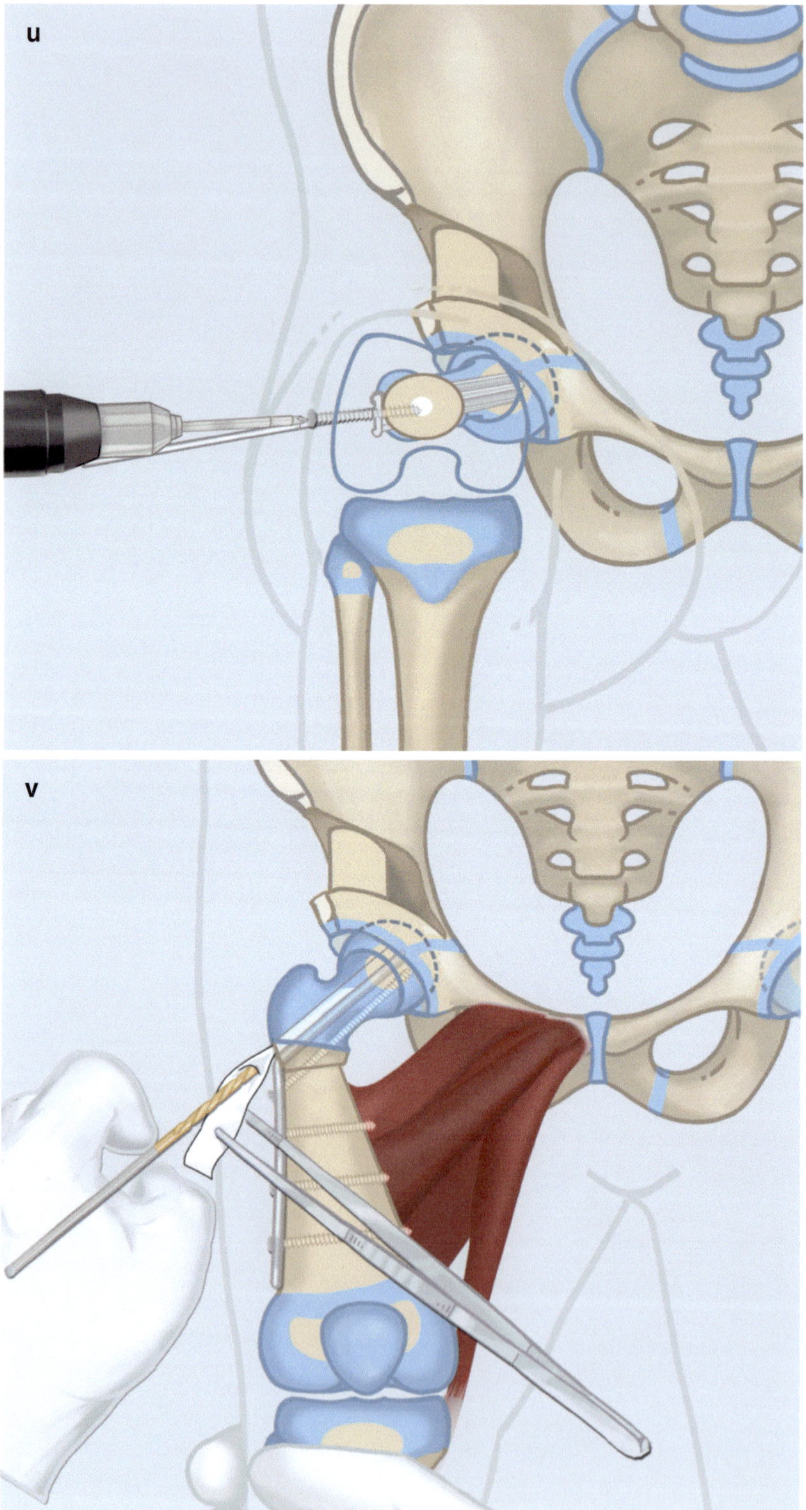

Fig. 35.8 (continued)

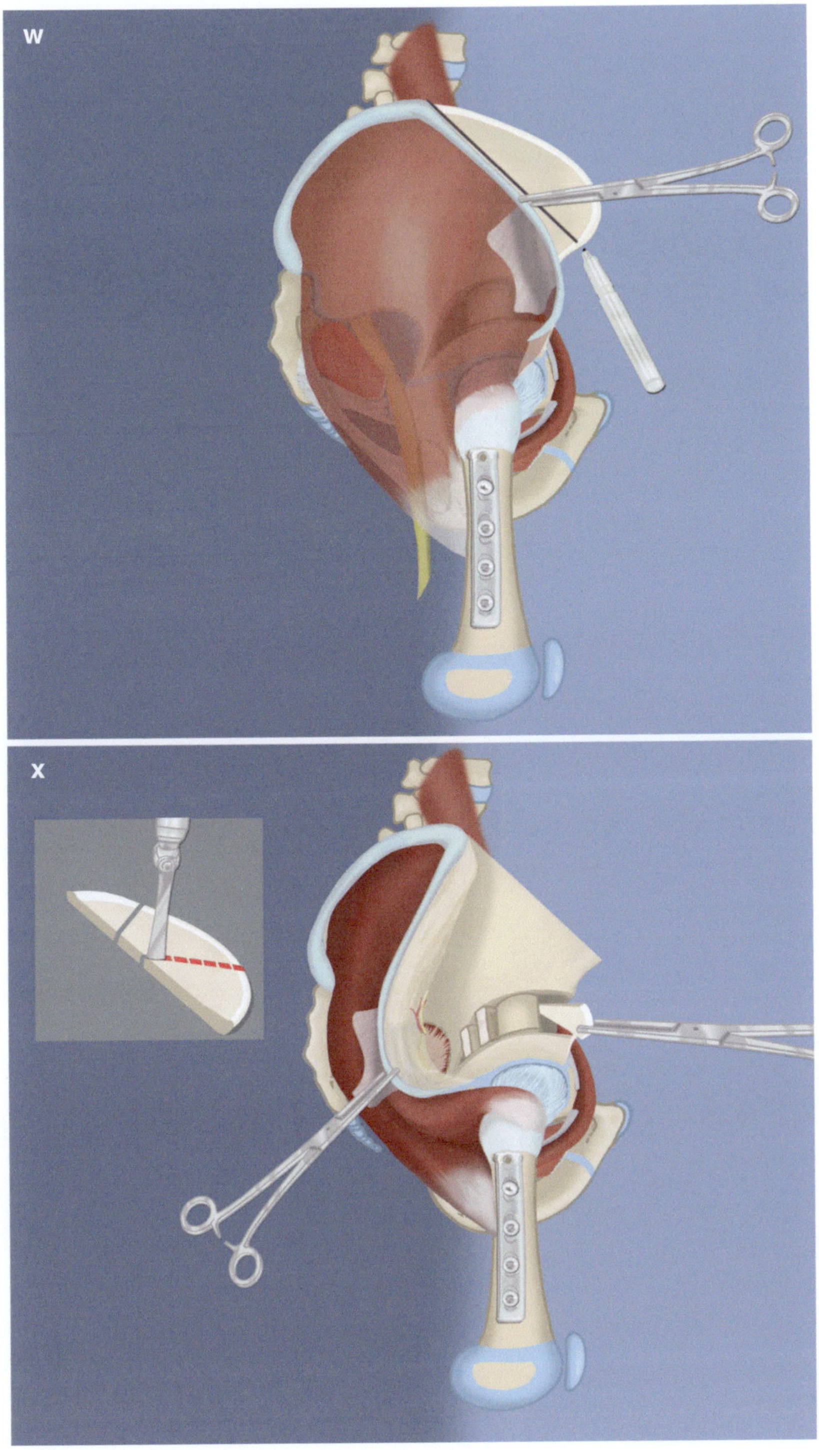

Fig. 35.8 (continued)

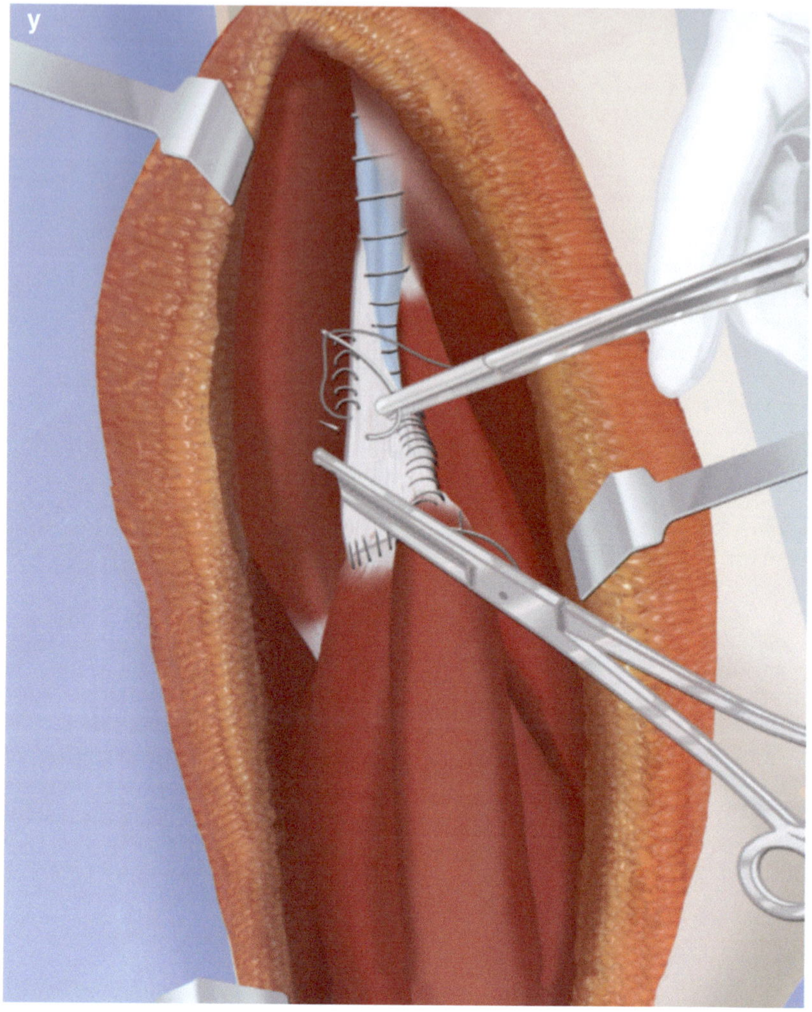

Fig. 35.8 (continued)

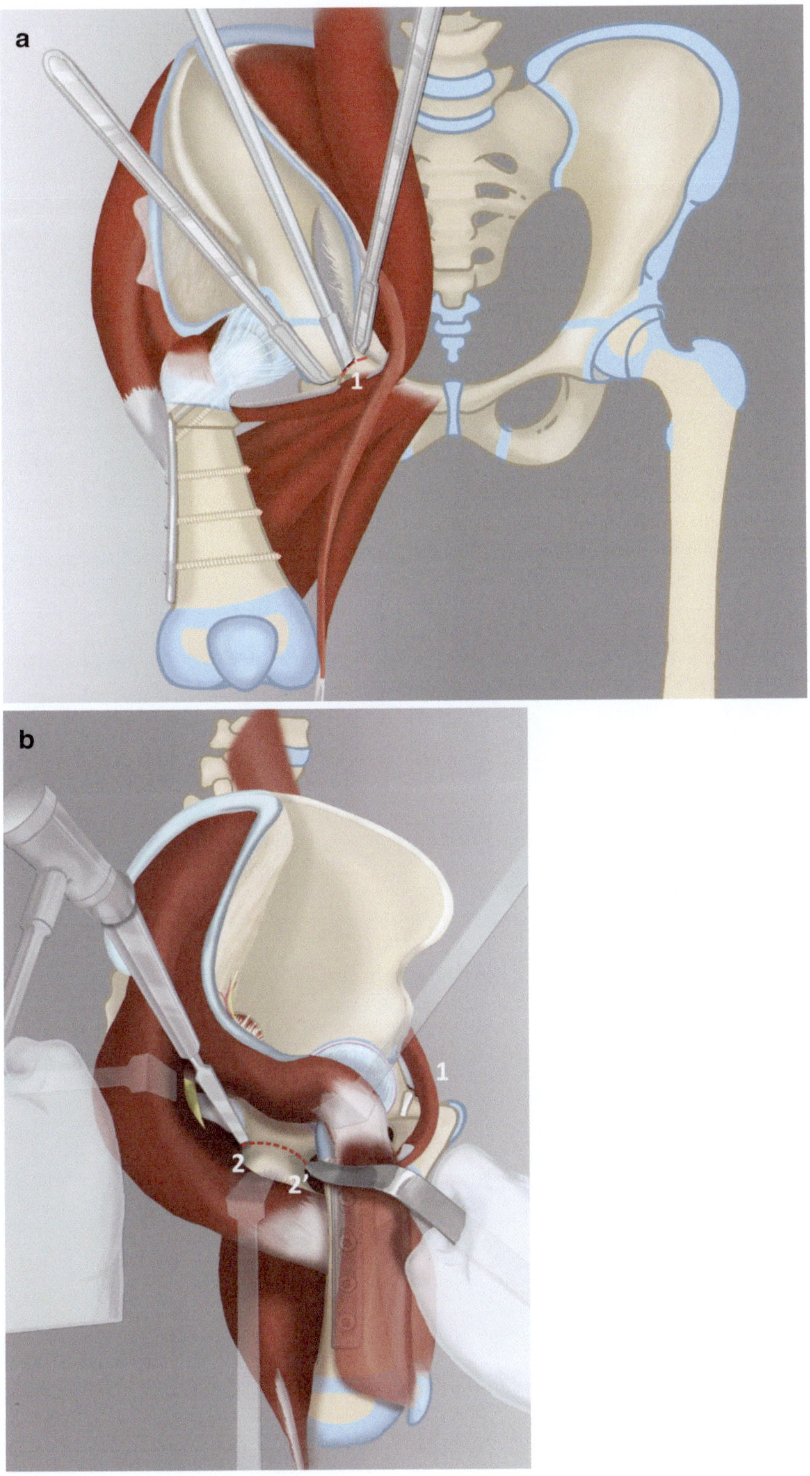

Fig. 35.9 (**a–o**) Periacetabular triple osteotomy: see steps of surgery corresponding to each figure. (© 2014 The Paley Foundation, with permission. All rights reserved)

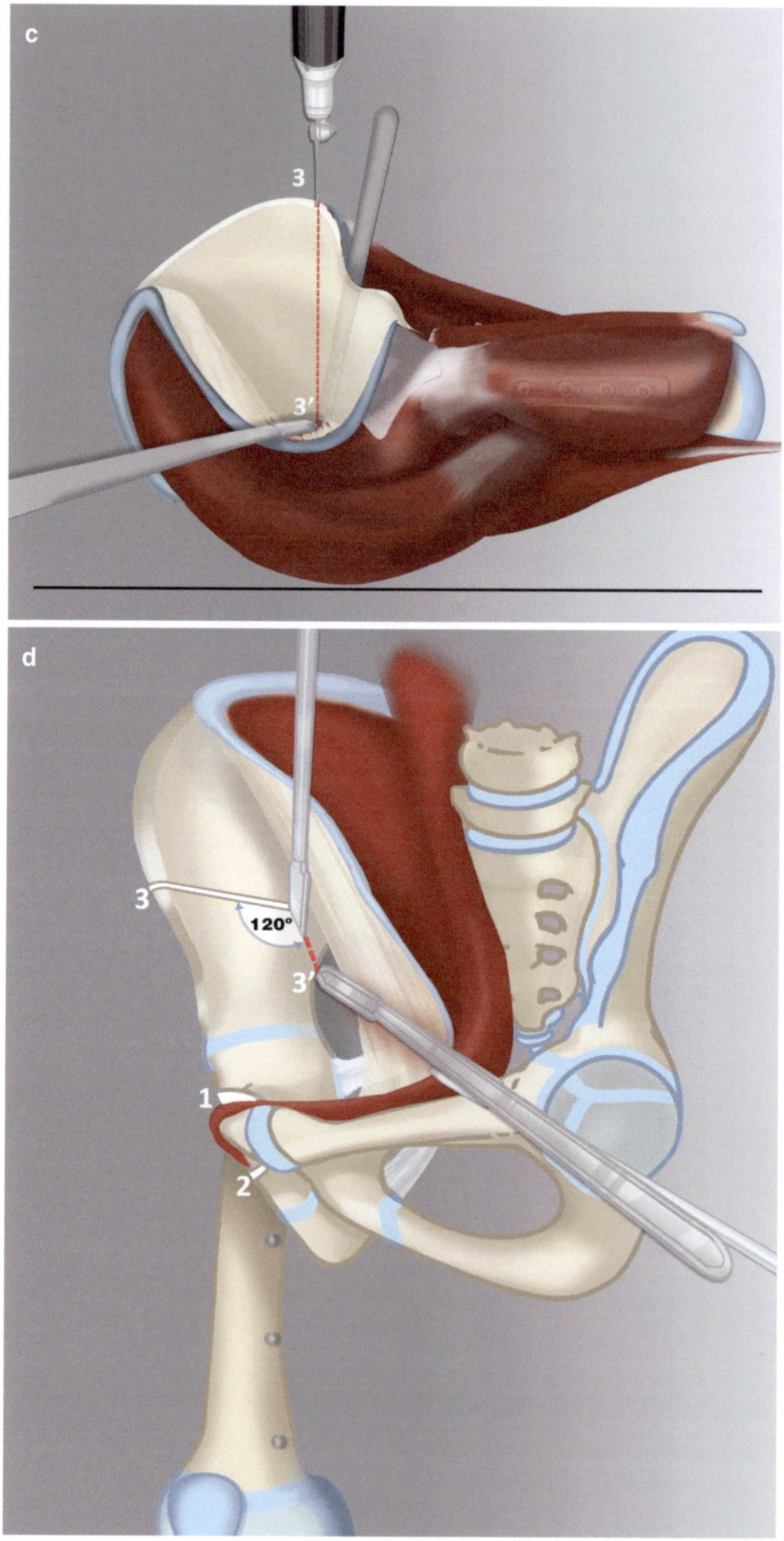

Fig. 35.9 (continued)

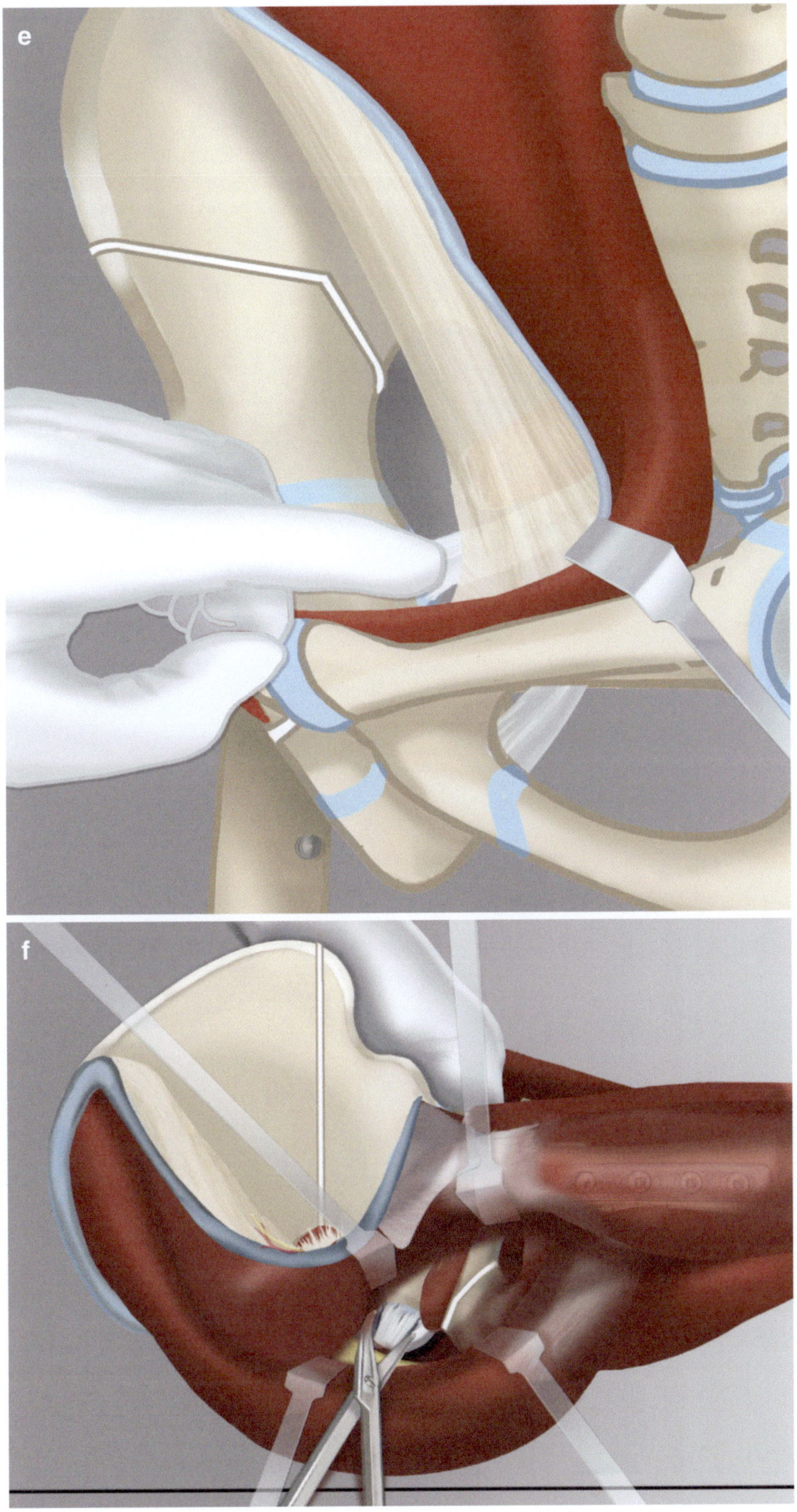

(continued)

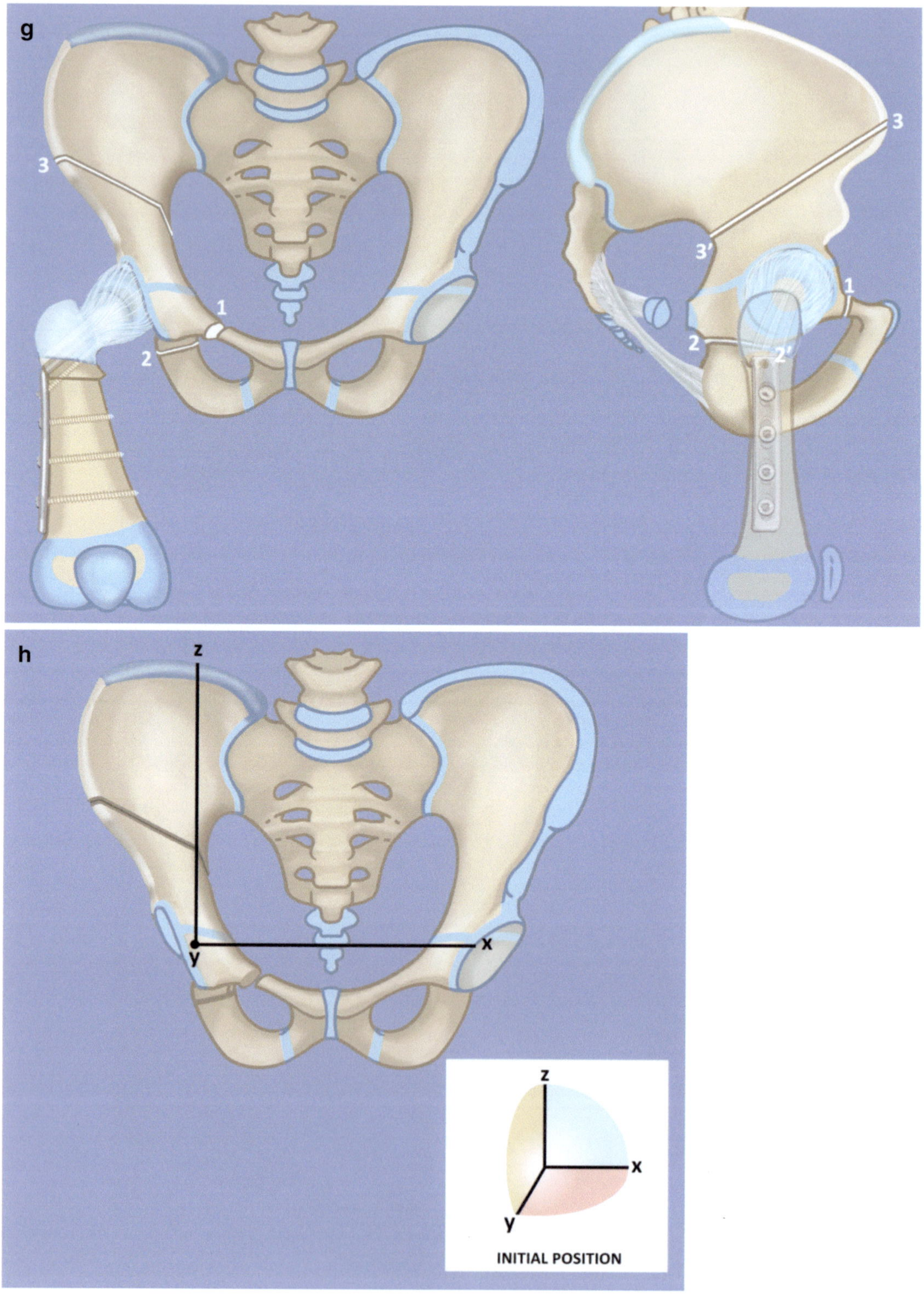

(continued)

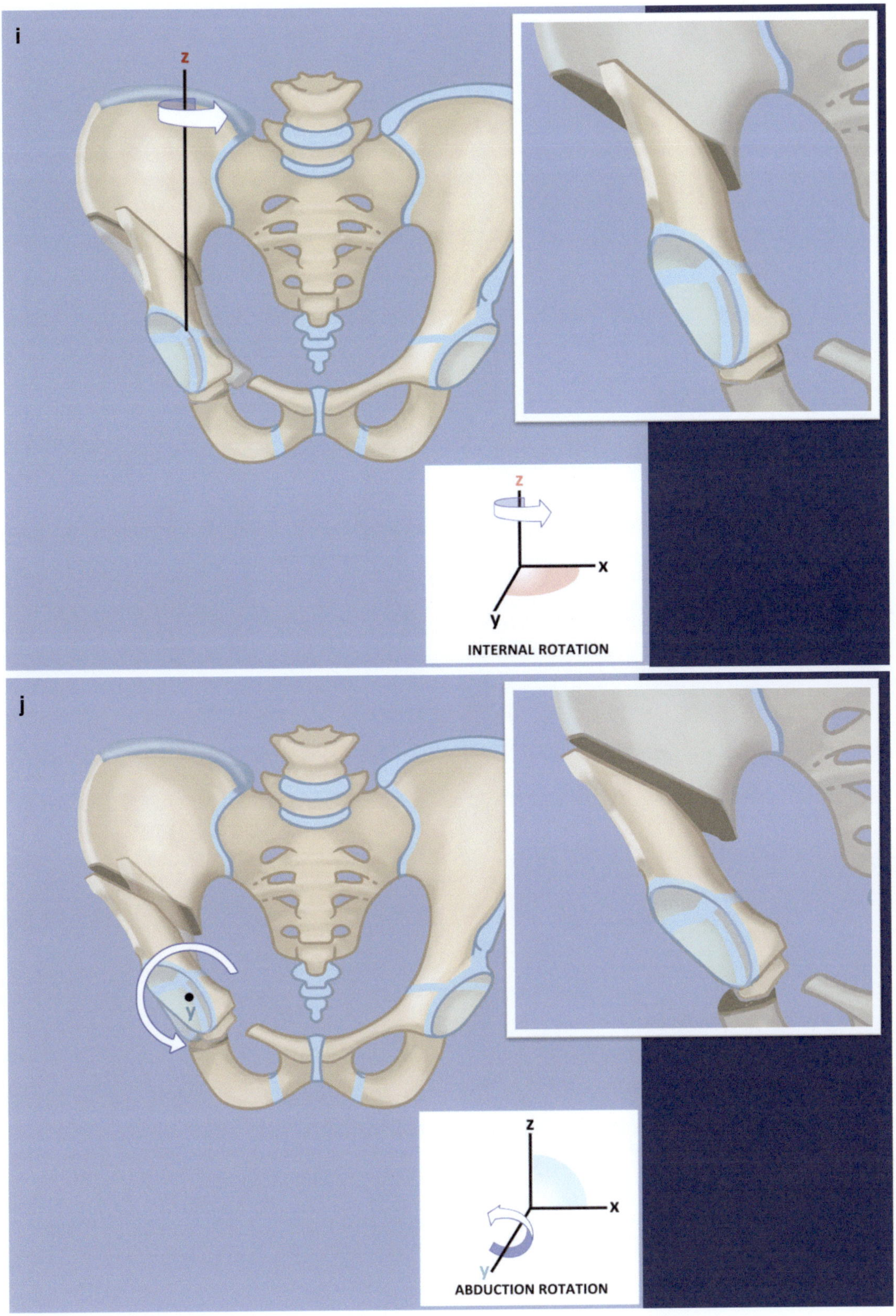

Fig. 35.9 (continued)

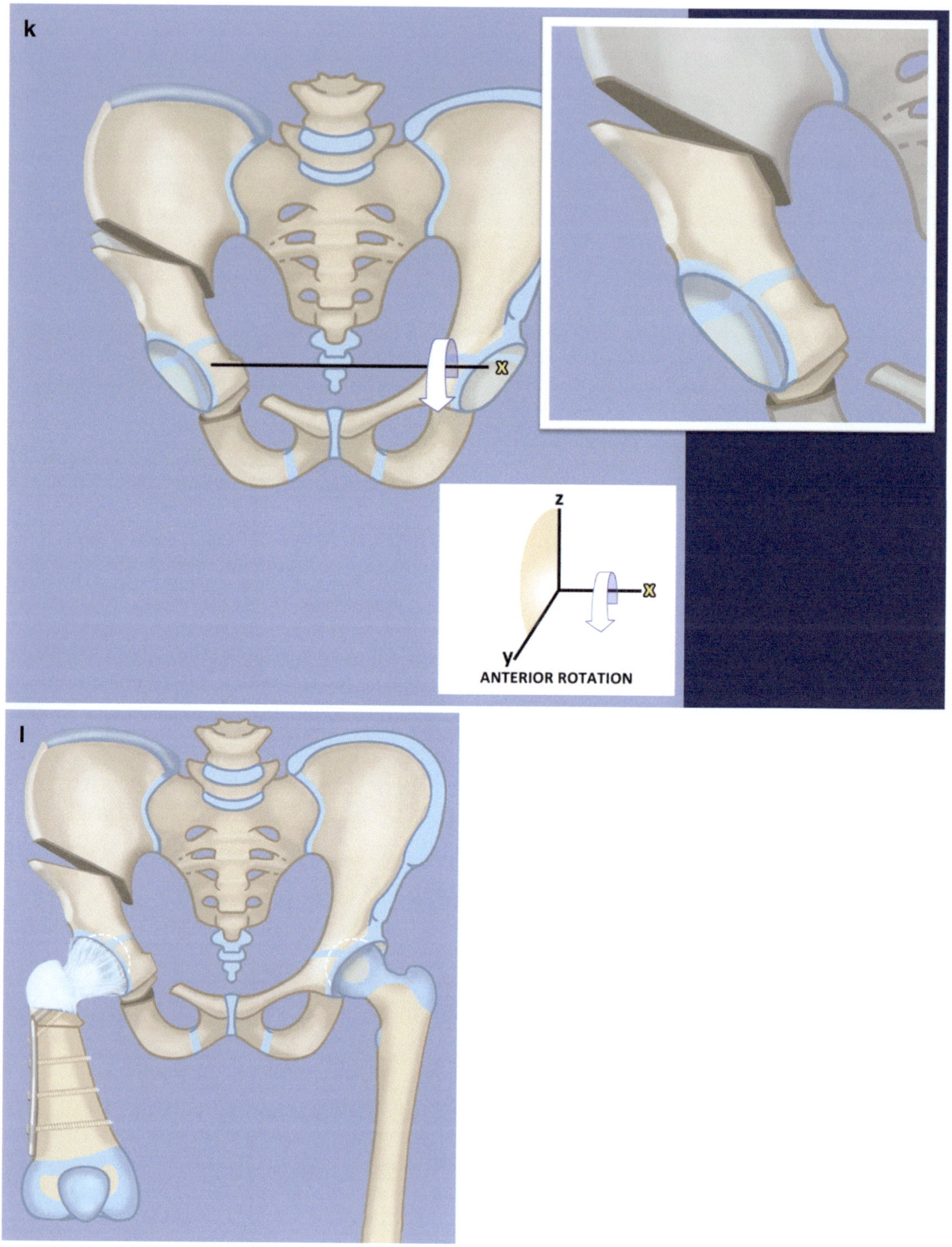

Fig. 35.9 (continued)

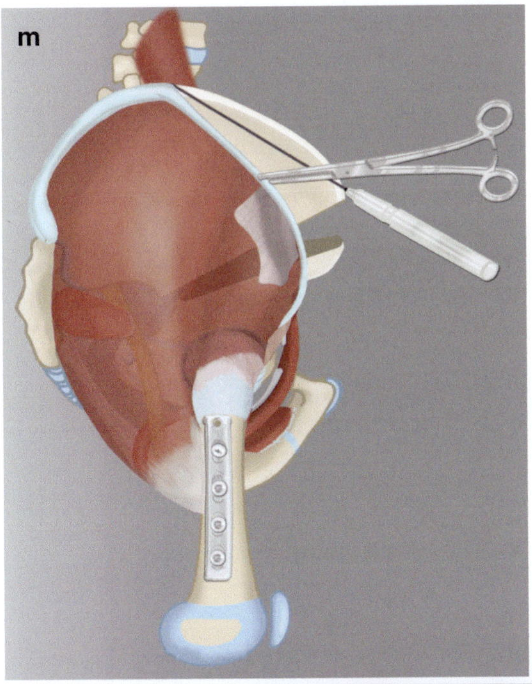

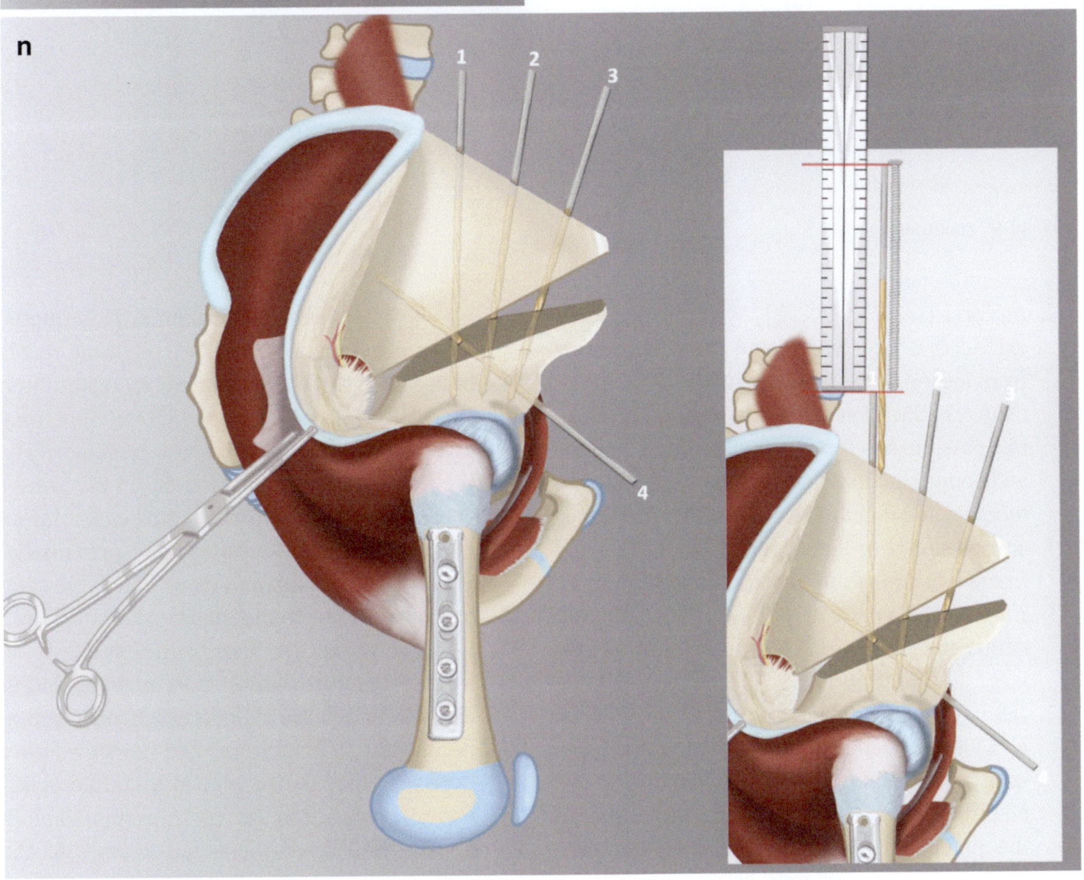

Fig. 35.9 (continued)

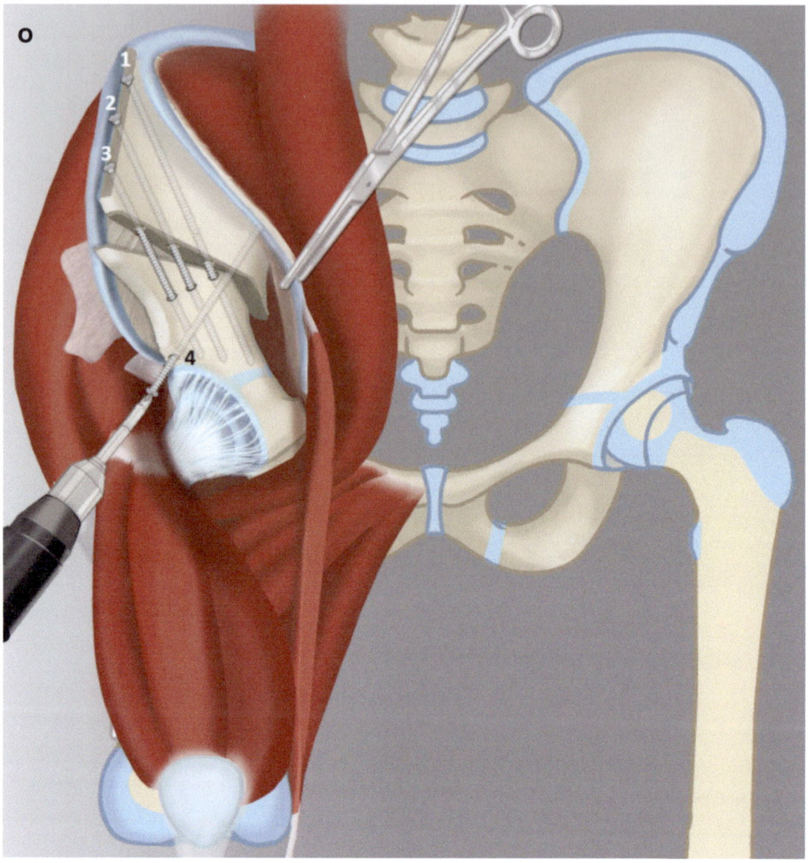

Fig. 35.9 (continued)

2. *Incision (see Fig. 35.7b).* With the leg fully extended, a long mid-lateral incision is made from the top of the iliac crest to the tibial tuberosity. The incision is kept as straight as possible, passing over the proximal femoral "bump" and continuing longitudinally towards Gerdy's tubercle and the tibial tubercle. The incision is carried down to the depth of the underlying fascia lata and iliotibial band.
3. *Flap elevation (see Fig. 35.7c).* The subcutaneous tissues and skin are elevated as one large flap anteriorly and posteriorly off the fascia of the thigh and pelvic region. The fat is adherent to the fascia and should be dissected preferably with an electrocautery. The electrocautery should be held flat, parallel to the plane of dissection. This can be quite technically difficult until one learns how to separate the fat without perforating the fascial layer or leaving fat behind. It is important not to incise or damage the fascia if it is being used for knee ligament reconstruction (SUPERknee procedure). Dissection may also be carried out with scissors. Anteriorly, the flap is extended just medial to the Smith-Peterson interval between the tensor fascia lata (TFL) and sartorius) proximally. Posteriorly, the subcutaneous flap is elevated to just posterior to the intermuscular septum. Distally, reflect the flap to the patella if no ligament reconstruction is to be done, and to the patellar tendon if ligament reconstruction is needed. The fascia lata is now fully exposed from the patella to a couple centimeters posterior to the intermuscular septum distally and from the anterior edge of the TFL to the mid gluteus maximus proximally.

4. *Fascia lata release (see Fig. 35.7d, e)*. The fascia is incised at the TFL-sartorius interval making sure to stay on the TFL side in order to avoid injury to the lateral femoral cutaneous nerve. The fascial incision is extended distally to the lateral border of the patella ending at the tibia. The posterior incision of the fascia lata starts distally and posterior at the intermuscular septum and extends proximally to overlie the gluteus maximus in line with the incision. The gluteus maximus (GMax) should be separated from the overlying fascia anterior to the posterior fascial incision. The fascia should be retracted anteriorly and away from the underlying muscle, while the GMax should be dissected off of the fascia and the intermuscular septum that separates it from the TFL. The GMax should not be split in line with the fascial incision to avoid denervating the muscle anterior to the split. It can now be reflected posteriorly to allow exposure of the greater trochanter, piriformis muscle and sciatic nerve.

   If knee ligamentous reconstruction is planned, the fascia lata is cut proximally and anteriorly at the musculotendinous junction. The fascial cut should be a step cut or sloped posteriorly and proximally to include a longer fascia segment posteriorly from the fascia that was dissected off of the GMax. The fascia lata is reflected distally to Gerdy's tubercle. The TFL can be left in place without further dissection. It does not have to be separated from the underlying gluteus medius (GMed). The two muscles are often adherent to each other, and it may be difficult to differentiate the muscle fibers. The distinguishing feature is that the GMed fibers insert on the greater trochanter while the TFL does not. The distal fascia lata becomes the iliotibial band and blends with the underlying lateral knee capsule, which may be partially reflected with the iliotibial band. The fascia should be mobilized all the way until Gerdy's tubercle. The fascia can then be divided into two halves using a straight pair of scissors. It should be kept moist while the rest of the surgery proceeds. The two limbs of the fascia are ready for later use in the SUPERknee procedure.
5. *Hip flexion contracture releases (see Fig. 35.7f, g)*. The dissection is carried beneath the sartorius to find the rectus femoris tendon. The rectus femoris tendon insertion is identified at the anterior inferior iliac spine. The constant ascending branch of the lateral femoral circumflex artery and vein is cauterized prior to cutting the tendon. The conjoint rectus femoris tendon (distal to the split into reflected and direct heads) is cut and allowed to retract distally. Care should be taken not to go too distal on the rectus femoris to avoid injury to its innervating branch of the femoral nerve. In the more dysplastic and deformed cases the entire femoral nerve may be lying immediately adjacent to the rectus femoris tendon especially if there is a lot of upward migration of the proximal femur. Just medial to the rectus is the iliopsoas muscle. The iliocapsularis muscle (capsular origin head of iliopsoas muscles) can also be seen here. The femoral nerve lies on the antero-medial surface of the iliopsoas muscle. Before looking for the psoas tendon, the femoral nerve should be identified and decompressed below the inguinal ligament. The posterior aspect of the iliopsoas muscle belly is now elevated from lateral to medial. The psoas tendon is located on the posteromedial surface in the substance of the muscle. The tendon is exposed and cut. Any remaining flexion contracture of the hip is due to the gluteus medius and minimus (the part of these muscles originating anterior to the center of rotation of the femoral head in the sagittal plane), and the anterior fascia of thigh. The release of the gluteus medius and minimus muscles is accomplished by the abductor muscle slide technique (see step 7). If the anterior thigh or sartorius fascia are still tight, they can also be released, taking care not to injure the lateral femoral cutaneous nerve, which should be identified and decompressed under the inguinal ligament.
6. *External rotation contracture release (see Fig. 35.7h)*. The piriformis tendon is con-

tracted and prevents internal rotation of the hip. It should be released off of the greater trochanter. To gain access to see this tendon, the gluteus maximus muscle must be retracted posteriorly. It can be left attached at its distal insertion on the femur. It can be swept posteriorly as a large sheet of muscle. The greater trochanter can be identified by palpation. The gluteus medius muscle posterior border is very distinct and proceeds down to the greater trochanter where it inserts. Deep to the medius is the gluteus minimus, and just distal to the minimus is the piriformis muscle. Its tendon can be palpated through its muscle. It may be difficult to identify the piriformis from the minimus. Care should be taken to avoid dissection at the distal border of the piriformis tendon. This is where the medial femoral circumflex branch anastomoses with the inferior gluteal artery branch. To get good visualization it is helpful to have an assistant lift up the patient using a sharp Senn retractor (also known as a *cat's paw* retractor). The sharp end is inserted into the posterior edge of the bump on the femur and the femur is pulled anteriorly (almost like lifting the hip off, of the table with this retractor). The entire piriformis is transected about 1 cm from its insertion onto the trochanter. The sciatic nerve can be identified and if necessary decompressed. It is more posterior and medial to the trochanter and runs deep to the piriformis.

7. *Abductor muscle slide (see Fig. 35.7i)*. The abductors may not appear to be tight on first inspection because of the coxa vara. Adduction into a true AP of the hip, with the neck oriented normally in the acetabulum, is now restricted by the gluteus medius and minimus since the fascia lata has already been cut. Furthermore, the Dega osteotomy, which lengthens the height of the ilium, makes the abductors even tighter. The abductors should be detached at their origin and not their insertion. This avoids changing the muscle-tendon length ratio and avoids weakening the hip abductors, avoiding a lurch or Trendelenburg gait.

   The subcutaneous tissue flaps should be elevated to provide adequate exposure to the iliac crest apophysis. There is a tendency to have inadequate posterior exposure, and the flaps should be elevated just beyond the highest lateral point of the apophysis. The anterior extent is the anterior superior and inferior iliac spines, which has been exposed for the release of the rectus femoris tendon. The abdominal external oblique muscles are partially released off of the entire length of the apophysis. Split the cartilagenous apophysis from the anterior inferior iliac spine to the anterior superior iliac spine, and then continue posteriorly spliting from anterior to posterior along the iliac crest. This should be done with a #15 blade. To know where to split, pinch the apophysis between thumb and index finger of the hand not holding the knife. Stay in the middle of the apophysis along its entire length, pushing down hard with the knife blade until one feels bone. Using a periosteal elevator, pop off the apophysis from the ilium. This should be done at multiple sites to get the entire apophysis to peel back as a unit from the ilium. The apophysis and lateral periosteum are reflected distally, thus relaxing the abductor muscles. The medial half of the apophysis is reflected medially with the iliacus muscle. Since some of the abductors act as flexors of the hip, the abductor slide helps eliminate any remaining flexion deformity of the hip. Furthermore, the iliacus muscle slide also relaxes any residual tension in the iliopsoas.
8. *Elevation of quadriceps (see Fig. 35.7j)*. The quadriceps are now elevated off of the femur in a subperiosteal fashion. Since the femur is so short, the exposure may extend as far as the distal femoral physis. The perforator vessels need to be cauterized as the quadriceps is detached from the linea aspera. Proximally, the vastus lateralis should be elevated off of part of the cartilage of the greater trochanteric apophysis by sharp dissection. Stay anterior to the gluteus maximus tendon which does not need to be dissected from the femur.

9. *Arthrogram (see Fig. 35.8a).* A hip arthrogram is now performed using a 20 gauge spinal needle. With the trocar inside, the needle is placed into the hip joint from the anterolateral side. Traction of the femur may facilitate placement. Once the needle appears to be in the joint on the image intensifier, the trocar is removed and normal saline is injected. If the needle is in the joint the saline should go in with little pressure, and when the syringe is removed from the needle, the saline should drip back out. These signs confirm that the needle is in the joint space. The arthrographic dye can now be injected into the hip joint to outline the femoral head, acetabulum, and femoral neck. The reason for this two step arthrogram is that if a false injection of dye occurs, it will obscure the visualization of the hip joint. The two step method is a more secure way of confirming intra-articular needle placement.
10. *Guide wire insertion (see Fig. 35.8b–d).* Since the abduction, flexion, and external rotation contractures have all been released, the femoral head and neck can now be placed in a neutral orientation to the pelvis by extending and maximally adducting the lower limb across the opposite leg. A guide wire should now be drilled up the center of the femoral neck to guide the insertion of a fixed angle fixation device. Since the femoral neck is unossified and short, it is very difficult to drill a guide wire at the correct angle up the femoral neck. The goal is to create a 130° neck-shaft angle and a medial proximal femoral angle (MPFA) of 85° (see Fig. 35.8d). In the normal femur, the angle between the neck-shaft line and the tip of the greater trochanter to center of femoral head line is 45°.

    The first guide wire is inserted from the tip of the greater trochanter to the center of femoral head (see Fig. 35.8b). Since the tip of the trochanter is cartilaginous in young children, it cannot be seen radiographically. The tip of the trochanter is located by palpation using the wire tip. From this point, the wire is then drilled towards the center of the femoral head as shown in the arthrogram. The image intensifier is placed into the lateral view and the leg rotated until a bull's-eye of three concentric circles is seen. This is formed by the overlapping dye shadows: the outermost circle is the femoral head, the middle circle is the femoral neck, and the inner circle is the ossific nucleus of the femoral head. A second wire should be drilled into the center of the bull's-eye at a 45° angle to the first wire (see Fig. 35.8c). Using a depth gauge or another wire of the same length as the second wire, measure the amount of wire inside the femoral neck by placing it alongside the second wire and measuring the difference in length between the two wires. This will be the length of the blade of the blade plate to be used. The position of the neck wire can also be confirmed by flexing the hip to 90° and looking at a frog-leg lateral of the neck.
11. *Blade plate insertion (see Fig. 35.8e–h).* The cannulated chisel for the blade plate should now be hammered up the femoral neck guided by the second guide wire (see Fig. 35.8e). The chisel should be rotated until it is perpendicular to the posterior aspect of the greater trochanter (see Fig. 35.8f). This will guide it to the correct angle in the sagittal plane. Tap the chisel out of the femur and reinsert the guide wire in its previous position. Insert the appropriate length 130° blade plate over this wire to the depth of the bend of the plate (see Fig. 35.8g). Make sure on the image intensifier that the tip of the blade is not too deep into the femoral head. Check its position on AP and lateral planes, as well as using the approach-withdrawal technique with live fluoroscopy to ensure that the blade is not advanced too close to the articular surface of the femoral head. If the blade is suspected of being too long, then replace it with one with a shorter length. Furthermore, if plate placement is off-center, there is greater risk of protrusion into the joint. The posterior edge of the plate should be parallel to the back of the greater trochanter. The femur diaphysis is usually flexed to the plate (see Fig. 35.8h).

12. *Subtrochanteric osteotomy (see Fig. 35.8i, j).* The femur should be cut perpendicular to the shaft of the plate, starting just below the bend in the plate (see Fig. 35.8i). This cut should be below the level of the greater trochanter cartilage. To guide this cut, drill a wire perpendicular to the plate. Keep the plane of the saw blade perpendicular to the plate in all planes. The width of the perpendicular cut surface should be as wide as the femoral diaphysis. A second subtrochanteric osteotomy should be made oriented less than 90° to the first osteotomy towards the base of the femoral neck to remove the bone protruding medially (Fig. 35.8j). The femoral head and neck can be manually tested for any residual impingement, removing any blocks to achieving 90° of hip flexion. The antero-medial corner often needs to be excised to prevent impingement.
13. *Periosteum release (see Fig. 35.8k–m).* After the second osteotomy, the distal femur is easily exposed and the surrounding periosteum is peeled off circumferentially. Medially, it is very thick and restricts correction of the varus and rotation deformity. Cut the periosteum transversely around the femur, carefully separating it from the surrounding muscle (see Fig. 35.8k). Be careful to avoid injury to the profunda femoris and its perforators, which pass immediately under the periosteum. Cutting the periosteum allows the thigh to stretch longitudinally, reducing the amount of shortening required of the femur. The hip adductors become the main tether to the length of the femur (see Fig. 35.8l). The anteromedial corner of the femur should be resected to prevent impingement in flexion (see Fig. 35.8m).
14. *Pelvic Osteotomy: Option 1—Paley Modified Dega Osteotomy (Paley-Dega) (see Fig. 35.8n, o).* It is preferable to perform the pelvic osteotomy at this juncture since it can affect the amount of femoral shortening and rotation. The iliac periosteum is reflected back to the edge of the acetabulum and to the sciatic notch. The periosteum should also be dissected off the anterior wall of the sciatic notch, feeling for the soft cartilage of the triradiate cartilage as it separates the ilium from the ischium. Using the image intensifier, a guide wire is drilled approximately 2 cm proximal to the lateral edge of the acetabulum towards the triradiate cartilage medially. Start the osteotomy posteriorly parallel to the sciatic notch anterior border. Start near the triradiate cartilage and continue proximally. Stay only a few millimeters anterior to the sciatic notch at the distal end of this limb of the cut. Curve anteriorly towards the guide wire and incline the cut medially towards the triradiate parallel to the guide wire (see Fig. 35.8n). The osteotomy remains unicortical except at the most anterior end where it exits anteriorly as the osteotomy heads towards the pubic eminence. The osteotomy never exits through the medial wall. This is the Paley Modification. The original Polish Dega osteotomy exits through the medial wall and heads towards the top of the sciatic notch. The Paley-Dega truly hinges on the triradiate cartilage medially and posteriorly. The osteotomy is levered distally to bring the roof of the acetabulum down. A laminar spreader is used to distract the osteotomy (see Fig. 35.8o). The posterior vertical limb of the osteotomy extending down to the triradiate cartilage at the ischium allows for greater bending and greater lateral coverage. It is a myth that the Dega osteotomy gives posterior coverage since the posterior lip is part of the ischium and this osteotomy is only iliac. The original Dega, as well as subsequent publications of this osteotomy, goes through the inner table of the pelvis, especially anteriorly and heads for the upper end of the sciatic notch. The Paley-Dega is unicortical and extends farther posterior and distal to also hinge near the triradiate at the level of the ischium. In this manner, there is true hinging in a three dimensional way near the triradiate. Even the anterior part of the cut does not exit the cortex and extends to the triradiate junction between the ilium and pubis. The bump

under the buttocks should be removed at this stage. This allows one to assess the coverage of the femoral head in the frontal plane. The laminar spreader can be distracted as needed to gain additional coverage and reorientation of the acetabular sourcil. The laminar spreader should be kept posterior to avoid increasing the anterior coverage and creating impingement. The dysplasia of the acetabulum in CFD cases is postero-lateral [2, 3]. The Dega osteotomy only provides lateral coverage. At this point, the femoral shortening should be carried out and the excised bone segment cut to fit the opening wedge gap of the pelvic osteotomy. Additional bone from the iliac crest, which is resected during the abductor slide, may be inserted to fill the remaining space.

Pelvic Osteotomy: Option 2—Paley Modification of Periacetabular Triple Osteotomy (Paley PATO) (Fig. 35.9). Pubis: The pubis is exposed subperiosteally by reflecting the medial iliac apophysis and periosteum more medially. The triradiate cartilage arm at the pubis is exposed and the dissection carried out just distal to it. The superior pubic ramus can be cut under direct vision under the protection of two Hohmann retractors with an osteotome (see Fig. 35.9a). Ischium: The ischium is exposed by returning to the back of the femur and finding the sciatic nerve again. The nerve is followed to the ischium. To avoid stretching the nerve, do not place a retractor between the nerve and the ischium. A Hohmann retractor can be placed anterior to the ischium. Subperiosteal elevation of the ischial periosteum is carried out. The ischium should be cut under direct vision near the junction where it forms the inferior wall of the acetabulum, distal to the triradiate cartilage (see Fig. 35.9b). Ilium: The ilium is cut with a saw from the anterior superior iliac spine towards the apex of the sciatic notch laterally (Fig. 35.9c). Medially it aims for the junction of the true and false pelvis in line with the sciatic notch (see Fig. 35.9d). As the cut reaches the junction of the true pelvis, an osteotome is used to change the angle of the cut (see Fig. 35.9d). The osteotome is about 120° to the saw cut. This bend in the cut rounds off the corner of the distal segment and creates a spike of bone on the proximal segment. This increases the surface area and creates a posterior buttress while making the distal segment rotate more easily with less distraction. This third bone cut completes the triple osteotomy (see Fig. 35.9e). Sacrospinous ligament release: For large corrections, it is important to release the tether of the sacrospinous ligament. In particular this ligament limits the amount of internal rotation used to achieve posterior coverage and the abduction used to achieve supero-lateral coverage. This ligament can be palpated after dissecting the medial iliac periosteum off of the quadrilateral plate inside the true pelvis. A finger can be placed on the tip of the ischial spine, and the ligament is then felt (Fig. 35.9e). Using proprioception, a finger from the other hand can be used to palpate the finger that is on the ligament. Make sure the sciatic nerve, which can be visualized laterally, is not in the way. With the ligament isolated in this manner, it can be cut with a blunt pair of curved Mayo scissors from the lateral side, cutting directly onto one's own finger (Fig. 35.9f) To make this easier to visualize, the acetabular bone segement can be rotated internally to deliver the spine more laterally (Fig. 35.9g). Since CFD is associated with a hypoplastic acetabulum, there is usually posterior as well as lateral deficiency. To gain posterior and lateral coverage, the acetabular segment should first be rotated internally along the long axis of the body (z-axis) (Fig. 35.9h-i). This moves the posterior lip laterally increasing the posterior coverage. The second manipulation is to rotate the acetabular segment laterally (abduction) to increase lateral coverage (y-axis) (Fig. 35.9j). These two movements decrease the anterior coverage. It is therefore essential to rotate the acetabular fragment anteriorly (flexion) to restore anterior coverage (x-axis) (Fig. 35.9k-l). To rotate internally, a lion-jaw bone clamp is placed antero-posteriorly, superior to the acetabulum and the bone fragment rotated internally. It can also be placed around the pubis to lever the acetabulum laterally. If the acetabular fragment does not move sufficiently, then each osteotomy sites should be checked for completeness. The ischial osteotomy is often the culprit, and the periosteum around the ischium may need to be divided. Fixation of the triple osteotomy is achieved using long 3.5 mm screws from the ilium to the acetabular fragment. However, because of the abductor slide, the proximal part of the iliac wing must be resected prior to screw fixation. The level of resection is determined by pulling up the apophysis with the femur held in a neutral position (see Fig. 35.9m). The bone proximal to the level the apophysis should be resected (see Fig. 35.9n). Four equal length drill bits are used to fix the osteotomy, three antegrade and one retrograde. A same sized drill bit is used to compare lengths with the drill bits inside the bone to determine the screw lengths (see Fig. 35.9n). One by one, the drill bits are removed, and replaced with solid, non-cannulated screws, making sure that they do not enter the triradiate cartilage or the hip joint (see Fig. 35.9o).

15. *Femoral shortening (see Fig. 35.8p–r)*. The distal femur is now mobile and can be corrected into valgus and rotated internally. The distal femur is too long to fit end-to-end with the proximal femoral cut. The two ends should be overlapped, and a mark should be made at the point of overlap (see Fig. 35.8p). The distal femur should be shortened at this level. A wire is drilled perpendicular to the femur at the level of the osteotomy and a saw is used to cut, using frequent irrigation to prevent heat necrosis (see Fig. 35.8q). The segment of bone is kept moist on the back table for use as bone graft for the Dega osteotomy. This is usually a trapezoid shaped piece about 2–5 cm long (see Fig. 35.8r).
16. *Bone grafting Dega osteotomy (see Fig. 35.8r, s)*. The segment of bone from the femoral shortening is cut to the dimensions needed to support the opening wedge Dega osteotomy (see Fig. 35.8r). The dimension of the graft needed is measured from the size of the opening wedge base using a caliper. A trapezoidal shaped graft is then fashioned from the femoral shortening segment. It is inserted into the pelvic osteotomy to support and stabilize it (see Fig. 35.8s).
17. *Distal femur fixation and internal rotation (Fig. 35.8s–v)*. The femur is now brought to the plate (see Fig. 35.8s). The bone ends should oppose without tension. The femur is internally rotated to correct the external torsion deformity. To adjust the femur to the correct anteversion, the guide wire should be reinserted into the cannulation of the plate to show the orientation of the femoral neck. The knee should be flexed to 90° and the angle between the wire and the frontal plane of the femur as judged by the perpendicular plane to knee flexion is observed (see Fig. 35.8t). This wire should appear at least 10° anteverted, relative to the knee. The most distal hole in the plate can now be drilled with the femur held in this rotation (see Fig. 35.8u). The drill hole should be made at the distal edge of the hole to compress the osteotomy with screw insertion. Two more screw holes are drilled and screws are inserted. The most proximal hole in the plate is designed to drill parallel to the blade of the plate and secures the plate to the proximal femur. The wire in the cannulated hole can be used to guide the drill bit. In type 1b cases, the blade of the plate and the oblique screw goes across the proximal physis and into the femoral head (see Fig. 35.8v). In type 1a cases with a horizontally oriented growth plate, neither the blade nor the screw should cross the growth plate of the upper femur. In type 1a cases with a vertically oriented growth plate, the blade but not the screw should cross the physis.
18. *Bone Morphogenic Protein2 (BMP2) insertion (see Fig. 35.8v)*. In type 1b neck cases, BMP should be inserted into the upper femur to induce ossification of the cartilaginous neck of the femur. A wire is drilled proximal and parallel to the guide wire in the cannulation of the plate. A 4.0 mm hole is then

drilled over this guide wire. The drill hole should extend all the way to the ossific nucleus. BMP-2 (Infuse, Wright Medical, Memphis TN, USA) is then prepared on collagen sponges. Radiocontrast dye can also be applied to the collagen sponges. The sponges are loaded into a metal tube whose outer diameter is 4 mm (Craig needle biopsy set). This cannula is then inserted into the drill hole. Using a blunt trochar the sponge is pushed out of the tube inside the femoral neck. Using the image intensifier it is possible to see the sponge in the unossified neck due to the radiocontrast dye on the sponge. It should be emphasized that such use of BMP2 (Infuse implant) is an off label use of this product since the product is not FDA cleared in children. Usually two sponges are used in one drill hole. Bone wax is used to seal the lateral entry hole to prevent leakage of BMP2 and heterotopic ossification.

19. *Iliac wing osteotomy (see Fig. 35.8w, x).* After the pelvic osteotomy, the apophysis should be sutured back together. Due to the abductor muscle contracture, the lateral apophysis cannot reach the top of the iliac crest. Part of the crest has to be resected to allow repair of the apophysis. Putting traction on the lateral apophysis with the femur held in a neutral position, one can mark the level to which the apophysis can reach. A saw is used to cut and remove the proximal part of the iliac wing, effectively a shortening osteotomy of the ilium. The removed bone is used as graft for the Dega osteotomy (see Fig. 35.8x). It can also be used as a bone graft around the subtrochanteric femoral osteotomy. The apophysis is then repaired with a running #1 Vicryl suture. The medial and lateral halves of the apophysis should be well opposed to avoid a bifid iliac wing. The external abdominal muscles should be advanced and repaired over the apophysis as a separate layer to avoid an abdominal wall hernia (see Fig. 35.8y).
20. *Muscle repairs and transfers (see Fig. 35.8y).* The rectus femoris muscle is sutured to the TFL. This restores its pelvic origin while lengthening this muscle at the same time. The interval between the TFL and the sartorius is closed, carefully avoiding suturing the lateral femoral cutaneous nerve. The quadriceps is sutured to the region of the linea aspera. Finally, the gluteus maximus is advanced back to the posterior border of the TFL.
21. *Closure.* If no knee releases or reconstruction are required, the fascia lata should be resected from Gerdy's tubercle. The incision can now be closed. Since there is no fascia lata, the deepest layer is the subcutaneous fat layer, called the "underlayer". One medium-sized drains are placed, exiting anterosuperiorly. The drain is secured with a clear adhesive sterile dressing (e.g. Tegaderm, 3M Medical, St. Paul MN, USA). It is important to close the wound in a fashion that the opposite layers get sutured at the same level. The deep edges of the subcutaneous underlayer are brought together with a running #1 braided absorbable suture. The Scarpa's fascia is closed with a running 2-0 braided absorbable suture. The deep dermal layer is closed with a running 3-0 braided absorbable suture, and the skin is closed using a subcuticular 4-0 monofilament suture. Dermabond™ may be used, and sterile dressings are applied.

    Final radiographs are taken: an AP pelvis and lateral knee, both including the femur. The patient is then placed into a one legged spica cast. The operative limb should be placed in full hip and knee extension with the foot and ankle left free. The cast should be bivalved to allow for swelling, before leaving the operating room.
22. *Postoperative Course*: Parents are educated on cast care, hygiene and how to transport the child in the cast. The bivalved spica cast can be converted into a removable cast after about 1 week. The patient can then start gentle passive flexion and extension of the hip from 0° to 90°, as well as passive abduction. The patient remains non-weight bearing for 6 weeks. After that the spica cast is discon-

tinued. The patient is progressed to full weight bearing. Dbony healing, then the patient is progressed to full weight bearing, gait training, strengthening, and active and passive range of motion. The end goal is to restore the child to normal function before they proceed with limb lengthening.

SUPERhip Procedure for Paley Type 1b Subtrochanteric Type

The following steps are modified when treating a subtrochanteric type 1b. The deformity is often of greater magnitude and the bump more prominent. When elevating the quadriceps open the interval between the quads and the gluteus medius. This allows the quadriceps to be lifted off of the sharp bump of the subtrochanteric region. The next difference is taking down the subtrochanteric delayed ossification site (which is like a stiff pseudarthrosis site. Instead of inserting the guide wires first, break up the stiff pseudarthrosis line and separate the bone ends. Allow the distal fragment to be freed from the periosteum. This untethers the proximal femoral segment, which now becomes more mobile. Since the femoral shaft has been removed from the proximal segment the best way to manipulate it is to apply a clamp (e.g., lion jaw) to its distal end. The guide wires can now be inserted to find the center of the femoral neck and the cannulated chisel followed by the blade plate inserted. The proximal femur needs an osteotomy perpendicular to the plate to establish a proximal bone healing surface. The rest of the procedure is as for the neck type except that no BMP or neck drill hole are needed in these cases.

SUPERhip2 Procedure (Figs. 35.10, 35.11, and 35.12)**: For Paley Type 2a or 2b CFD** (see Fig. 35.10a) [2, 4, 5, 9, 10]

1. *Incision and initial dissection*. Use the same anesthesia, preparation, positioning and incision as for the SUPERhip procedure described previously. Create the same subcutaneous flap and exposure and resection of the fascia lata and iliotibial band. Release the rectus femoris tendon and decompress the femoral nerve as previously described.
2. *Psoas tendon*. Identify and dissect but do not release the psoas tendon (see Fig. 35.10b).
3. *Anterior exposure*. Separate the vastus muscles from the hip abductors anteriorly to help expose the anterior hip capsule (see Fig. 35.10b).
4. *Gluteus maximus*. Release the gluteus maximus tendon off of the femur and reflect this muscle posteriorly (see Fig. 35.10c).
5. *Sciatic nerve decompression*. Identify and free the sciatic nerve (see Fig. 35.10d).
6. *External rotators*. Release all of the external rotators off of the back of the femur. Also release the piriformis tendon off of the trochanter (see Fig. 35.10d, e).
7. *Psoas tenotomy*. Follow the psoas tendon to its insertion on the back of the femur. Release this tendon off of the femur. Try and preserve the medial femoral circumflex vessel and its ascending branch. Tag the psoas tendon for later transfer (see Fig. 35.10e, f).
8. *Hip abductors*. Release the gluteus medius and minimus tendon attachments from the greater trochanter and reflect them proximally (see Fig. 35.10g).
9. *Femoral neck fibrous anlage*. Identify the femoral neck analge, which travels from the femoral head to the greater trochanter (see Fig. 35.10h, i). Resect this thick structure (see Fig. 35.10j).
10. *Hip capsule superior*. Make a very small incision into the hip capsule superiorly (see Fig. 35.11a).
11. *Femoral head mobility*. Confirm that the femoral head is either mobile or fused (see Fig. 35.11a).
12. *Hip capsule inferior*. Make a larger inferior capsular incision in the hip capsule (see Fig. 35.11b).
13. *Transverse acetabular ligament*. Cut this ligament (see Fig. 35.11b)
14. *Ossific nucleus*. If the femoral head is mobile, cut down to the ossific nucleus (see Fig. 35.11b).

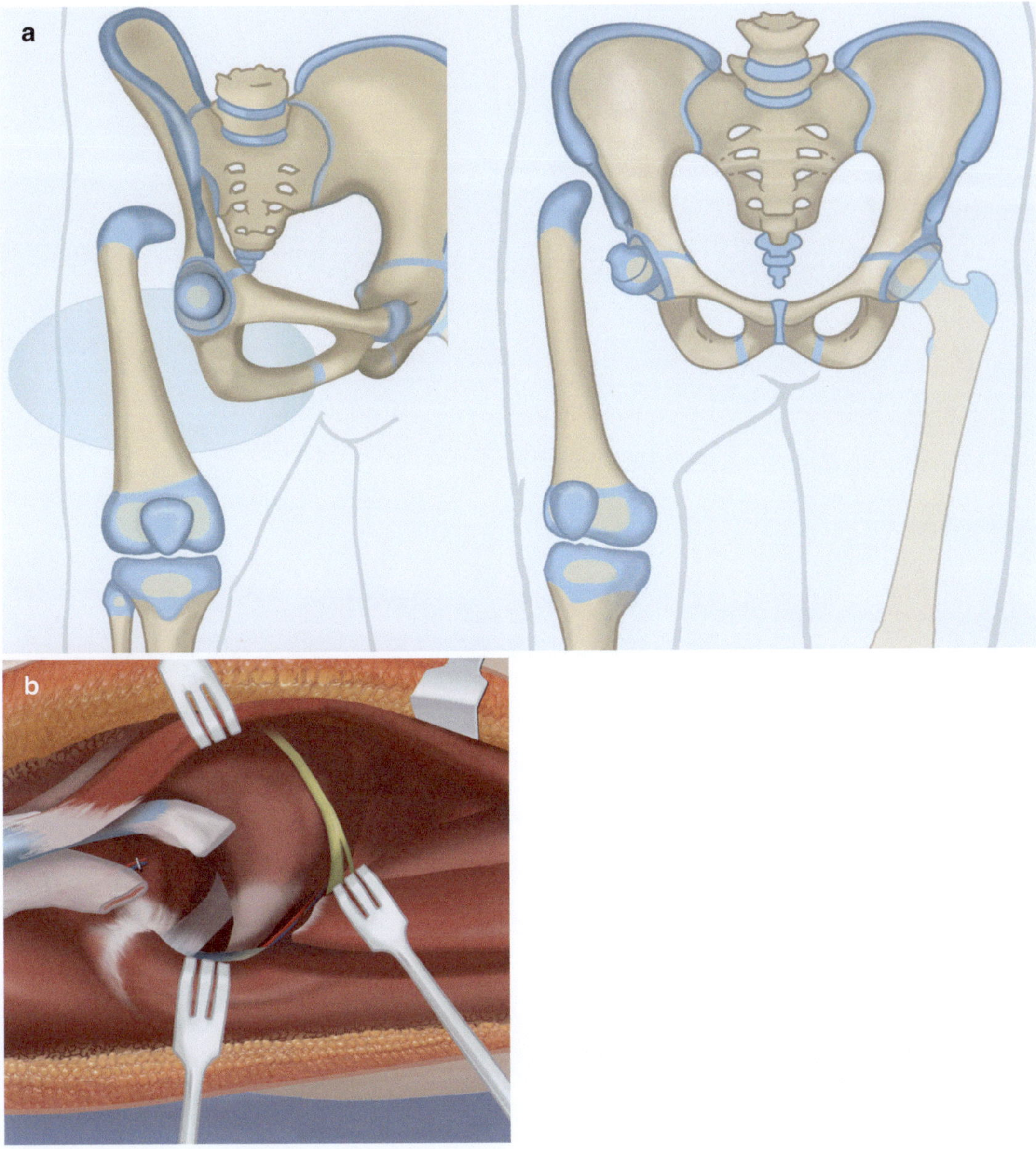

Fig. 35.10 (**a–j**) SUPERhip2 procedure soft tissue releases: see steps of surgery corresponding to each figure.

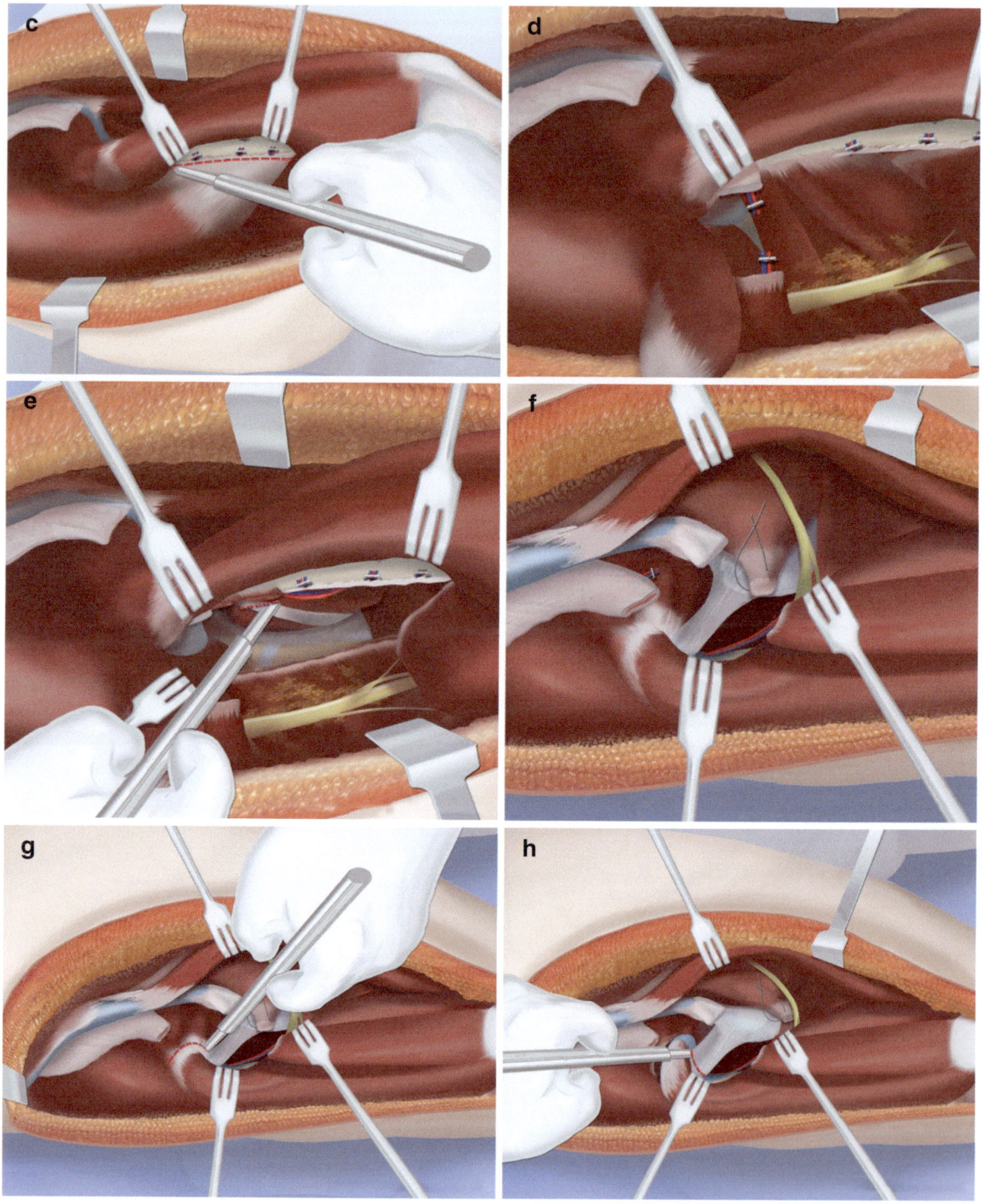

Fig. 35.10 (continued)

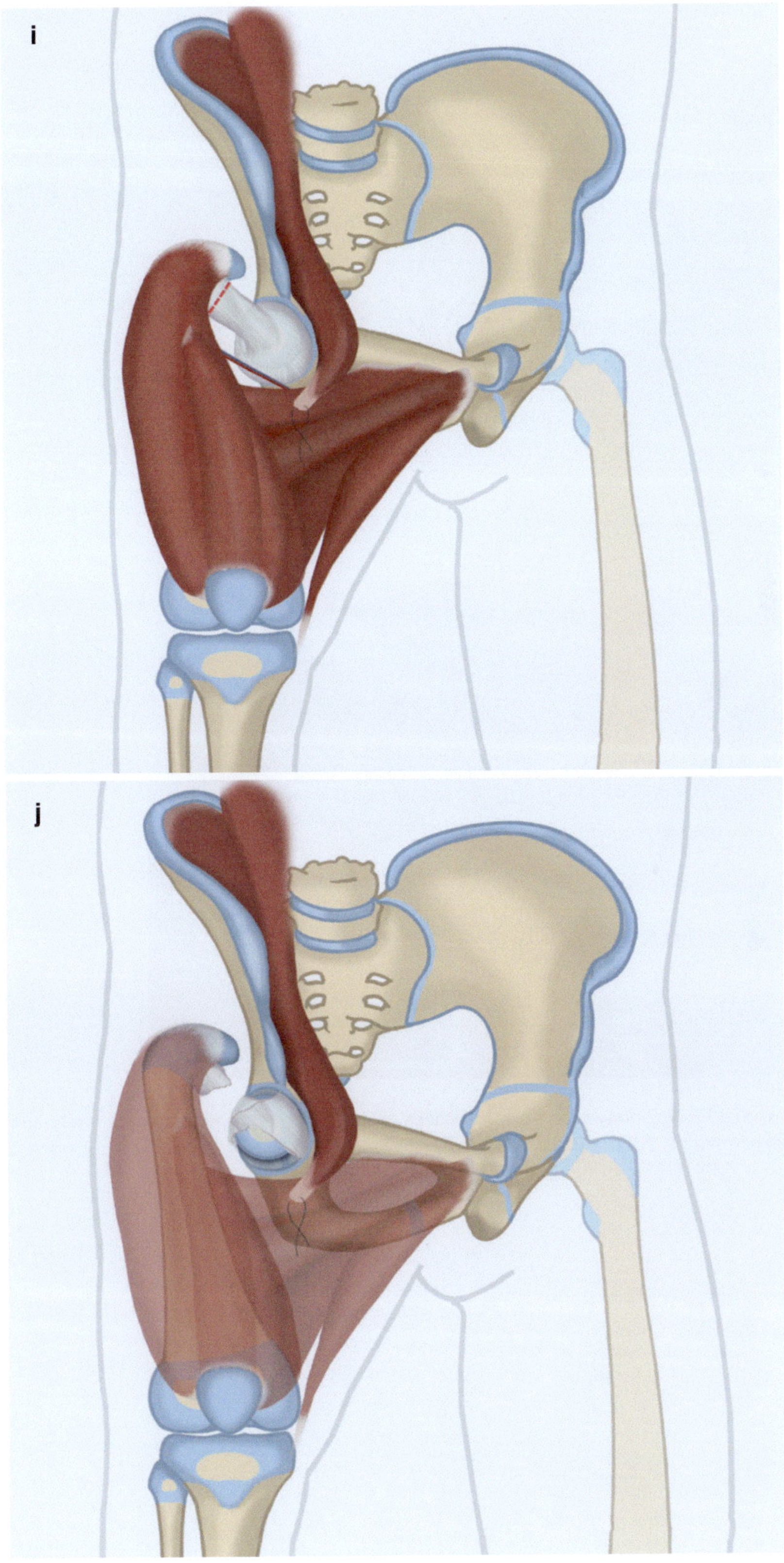

Fig. 35.10 (continued)

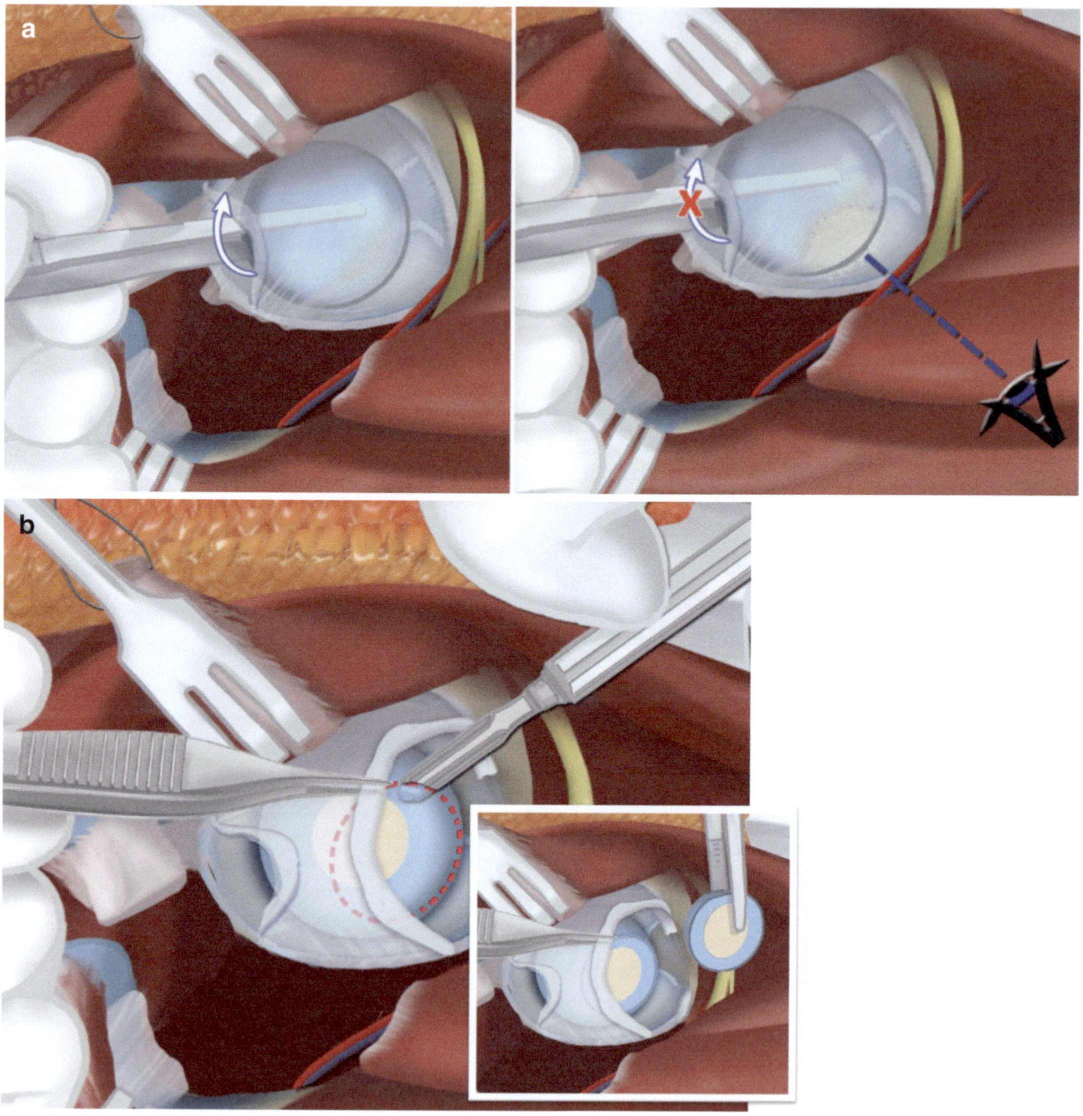

Fig. 35.11 (**a–x**) SUPERhip2 bony procedures: see steps of surgery corresponding to each figure. (© 2014 The Paley Foundation, with permission. All rights reserved)

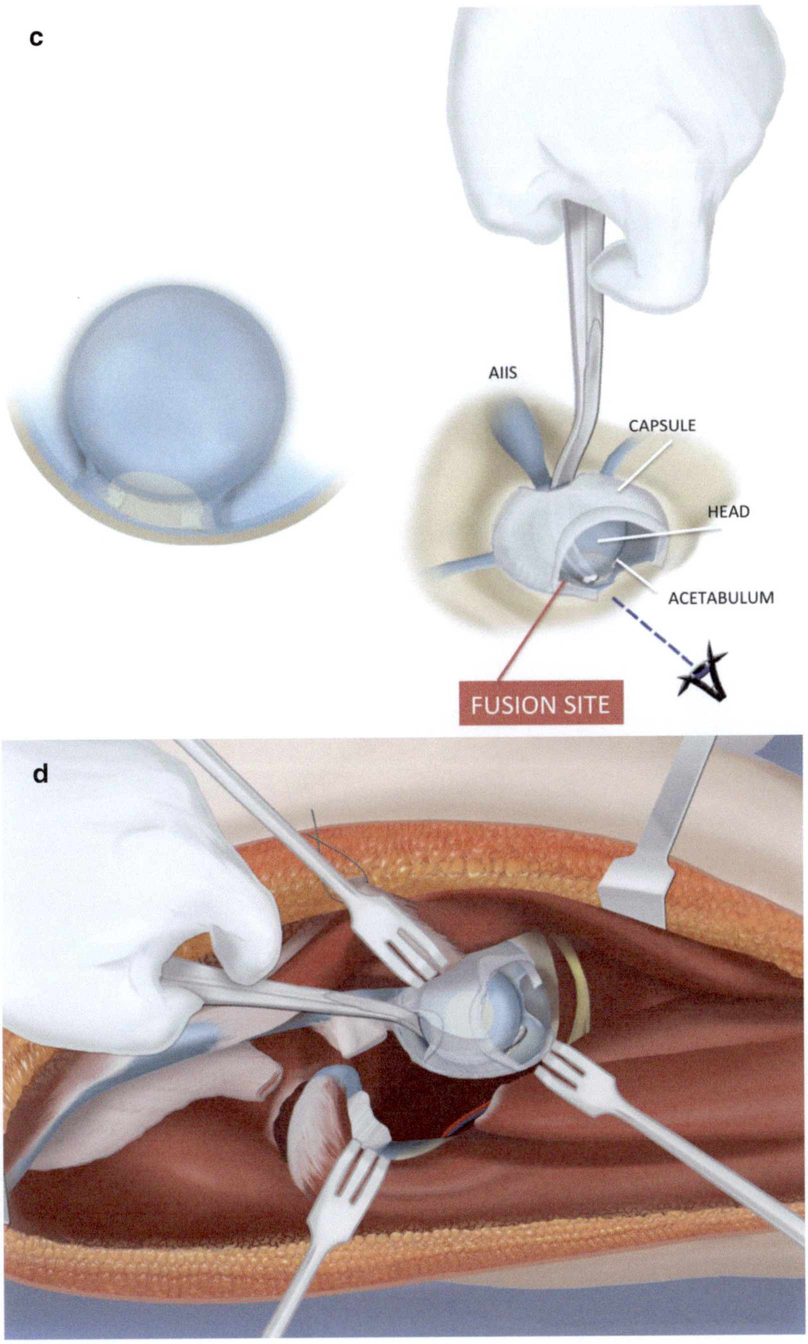

Fig. 35.11 (continued)

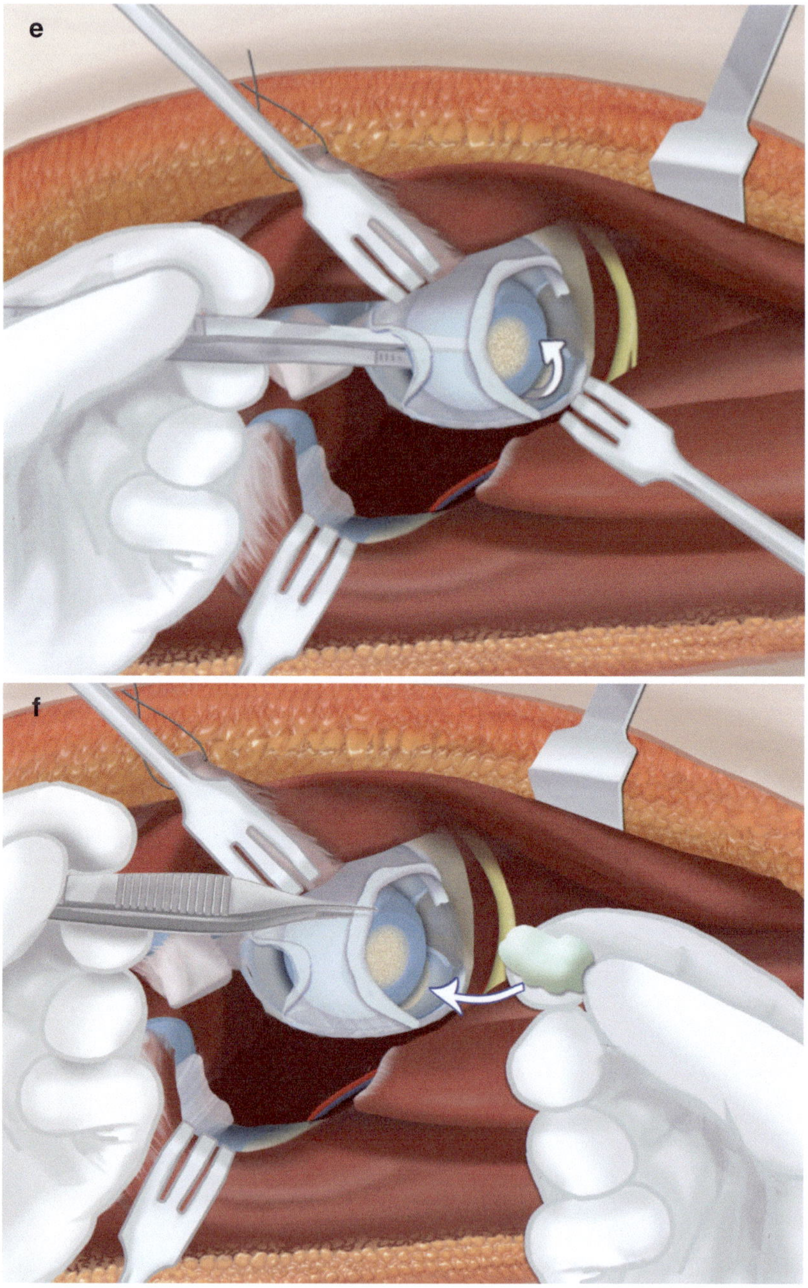

Fig. 35.11 (continued)

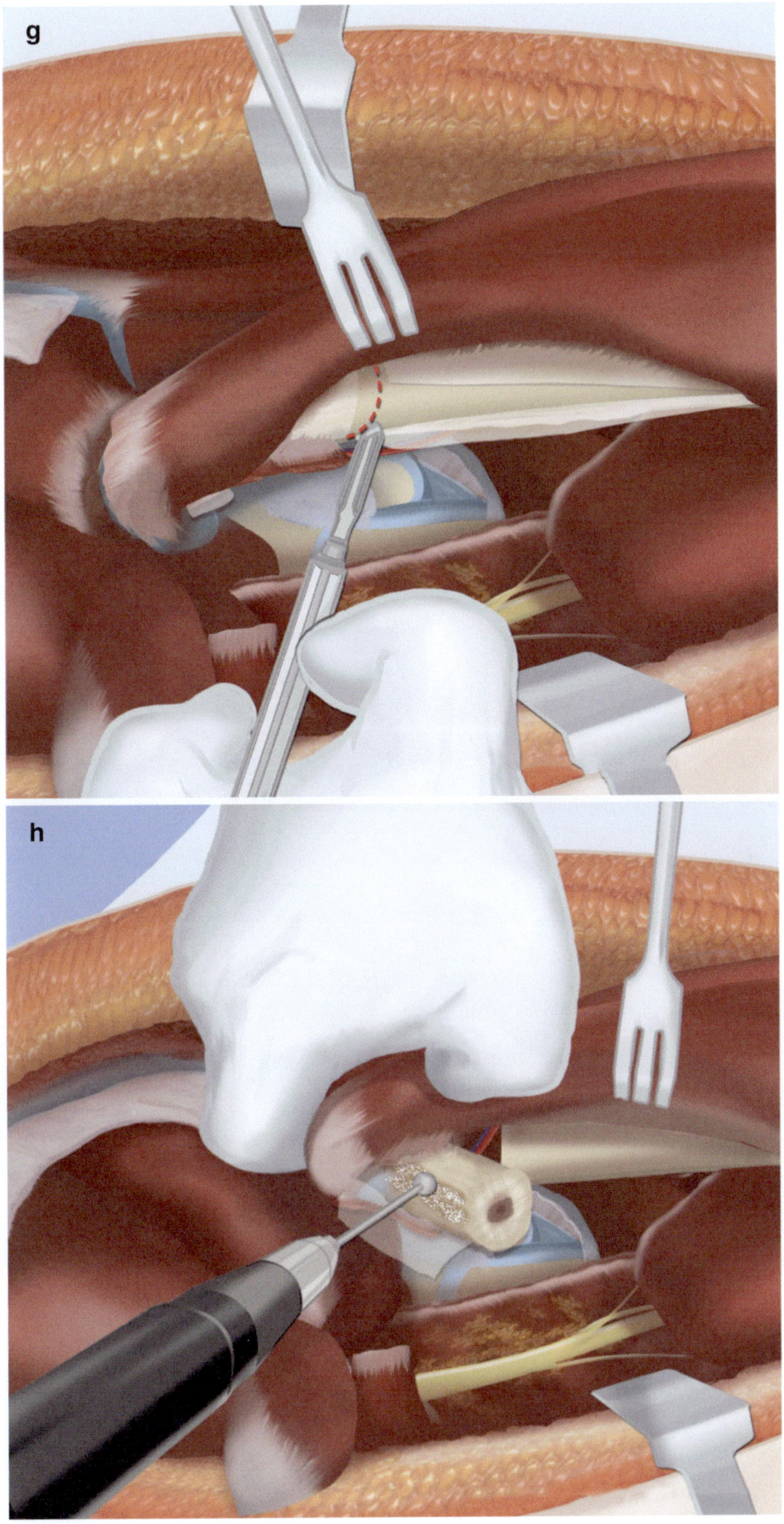

Fig. 35.11 (continued)

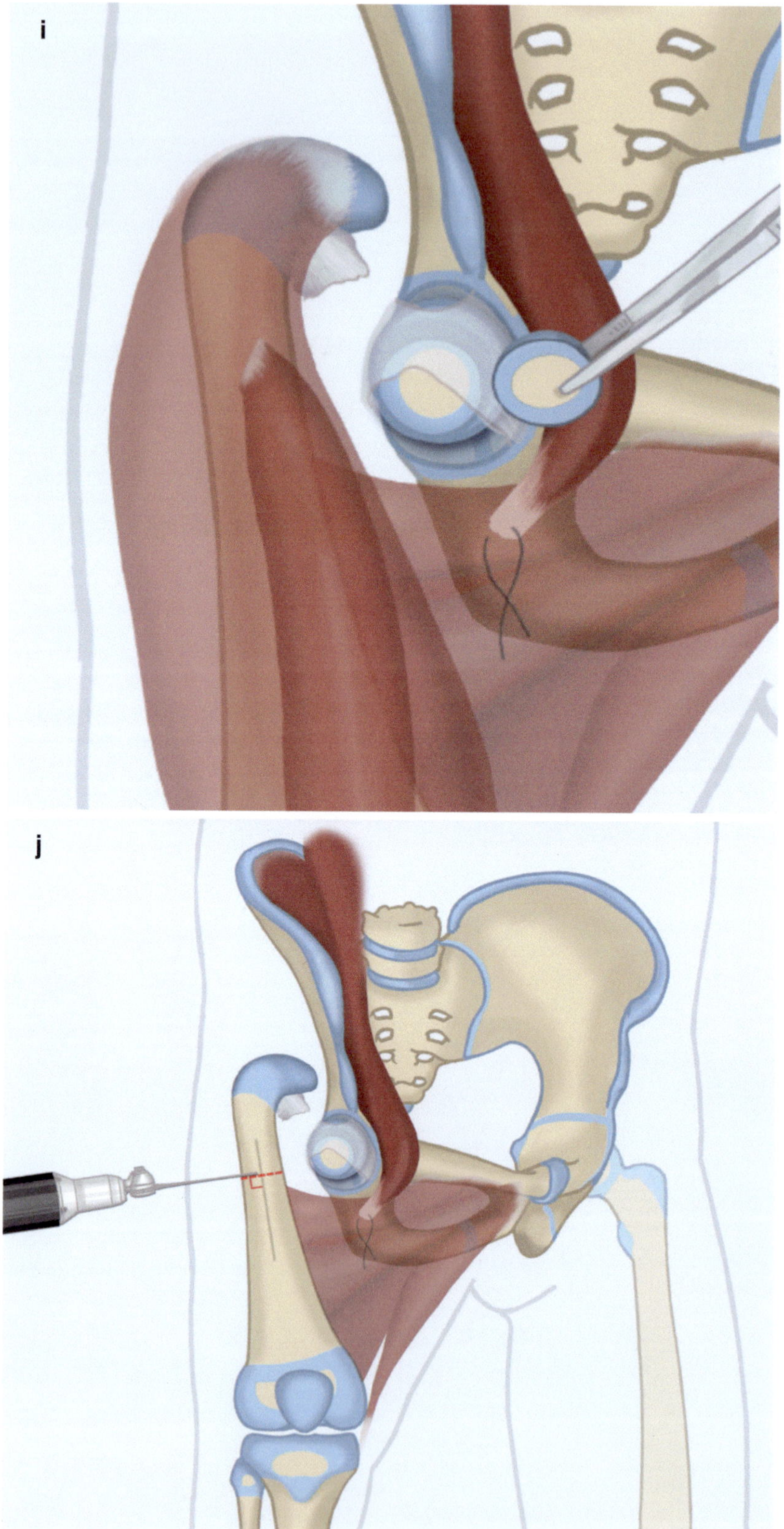

Fig. 35.11 (continued)

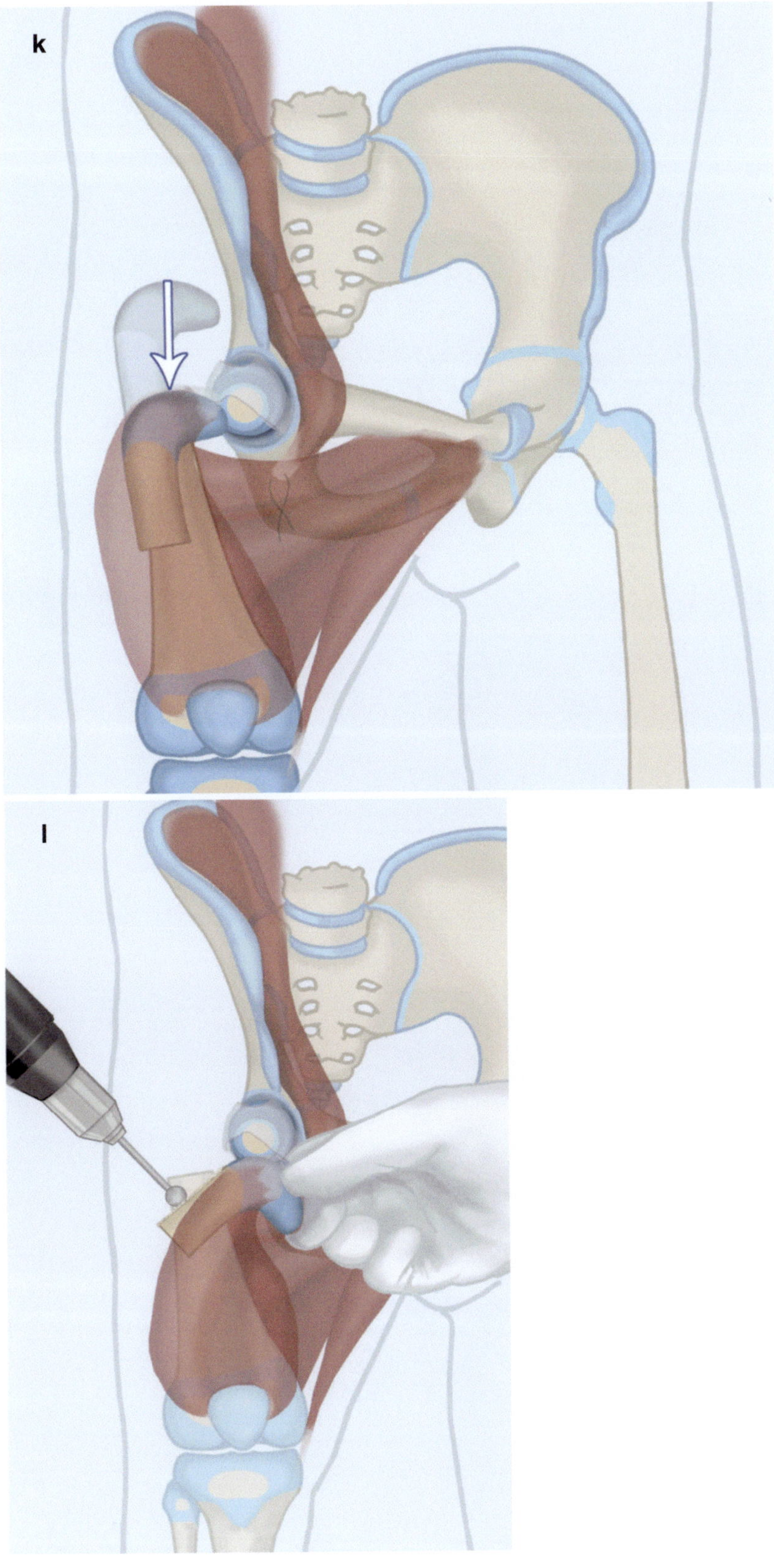

Fig. 35.11 (continued)

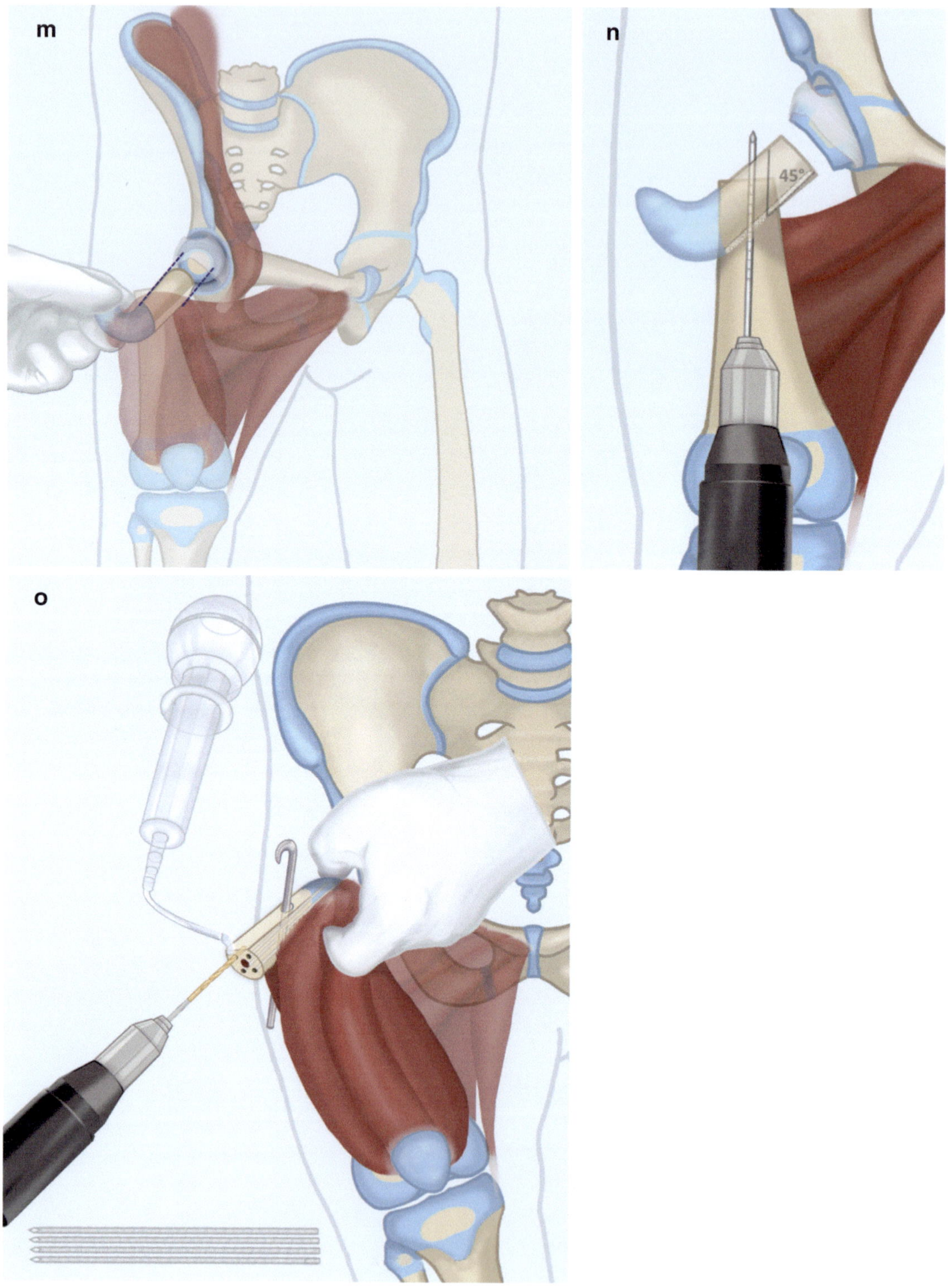

Fig. 35.11 (continued)

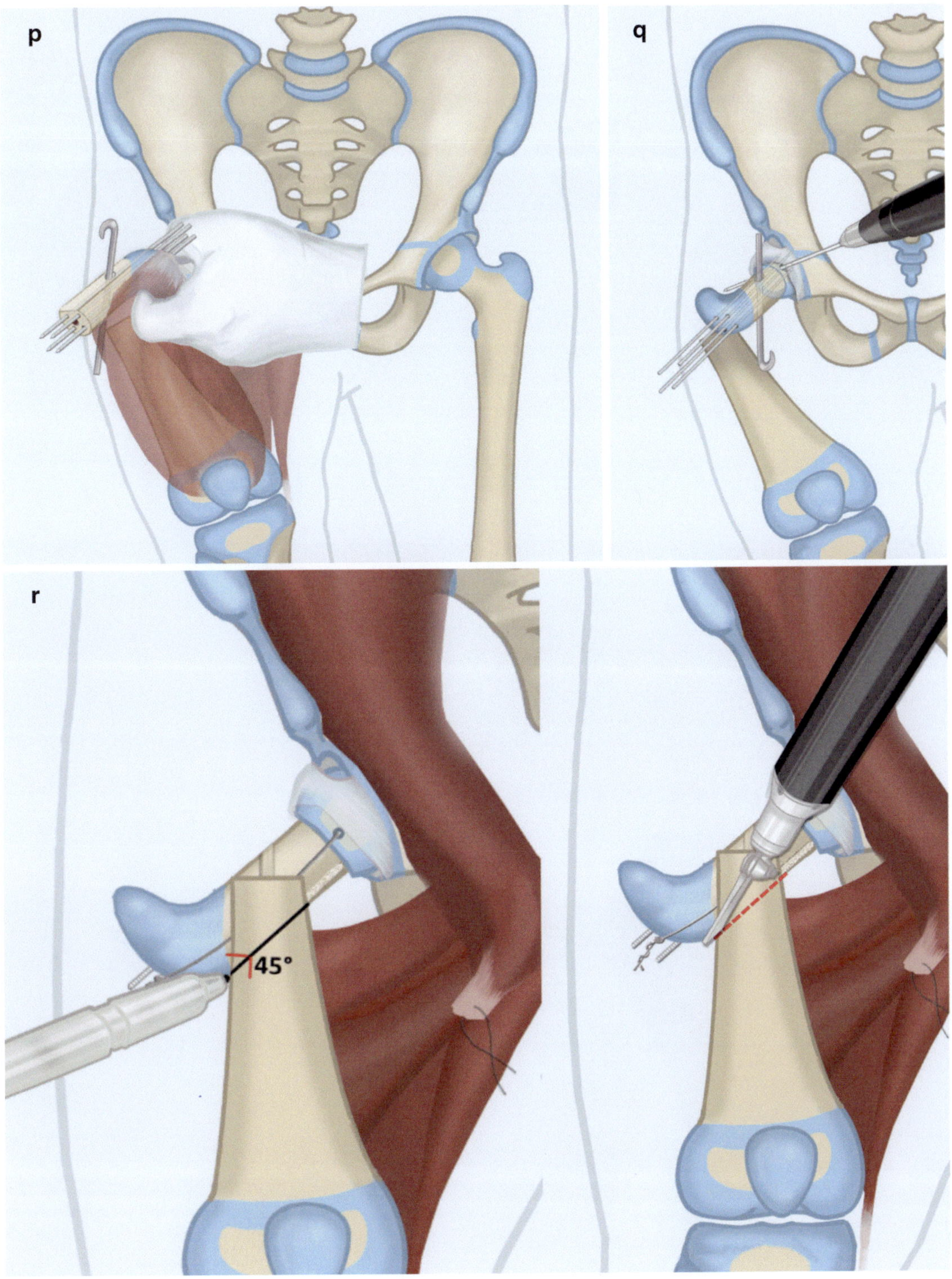

Fig. 35.11 (continued)

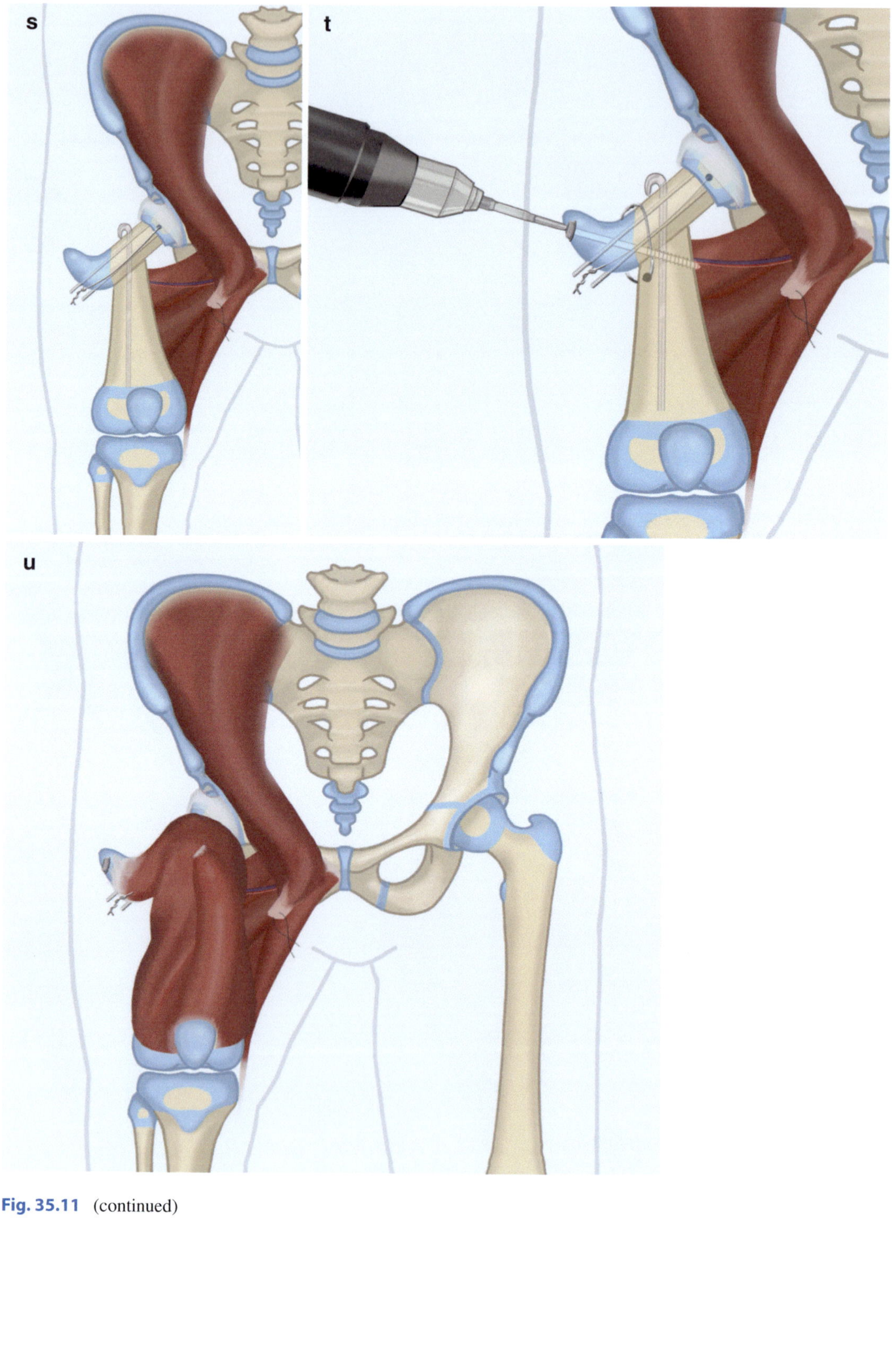

Fig. 35.11 (continued)

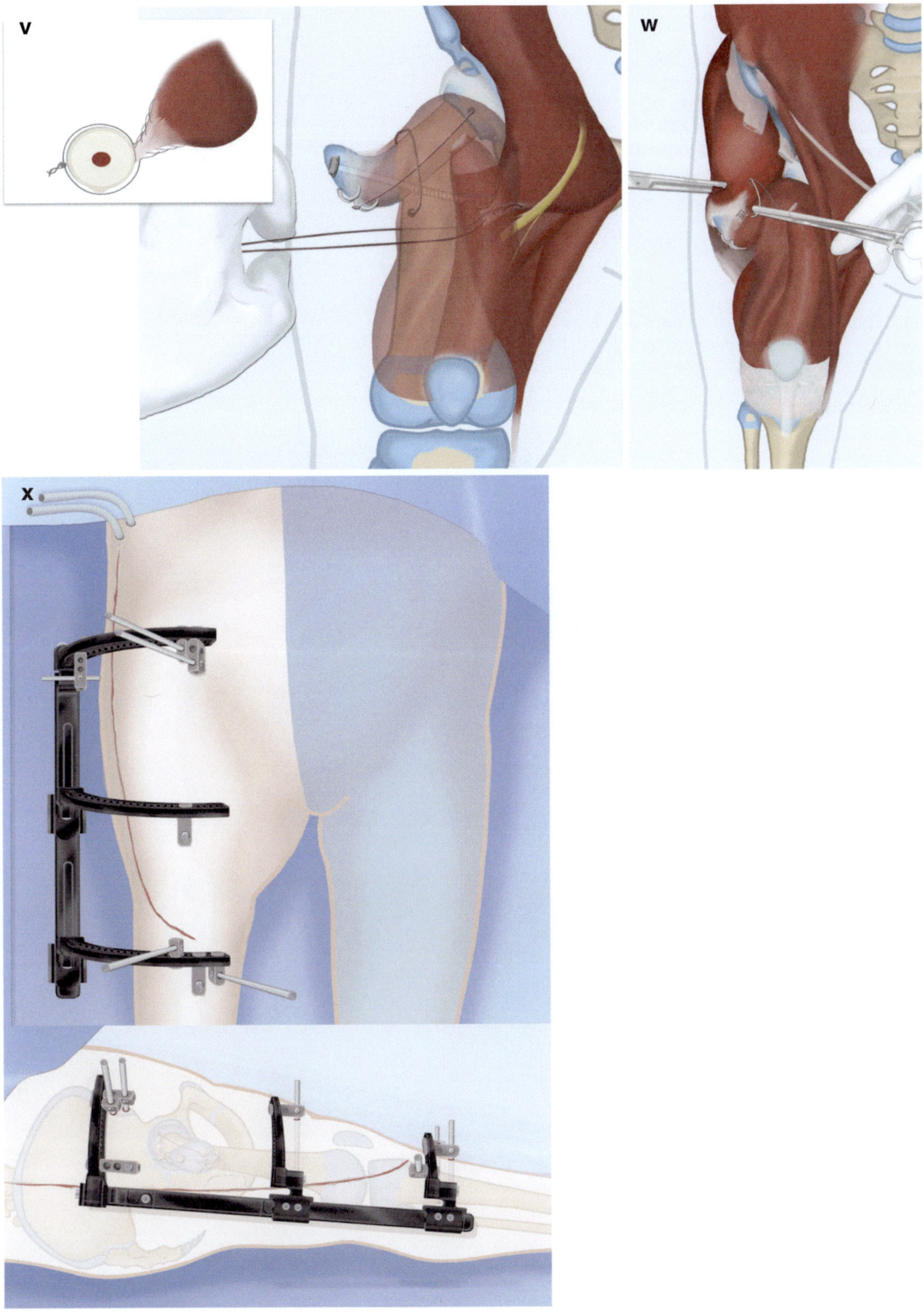

Fig. 35.11 (continued)

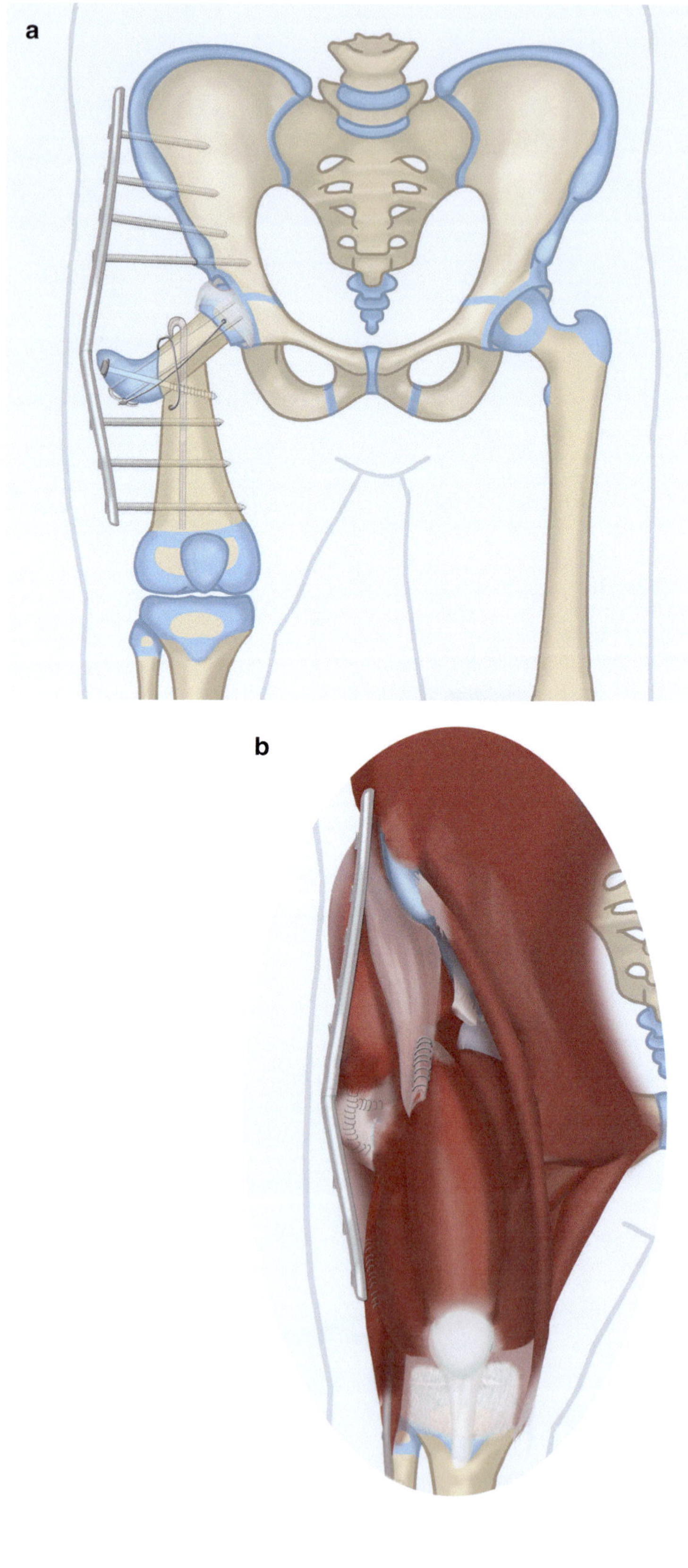

Fig. 35.12 (**a**, **b**) Use of an internal external fixator to temporarily arthrodese the hip. See steps of surgery corresponding to each figure. (© 2014 The Paley Foundation, with permission. All rights reserved)

15. *Break fusion site*. If the femoral head has a fusion site, identify the location of this site (opposite the ischium) and break this fusion using a small curved instrument (see Fig. 35.11c, d). Place bone wax on the exposed bone of the acetabulum and rotate the exposed bone of the femoral head outward (see Fig. 35.11e, f).
16. *Quadriceps elevation*. The quadriceps muscle is the vascular pedicle of the new femoral neck (see Fig. 35.11g). Therefore care should be taken to minimize dissection of this muscle off of the upper femur. The quads can be removed at the linea aspera and off the lateral wall of femur. It should not be dissected subperiosteally off of the anterior or medial aspects of the femur (see Fig. 35.11h).
17. *Femur osteotomy*. The femur can now be cut in the subtrochanteric region. The lateral wall of the femur is burred flat (see Fig. 35.11h).
18. *Remove bump*. The bump under the ischium can now be removed.
19. *Femoral neck mobilization*. The only tether at this point on the new femoral neck should be the quadriceps muscle and the femoral nerve (see Fig. 35.11m).
20. *Pre-drill femoral neck*. Pre-drill a 3.2 mm hole at 45° to the femoral neck as lateral as possible and as central as possible (see Fig. 35.11n). Insert a temporary 3.2 mm Rush rod and then predrill the femoral neck with three or four 1.5 mm cortical drill holes (see Fig. 35.11o). Insert two threaded and two nonthreaded k-wires (see Fig. 35.11p).
21. *Circlage wire*. Insert one 20 guage wire through the femoral head (see Fig. 35.11q).
22. *Femoral neck to head connection*. Reduce the femur to the femoral head and advance the 4 wires into the femoral head to gain fixation. Pass the circlage wire under the quads and secure it by twisting the wire to compress the neck to the head.
23. *Knee flexion contracture*. If the knee joint has a flexion contracture a posterior capsulotomy with peroneal nerve decompression and biceps and gastrocnemius tendon releases is done. After the knee is fully straight it is pinned. This affects the amount of femoral shortening.
24. *Distal femur shortening osteotomy*. Overlap the bone ends and mark a 45° line to cut the femur. Internally rotate the distal femur 10° so that the cut is anteverted. Make the cut so that it shortens sufficiently to allow the bone ends to come to be reduced (see Fig. 35.11r).
25. *Rush rod length*. Pre-measure the length of the rod by predrilling into the distal femur. Cut a rod to the correct length.
26. *Insert Rush rod*. Insert the Rush rod antegrade to reduce and fix the neck to the shaft (see Fig. 35.11s).
27. *Second circlage*. Add another circlage to fix the trochanter to the femur. Make sure it passes under the quadriceps so as not to strangulate the muscle pedicle (see Fig. 35.11t).
28. *More fixation*. A screw can also be added between the trochanter and the femur (see Fig. 35.11t).
29. *Psoas transfer*. Pass the psoas tendon distally and fix to the femur with a suture (see Fig. 35.11u, v).
30. *Reattach abductors*. Suture the abductor tendon to the greater trochanter. If it does not reach then do an abductor slide (see Fig. 35.11w).
31. *Temporary arthrodesis of hip with external fixation*. At this juncture decide how to temporarily arthrodesis the hip with either external fixation (see Fig. 35.11x) or internal fixation (see Fig. 35.12). With external then the wound is closed first and three pins are inserted into the pelvis, one in the femur and three in the tibia (see Fig. 35.11x).
32. *Temporary arthrodesis of the hip with internal fixation*. This is done using a locking plate to span the hip with locking screws into the lateral wall of the ilium and the femur (see Fig. 35.12).

33. *Removal of temporary arthrodesis fixation.* The temporary arthrodesis of the hip, external or internal, remains in place for 4 months and is then removed. By then union should have occurred both at the subtrochanteric osteotomy site and the femoral head neck junction.

Postoperative Imaging

Case 1 Plain radiographs are taken after the SUPERhip procedure to evaluate the healing of the pelvic osteotomy and femur osteotomy (see Fig. 35.3e). Subsequent lengthening surgery a year later is followed with plain radiography (see Fig. 35.3f, g) and clinically (see Fig. 35.3h).

Case 2 Plain radiographs are taken after the SUPERhip procedure to follow the ossification of the femoral neck and healing of the pelvic and femoral osteotomies. Standing radiographs also follow the progression of growth and discrepancy (see Fig. 35.4d–f). A year later the femur can be lengthened (see Fig. 35.4g, h). Several years later it can be lengthened a second time (see Fig. 35.4i, j).

Case 3 Plain radiographs are taken after the SUPERhip procedure to follow the healing and growth of the femur (see Fig. 35.5c). Femoral lengthening can be done one or more years later (see Fig. 35.5d, e).

Case 4 Plain radiographs are followed during the temporary arthrodesis period (usually 4 months) to assess for union at the subtrochanteric osteotomy and at the femoral head-neck junction (see Fig. 35.6c). The temporary arthrodesis external fixator is removed once union is achieved and growth and discrepancy are followed with standing radiographs (see Fig. 35.6d). Radiographs to follow lengthening and the hip are done at intervals (see Fig. 35.6e, f).

Pearls and Pitfalls

SUPERhip

- Pay careful attention to soft tissue handling, making sure the subcutaneous flaps are cleanly dissected to preserve their integrity and prevent fat necrosis.
- The lateral femoral cutaneous nerve is usually found just under the sartorius fascia and originates from deep to the inguinal ligament.
- The femoral nerve lies on the anteromedial side of iliopsoas muscle. The tendon lies posteromedial.
- Do not dissect distal or deep to the piriformis tendon to avoid interrupting the inferior gluteal anastomosis with the medial femoral circumflex artery.
- The apophysis should be split with a single continuous cut, pushing hard down to bone. Multiple passes will piecemeal the apophyseal cartilage.
- Palpate the back of the greater trochanter while placing the chisel and blade plate to make sure they stay perpendicular to its posterior border in the sagittal plane.
- The extent of the flexion and adduction deformity should be fairly evident by the orientation of the blade plate to the uncut femur. Greater than 45° of flexion deformity and up to 90° of varus deformity is not uncommon.
- Test the flexion of the hip and if obligatory external rotation occurs it is due to femuroacetabular impingement. This requires shaving more bone off of the anteromedial aspect of the proximal femur (see Fig. 35.8m). This can weaken the cartilage bone connection between the femoral epiphysis and the subtrochanteric bone. To protect this a circlage wire can be used between the greater trochanter and the bone (drill anteroposterior into the cartilagenous trochanter and the bone for passage of the wire).
- Place the guide wire in the cannulated plate to help guide the rotational correction, BMP hole placement, and determining femoral anteversion

- Make sure that the hole drilled for BMP2 insertion does not connect with the hip joint. Also make sure to plug the lateral entry hole with bone wax. This will prevent heterotopic ossification.
- Placement of the guidewire into the center of the femoral neck is perhaps the most difficult step. Incorrect placement will cause the blade of the plate to be maloriented or even to be intra-articular. If you meet a lot of resistance when introducing the cannulated chisel it may mean that the chisel is not following the guide wire and is notching or bending this wire.
- It is important to shorten the femur adequately to avoid dislocation or stiffness of the hip joint.
- For the Paley modification of the Dega, be careful not to enter the hip joint or the triradiate cartilage with the posterior distal part of the cut. This can be avoided by staying as close to the sciatic notch as possible and not going to distal. Do not cut across the triradiate cartilage otherwise a partial growth arrest may occur.

SUPERhip2

- Do not strip the quadriceps off of the upper femur except on the lateral side. The quads are the vascular pedicle of the new neck.
- Do this procedure at an older age than the SUPERhip. The SUPERhip can be done as young as age 2. The SUPERhip2 should be deferred to age 3 or 4 depending on the size of the femur.
- Despite best efforts union of the neck to head site may not occur.
- Despite best efforts the femoral head may fuse back to the acetabulum.
- This procedure is technically extremely difficult and is one order of magnitude harder then the SUPERhip procedure. Become proficient at the SUPERhip before considering taking on an SUPERhip2.

Indications and Contraindications (Table 35.1)

Table 35.1 SUPERhip and SUPERhip2 procedures for congenital femoral deficiency: Surgical indications and contraindication

Indications
The SUPERhip procedure is indicated for Paley type 1 congenital femoral deficiency (CFD) where there is a marked coxa vara (real or apparent) and the other associated deformities. Most patients who need the SUPERhip have Paley type 1b. There is a subgroup of Paley type 1a referred to as $1a_3$ that have similar deformities to the type 1b without the delayed ossification of the neck or subtrochanteric regions. Another indication are the congenital coxa vara patients. They all have an associated abduction contracture. The abductor slide and TFL release are essential in order to be able to fully correct the coxa vara. Bone morphogenic protein may help, especially in the congential coxa vara that has the inverted Y delayed ossification region
Other conditions that lead to chronic severe deformation of the proximal femur such as fibrous dysplasia, osteogenesis imperfecta, rickets, and certain dysplasias are also good indications for part or all of this technique
The SUPERhip2 procedure is indicated primarily for patients with CFD type 2a or 2b. While it can be used for CFD type 3, those patients have such severe discrepancy that they are better candidates for a rotationplasty than for a SUPERhip2
SUPERhip2 can also be used for other situations with a femoral neck nonunion but with preservation of the femoral head. These can include post-traumatic, post-infectious, and post tumor resection
While most patients undergoing this procedure are doing so as a preparatory surgery to limb length equalization surgery, the SUPERhip procedure is still indicated in patients who choose to have a Syme's amputation for Paley type 1b. While the amputation with prosthetic fitting will obviate the need for limb length equalization surgery, it does not address the hip deformity and the limitations and problems created by this deformity, including more problematic and bulky prosthetics, late arthritis of the hip, limitation of abduction and other range of motion and cosmetic. The SUPERhip is still an excellent option in these patients notwithstanding the Syme's amputation
Contraindication
Perhaps the one contraindication for a SUPERhip procedure is if one is considering performing a rotationplasty at a later time. The amount of dissection for the SUPERhip procedure is quite large. A previous SUPERhip dissection can complicate the viability of the skin and muscle flaps created with rotationplasty

Acknowledgements The author wishes to thank Pamela Boullier Ross, who created all of the illustrations used in this chapter. The author would also like to thank the Paley Foundation for funding the cost of the illustrations and for giving permission to Springer for their use in this chapter.

References

1. Paley D. Lengthening reconstruction surgery for congenital femoral deficiency. In: Herring JA, Birch JG, editors. The child with a limb deficiency. Rosemont, IL: American Academy of Orthopaedic Surgeons; 1998. p. 113–32.
2. Paley D, Chong DY, Prince DE. Congenital femoral deficiency reconstruction and lengthening surgery. In: Sabharwal S, editor. Pediatric lower limb deformities, principles and techniques of management. Heidelberg: Springer; 2016. p. 361–425.
3. Eidelman M, Jauregui JJ, Standard SC, Paley D, Herzenberg JE. Hip stability during lengthening in children with congenital femoral deficiency. Int Orthop. 2016;40(12):2619–25.
4. Paley D. Treatment of congenital femoral deficiency. In: Weisel SW, editor. Operative techniques in orthopaedic surgery. 2nd ed. Philadelphia: Lippincott Williams & Wilkins; 2015. p. 1532–51.
5. Paley D, Guadro F. Lengthening reconstruction surgery for congenital femoral deficiency. In: Kocaoğlu M, et al., editors. Advanced techniques in limb reconstruction surgery. Berlin: Springer; 2014. p. 245–99.
6. Paley D, Robbins CA. Congenital femoral deficiency: Paley type 1b and Paley type 1c. In: Rozbruch R, Hamdy R, editors. Limb lengthening and reconstruction surgery case atlas. Cham: Springer; 2015. p. 395–404.
7. Paley D, Standard SC. Lengthening reconstruction surgery for congenital femoral deficiency. In: Rozbruch SR, Ilizarov S, editors. Limb lengthening and reconstruction surgery. New York: Informa; 2007. p. 393–428.
8. Paley D, Standard SC. Treatment of congenital femoral deficiency. In: Wiesel S, editor. Operative techniques in orthopaedic surgery. Philadelphia: Lippincott Williams & Wilkins; 2010. p. 1202–23.
9. Paley D. Progress in and from limb lengthening. In: Current progress in orthopedics. Mumbai: Tree Life Media, Kothari Medical Subscription Services Pvt Ltd; 2014. p. 55–80.
10. Paley D, Robbins CA. Congenital femoral deficiency: Paley type 2a. In: Rozbruch SR, Hamdy R, editors. Limb lengthening and reconstruction surgery case atlas. Cham: Springer; 2015. p. 405–20.

36 Hip Arthrodesis Using Surgical Hip Dislocation and Subtrochanteric Osteotomy

Neil Saran

Introduction

Severe painful arthrosis in adolescent patients is a difficult dilemma. The surgical treatment options include total joint replacement or hip arthrodesis. As the longevity of hip replacements continues to improve, the option of hip replacement looks enticing. However, the long-term outcomes of joint replacements in adolescent patients still remain concerning. As such an argument can be made that in adolescent patients with severe painful degenerative joint disease of the hip, arthrodesis remains the preferred treatment option. Short-term problems with hip arthrodesis include nonunion, malalignment, and limb length discrepancy. Long-term problems include degenerative low back pain and ipsilateral knee pain as well as a difficult conversion to total hip arthroplasty. While the short-term problems can be minimized using the approach described in this chapter, the long-term problems of adjacent segment degenerative joint disease cannot and may in fact necessitate future conversion to total hip arthroplasty. Avoiding the use of complex plating techniques and minimizing trauma to the abductor musculature during the hip arthrodesis are important factors to consider for future total hip arthroplasty.

N. Saran (✉)
Department of Orthopaedic Surgery, Shriners Hospital for Children Canada, Montreal, QC, Canada

Department of Paediatric Surgery, The Montreal Children's Hospital, Montreal, QC, Canada

Division of Orthopaedic Surgery, Department of Surgery, McGill University, Montreal, QC, Canada
e-mail: neil.saran@mcgill.ca

Brief Clinical History

The patient (12-year-6-month-old female) presented to our clinic 6 months after a pinning for a slipped capital femoral epiphysis (SCFE) with chondrolysis and a very stiff hip. She underwent removal of the SCFE screw and a steroid injection of the hip joint followed by physiotherapy and anti-inflammatory medications. Over the following 6 months, her hip pain and functional limitations worsened. At the 1 year mark, she could no longer walk without crutches due to hip pain. Her range of motion at this time revealed a flexion contracture of 35°, a hip flexion arc of no more than 25°, abduction of 20°, adduction of 10°, and a rotation arc of 10°. In addition, she had a limb length discrepancy of about 2.5 cm. Her preoperative radiographs revealed an aspherical femoral head and acetabulum with severe joint space narrowing (Fig. 36.1).

R. C. Hamdy, N. Saran (eds.), *Pediatric Pelvic and Proximal Femoral Osteotomies*,
https://doi.org/10.1007/978-3-319-78033-7_36

Preoperative Imaging

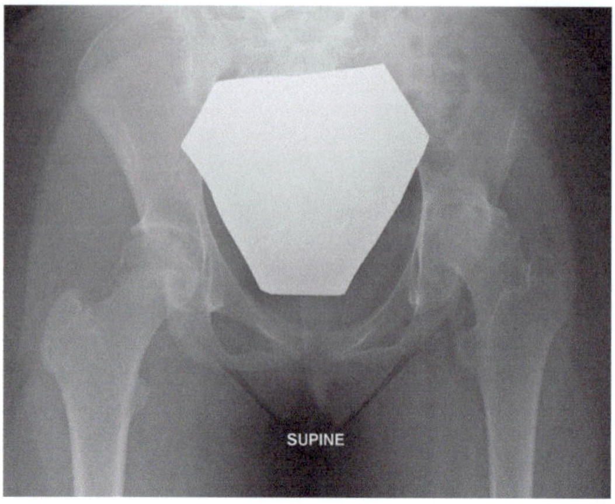

Fig. 36.1 Anteroposterior pelvis radiograph reveals severe joint space narrowing of the right hip. The femoral head and acetabulum are aspherical

Goals of Treatment

- Obtain a robust fusion of the hip joint without disturbing the abductors.
- Achieve optimal fusion position.
- Lengthen the limb to optimize limb length discrepancy for fused hip.

Treatment Strategy

The treatment strategy entails obtaining an adequate fusion of the hip with the leg in a functional position with minimal disruption of the abductor mechanism. In order to achieve optimal surface preparation for the fusion, the surgical hip dislocation approach [1] is chosen as it gives excellent exposure of the femoral head and acetabulum. Furthermore, this approach is abductor sparing. Rigid compressive fixation is achieved with partially threaded cannulated screws without the need for complex plating techniques that can further compromise the abductor mechanism either during the initial surgery or at the time of conversion to a total hip. An offloading osteotomy is performed to decrease the lever arm and moment on the hip fusion fixation and thus allow for an adequate fusion and minimize the risk of nonunion [2]. An iliofemoral fixator is applied to stabilize the osteotomy. The external fixator consists of a hinge at the offloading osteotomy site and a rail to allow for realignment and lengthening to ensure that the limb length discrepancy is less than 2 cm at the end of treatment.

Surgical Details

The setup and approach are the same for a surgical hip dislocation (described in Chap. 24, “Combined Osteotomy and Osteoplasty for Healed Slipped Capital Femoral Epiphysis Deformity”), with the exception of the trochanteric osteotomy. The only difference here is that the distal extent of the osteotomy should be limited if at all possible to better facilitate positioning of the screws that will be used to fix the arthrodesis site.

Surface Preparation

The use of acetabular reamers for the acetabulum and humeral head resurfacing reamers for the femoral head enables an excellent surface preparation. Once the femoral head is dislocated, the acetabulum is lightly reamed, starting with a small reamer and gradually increasing the size until there is punctate bleeding throughout.

The femoral head is reamed starting with a large diameter reamer gradually decreasing to 2 mm less than the acetabulum (Fig. 36.2). The femoral head reamings are kept and are used as bone graft. The joint is then irrigated and packed with a small amount of the femoral head reamings. The femoral head is then relocated into the acetabulum.

Positioning for Fusion

At this stage, the leg is positioned in 20–30° of hip flexion, 5° of adduction, and 5–10° of external rotation. The leg must stay in this position until the external fixator is on; therefore, sponge blocks are used to maintain this position.

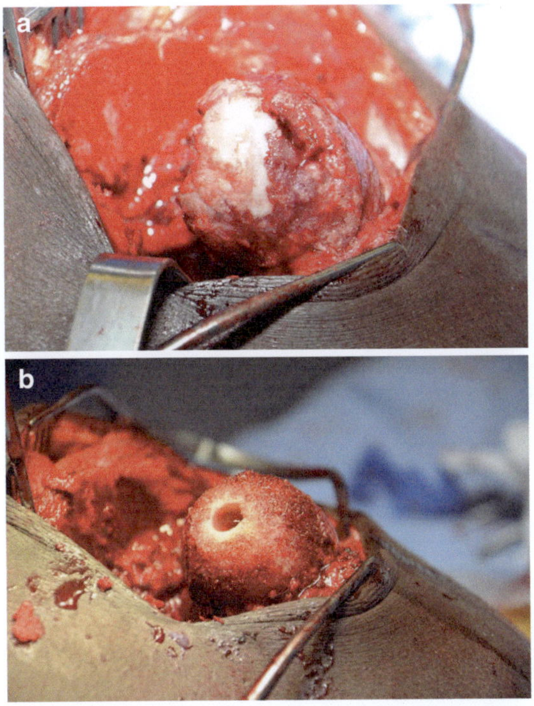

Fig. 36.2 Intraoperative photos of the femoral head before (**a**) and after (**b**) it has been prepared using humeral head reamers from a similar case

Fixation of the Hip Joint

Under fluoroscopy, two guide wires for 7.0 or 7.3 mm cannulated screws are placed from the proximal femur at the distal edge or just outside of the trochanteric osteotomy site into the supraacetabular bone transfixing the hip joint. The screws should be kept as low as possible in the supraacetabular bone to leave plenty of room for the supraacetabular external fixator pins. A partial threaded cannulated screw is placed to obtain compression followed by another partially or fully threaded cannulated screw to add rotational control and further rigidity to the fixation (Fig. 36.3). The hip capsule is closed with 1-0 Vicryl suture.

Trochanteric Fixation

The trochanter is brought back to its original position and transfixed using two 3.5 or 4.5 mm cortical screws (Fig. 36.4).

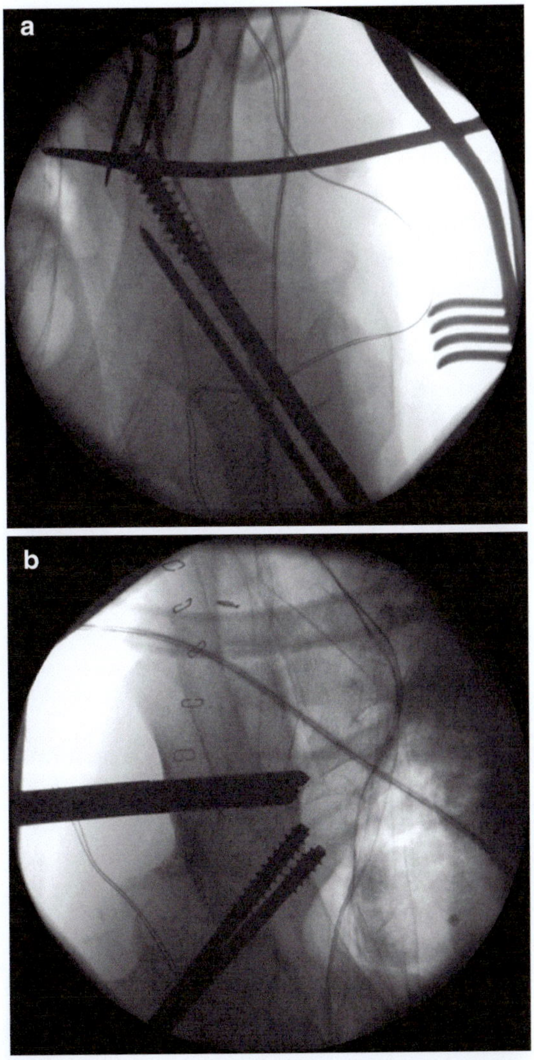

Fig. 36.3 (**a**) Fluoroscopic view showing a partial threaded screw being inserted, crossing the hip joint to obtain compressive fixation of the arthrodesis site. A second screw will be inserted over the guide wire seen on the image. (**b**) Fluoroscopic view of a similar case showing better screw placement that will enable improved placement of the supraacetabular external fixator pins

Iliofemoral External Fixator

Three 6 mm external fixator pins are placed from lateral to medial in the supraacetabular bone just above the hip fusion fixation screws through 1 cm skin incision. Cannulated external fixation pins can be useful in that they can be repositioned if necessary prior to placement of the actual external fixation pins. There should be no contact between the external fixation pins and the hip fusion screws.

An iliofemoral external fixator is then assembled with a ball-hinge placed at the location of the offloading subtrochanteric osteotomy site 1–2 cm below the cannulated screw insertion site and a rail distally along the femur.

Three 6 mm external fixation pins are placed from lateral to medial in the distal femoral diaphysis through 1 cm incisions through the iliofemoral external fixator. These pins should be placed perpendicular to the mechanical axis of the femur, should lengthening be desired. The frame may need to be adjusted to ensure that this is feasible. The frame is then tightened in place and removed from the pins to facilitate execution of the subtrochanteric osteotomy.

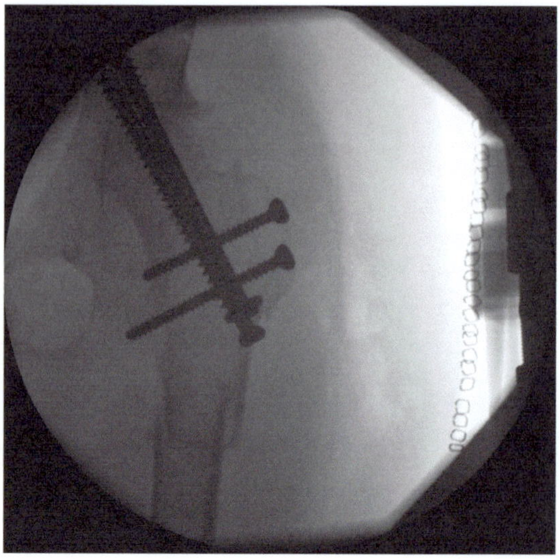

Fig. 36.5 Fluoroscopic view showing alignment of the subtrochanteric osteotomy once fixator is assembled

Subtrochanteric Osteotomy

A low energy oblique osteotomy is performed 2 cm below the cannulated screws used to transfix the hip joint (see Fig. 36.4). The osteotomy is performed by creating multiple drill holes and completed with an osteotome. The osteotomy is made in an oblique fashion to maximize surface area for improved healing.

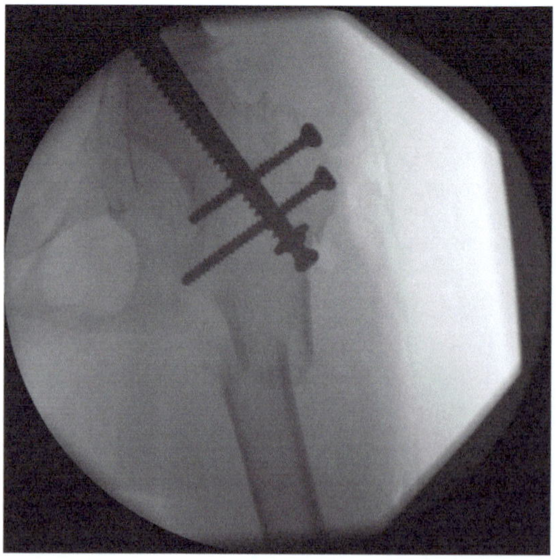

Fig. 36.4 Fluoroscopic view showing trochanter fixed with two screws. The subtrochanteric osteotomy is located approximately 2 cm below the arthrodesis screws

The vastus lateralis is then reapproximated, followed by the iliotibial band, tensor fascia, subcutaneous tissue, and skin.

The external fixation rail is then reassembled onto the pins. Fluoroscopy is used to realign the osteotomy site and the frame is tightened to the pins (Fig. 36.5).

Realignment of the Limb

Once the dressing has been placed, the patient is repositioned in the supine position and the position of the limb is reassessed. If required, repositioning of the limb can be performed through the subtrochanteric osteotomy by manipulating the ball joint.

Postoperative Realignment of the Limb and Lengthening

Lengthening is started on postoperative day 7 at 1 mm/day until the limb is approximately 1 cm shorter than the opposite side.

At 10 days postoperatively, the patient is assessed by an occupational therapist and physiotherapist to help decide on whether or not the hip fusion position is adequate. At this point, if required, further adjustments can be made through the osteotomy site in regard to flexion/adduction/rotation, and the ball joint is cemented to prevent drift into adduction and extension (Fig. 36.6).

The patient is kept non-weight bearing. A computed tomography (CT) scan is performed at 3 months to assess both the hip fusion and the subtrochanteric osteotomy (Fig. 36.7). If there is minimal healing on the CT scan, the scan is repeated in 4–6 weeks. Weight bearing is started once the scan shows evidence of bony union at the hip joint, and the frame is removed 4–6 weeks after there is adequate callous at the lengthening site (Fig. 36.8).

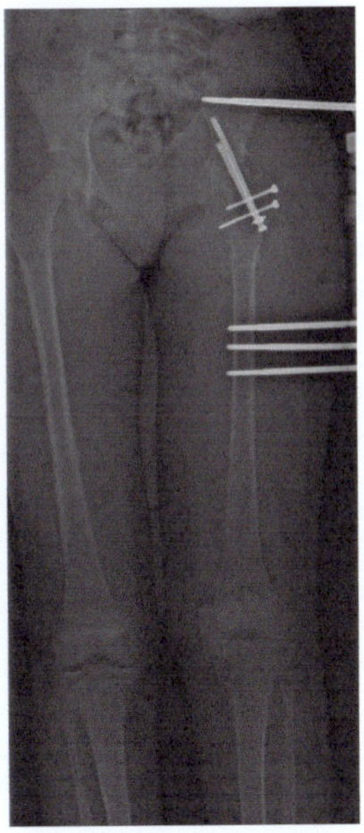

Fig. 36.6 Standing anteroposterior radiograph of both femora with a 2 cm lift under the left leg shows overall good alignment in the immediate postoperative period

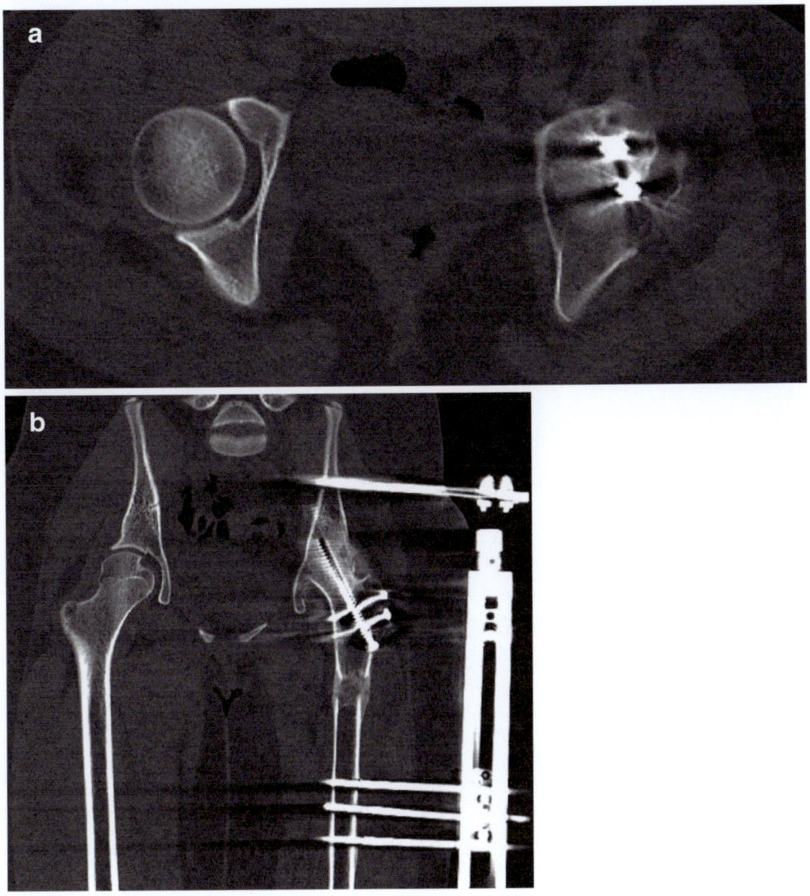

Fig. 36.7 Computed tomography images at 3 months showing consolidation of the arthrodesis site on axial (**a**) and coronal (**b**) planes. The coronal plane also shows the regenerated bone at the subtrochanteric osteotomy site, which has gained approximately 1.5 cm in length and is healing nicely

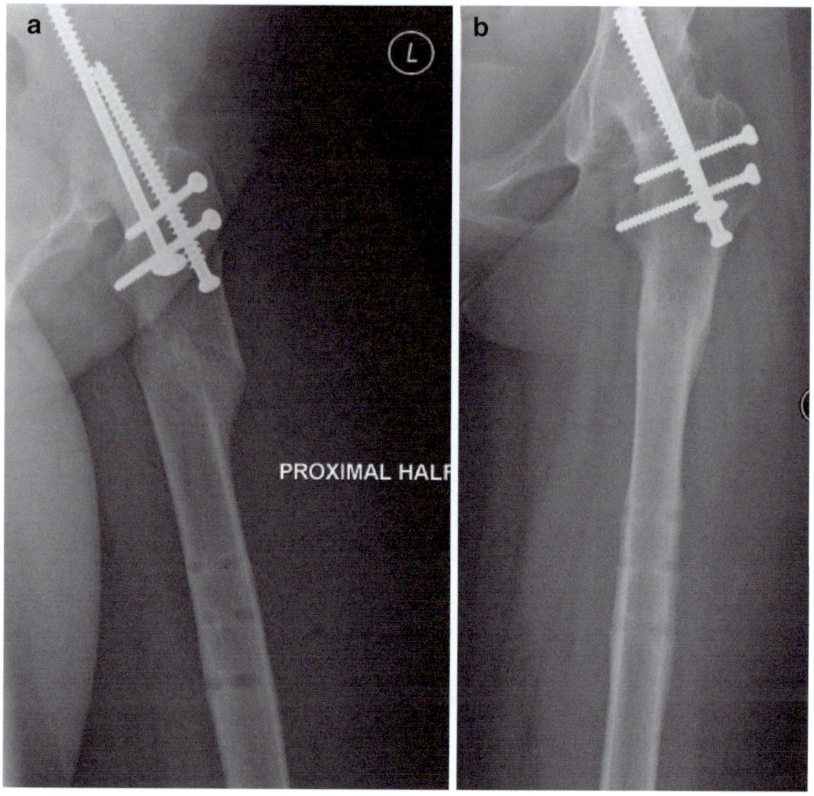

Fig. 36.8 Left hip anteroposterior (**a**) and lateral (**b**) radiographs showing consolidation of the subtrochanteric osteotomy and hip arthrodesis taken 2 months after frame removal and 6 months postoperative

Postoperative Imaging

At 2-year follow-up (age 15), the patient was participating with her gym class in sports, including volleyball, soccer, and basketball, albeit at a decreased level compared to her peers. She has a 1 cm limb length discrepancy and no hip pain. She has occasional mild low back pain that is not yet bothersome. She has no knee pain. She can walk without limit. Her radiographs reveal an excellent consolidation of the fusion and subtrochanteric osteotomy (Fig. 36.9).

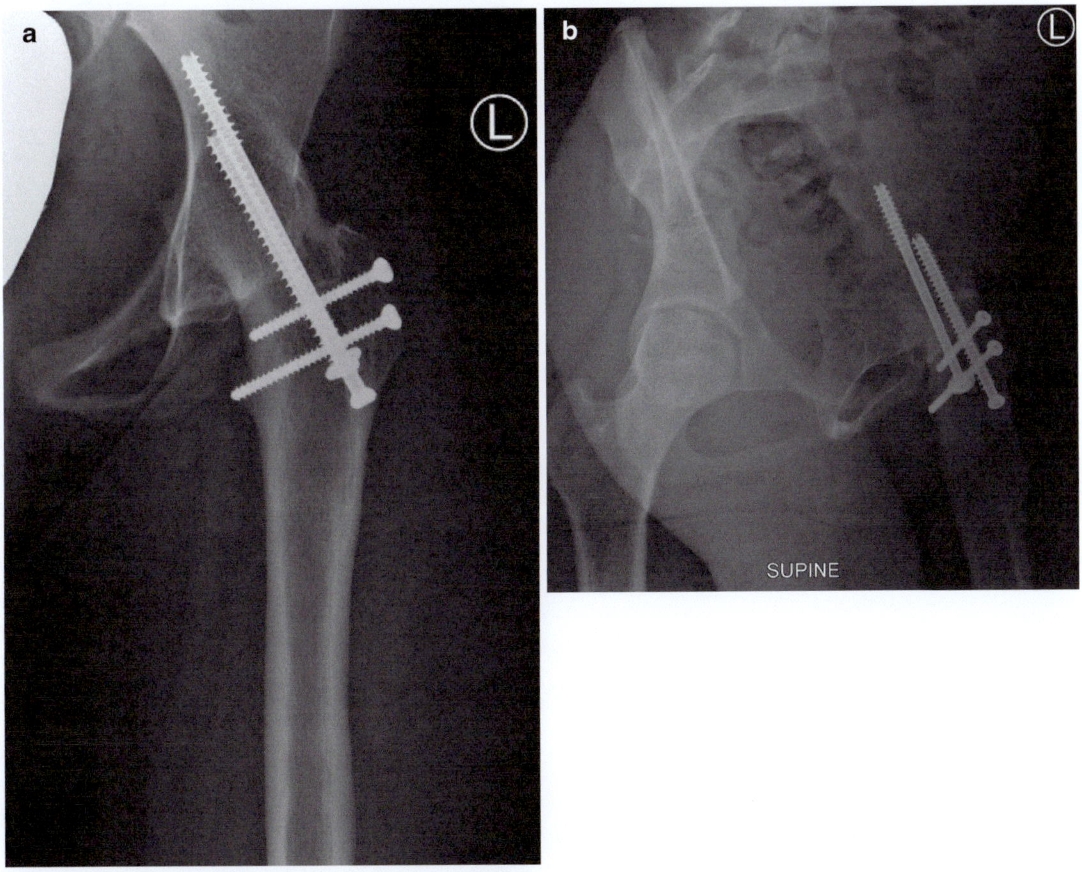

Fig. 36.9 Left hip anteroposterior (**a**) and lateral (**b**) radiographs showing a solid fusion of the hip and remodelling of the femoral osteotomy site at 2 years postoperative. (**c**) Standing anteroposterior full length lower extremity radiographs taken with a 1 cm lift reveal an overall good alignment with perhaps slightly excessive adduction

Fig. 36.9 (continued)

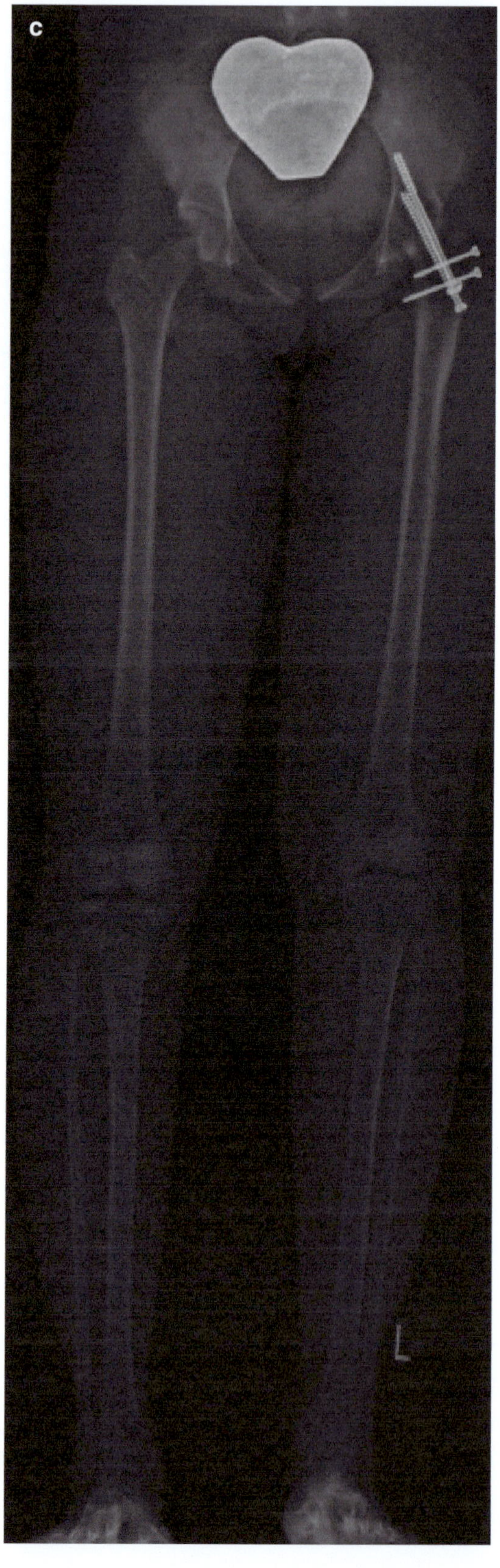

Pearls and Pitfalls

- The keys to a good outcome after a hip fusion are obtaining union, ensuring adequate alignment of the leg, and minimizing leg length discrepancy to <2 cm.
- The fusion position is 20–30° of hip flexion, 5° of adduction, and 5–10° of external rotation.
- The trochanteric osteotomy should not extend too distally, as this will result in a more challenging placement of the hip fixation screws.
- The fixation of the joint should be carefully templated along with the placement of the external fixator pins in the supraacetabular region. The hip fixation screws should remain as low in the supraacetabular bone as possible while allowing for a partially threaded screw to completely cross the joint. This will allow for stronger supraacetabular external fixation.
- The main problem postoperatively is drift of the osteotomy alignment through the ball-hinge into adduction and extension. In order to avoid this, the hinge can be cemented; however, this precludes any future realignment. Another approach is to monitor the alignment on a weekly basis and adjust it in clinic as necessary during the first 6 weeks of treatment. In addition, pillows should be kept under the leg whenever the patient is in the supine position to decrease the tendency towards extension.

Indications and Contraindications (Table 36.1)

Table 36.1 Hip arthrodesis using surgical hip dislocation and subtrochanteric osteotomy: surgical indications and contraindications

Indications
Painful severe joint disease in adolescent patient
Adolescent patient that is not a candidate for total hip arthroplasty
Young active labourer with painful stiff hip
Relative contraindications
Active avascular necrosis of femoral head (may increase risk of pseudarthrosis)
Contraindications
Potential polyarticular involvement (especially contralateral hip, lumbar spine or ipsilateral knee)
Osteoporosis
Active infection

References

1. Ganz R, Gill TJ, Gautier E, Ganz K, Krügel N, Berlemann U. Surgical dislocation of the adult hip: a technique with full access to the femoral head and acetabulum without the risk of avascular necrosis. J Bone Joint Surg Br. 2001;83(8):1119–24.
2. Benaroch TE, Richards BS, Haideri N, Smith C. Intermediate follow-up of a simple method of hip arthrodesis in adolescent patients. J Pediatr Orthop. 1996;16(1):30–6.

37 Combined Periacetabular and Proximal Femoral Osteotomies for Healed Perthes

Perry L. Schoenecker and John C. Clohisy

Introduction

Following the occurrence and healing of Legg-Calve-Perthes (LCP) in childhood, residual hip joint deformity of variable severity can occur, which is characterized by morphological features of both femoral acetabular impingement (FAI) and variable secondary relative acetabular deficiency. The femoral head is enlarged and aspherical and characteristically pathologically impinges against the acetabulum in hip flexion, in internal rotation in flexion and abduction. It also typically impinges in adduction. The femoral neck is relatively short, the greater trochanter high riding resulting in a functional coxa vara. The high-riding trochanter also potentiates both abductor insufficiency and extra-articular impingement. Secondarily, the acetabulum variably remodels in response to its long-standing articulation with a post-Perthes enlarged aspherical femoral head. If the acetabulum is dysplastic, both femoral head instability and labral-chondral rim overload can occur.

P. L. Schoenecker (✉) · J. C. Clohisy
Shriners Hospitals for Children, St. Louis, MO, USA

St. Louis Children's Hospital, St. Louis, MO, USA

Barnes-Jewish Hospital, St. Louis, MO, USA

Department of Orthopaedic Surgery, Washington University School of Medicine, St. Louis, MO, USA
e-mail: pschoenecker@shrinenet.org; clohisyj@wudosis.wustl.edu

Residual post-Perthes hip joint deformity can become symptomatically problematic in mid-adolescence with both restricted painful hip motion and discomfort while walking or running. Recently it has been shown that comprehensive correction of the complex problematic post-Perthes deformity (FAI impingement and acetabular dysplasia) can be achieved in order to preserve the hip joint. Following comprehensive correction, patients have experienced both resolution of hip joint pain and increased hip joint flexibility with a marked improvement in hip joint function.

Brief Clinical History and Preoperative Xrays

Patient is a 16-year-6-month-old male who had been treated for acute Legg-Calve-Perthes (LCP) (Fig. 37.1) at 7 years of age who presents now with a 1-year history of progressive left hip pain. Previously he had actively participated in high school sports but recently curtailed participation because of both groin and trochanteric pain (Fig. 37.2). On examination there is less than one-half inch leg length discrepancy (left being shorter than right) and positive Trendelenburg sign on the left. Range of motion of his right hip was 0–95° flexion with 10° internal rotation and 35° of external rotation in flexion, 35° abduction, 20° adduction, and a negative anterior impingement test. Range of motion of

R. C. Hamdy, N. Saran (eds.), *Pediatric Pelvic and Proximal Femoral Osteotomies*,
https://doi.org/10.1007/978-3-319-78033-7_37

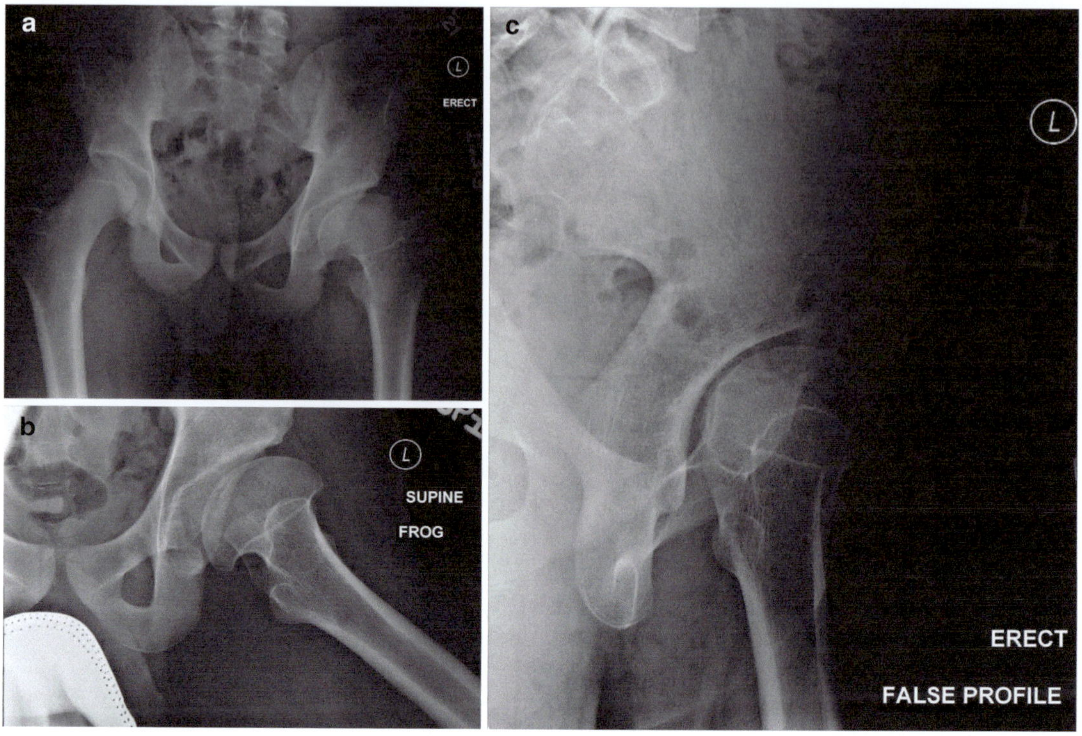

Fig. 37.1 (**a**) Anteroposterior, (**b**) frog lateral, and (**c**) false profile radiographs: note enlarged, aspherical femoral head; the femoral neck is relatively short and the greater trochanter high riding; the acetabulum is dysplastic; there is an increased Tönnis angle and decreased lateral and anterior coverage

the involved left hip was 0–90° flexion with 0° internal rotation and 20° external rotation in flexion, 25° abduction, and 15° adduction. The interior impingement test was very positive. Radiographs of the left hip demonstrated left hip coxa magna deformity with asphericity, a relative short neck, and high-riding trochanter. The acetabulum had become dysplastic though relatively congruent with the femoral head, Tönnis angle 21°, lateral center-edge angle (LCEA) 20°, anterior center-edge angle (ACEA) 5°, and lateral extrusion index (% head uncovered) 30%. The Tönnis arthritic grade was 0. The femoral head was circumferentially enlarged and aspherical and the acetabulum dysplastic on both anterior posterior and false profile views. A surgical approach that included an extensive proximal femoral reconstruction and anticipatedly acetabular reorientation was planned.

Goals of Treatment

The principles of treatment include:

- Eliminating femoroacetabular impingement by extensively reconstructing the proximal femur by removing the large cam deformity
- Improving abductor function and decreasing lateral trochanteric impingement by transferring the trochanter distally, which relatively increases the femoral neck length
- Restoring hip stability and femoral head coverage by redirecting the dysplastic acetabulum

Treatment Strategy

We have found that concomitant correction of both the cam and, as necessary, acetabular dysplasia pathology can be accomplished at the same setting and that doing so facilitates a patient's rehabilitation from comprehensive correction of all aspects of deformity. The hip joint is approached through the transtrochanteric surgical hip dislocation (SHD) which gives full access to the proximal femur and acetabulum. This approach provides the surgeon the ability to reconstruct deformity of all aspects of the hip joint. The large aspherical femoral head can be effectively reduced in size and recontoured with a peripheral osteochondroplasty. The trochanter is reattached distally, which effectively lengthens the functional femoral neck. The acetabulum is inspected; the labral-chondral complex reattached or debrided as necessary. The Bernese periacetabular osteotomy (PAO) allows for redirection of the acetabulum rather precisely to optimize coverage and minimize any potential iatrogenic-induced impingement. A surgical team approach facilitates performing both of these extensive procedures at the same surgical setting. In the end, improved flexibility in both daily and athletic activities predictably occurs given appropriate patient selection.

Surgical Details

Surgical Hip Dislocation

The proximal femoral and intra-articular hip joint post-Perthes deformity is addressed first. The patient is positioned in the lateral decubitus position optimally stabilized with a peg board support (see Fig. 37.2). The hip joint is exposed through the SHD approach. The lateral fascia and gluteus

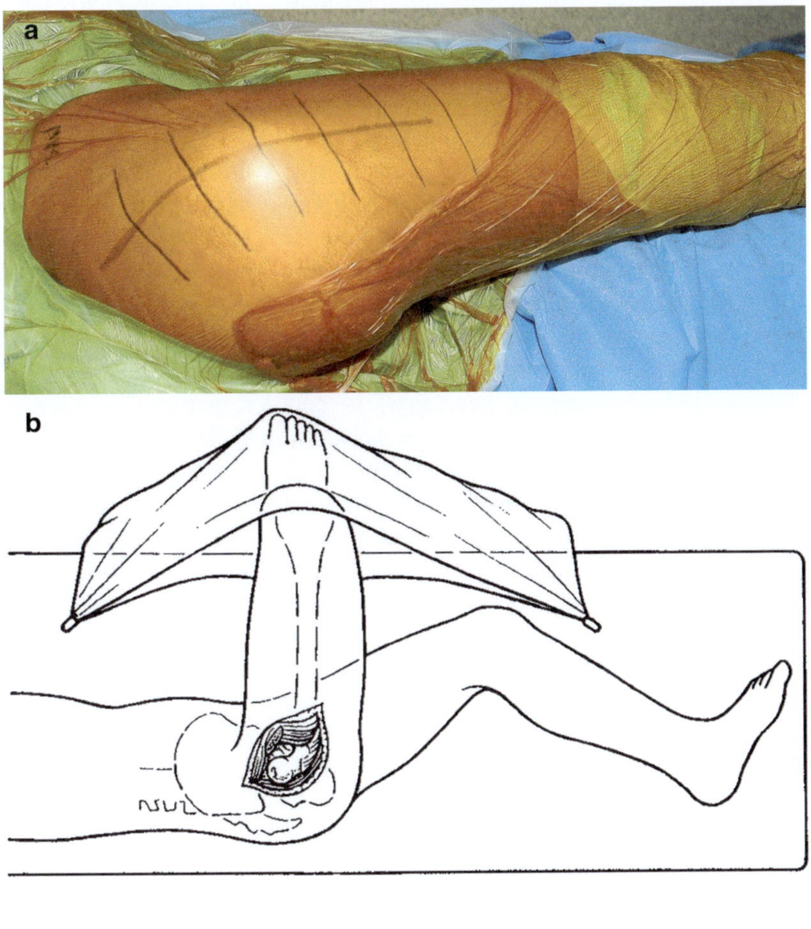

Fig. 37.2 (**a**) Intended incision for performing surgical hip dislocation and (**b**) diagram demonstrating dislocation of right hip following capsulotomy, flexion, and external rotation of right hip joint and cutting the ligamentum teres

maximus are longitudinally incised, and the piriformis tendon is identified at its attachment to the proximal greater trochanter. The trochanter is osteotomized from posterior to anterior, ideally through the most lateral attachment of the piriformis to the greater trochanter base. This will protect the lateral retinaculum containing the terminal branches of the medial circumflex artery as those vessels enter into the lateral femoral neck. The vastus muscle (lateralis and intermedius) and gluteus medius and minimus muscles proximally are together with the trochanter reflected medially to the reflected head of the rectus muscle exposing the hip capsule. The capsule is incised in a Z fashion and the femoral head dislocated by variably flexing, externally rotating, and adducting the leg. The ease of being able to dislocate the hip with residual Perthes deformity is variable; it may be difficult to dislocate given a relatively tighter hip capsule with a shorter femoral neck and long-standing deformity. Continued manipulation and a firm push in a posterior direction can be helpful. The ligamentum teres must be transected.

Once dislocated, the entire femoral head and acetabulum can be inspected (Fig. 37.3). Labral morphology varies, often enlarged with significant labral-chondral instability. Acetabular cartilaginous surface lesion (chondromalacia and also focal lesions) is more likely to be present in relatively more severely impinged hips. Small and/or superficial flap tears are appropriately debrided sharply. Microfractures are performed on full thickness defects. Labral repair, if necessary, is performed later, after completing the proximal femoral osteochondroplasty and relative neck lengthening. The surface of the entire femoral head is inspected for focal surface lesions and/or discoloration. Typically there will be demarcated areas with a light pinkish discoloration on the femoral head articular surface (no doubt secondary to areas of high joint stress) anterolaterally and similarly around the fovea. Small superficial defects are sharply debrided and focal small full thickness defects microfractured. The hip is examined in flexion, internal rotation in flexion, and abduction, noting areas of pathological impingement (anteriorly, anterolaterally, and laterally). The osteochondroplasty reshaping of the relatively large femoral head is outlined initially with a 15 mm curved osteotome raising contiguous flaps of cartilage and bone. The resection starts proximally and typically includes that portion of the femoral head that pathologically impinges against the acetabulum (impingement grooves, bumps, and/or portions of the pinkish discolored cartilage and underlying bone). Typically the largest resection is performed anterolaterally and extending also posteriorly (and proximally) to the lateral retinaculum (Fig. 37.4). A fine-tipped Doppler probe is used to identify (if possible) the pulse in the lateral retinaculum. The bone removal is extensively contoured and completed using a high-speed burr.

The short femoral neck and prominent trochanter deformity are corrected by resecting the proximal trochanteric base and then later reattaching the trochanter distally, which achieves relative lengthening of the femoral neck (Fig. 37.5). The proximal trochanteric base is resected with a meticulous technique utilizing the extended retinaculum technique developed by Ganz; the periosteum and external rotators are dissected away from the proximal base of the trochanter. Again, detection of the terminal branches of the medical circumflex vessel within the lateral retinaculum with the Doppler probe is very helpful in assuring a safe resection. The trochanter bony base is carefully excised in a piecemeal manner off of the surrounding soft tissues (Fig. 37.6). The extent of the proximal trochanter base resection is estimated by examining a preoperative anteroposterior hip x-ray. The proximal extent of the distally reattached trochanter should be on a horizontal line connecting the tip of the reattached trochanter and center of the femoral head. The anterior lateral trochanteric base prominence often impinges against the acetabulum. It is removed by sculpting with a burr,

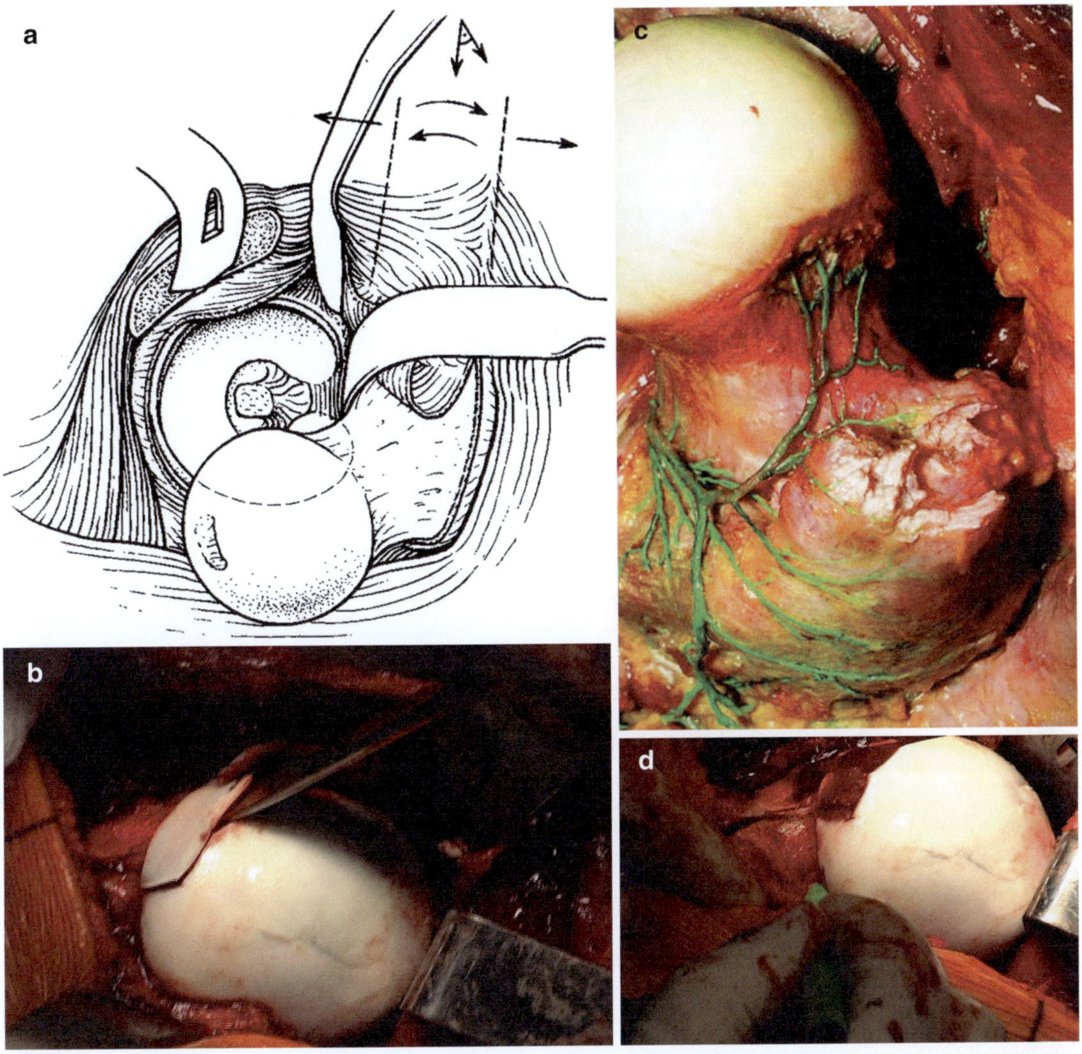

Fig. 37.3 (**a**) Diagram demonstrating anterolateral femoral head dislocation allowing for access to the entire hip joint; (**b**) curved osteotome elevation of osteocartilaginous flaps from anterolateral proximal femur; (**c**) photo of cadaver dissection and injection showing terminal branches of medical circumflex vessel entering into the lateral head neck junction; (**d**) marking site of same vessel location intraoperatively

developing a smooth gradual contour from the base of the trochanter extending proximally to the head neck resection.

The hip is reduced and assessed for any residual areas of impingement of the anterolateral femoral head and neck and the base of the trochanter against the rim of the acetabulum (Fig. 37.7). Similarly, a decision is made at this time regarding relative hip instability. The hip is tested for posterior instability in flexion/adduction and internal rotation and anterior instability in extension and external rotations. Noted subluxation, major head displacement, or frank dislocation suggests the need for performing a PAO. Typically hips with a preoperative relatively dysplastic acetabulae will be relatively unstable on the table following osteochondroplasty. These hips also usually have motion sufficient to

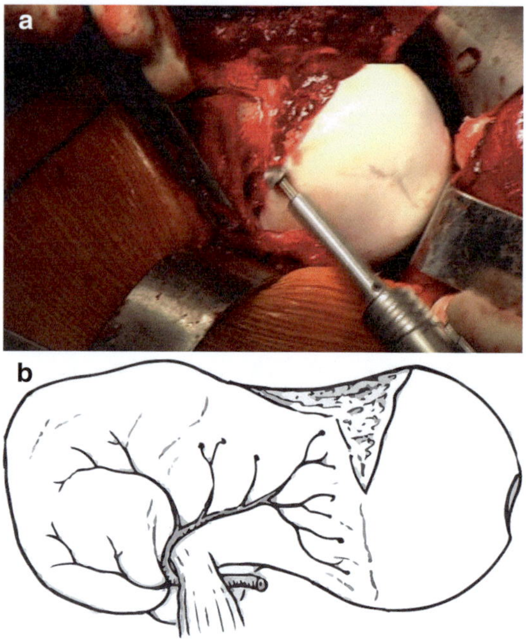

Fig. 37.4 (**a**) Extending the osteochondroplasty with a 65 mm power burr posteriorly (**b**) but proximal to and above vessel entrance into the proximal femur

tolerate a PAO to enhance stability. If needed we typically proceed with the PAO at the same setting (Fig. 37.8).

Having completed the bone reshaping of the proximal femur, the labral-chondral complex is repaired as necessary. Often the unstable hypertrophied anterolateral labrum can be securely reattached to the anterolateral surface of the acetabular rim with #2 suture anchors (typically 2 or 3 in number). The capsule is loosely reapproximated and the trochanter optimally advanced and securely reattached with two or three large fragment cortical screws as confirmed with the C-arm. The wound is closed in layers.

Periacetabular Osteotomy

If a PAO is to be done, the patient is repositioned still on the x-ray translucent table in a supine position, reprepped, and draped. The pelvis is exposed anteriorly through a modified Smith-Peterson approach. The rectus muscle typically is

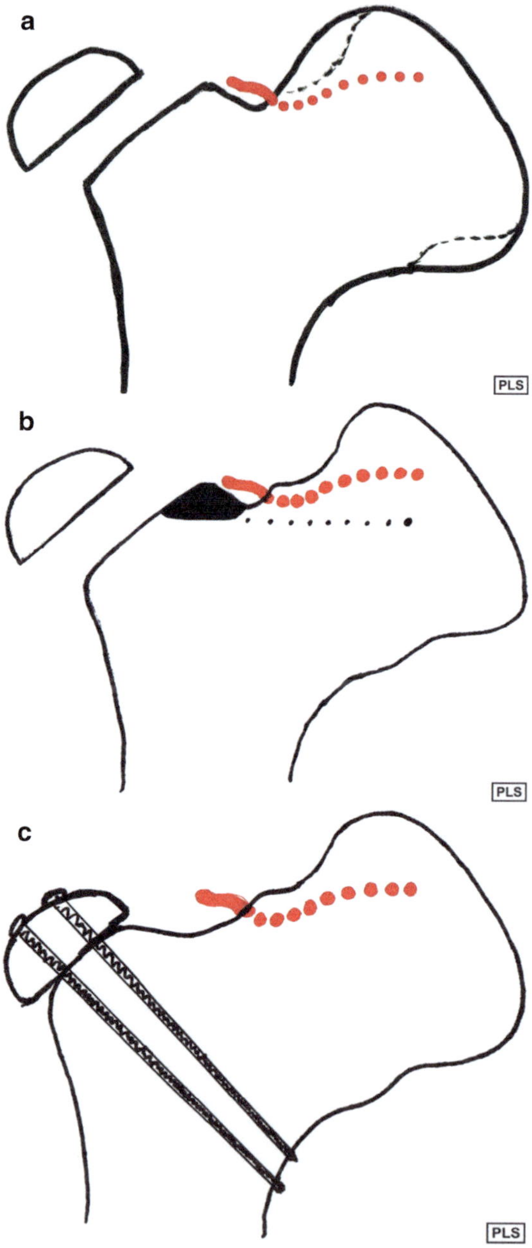

Fig. 37.5 (**a**) Diagramatic illustration of trochanteric osteotomy, avoiding injury to medial circumflex vessels entering the proximal femur and intended lines of head neck osteochondroplasty; (**b**) *dotted line* shows the planned extent of necessary resection of proximal aspect of the base of the trochanter (*solid black*), so when reattached later, the proximal edge of the trochanter will be at the same level as the center of the head; (**c**) following completion of above and distal reattachment of the trochanter effecting a relatively lengthening of the femoral head

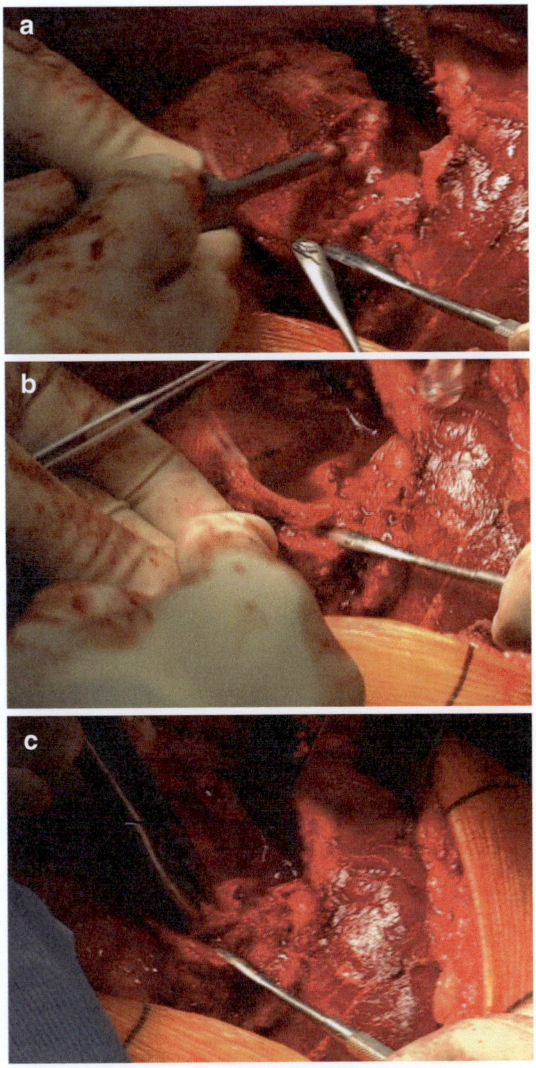

Fig. 37.6 (**a**) Resecting proximal portion of trochanteric base; (**b**) reflection of short external rotators (and vessel); (**c**) completion of resection

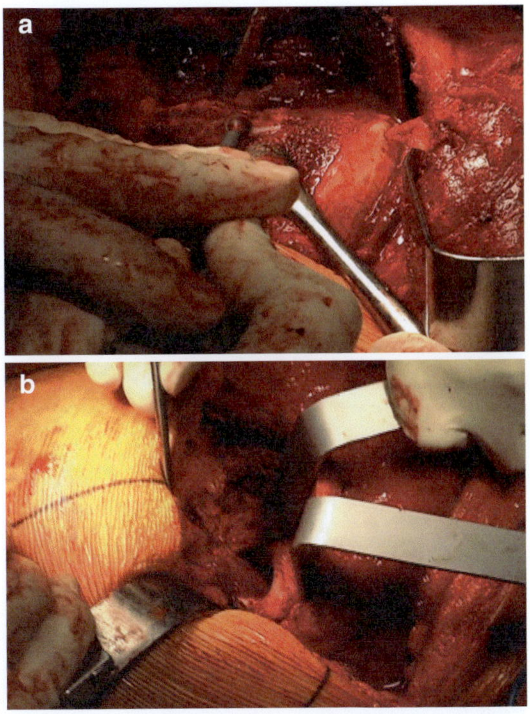

Fig. 37.7 (**a**) Final resection to affect a smooth contouring from base of trochanter to femoral head reestablishing a more normal offset; (**b**) hip flexion/internal rotation now possible without impingement

not transected. The Bernese PAO is completed with four orthogonal cuts. (Fig. 37.9) In performing the ischial (first cut) and/or the superior public ramus (second cut), the surgeon must be cognizant that a capsulotomy had been done during the previously completed surgical hip dislocation; it is possible to inadvertently enter the hip joint in performing the first or second cuts. Once the acetabular fragment is mobilized, it is redirected so as to optimize coverage laterally and anteriorly, medialize as indicated, and assure version is correct (Figs. 37.10 and 37.11). Having completed the extensive osteochondroplasty, the markedly improved hip range of motion greatly facilitates the ease of redirecting the acetabulum. This both enables correction of the hip instability and preserves satisfactory functional range of motion. In the end, correction obtained is adjusted so as to assure there is at least 90° flexion and 25° abduction. Having obtained satisfactory coverage, the acetabular fragment is securely fixed utilizing large fragment screws. The amount of correction achieved depends on the flexibility of the hip.

Patients are mobilized on postoperative day 1, using touchdown weight bearing and discharged on postoperative day 2 or 3. Follow-up radiographs are obtained at 4 weeks postoperatively and weight bearing advanced as tolerated. Typically by 6–8 weeks, early healing of both osteotomies will be demonstrated on radiographs. Patients are instructed and monitored on a comprehensive

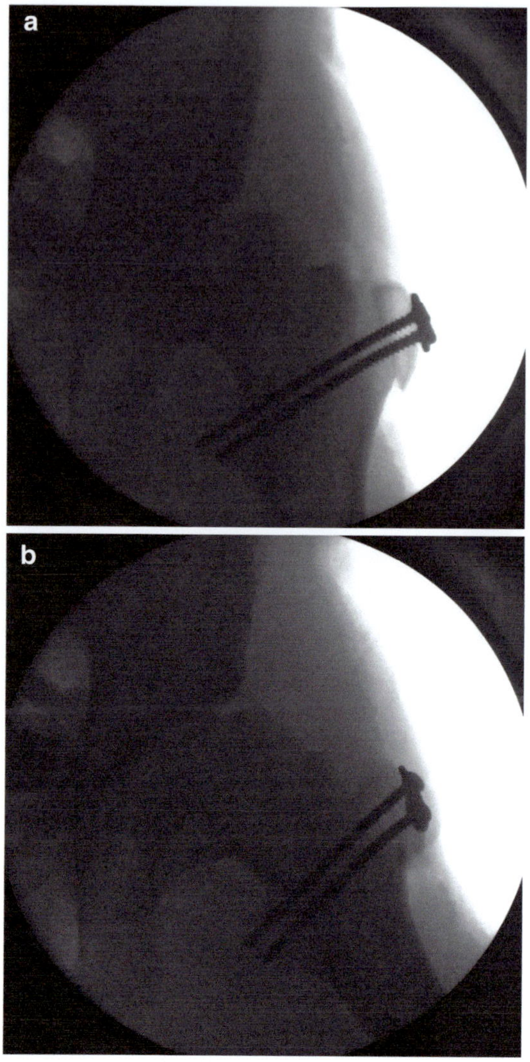

Fig. 37.8 (**a**) Intraoperative anteroposterior fluoroscopy after proximal femoral osteochondroplasty and distal transfer of the trochanter, congruent articulation with deficient lateral coverage; (**b**) hip abduction (simulates) potential improved coverage effect of performing a periacetabular osteotomy

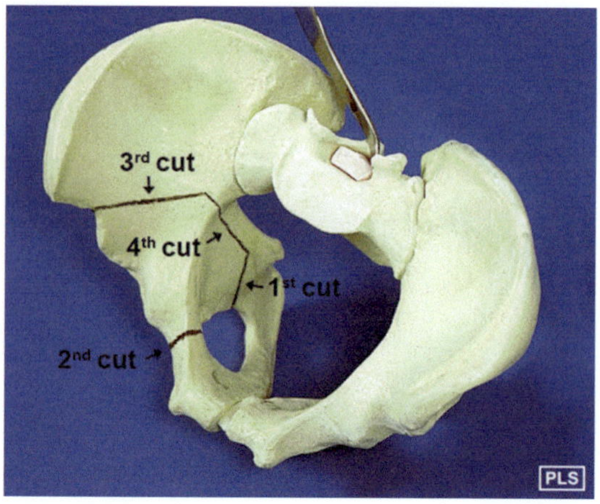

Fig. 37.9 *Arrow* at site of ischial (*first cut*) starting anteriorly and directed posteriorly (distal to the acetabulum) ending within the ischium at the mid-base of the ischial spine. *Arrow* at site of superior: pubic ramus (*second cut*) directed in an anterior to posterior and ideally directed lateral to medial plane. *Arrow* at site of iliac (*third cut*) directed from lateral to medial started just distal to the anterior superior iliac spine (ASIS) and ending lateral to the pelvic brim at level corresponding to the middle of the sciatic notch. *Arrow* at site of posterior column (*fourth cut*) starting at the medial extent of the iliac (*third cut*) and directed at angle of 120° from the iliac cut down the posterior column, connecting with the first ischial cut

rehabilitation program, including strengthening throughout postoperative months 2–6. Recreational activities may be resumed postoperatively at 6 months. Return to competitive sports is discouraged postoperatively until 9–12 months. The comprehensive correction of all aspects of the complex post-Perthes deformity optimizes the potential for achieving the desired outcome of both increased joint mobility and stability and, most importantly, relief from functional pain.

Pearls and Pitfalls

- Patient selection is essential. Patients with problematic symptoms (pain and stiffness that notably limit activity and radiographic post-Perthes deformity with minimal evidence of arthritis) have the optimal chance of achieving a desired outcome. Joint motion improves, stability is achieved, and patients have relief from functional hip pain. This extensive procedure is not indicated in patients with post-Perthes hip deformity but without notable complaints of pain and/or functional limitations. Similarly, it is contraindicated in patients with severely restricted and painful

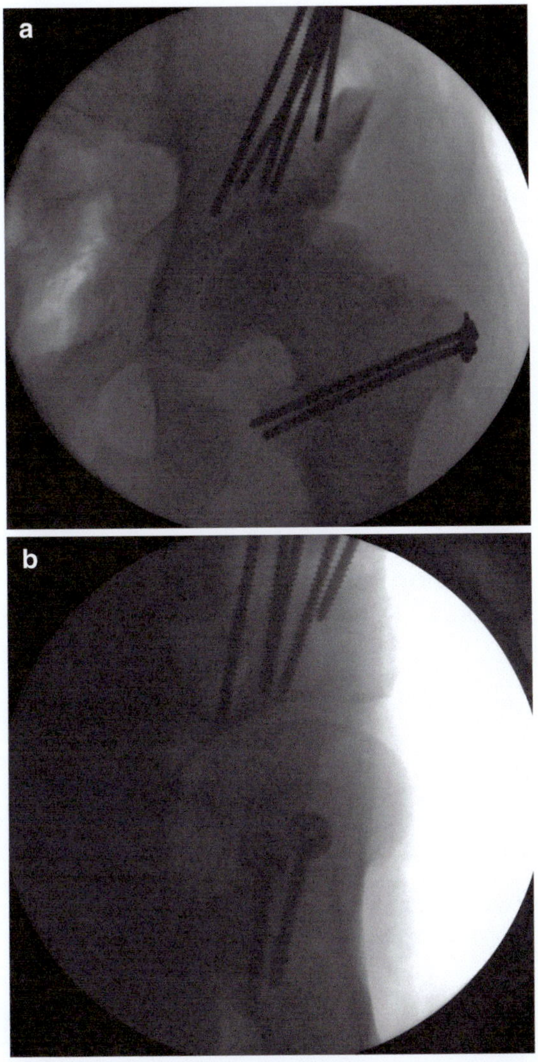

Fig. 37.10 (**a**) Anterior posterior view post-completion of a periacetabular osteotomy showing improved lateral coverage; (**b**) improved anterior coverage noted on false profile view

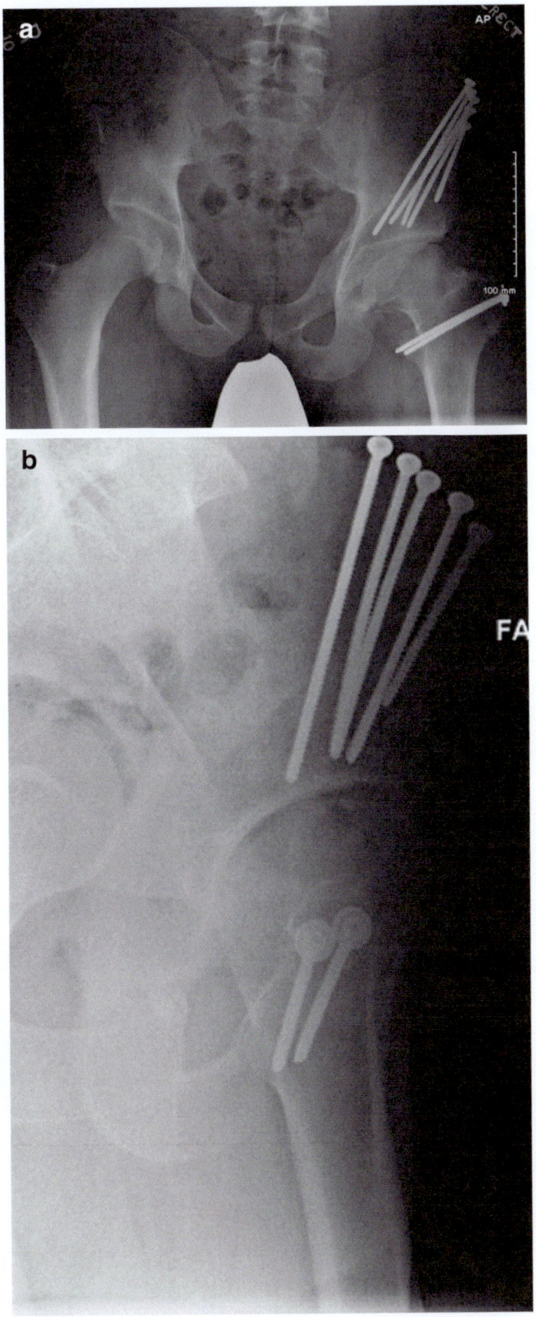

Fig. 37.11 (**a**) Anterior posterior and (**b**) false profile radiographs: periacetabular osteotomy and trochanter osteotomies are head; coverage improved both laterally and anteriorly, congruent articulation; patient has returned to full activities

motion. If performed in patients with notable preoperative arthritis findings (stiff and painful on exam and, for instance, Tönnis arthritic type II x-ray changes), worsening problematic postoperative joint stiffness may preclude a satisfactory clinical outcome.

- It is necessary to first perform the surgical hip dislocation and capsulotomy (for purposes of achieving a proximal femoral reconstruction and labral-chondral repair). Later when doing the PAO, caution must be taken in performing either the infra-acetabular ischial (first cut) or second superior pelvic ramus cut (second cut) to assure the osteotome is not inadvertently inserted into the hip joint injuring the acetabular labrum.

- We are less aggressive in obtaining correction deficiency with post-Perthes deformity than we are in the treatment of primary acetabular dysplasia. Following K-wire fixation of the redirected acetabulum, it is critical to carefully examine hip motion; coverage achieved must be adjusted so as to assure there is at least 90° flexion and 25–30° abduction. Relative overcorrection carries a high risk of further impingement pain for the patient.
- In some hips it is sometimes questionable preoperatively as to whether a PAO will be needed to stabilize relative hip instability noted after performing a capsulotomy and reducing the size of the femoral head. We initially staged the PAO weeks after reconstructing the proximal femur. We soon found it relatively easier on the patient and quite technically possible to, if necessary, always perform the two procedures at the same setting. With time, our technique has improved; the time necessary to complete both procedures is notably less as is blood loss. We now always plan to perform as indicated both procedures when indicated at the same setting.

Indications and Contraindications (Table 37.1)

Table 37.1 Combined periacetabular and proximal femoral osteotomies for healed Perthes: surgical indications and contraindications

	Indications	Contraindications
Range of motion (ROM)	0–90° extension/flexion >30° combined rotation >30° combined abduction/adduction	<90° flexion <30° combined rotation >30° combined abduction/adduction
Pain	Relatively pain free throughout mid-arc on ROM assessment; painful more so at end points	Painful during much of mid-arc as well as end points
Radiographic evidence of arthritis	<Tönnis 1	>Tönnis 1
Stulberg classification (i.e., congruency)	I–III, ±IV	V
Age	<25 (maybe older for a physiologic outlier)	>25

Suggested Reading

Clohisy JC, Nepple JJ, Pashos G, Schoenecker PL. What are the factors associated with acetabular correction in Perthes-like hip deformities? Clin Orthop Relat Res. 2012;470(12):3439–45.

Clohisy JC, Ross JR, North JD, Nepple JJ, Schoenecker PL. Does surgical hip dislocation and periacetabular osteotomy improve pain in patients with Perthes-like deformities and acetabular dysplasia? Clin Orthop Relat Res. 2015;473(4):1370–7.

Ganz R, Gill TJ, Gautier E, Ganz K, Krügel N, Berlemann U. Surgical dislocation of the adult hip: a technique with full access to the femoral head and acetabulum without the risk of avascular necrosis. J Bone Joint Surg Br. 2001;83(8):1119–24.

Ganz R, Huff TW, Leunig M. Extended retinacular soft-tissue flap for intra-articular hip surgery: surgical technique, indications, and results of application. Instr Course Lect. 2009;58:241–55.

Gautier E, Ganz K, Krugel N, Gill T, Ganz R. Anatomy of the medial femoral circumflex artery and its surgical implications. J Bone Joint Surg Br. 2000;82(5):679–83.

Schoenecker PL, Lewis TR, Clohisy JC. Treatment of combined structural instability and FAI (Perthes deformities). In: Clohisy JC, Beaulé PE, Della Valle CJ, Callaghan JJ, Rosenberg AG, Rubash HE, editors. The adult hip: hip preservation surgery. Philadelphia: Wolters Kluwer; 2015. p. 605–20.

Femoral Head Reduction Osteotomy

38

Dror Paley and David S. Feldman

Introduction

Femoral head reduction osteotomy (FHRO) is the surgical treatment of choice for a misshapen (nonspherical) and enlarged (coxa magna) femoral head in a spherical acetabulum, most often occurring as a sequela of Legg–Calves–Perthes disease, but also arising secondary to skeletal dysplasia and avascular necrosis. Left untreated, the nonspherical femoral head will cause pain due to femoro-acetabular impingement and subsequent femoro-acetabular cartilage damage and labral tear.

The aim of the FHRO is to restore sphericity in a non-spherically shaped femoral head. This technique was originally concieved by Reinhold Ganz (2002) using a safe surgical dislocation technique with resection of the central third of the femoral head to convert an ellipsoid to a sphere again using osteotomies inclined with the femoral neck [1] (Fig. 38.1a, Fig. 38.2 (left)). It was modified by Paley (2011) both changing the orientation of the osteotomy to more horizontal to the femoral neck and including wedge resection for biplanar reduction compared to the parallel cuts proposed by Ganz [2, 3] (Fig. 38.1b, Fig. 38.2 (center)). Another recent FHRO (2016) (Fig. 2 (right)) is using an anterior approach, avoiding the piriformis fossa and hinging on the medial calcar [5].The alternative to FHRO is osteochondroplasty with relative neck lengthening [4]. This technique removes the lateral/anterior protuberance of the femoral head to reduce impingement, while preserving the central portion of the femoral head. The best indication for osteochondroplasty is when the lateral portion of the femoral head is nonspherical or has significant cartilage damage [4]. In most cases however, the central portion is the location of impingement and damage and the lateral portion is spherical and remains well preserved. The FHRO is indicated in these central impingement/damage cases since it does not make sense to resect the good lateral cartilage and preserve the damaged central cartilage.

D. Paley (✉) · D. S. Feldman
Paley Orthopedic and Spine Institute, St. Mary's Medical Center, West Palm Beach, FL, USA
e-mail: dpaley@paleyinstitute.org

Brief Clinical History and Imaging

Patient 1 (Fig. 38.3a–r) Fifteen-year-old girl with history of left-sided Perthes disease since age eight, treated non-operatively with rest, casting, and physical therapy. She developed left hip pain a year prior to presentation. The pain was brought on by activity and prolonged sitting. She had a mild lurch to the left, which got worse as the day progressed. On examination she had pain on flexion with internal rotation of the hip. The hip range of motion was: flexion 0–90°, internal rotation 5°, external rotation 45°, adduction 20°, and abduction 15°.

R. C. Hamdy, N. Saran (eds.), *Pediatric Pelvic and Proximal Femoral Osteotomies*,
https://doi.org/10.1007/978-3-319-78033-7_38

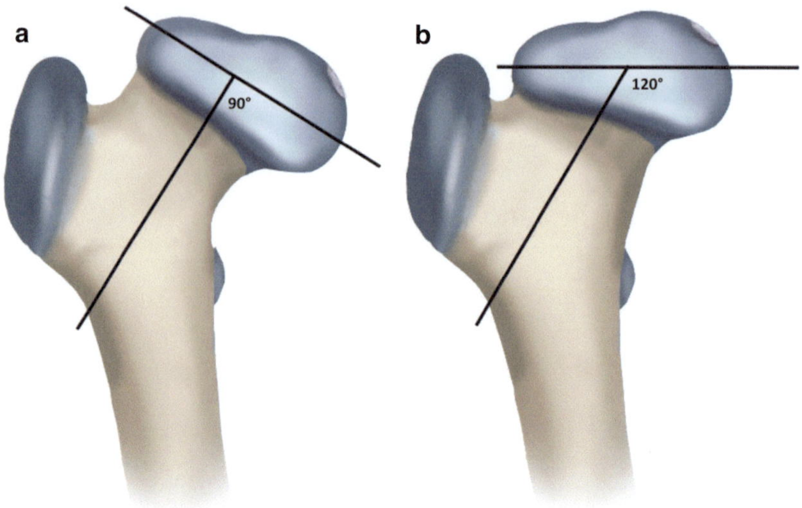

Fig. 38.1 (**a**) elongation of femoral head perpendicular to femoral neck; (**b**) elongaton of femoral head not perpendicular to the femoral neck (© 2017 The Paley Foundation, with permission. All rights reserved)

Patient 2 (Fig. 38.4a–m) Fourteen-year-old boy with history of right-sided Perthes since age 11 (see Fig. 38.2a), treated non-operatively by range of motion exercises. He became significantly disabled by the progressive collapse and misshapen femoral head. He had a significant antalgic lurch to the right. On examination his hip flexion was 0–90° with obligatory external rotation. He had 45° prone hip internal rotation and 10° prone hip external rotation. His hip abduction was 15°. He had a leg length discrepancy (see Fig. 38.4b).

Patient 1 Preoperative (AP) and frog pelvis radiograph demonstrated coxa magna with coxa breva and high greater trochanter (GT) (Fig. 38.3a). Her 3D CT scan demonstrated an enlarged femoral head with anterolateral extrusion of the femoral head from the confines of the acetabulum (Fig. 38.1b).

Patient 2 Preoperative radiographs (Fig. 38.4c, d) showed coxa magna, coxa breva, and a saddle shaped femoral head. The GT was overgrown. The acetabulum had not remodeled to the enlarged femoral head.

Goals of Treatment

- Convert an aspherical shaped femoral head to a spherical shaped femoral head.
- Eliminate any residual femoro-acetabular impingement by osteochondroplasty.
- Reduction of coxa magna to normal sized femoral head.
- Change from coxa breva to a relatively longer femoral neck.
- Advance the overgrown GT.
- Identify and repair labral tear.
- Restore normal femoral head coverage.

Treatment Strategy

- Determine preoperatively whether the elongation of the head is perpendicular to the femoral neck or not (Fig. 38.1a, b). For elongation perpendicular to the neck a Ganz type of FHRO is preferred (Fig. 38.2 (left)) while for elongation not perpendicular to the femoral neck the Paley type of FHRO is preferred. Then determine if it is a type A or type B

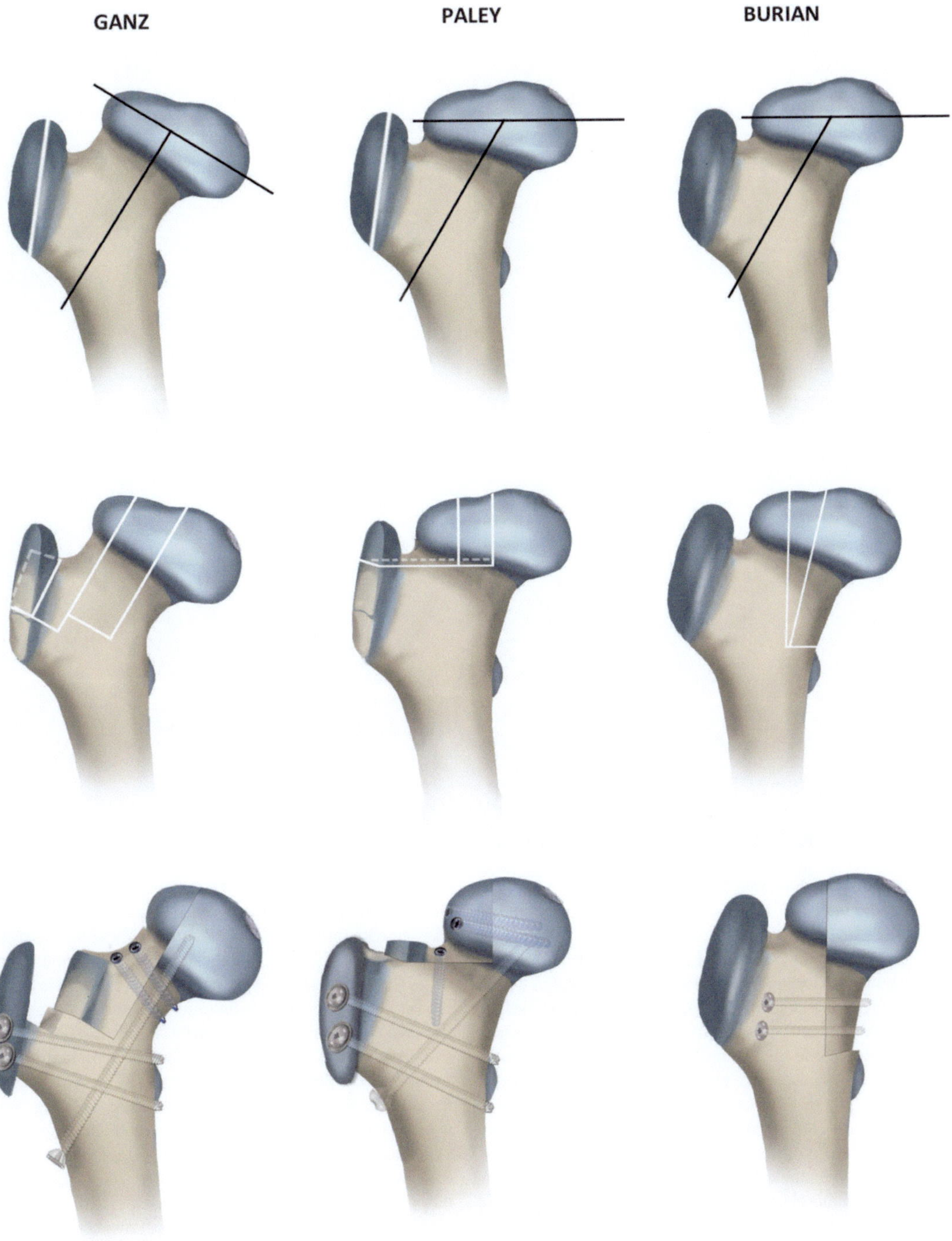

Fig. 38.2 (*left*) Ganz type of FHRO, (*center*) Paley type of FHRO, (*right*) Burian et al type of FHRO (© 2017 The Paley Foundation, with permission. All rights reserved)

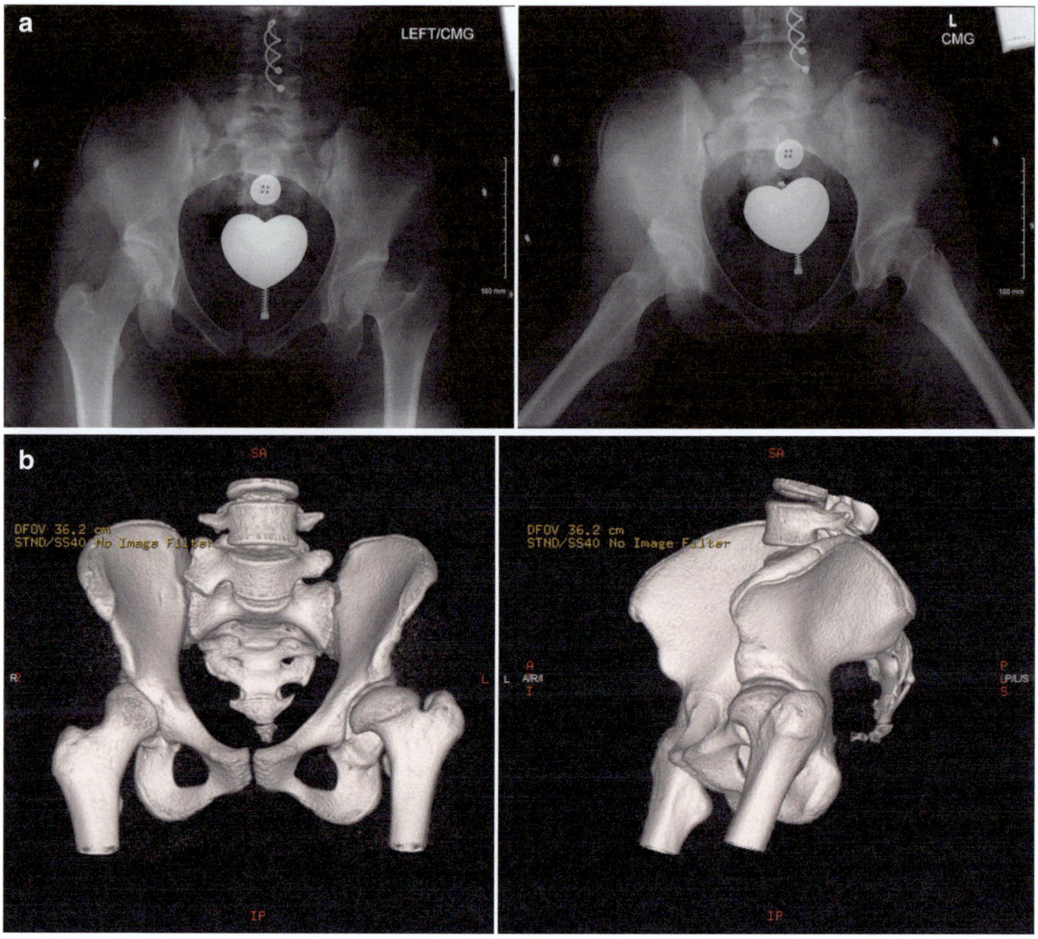

Fig. 38.3 (**a**) Preoperative anteroposterior (AP) and frog lateral radiographs of 15-year-old girl with coxa magna, coxa breva, and overgrown trochanter sequelae from previous Perthes. (**b**) 3D computed tomography AP and lateral views showing coxa magna and uncovered, elongated femoral head. (**c**) Postoperative AP radiograph showing healed femoral head reduction osteotomy with level of greater trochanter restored and relative neck lengthening. The femoral head coverage is inadequate and a periacetabular osteotomy (PAO) is required. (**d**) Final AP radiograph after femoral head reduction osteotomy and Ganz type PAO. There is excellent coverage of the femoral head. (**e**) AP femur radiograph after implantable limb lengthening to equalize limb lengths. The femoral head remains round, located, well covered and the hip shows and excellent joint space with no degeneration. (**f**) Intraoperative photograph showing superior view of femoral head after dislocation. The diameter of the femoral head is measured with a caliper. This is a Type A femoral head. (**g**) Intraoperative photograph showing acetabular sizer in place. (**h**) Intraoperative photograph showing femoral spherical template corresponding to acetabular size measured. The lateral side of the template is where the femoral head leaves the round. (**i**) Intraoperative photograph showing a caliper measuring the width of the medial femoral head at the point where the femoral head leaves the round. (**j**) Intraoperative photograph showing lateral part of femoral head measured for the remainder of the diameter of the femoral head after the planned reduction. This width is marked. (**k**) Intraoperative photograph showing the osteotomy lines for resection of the central portion of the femoral head. (**l**) Intraoperative photograph from anterior view of the femoral head showing the baseline osteotomy planned with the two superior osteotomy lines marked. This baseline extends to the trochanteric osteotomy laterally. (**m**) Intraoperative photograph showing the superior osteotomy is being made with a thin sagittal saw which is being cooled with water. (**n**) Intraoperative photograph showing the lateral fragment reduced to the medial fragment and being fixed with a headless variable pitch screw. Note that the posterior reduction is prioritized. (**o**) Intraoperative photograph showing the reduced femoral head with two headless screws in place. The posterior femoral head is very congruous and spherical. There is mild anterior incongruity. The lateral femoral protrudes anteriorly beyond the medial femoral head. (**p**) Intraoperative photograph showing the anterior femoral head incongruity. The spherical template rests on the posterior femoral head and demonstrates the step off. (**q**) Intraoperative photograph showing the excellent posterior congruity with no step off. (**r**) Intraoperative photographs showing the step off reduced by performing an anterolateral osteochondroplasty

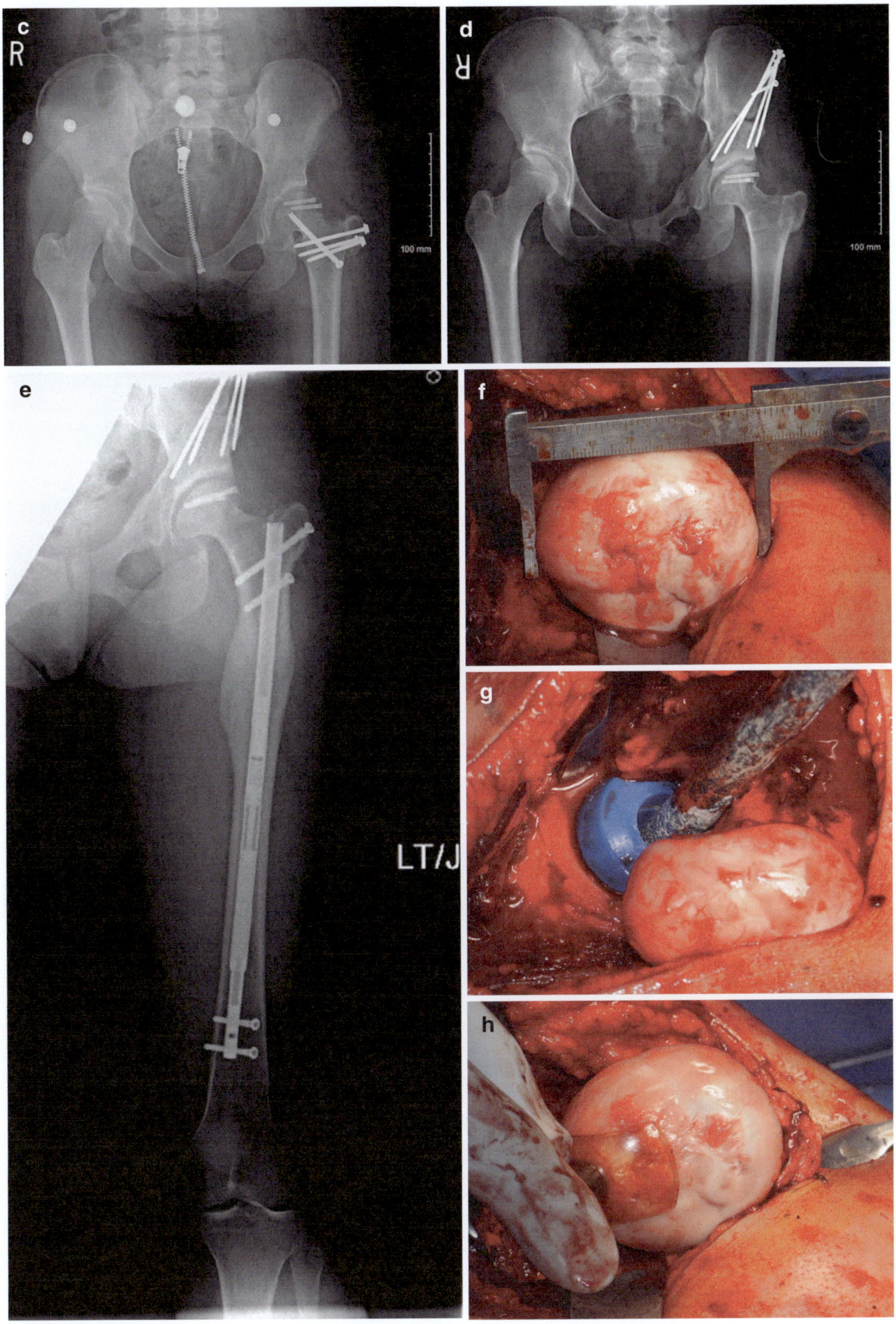

Fig. 38.3 (continued)

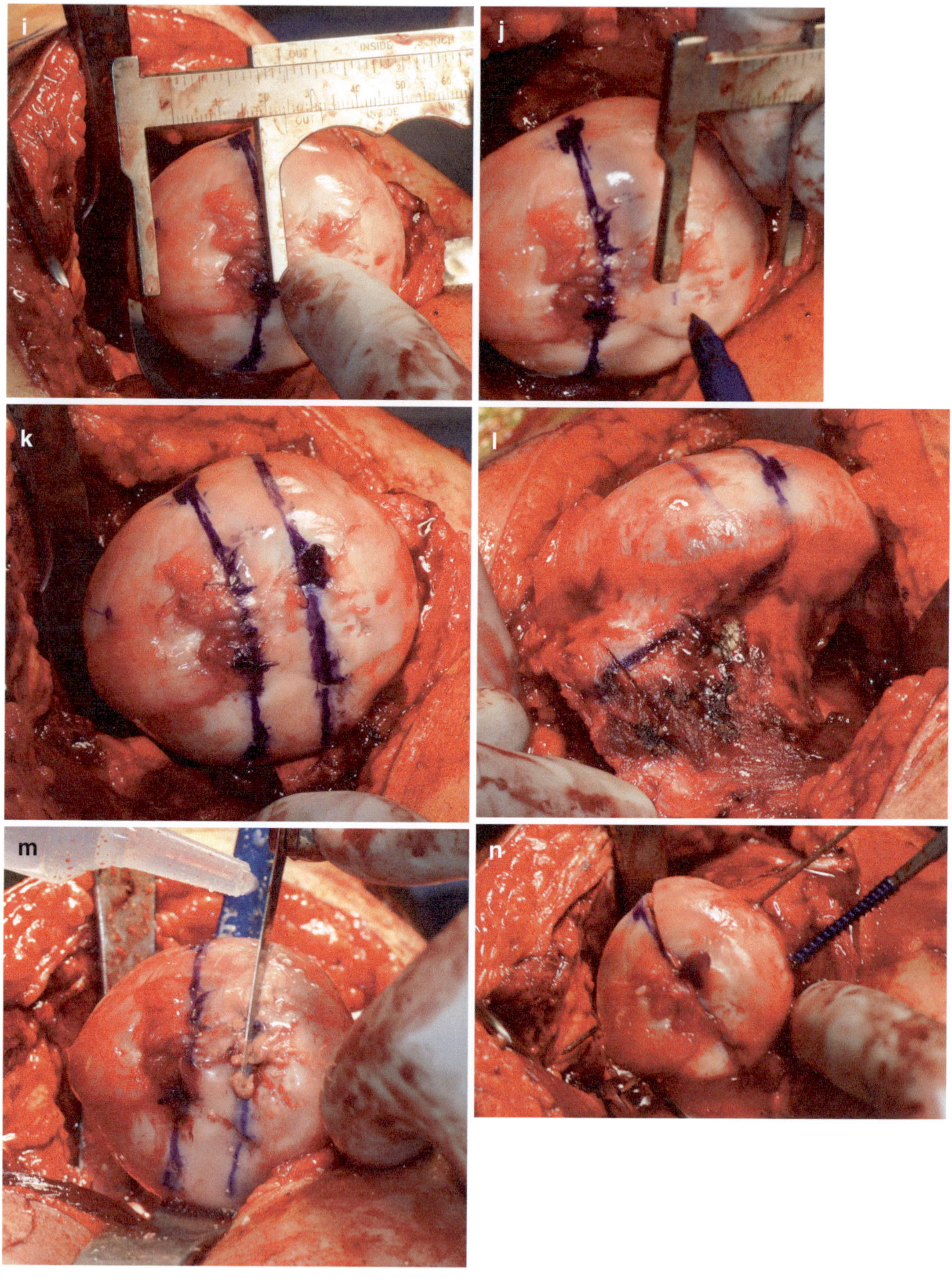

Fig. 38.3 (continued)

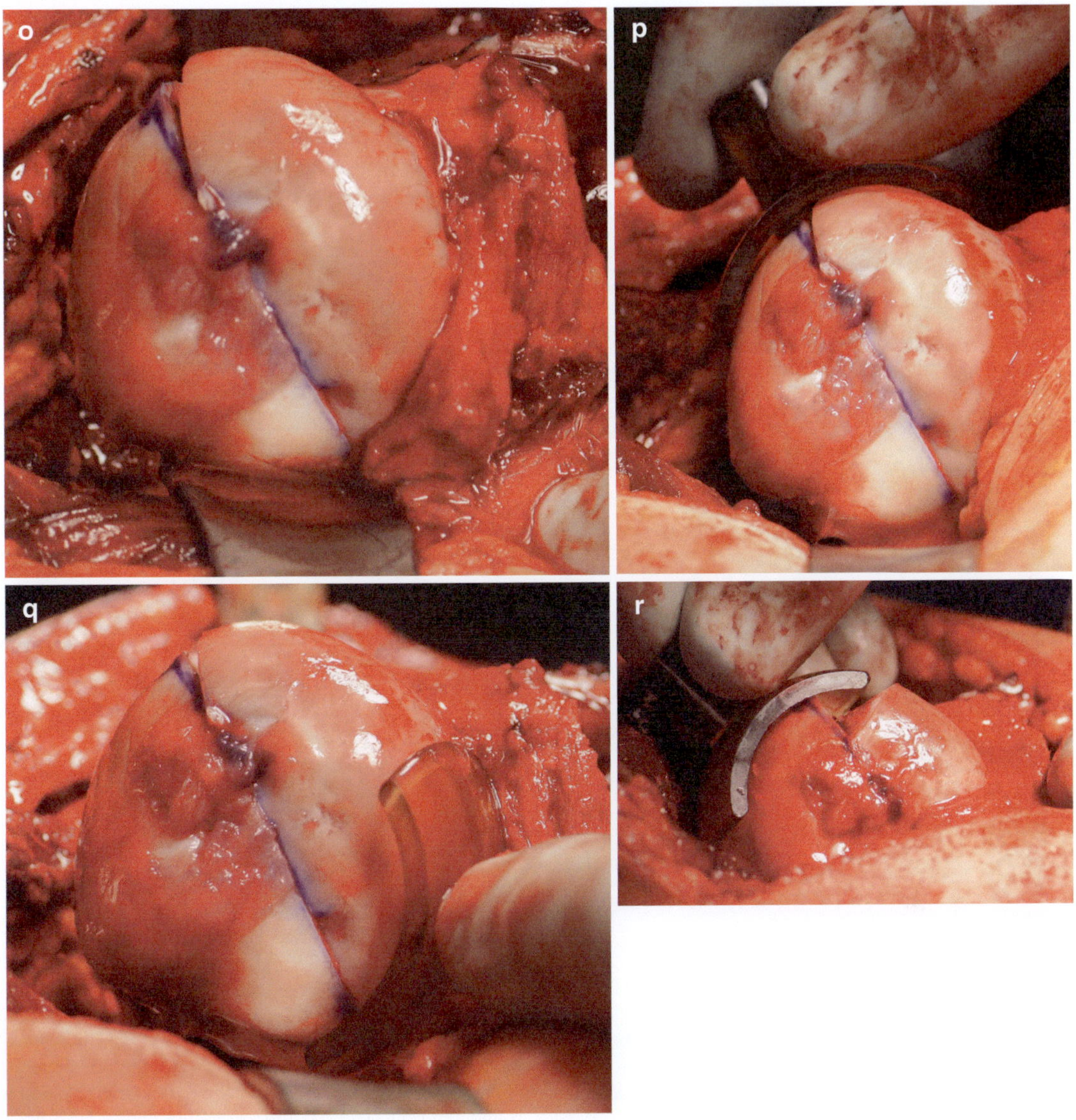

Fig. 38.3 (continued)

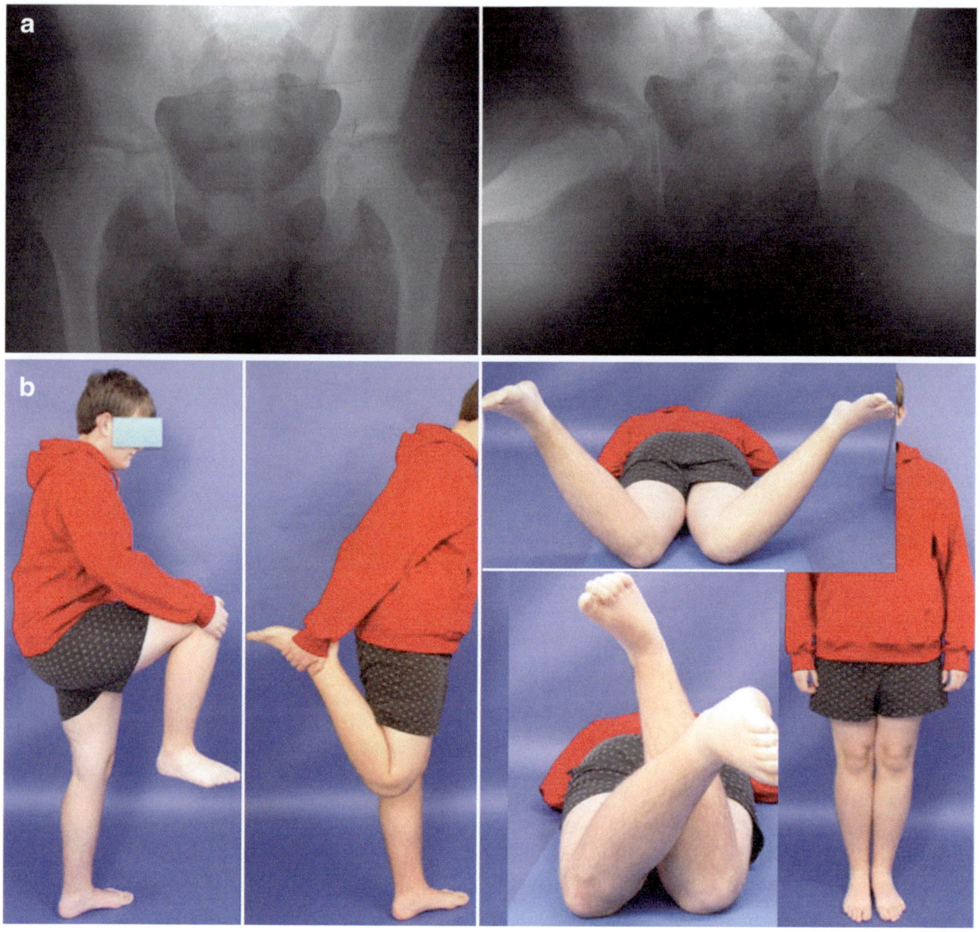

Fig. 38.4 (**a**) Anteroposterior (AP) and frog lateral radiographs of the pelvis at age 11 years, showing Perthes disease affecting the right hip. There is whole head involvement and early collapse with a break in Shenton's line. There is already coxa magna with extrusion of the femoral head (proximal and lateral migration) and the greater trochanter already appears to be overgrowing. (**b**) Preoperative photographs showing hip range of motion. There is excellent flexion and extension but limited external rotation. There is no photograph of his hip abduction but it is limited. (**c**) Preoperative AP radiograph (*right*) compared to postoperative AP radiograph (*left*) after femoral head reduction osteotomy (FHRO). (**d**) Preoperative frog lateral radiograph (*right*) compared to postoperative frog lateral radiograph (*left*) after FHRO. (**e**) Intraoperative photograph showing superior view of Type B femoral head. Note the large anterolateral bump. There is already significant damage to the central femoral head. Note that the lateral femoral head has excellent cartilage. (**f**) Intraoperative photograph showing superior view of the wedge shaped osteotomy resecting the anterior bump. (**g**) Intraoperative osteotomy showing superior view with the wedge removed. The wedge contains the most damaged cartilage. (**h**) Intraoperative photograph showing superior view of the osteotomy wedge closed, creating a round femoral head. (**i**) Intraoperative photograph from anterior view showing the femoral head is now spherical. The spherical template fits perfectly on the femoral head. (**j**) Postoperative hip range of motion 10 years after FHRO surgery and 6 years after leg lengthening surgery showing excellent range of motion with improved hip abduction and external rotation. The range of motion is now symmetric to the opposite side. Note there is no lurch or Trendelenburg when in single leg stance (*left*). (k–m) Ten-year follow-up radiographs show excellent preservation of the femoral head shape and location and no evidence of any degenerative changes in the joint

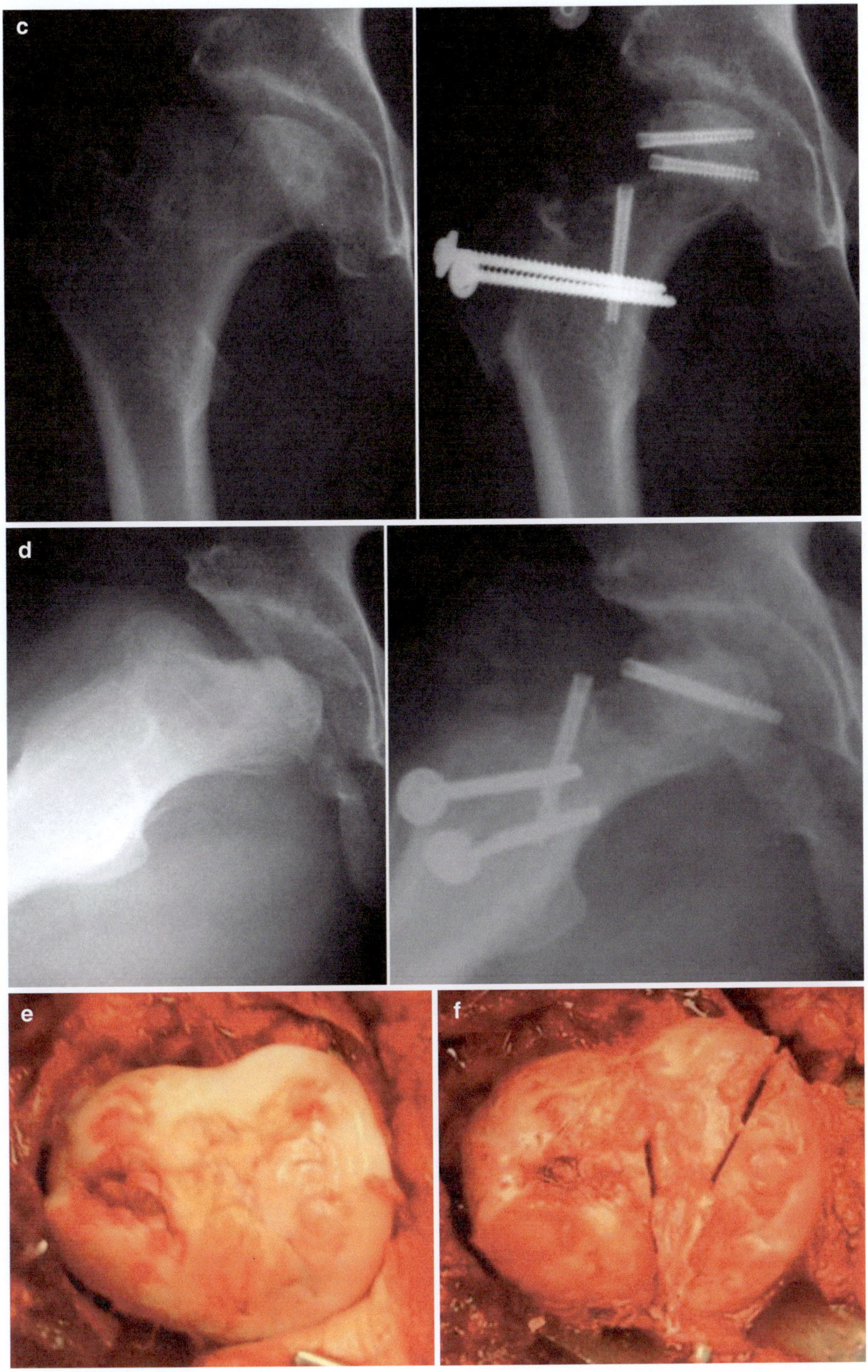

Fig. 38.4 (continued)

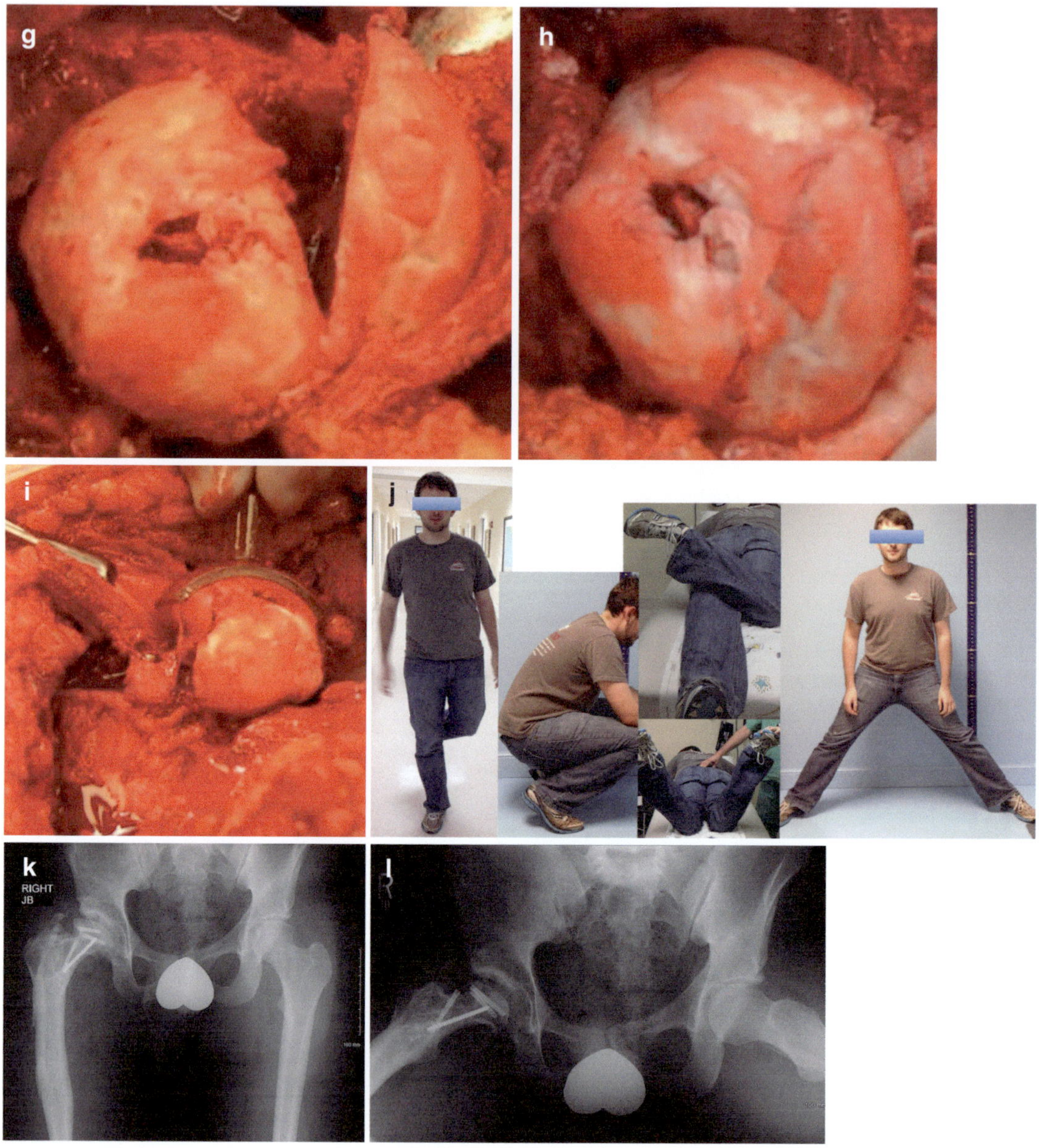

Fig. 38.4 (continued)

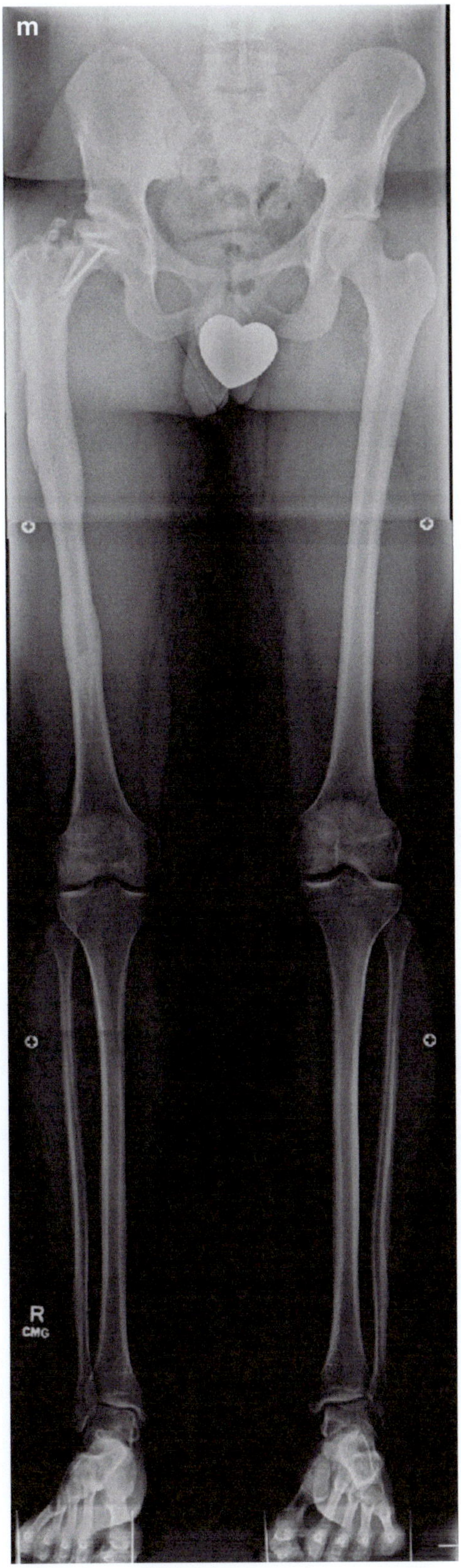

Fig. 38.4 (continued)

(Fig. 38.5). Type A requires a uniplanar reduction with parallel bone cuts, while type B requires a biplanar osteotomy with convergent bone cuts (wedge resection).

- Measure the opposite normal shaped femoral head and acetabulum and measure the ipsilateral femoral head and acetabulum.
- Determine the amount of reduction needed on AP and lateral views.
- Plan the amount of transfer needed to move the GT laterally and distally so that the tip of the GT is at the level of the center of the femoral head and is twice the radius of the femoral head away from the center of the joint.

Surgical Details of Femoral Head Reduction Osteotomy

Step 1: Anesthesia, Positioning and Draping An epidural is placed by the anesthesia service with a catheter running up the back on the non-operative side. A urinary catheter is inserted. The patient should be placed on their side on a beanbag on a radiolucent table in the lateral decubitis position with the operative side up. The ipsilateral arm should be appropriately padded and supported on an armrest. An axillary roll is utilized for the arm on the opposite side, and there is soft protection of boney prominences including the peroneal nerve as it crosses the fibular neck on the leg that is down. The entire operative side should be prepped and draped free from the nipple to the toes. The drapes should extend from the mid buttocks to the scrotal/labial-thigh fold. The lower limb should be completely free of the drapes. A sterile pocket should be created using drapes or a special pouch and fixed to the anterior side of the patient in line with the hip. Place a bump under the operative knee to abduct the operative hip.

Step 2: Incision and Fascia Lata Cut An approximately 15 cm long incision centered on the GT is made to and through the fascia lata (Fig. 38.4a). The fascia is separated from the gluteus maximus muscle anteriorly to reflect this muscle posteriorly (Fig. 38.6b, c). This avoids splitting and denervating the anterior portion of this muscle.

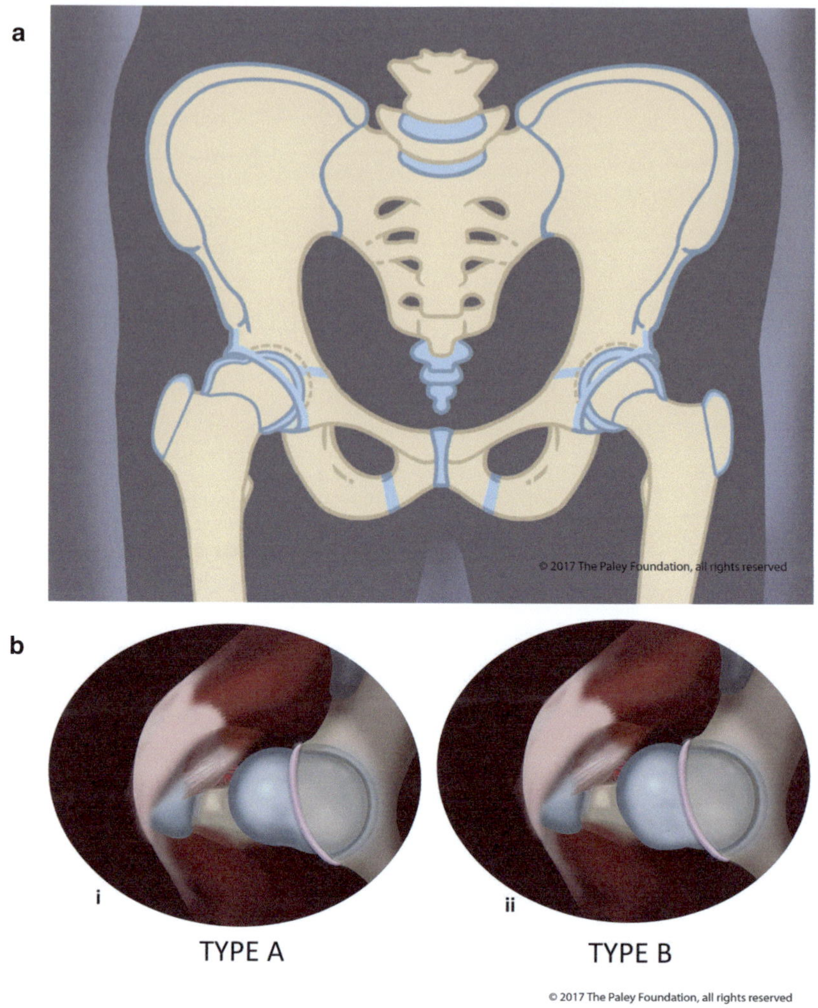

Fig. 38.5 (**a**) Illustration of saddle shaped right coxa magna, coxa breva with overgrown greater trochanter. The saddle part of the femoral head is where the femoro-acetabular impingement occurs. (**b**) Superior view of (i) Type A coxa magna with lateral elongation of femoral head and (ii) Type B coxa magna with lateral elongation with anterior protrusion (© 2017 The Paley Foundation, with permission. All rights reserved)

Step 3: Trochanteric Bursa and Piriformis Muscle Enter the trochanteric bursa (see Fig. 38.6c) and identify the inferior edge of the piriformis tendon and the posterior edge of the gluteus medius muscle (Fig. 38.7a). The posterior border of the gluteus medius is very distinct. The terminal branch of the inferior gluteal artery (which anastomoses with the medial femoral circumflex artery) runs along the inferior border of the piriformis muscle. Also identify the junction between the gluteus maximus tendon and the posterior edge of the vastus lateralis.

Step 4: Retract Gluteus Medius and Minimus Muscles Identify the junction of the gluteus medius and its underlying gluteus minimus and the superior border of the piriformis muscle (Fig. 38.7b). The gluteus medius is more superficial than the deeper piriformis. The piriformis is in a more superficial layer than the gluteus minimus. The border of these three muscles is nestled with each other such that the posterior border of the gluteus medius slightly overlies the superior border of the piriformis which slightly overlies the posterior border of the gluteus minimus. Separate the superior border of the piriformis

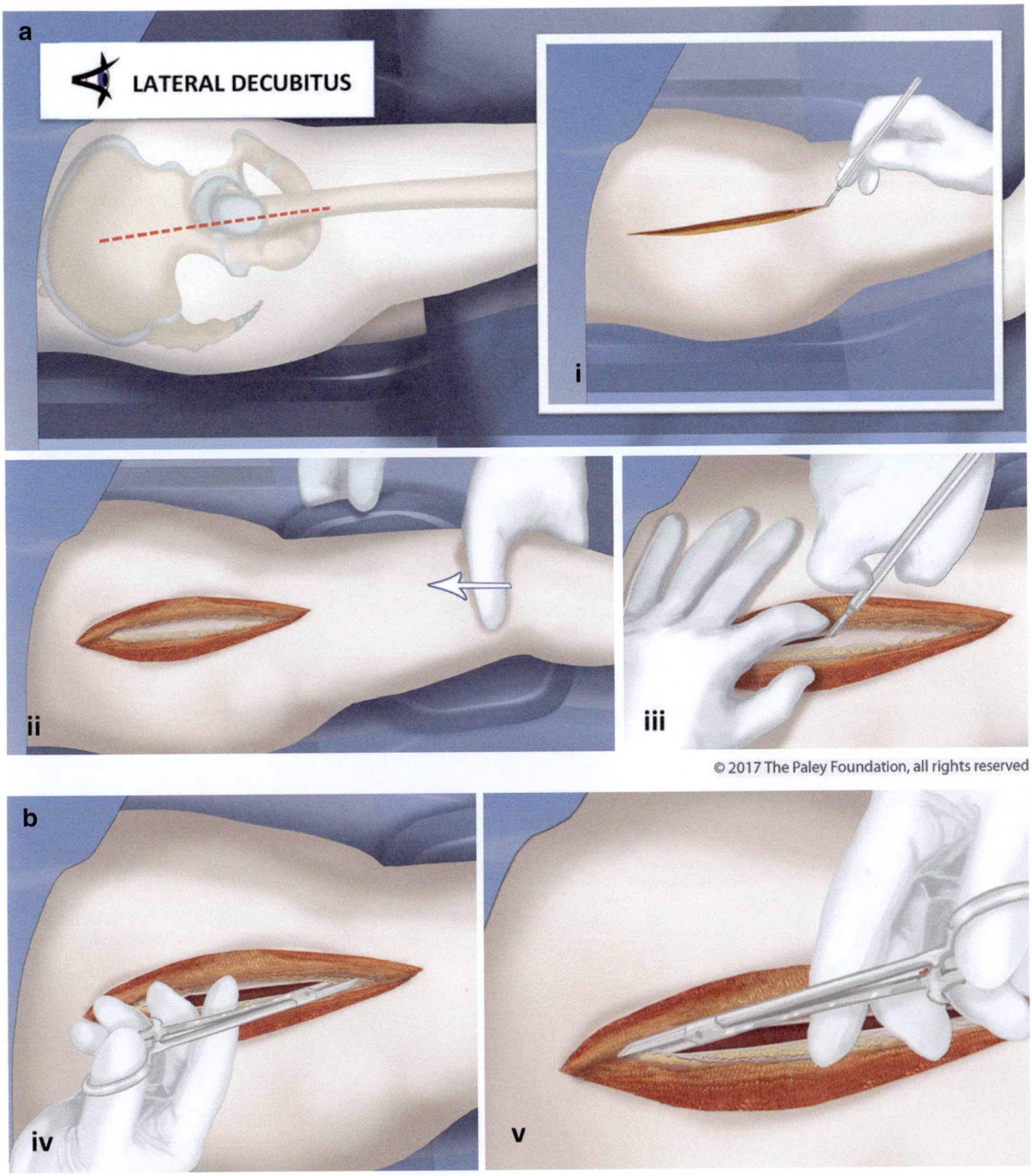

Fig. 38.6 (**a**) Lateral decubitis position with midlateral incision (i). The incision goes straight through skin, subcutaneous fat (ii) and fascia lata (iii). (**b**) The fascia is split longitudinally the entire length of the incision (iv, v) and then separated anteriorly from the underlying gluteus maximus. (**c**) The gluteus maximus is reflected posteriorly from its anterior edge so as not to split and denervate it (viii, ix). The trochanteric bursa is opened (x) to expose the greater trochanter (xi) (© 2017 The Paley Foundation, with permission. All rights reserved)

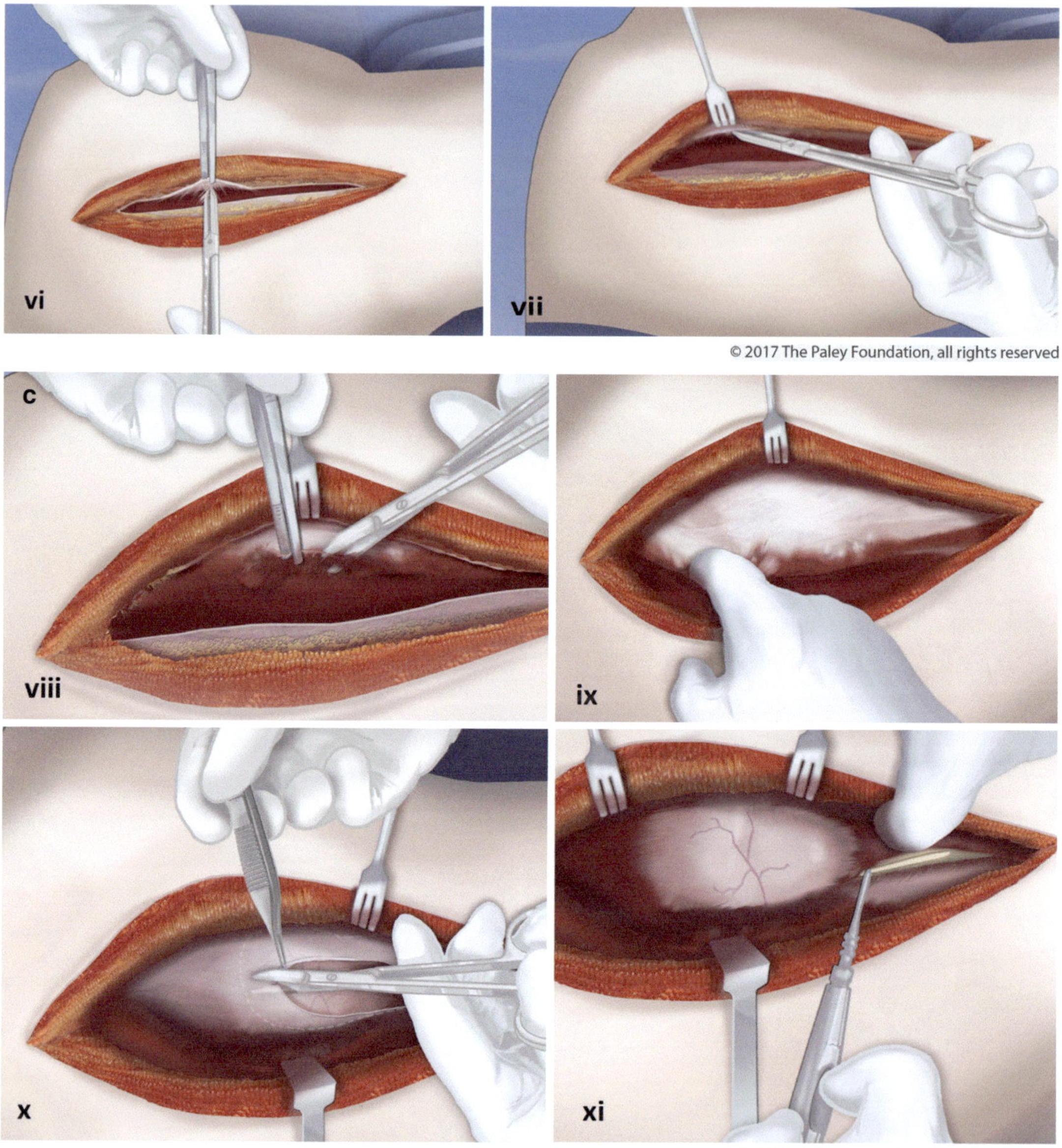

Fig. 38.6 (continued)

from the posterior borders of the two glutei. Undermine the gluteus minimus to find the interval between this muscle and the capsule. Insert a Z retractor into this interval to lift the glutei away from the capsule (Fig. 38.7c).

Step 5: Elevate and Retract the Vastus Lateralis Using a cautery elevate the posterior border of the vastus lateralis off the femur. This is just anterior to the GMax tendon. Insert a Hohmann elevator to elevate this muscle (see Fig. 38.7c).

Step 6: Cauterize the Posterior Border of the GT Connect a virtual line between the elevated vastus and the elevated glutei. Use a cautery to mark this line along the trochanteric ridge. This serves to cauterize the trochanteric vessels (Fig. 38.8a, b).

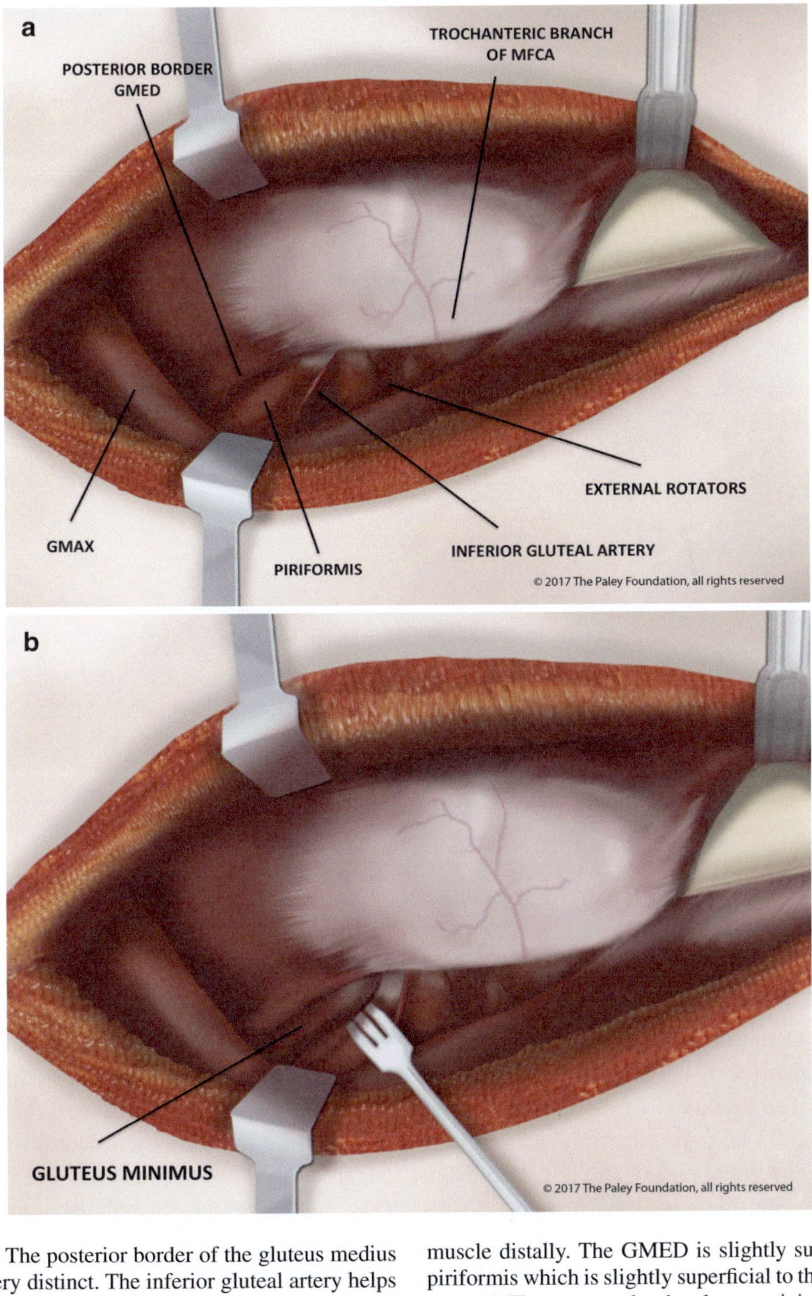

Fig. 38.7 (**a**) The posterior border of the gluteus medius (GMED) is very distinct. The inferior gluteal artery helps define the inferior border of the piriformis muscle. The trochanteric branch of the medial femoral circumflex artery is readily seen on the greater trochanter. The gluteus maximus tendon is seen inserting into the femur. The vastus lateralis muscle is lifted off of the femur. (**b**) The gluteus minimus can be seen by reflecting the piriformis muscle distally. The GMED is slightly superficial to the piriformis which is slightly superficial to the gluteus minimus. (**c**) The space under the gluteus minimus is dissected (i) so that a Z retractor can be inserted beneath it overtop the capsule (ii). The Z retractor is used to expose the underlying capsule (iii). A Hohmann elevator is lifting the vastus lateralis off the femur. (© 2017 The Paley Foundation, with permission. All rights reserved)

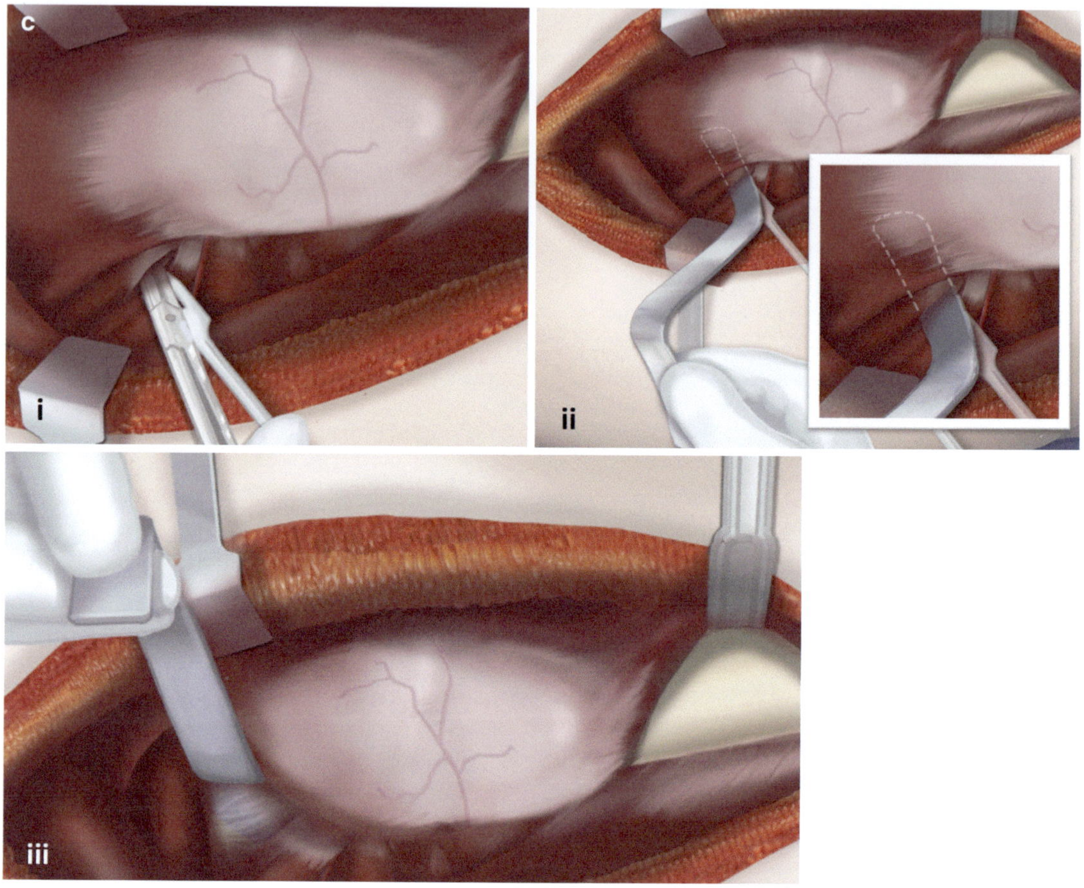

Fig. 38.7 (continued)

Step 7: GT Osteotomy Use a saw to cut from posterior to anterior along the trochanteric ridge (Fig. 38.8c). The thickness of the lateral portion of the GT should be approximately 1.5 cm (see Fig. 38.6b). The distal end of the cut should not penetrate the lateral femoral cortex to avoid subtrochanteric notching. The plane of this cut should be in line with the true lateral (maximum profile) of the GT notwithstanding the rotation at the knee.

Step 8: Cut the Soft Tissues Around the GT The soft tissues around the GT should be cut with a sharp serrated scissors. At the proximal end insert one leg of the scissors under the gluteal flap and the other end in the osteotomy (Fig. 38.8d). Orient the curve of the scissors concave medial to allow them to conform to the hip capsule and go around the corner anteriorly (Fig. 38.6e). Make sure that the piriformis muscle remains posterior to the scissors. The piriformis tendon should remain connected to the stable portion of the GT with no more than a third of it still attached to the mobile GT (see Fig. 38.8d). Release the piriformis off of the mobile GT. Distally, do the same placing one leg of the scissors between the femur and the vastus and the other leg inside the osteotomy (Fig. 38.8f). The two cuts will converge on each other.

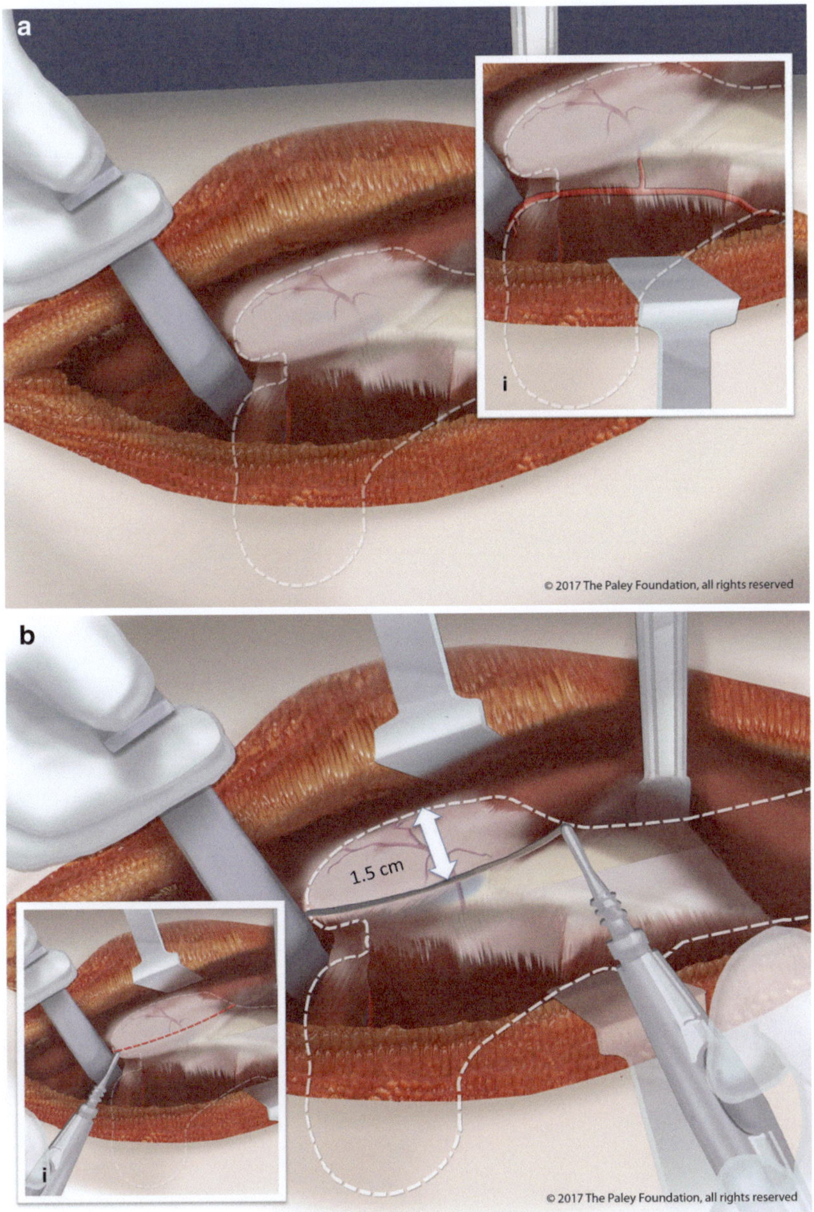

Fig. 38.8 (**a**) A lateral view of the greater trochanter is shown with the external rotator muscles inserting medial to the posterior trochanteric ridge. Underlying these running along the periosteum is the ascending branch of the medial femoral circumflex artery (i) as it courses towards the piriformis fossa and anastomoses with the inferior gluteal artery. (**b**) The line for the trochanteric osteotomy is marked with a cautery. This line is defined along the trochanteric ridge between the insertion of the vastus lateralis distally and the Z retractor proximally. The trochanteric artery is intentionally cauterized. The thickness of the trochanteric segment is 1.5 cm. (**c**) Osteotomy of the greater trochanter is carried out with an oscillating saw. (**d**) The mobile trochanter is mobilized by cutting the soft tissues on its superior, medial, and inferior sides. At the upper end any tendinous extension from the piriformis is released. (**e**) The superomedial side of the trochanter is released. (**f**) The inferomedial side of the trochanter is released (© 2017 The Paley Foundation, with permission. All rights reserved)

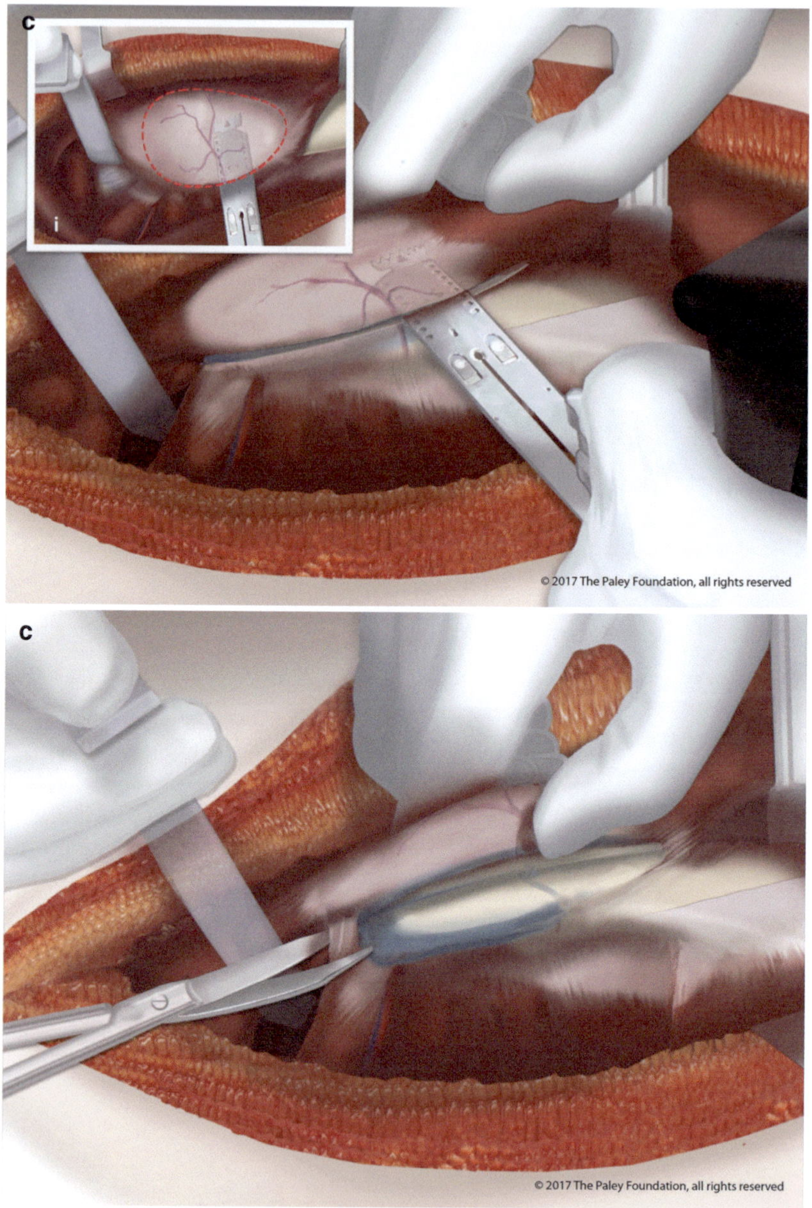

Fig. 38.8 (continued)

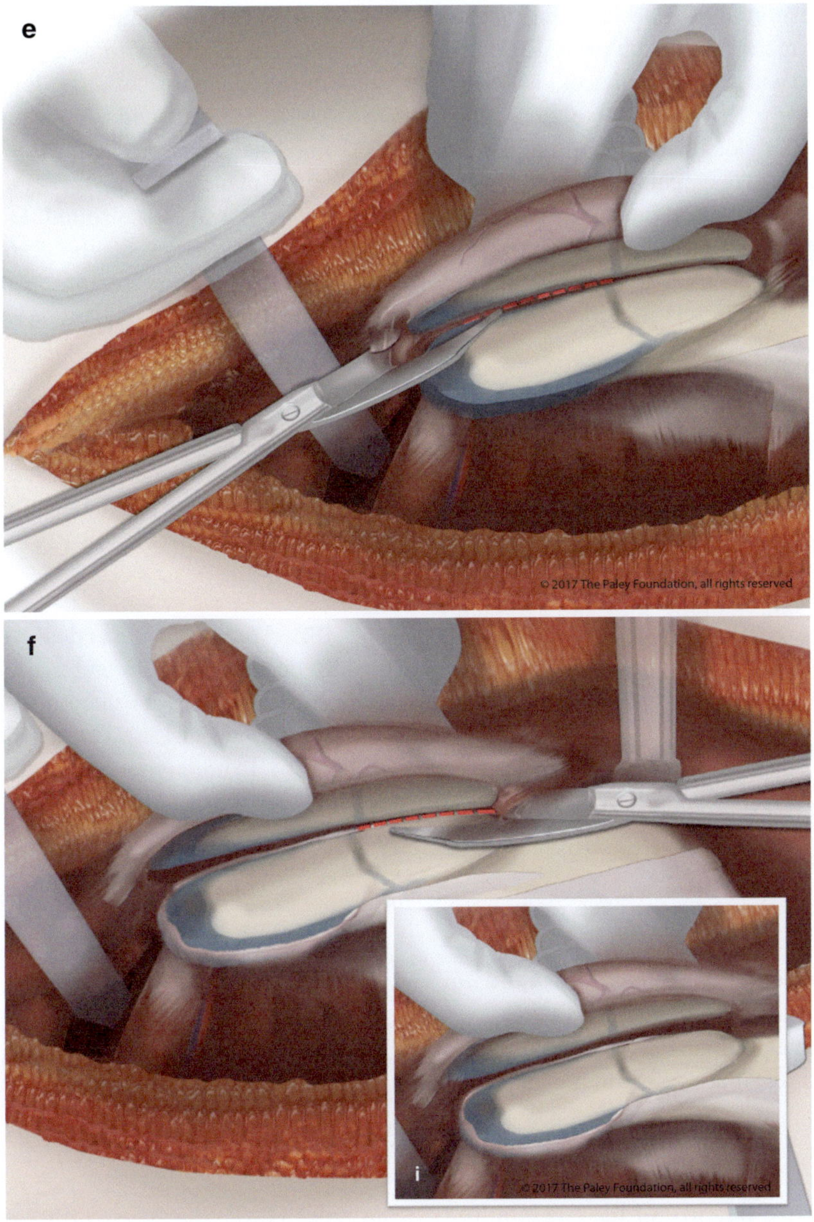

Fig. 38.8 (continued)

Step 9: Insert Two Hohmann Elevators Flex the hip and remove the bump from under the knee. Bluntly dissect under the muscle flap to the anterior inferior iliac spine (AIIS). Place a Hohmann elevator around the AIIS with care to stay between bone and muscle on the inside of the pelvis (Fig. 38.9a). Use a Cobb elevator to sweep the gluteus minimus muscle off of the capsule and lateral wall of the ilium. Impact a Hohmann elevator through the lateral wall of the ilium (Fig. 38.9b). These two elevators, which are 90° to each other, stay in place for the duration of the procedure.

Step10: Z Capsulotomy Make a Z-shaped capsulotomy. The intermediate limb of the Z (lateral to medial in line with the femoral neck) is located at 11 o'clock for a left hip and 1 o'clock for a right hip with 12 o'clock being the top of the hip joint (Fig. 38.9c). Take care not to cut the labrum (Fig. 38.7d). Make the distal limb of the Z anterolateral and the proximal limb poster-medial. Leave a cuff of capsule at both limbs in order to sew into and also to preserve the relationship of the capsule to the labrum.

Step 11: Cut Ligamentum Teres To be able to dislocate the hip cut the ligamentum teres with a long curved scissors (e.g., Jorgenson's) (Fig. 38.9e).

Step 12: Dislocate the Hip Flex and externally rotate the hip to dislocate it (Fig. 38.10).

Step 13: Resect the Ligamentum Teres Resect the remnant of the ligamentum both in the acetabulum and from the femoral head. Clean out the cotyloid notch from soft tissues (see Fig. 38.10).

Step 14: Inspect and Repair the Labrum Inspect the labrum with a blunt hook to look for a partial or complete labral tear. If the labrum is torn, resect and repair according to the pattern of the tear.

Step 15: Measure the Size of the Acetabulum Use spherical acetabular sizers to measure the diameter of the acetabulum (Fig. 38.11a).

Step 16: Size the Femoral Head Use femoral head spherical templates to assess the sphericity of different parts of the femoral head (Fig. 38.11b, c). Start with the acetabular size. The femoral head can be sized for its curvature in different planes. Mark the femoral head where the sizer leaves the round. Do the same for the lateral portion of the femoral head. Using this method the femoral head can be mapped for its sphericity.

Step 17: Retinacular Flap—Reduce the Hip into Joint Do a subperiosteal dissection of the posterior femur starting at the level of the lesser trochanter and working proximally up to the level of the piriformis fossa (Fig. 38.12).

Step 18: Mark the Vertical Osteotomy Lines Redislocate the hip and mark the osteotomy lines. There are two osteotomy patterns: (1) parallel cuts (Fig. 38.13a); (2) non-parallel cuts (Fig. 38.13b). In both types the length of femoral head medial and lateral to the medial and lateral osteotomy lines are the same. In both types the sum of the lengths of the two segments adds up to the size of the diameter of the acetabulum.

Step 19: Mark the Horizontal Baseline Osteotomy Line Mark this line distal enough to include the anterior part of the piriformis fossa but not too deep to narrow the femoral neck too much (see Fig. 38.13a, b).

Step 20: Mark the Vertical Central Head Osteotomies (Fig. 38.14a–e, Fig. 38.15a–e) Use a thin saw to make the horizontal cut first fol-

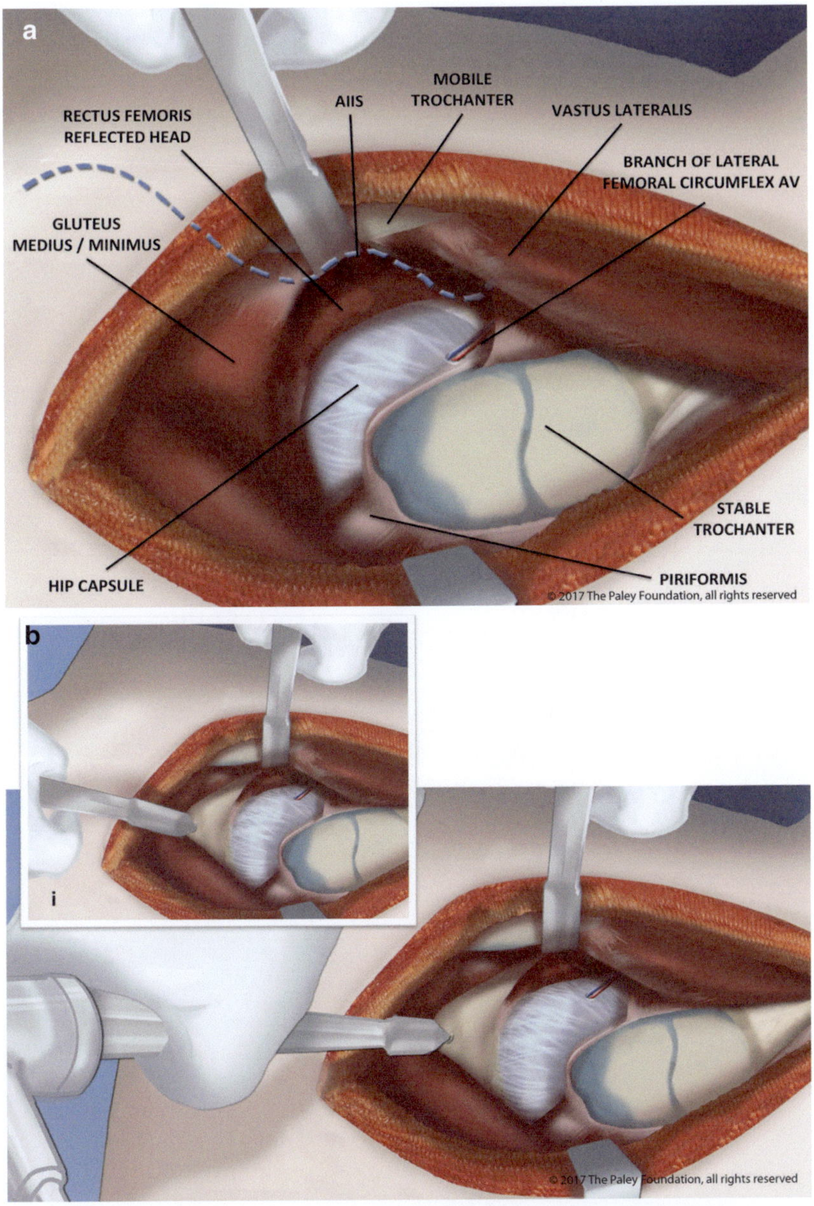

Fig. 38.9 (**a**) The hip is flexed and a Hohmann elevator is inserted around the anterior inferior iliac spine. The branch of the lateral femoral circumflex artery should be spared if possible. (**b**) The gluteus minimus is elevated off of the capsule and lateral ilium. A Hohmann elevator is impacted into the lateral ilium to help retract the soft tissues. The two Hohmann elevators are 90° to each other and should be retracted separately with separate hands in two different directions for best exposure. (**c**) The Z-shaped capsulotomy has the distal arm lateral and the proximal arm medial. It is shown for right and left hips. (**d**) The anterior part of the capsulotomy. (**e**) After the entire capsulotomy is completed the hip can start to be dislocated and the ligamentum teres cut with curved right angle scissors (i) (© 2017 The Paley Foundation, with permission. All rights reserved)

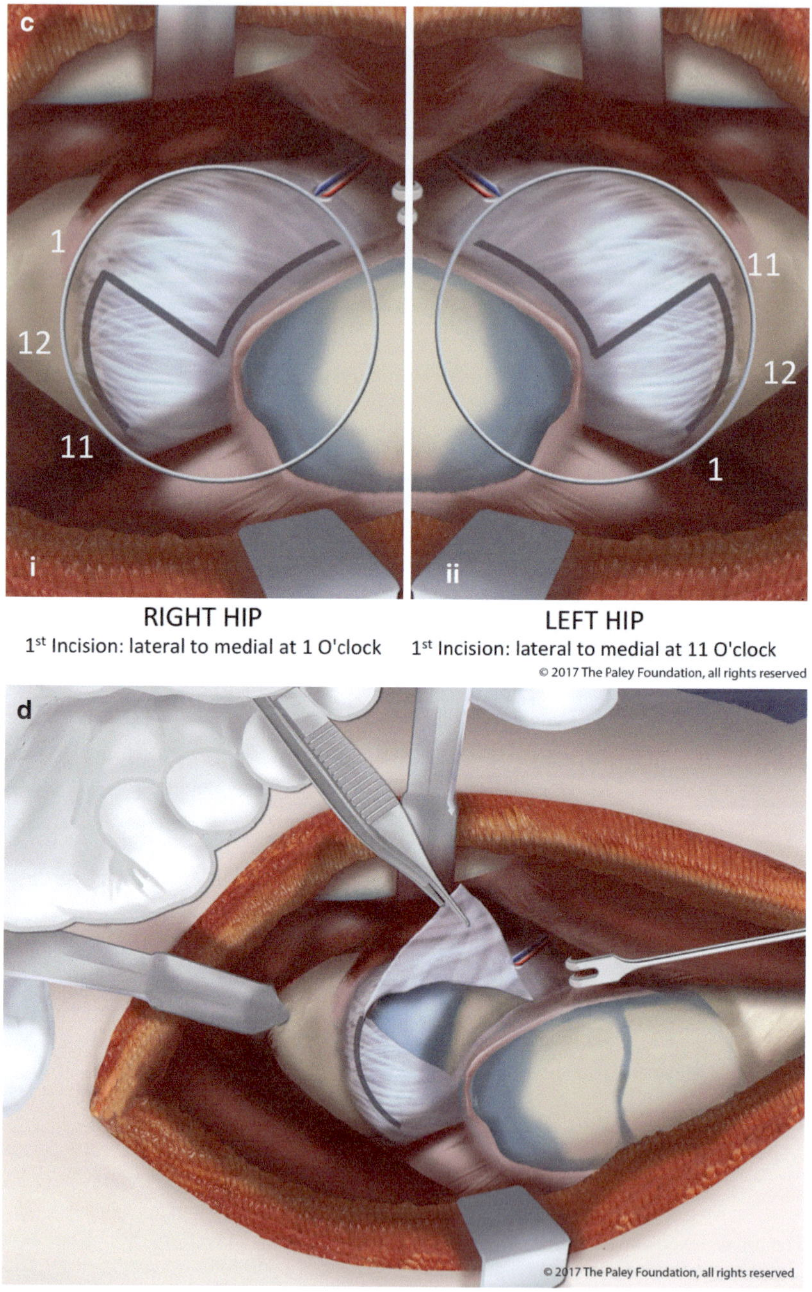

Fig. 38.9 (continued)

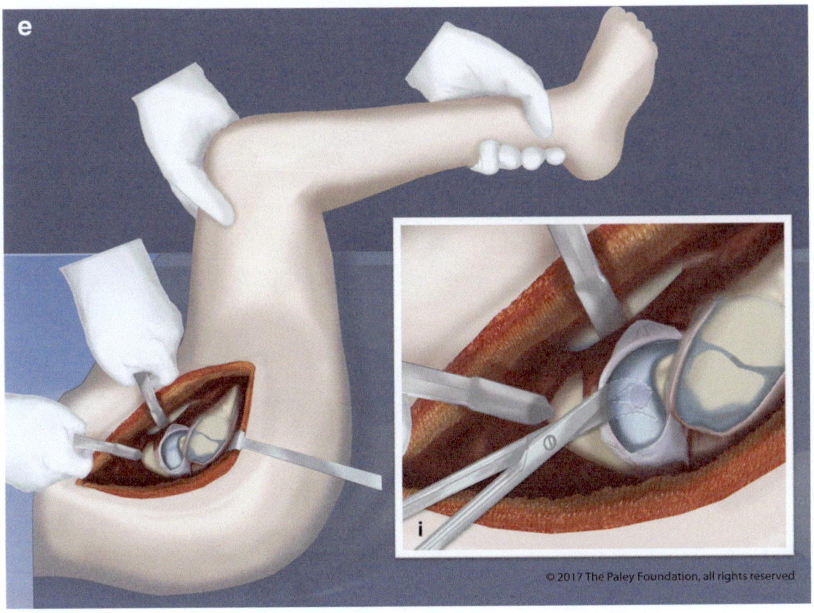

Fig. 38.9 (continued)

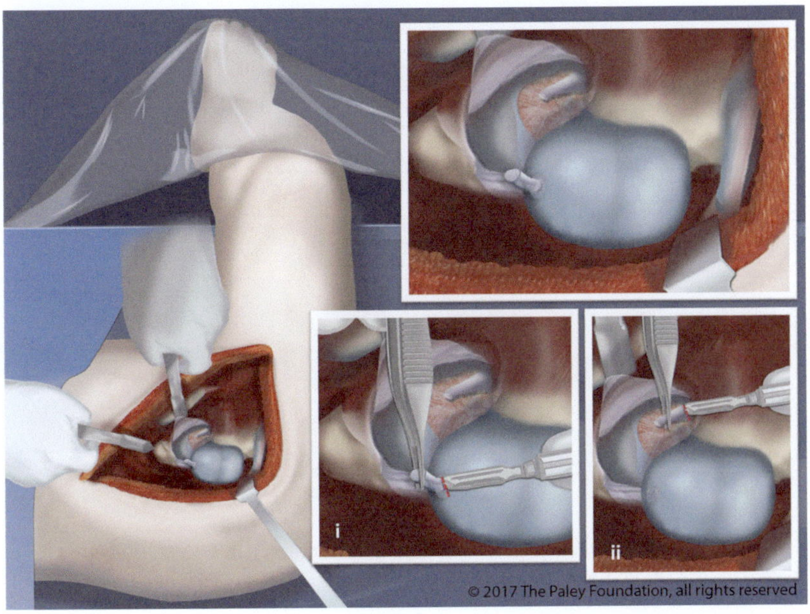

Fig. 38.10 The leg is crossed over the opposite leg and dropped into a sterile bag. The hip is now dislocated. The ligamentum teres and any pulvinar can be excised. The labrum can be probed for tears (© 2017 The Paley Foundation, with permission. All rights reserved)

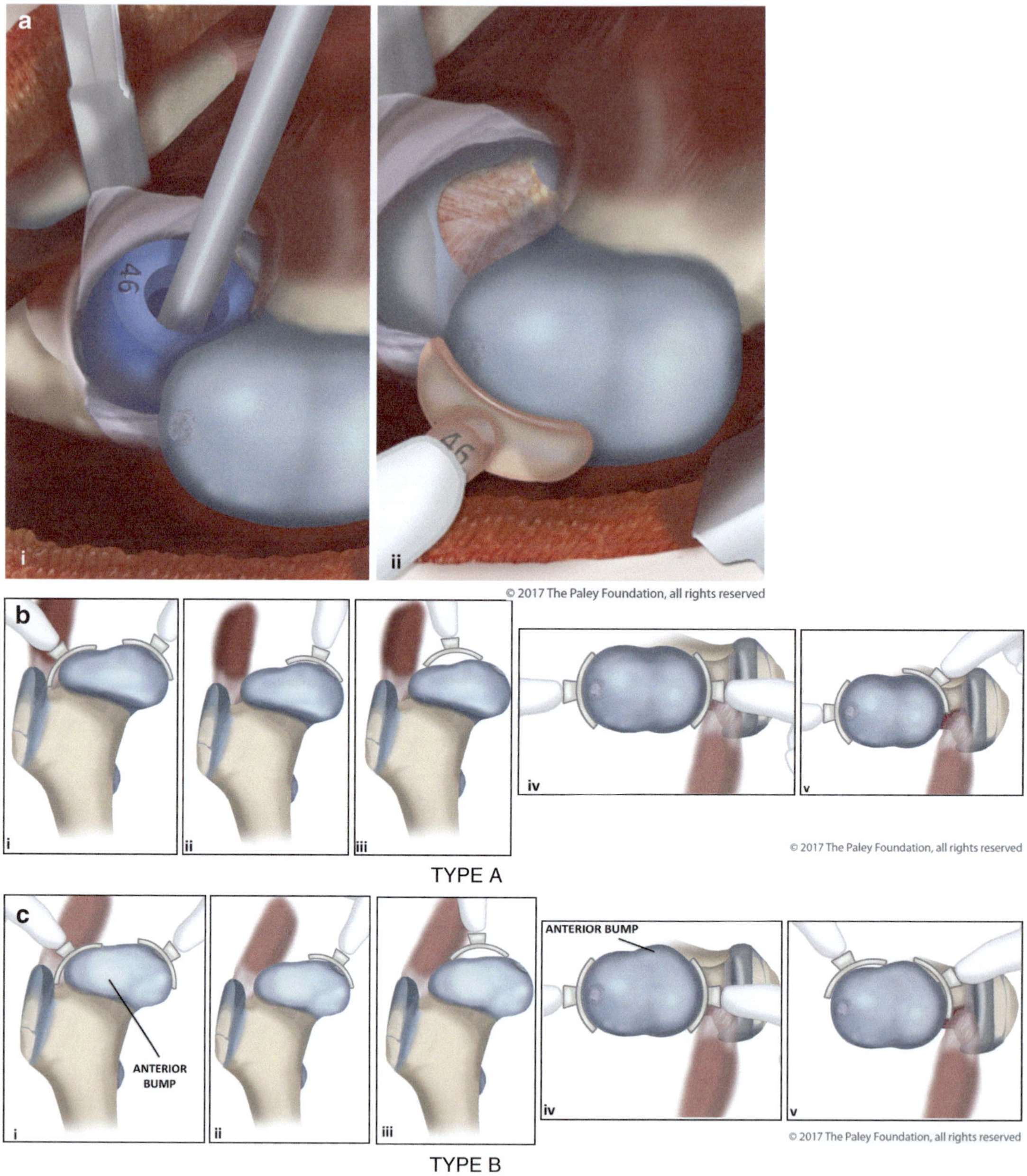

Fig. 38.11 (**a**) The acetabulum is sized (i). A femoral head template of the same size as the acetabulum (in this case 46 mm) is used to check the sphericity of the medial femoral head. (**b**) The femoral head is template along its medial and lateral sides as well as along its medial and lateral superior surfaces. It is important to note where the femoral head leaves the round. This is shown for Type A. (**c**) The same is done for a Type B case. Note the anterior bump and incongruity (© 2017 The Paley Foundation, with permission. All rights reserved)

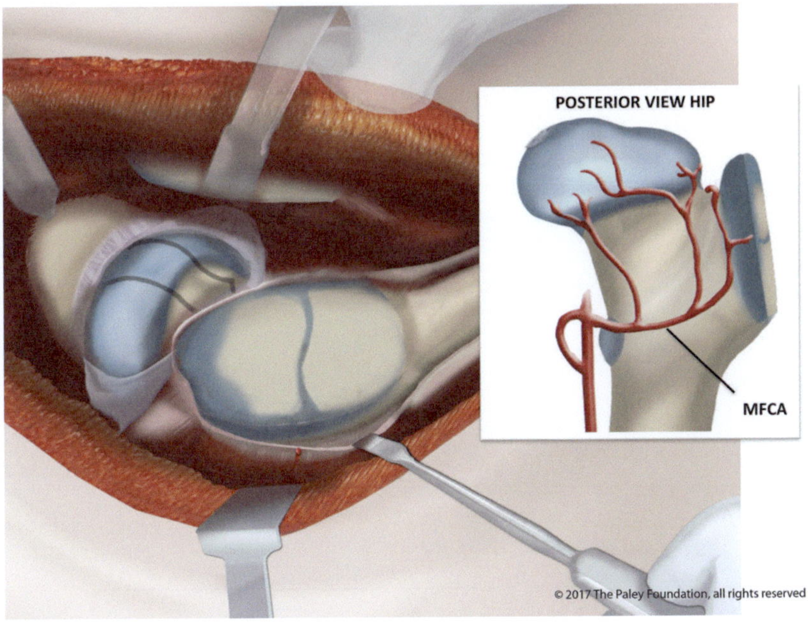

Fig. 38.12 The hip is reduced into joint again and the periosteum at the back of the femur is stripped carefully and extended proximally to help separate the retinaculum from the lateral femur. This moves the medial circumflex femoral artery away from the lateral femur (© 2017 The Paley Foundation, with permission. All rights reserved)

lowed by the two vertical cuts. Do not cut all the way to the back. After making most of the cut with the saw, complete the osteotomy with an osteotome. Crack the back of the osteotomy.

Step 21: Remove the Intercalary Segment Remove the middle segment (see Fig. 38.14e, see Fig. 38.15e).

Step 22: Mobilize the Lateral Segment Mobilize the lateral segment by lifting it from front to back hinging on the retinacular flap (Fig. 38.16a). Carefully strip the retinaculum off of the neck to remain on the mobile lateral segment. This allows it to move from lateral to medial to close the defect without tethering or tearing the retinaculum (Fig. 38.16b).

Step 23: Reduce the Femoral Head Adjust the lateral segment so that the posterior congruity is as perfect as possible (see Fig. 38.16b). If there is a step, make sure it is anterior.

Step 24: Fix the Femoral Head with Headless Screws Fix the segments with k-wires and then measure and drill over these and insert two parallel variable pitch headless screws (Fig. 38.17a). The variable pitch thread compresses the intra-articular osteotomy line.

Step 25: Insert a Third Headless Screw Perpendicular to the Osteotomy at the Base of the Lateral Fragment Drill a wire, cannulated drill, measure and then insert a headless screw (Fig. 38.18b).

Step 26: Osteochondroplasty Perform an osteochondroplasty on any incongruous anterior aspects of the femoral head.

Step 27: Insert Prophylactic Screw for Femoral Neck Drill a guide wire from the fovea retrograde into the femoral neck through the lateral femoral cortex. Measure and insert an antegrade cannulated screw up the femoral neck (Fig. 38.18c, d).

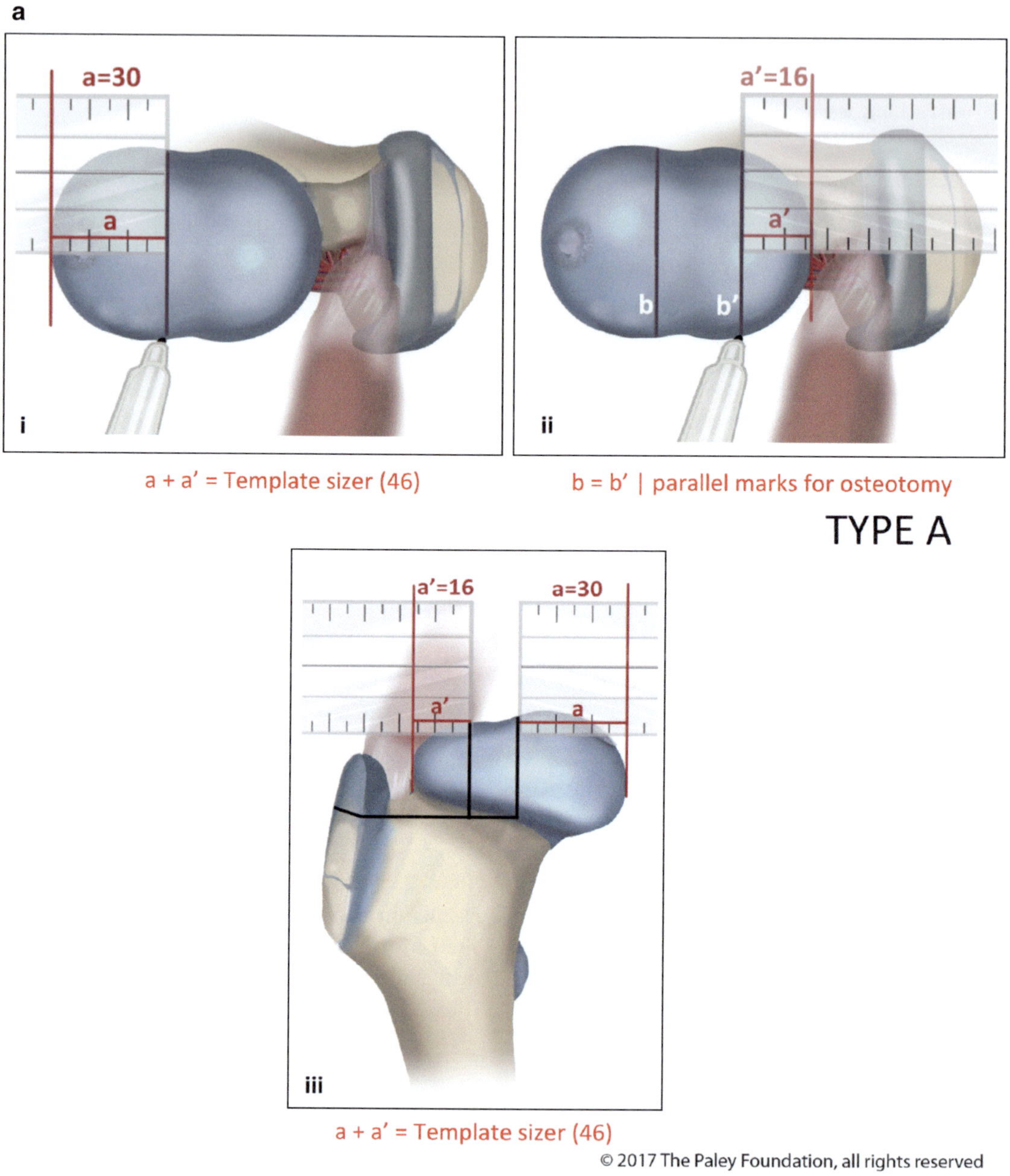

Fig. 38.13 (**a**) The femoral head is marked at the borders of where it leaves the round based on the femoral head spherical templates. Since the medial part measures 30 mm and since the total diameter of the reduced femoral head is 46 mm then the lateral segment should be 16 mm. Since the coxa magna is Type A the planned osteotomy lines are parallel. The baseline runs just below the ridge of the femoral head and distal to the anterior piriformis fossa. It is still superior to the most posterior piriformis fossa. The stable trochanter will be part of the lateral fragment. (**b**) For Type B the two lines are convergent posteriorly. The dimensions of the medial and lateral parts of the femoral head are the same as for Type A and add up to a 46 mm diameter femoral head (© 2017 The Paley Foundation, with permission. All rights reserved)

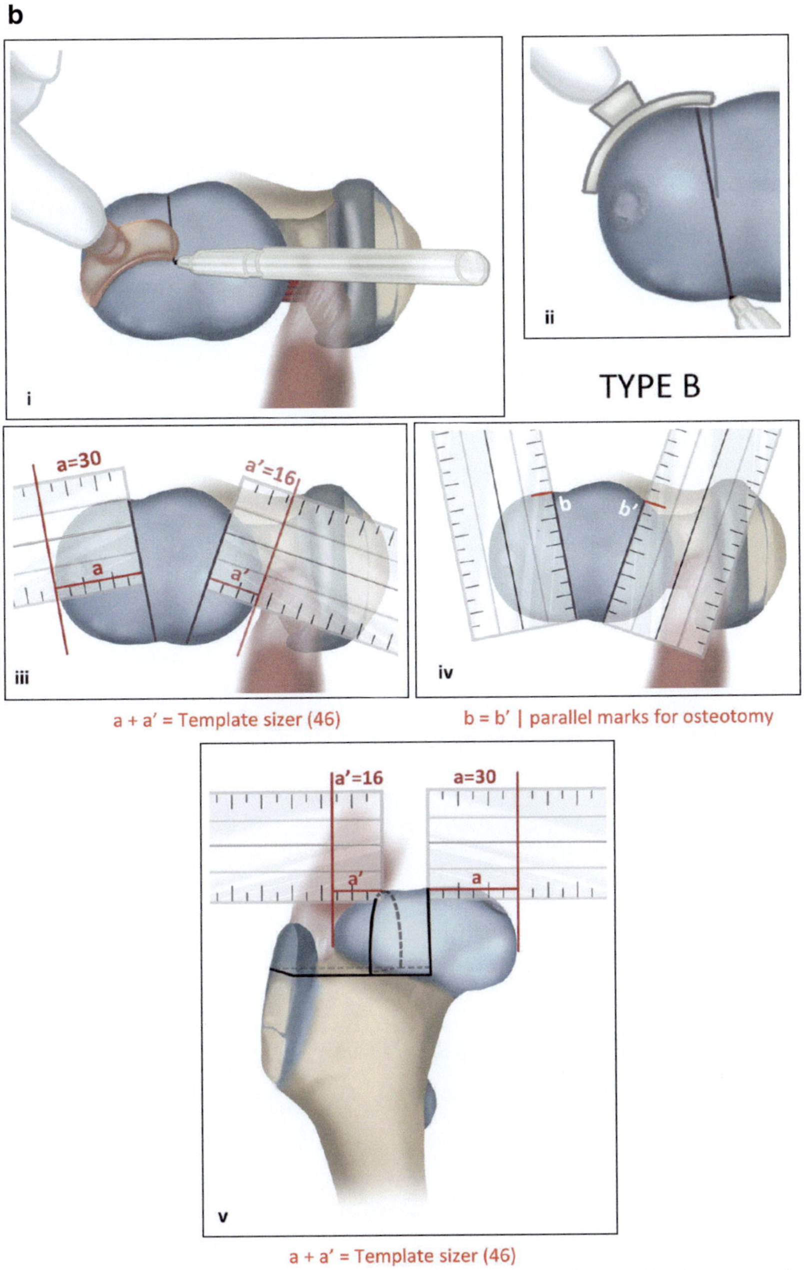

Fig. 38.13 (continued)

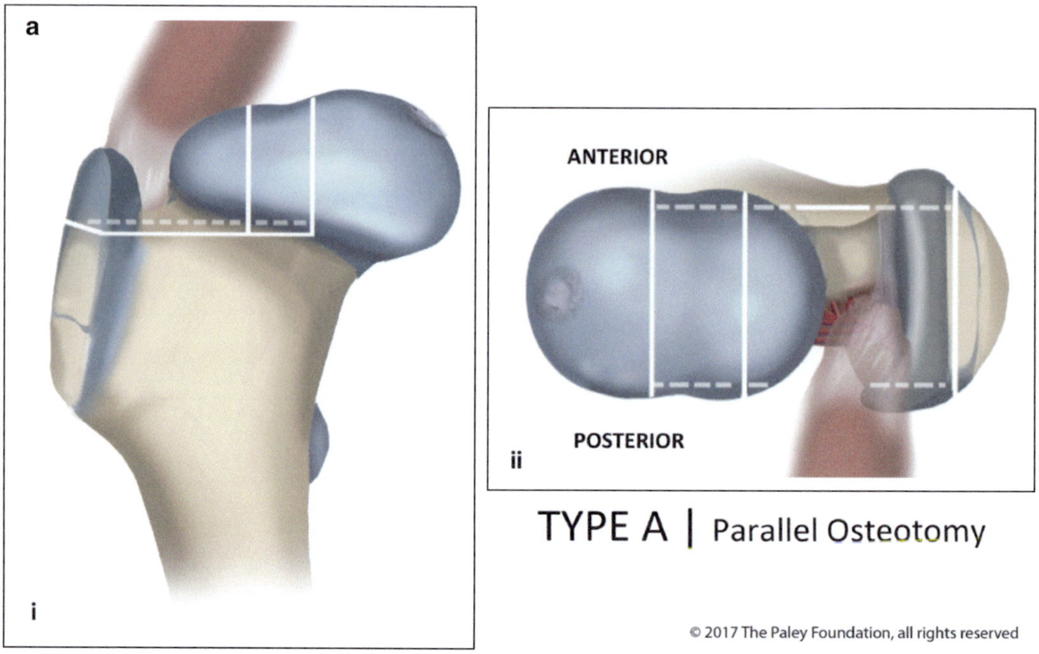

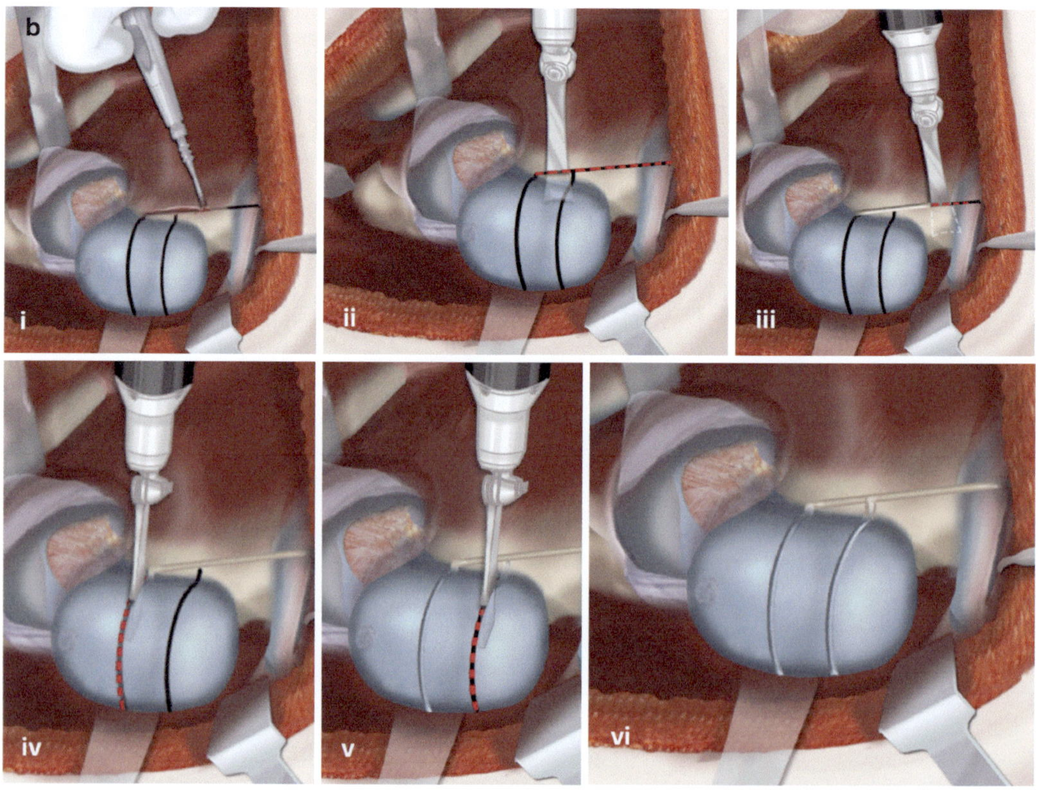

Fig. 38.14 (**a**) The osteotomy lines are *outlined in white*. (**b**) The cautery is used to mark the anterior baseline cut (i). A very thin saw is then used to make the horizontal baseline cut (ii, iii) and then the two parallel vertical cuts (iv, v, vi). (**c**) An osteotome is used to complete the posterior aspect of the osteotomies and to pry out the intercalary segment (i). (**d**) The fragment is sharply dissected off of any posterior retinacular tissues. (**e**) The intercalary middle segment is removed (© 2017 The Paley Foundation, with permission. All rights reserved)

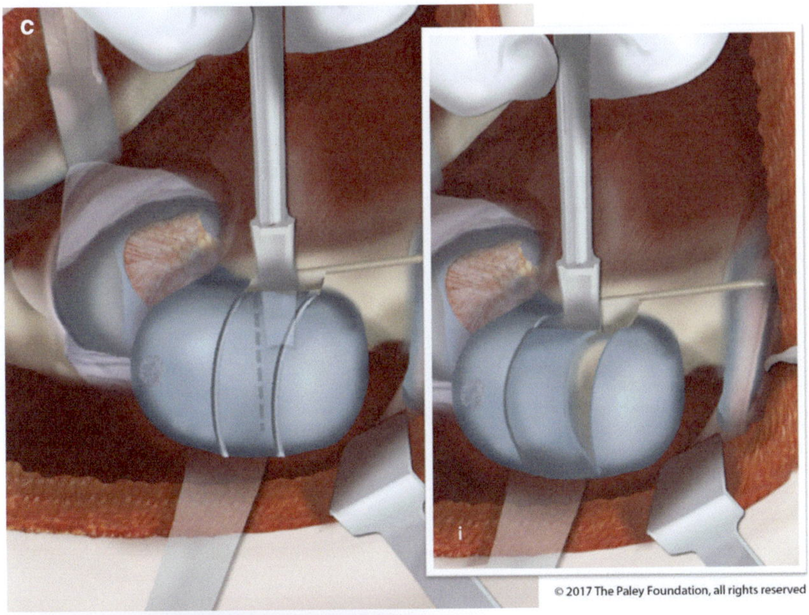

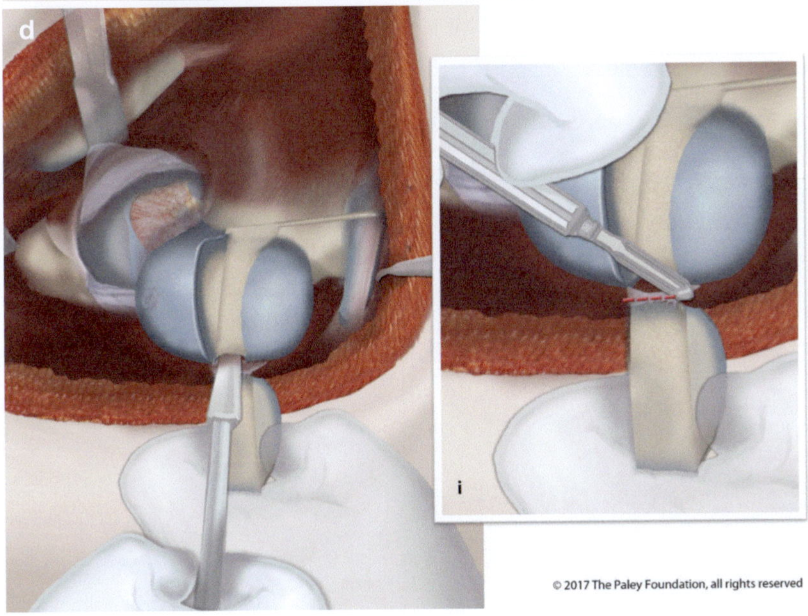

Fig. 38.14 (continued)

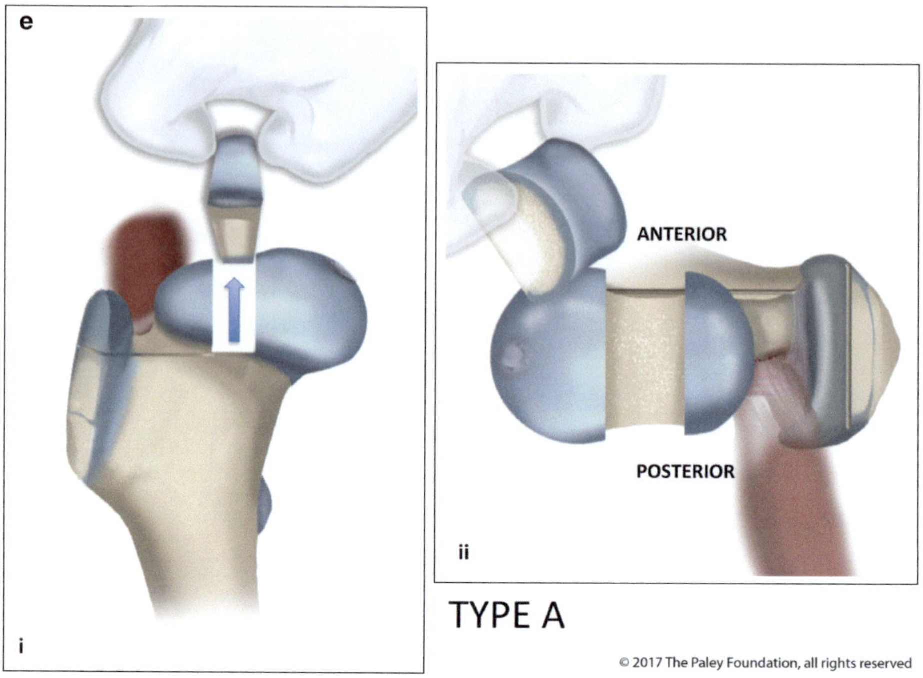

Fig. 38.14 (continued)

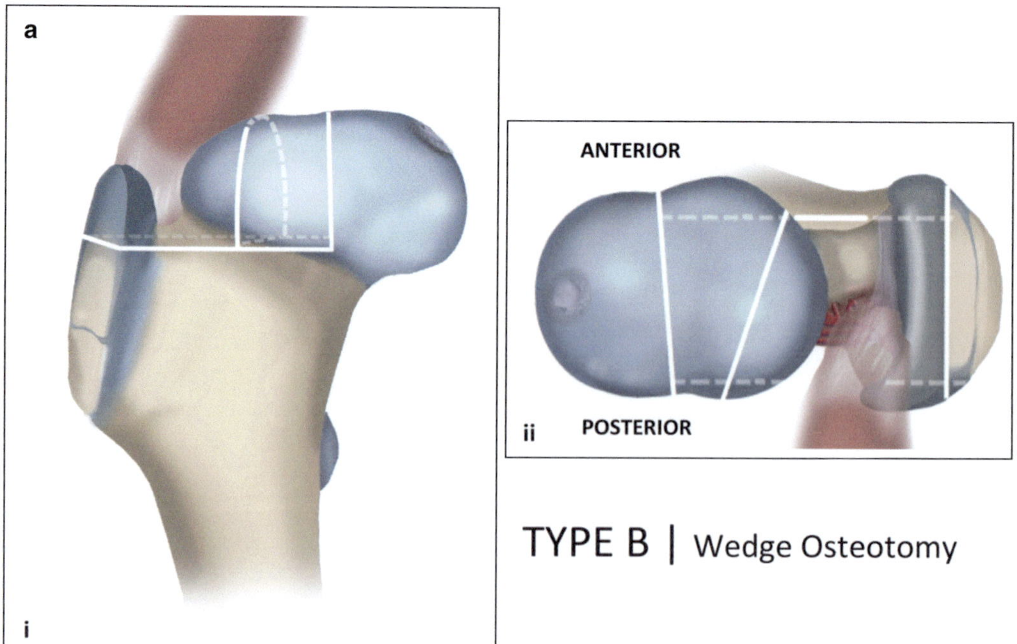

Fig. 38.15 (**a**) The osteotomy lines are *outlined in white*. (**b**) The cautery is used to mark the anterior baseline cut (i). A very thin saw is then used to make the horizontal baseline cut (ii, iii) and then the two nonparallel vertical cuts (iv, v, vi). (**c**) An osteotome is used to complete the posterior aspect of the osteotomies and to pry out the intercalary segment (i). (**d**) The fragment is sharply dissected off of any posterior retinacular tissues. (**e**) The intercalary wedge shaped middle segment is removed. This removes the anterior bump with it (© 2017 The Paley Foundation, with permission. All rights reserved)

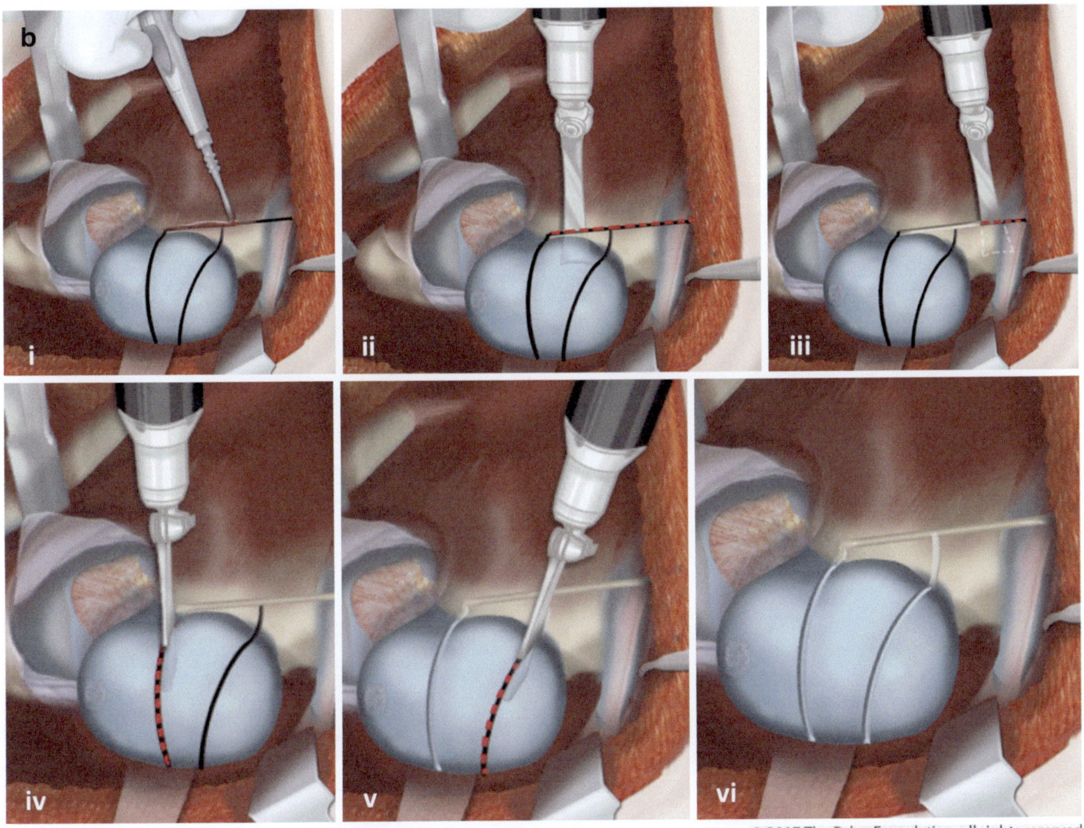

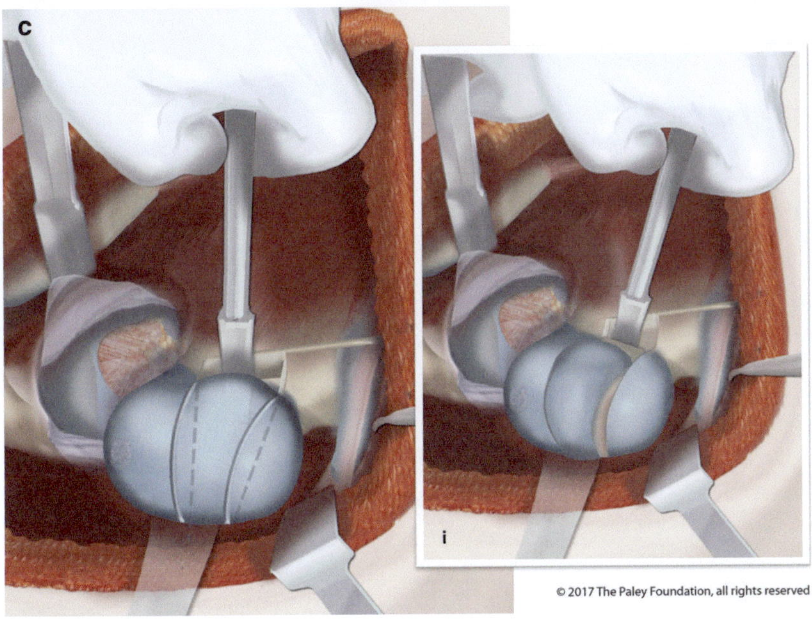

Fig. 38.15 (continued)

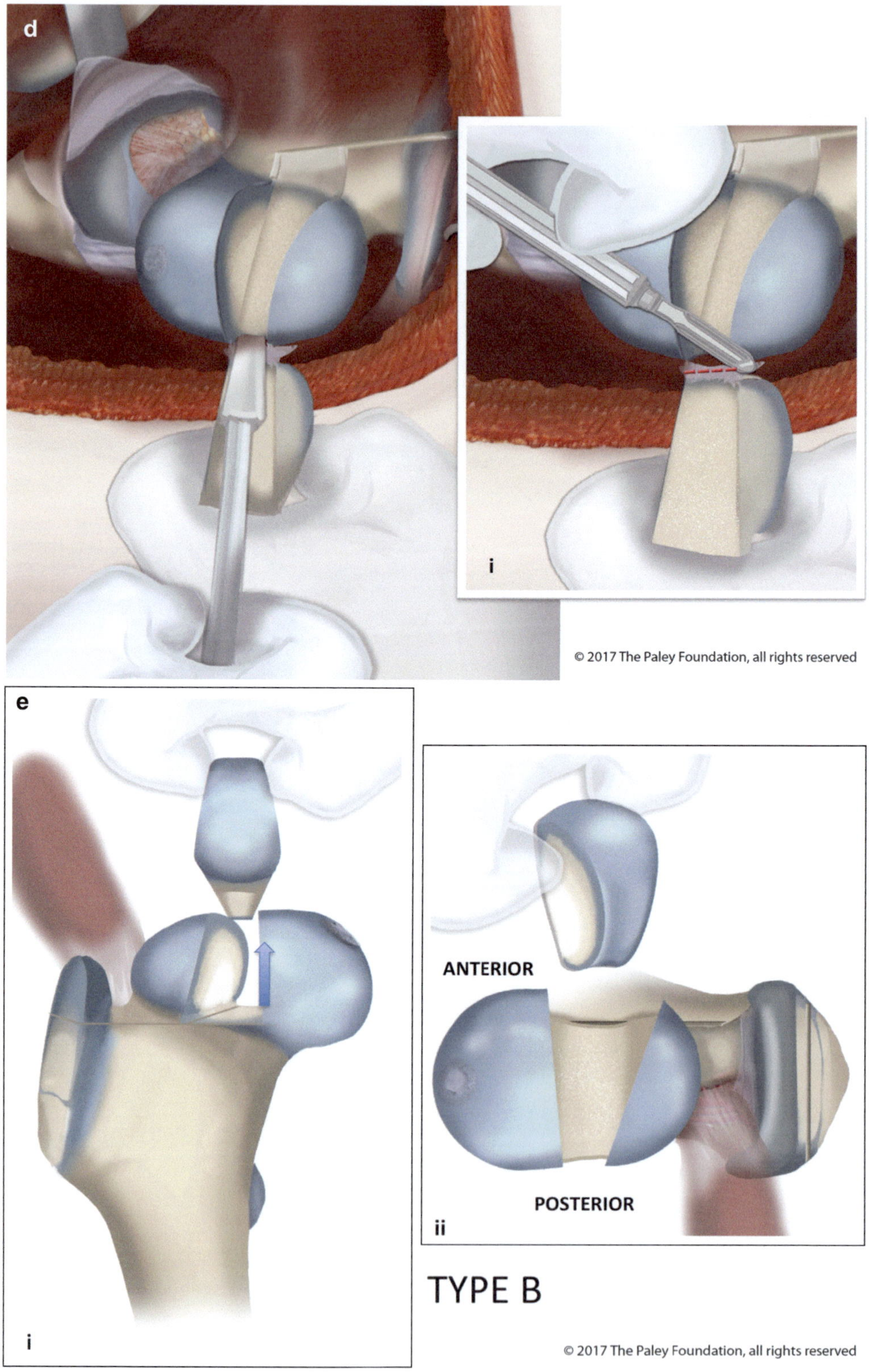

Fig. 38.15 (continued)

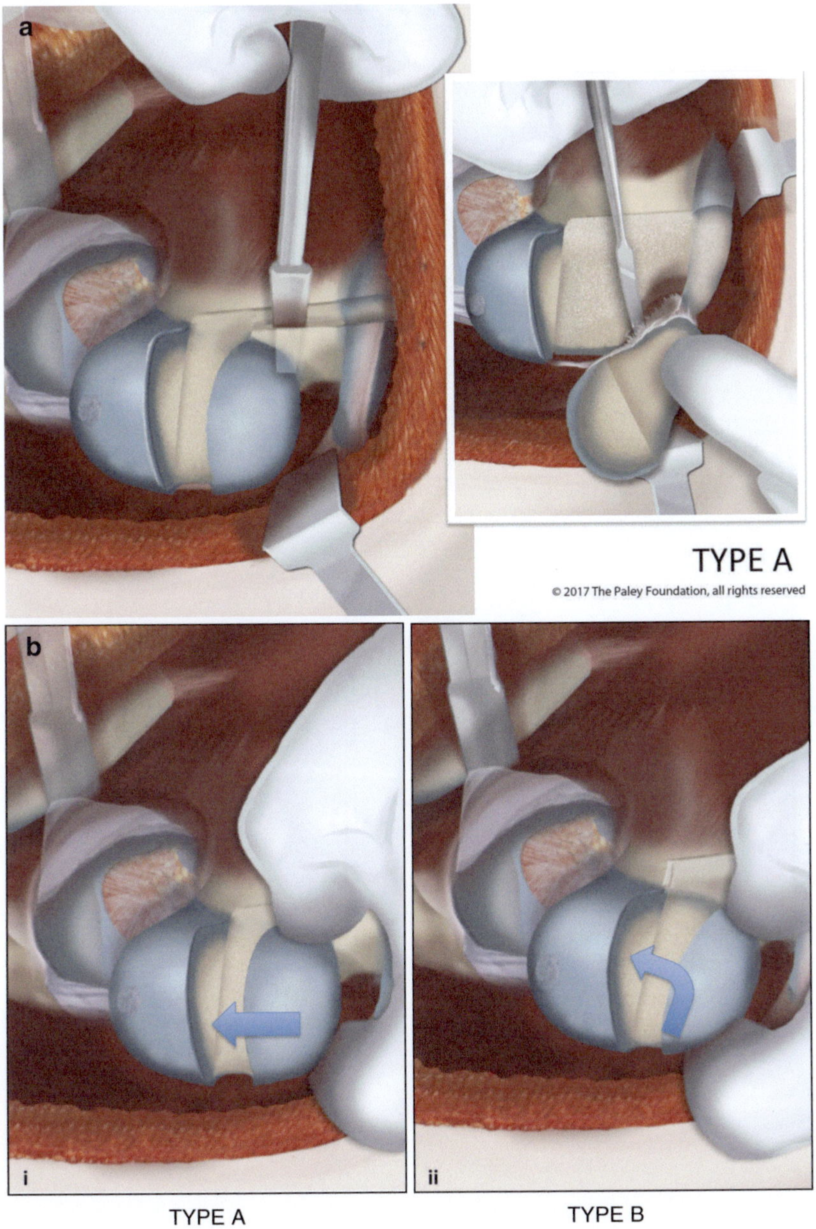

Fig. 38.16 (**a**) The lateral segment is mobilized posteriorly to connect this dissection with the original retinacular flap dissection. (**b**) The untethered lateral fragment can now be moved medially without putting tension on or tearing the retinacular flap. The trochanter moves medially with the segment which maintains the stability of the retinacular flap. This is shown for both Type A (*upper*) and Type B (*lower*) (© 2017 The Paley Foundation, with permission. All rights reserved)

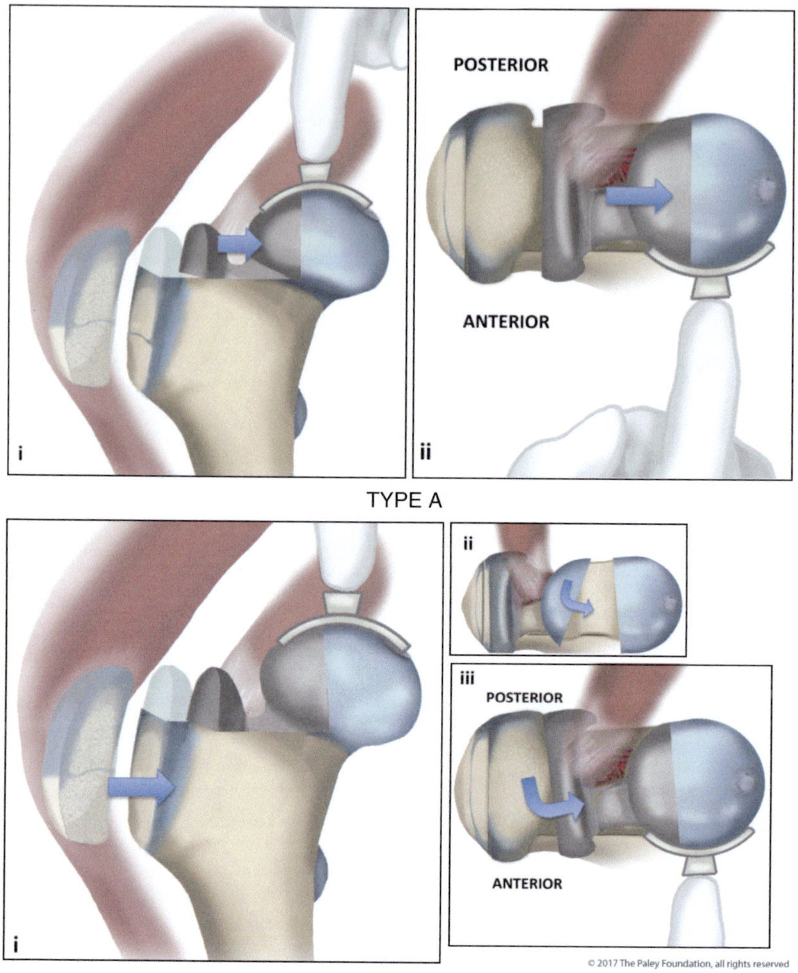

Fig. 38.16 (continued)

Fig. 38.17 (**a**) The lateral mobile femoral head is reduced to the stable medial femoral head. Priority should be given to matching the posterior aspects of the two parts since the anterior part can be shaved off with the osteochondroplasty method. Two wires are inserted in parallel to each other and perpendicular to the osteotomy line. After measuring and drilling, two variable pitch headless screws are inserted into the femoral head from lateral to medial. (**b**) A third headless screw is drilled and inserted perpendicular to the baseline osteotomy. (**c**) A wire is drilled from the fovea down the femoral neck and out the lateral side of the femur. A hole is drilled for a cannulated screw with a cannulated drill. (**d**) A cannulated screw is inserted to prevent fracture of the femoral neck (© 2017 The Paley Foundation, with permission. All rights reserved)

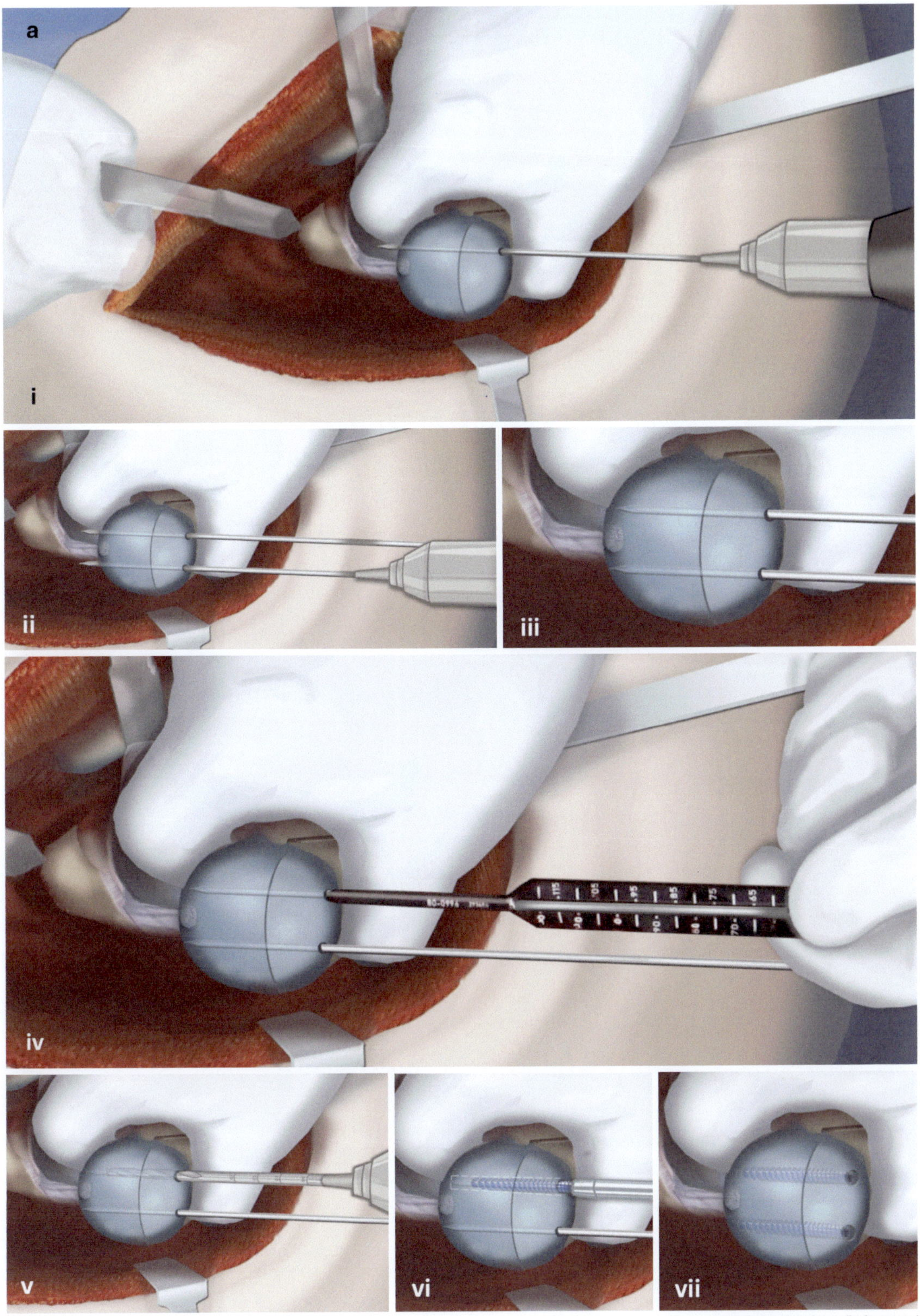
a
i
ii
iii
iv
v
vi
vii

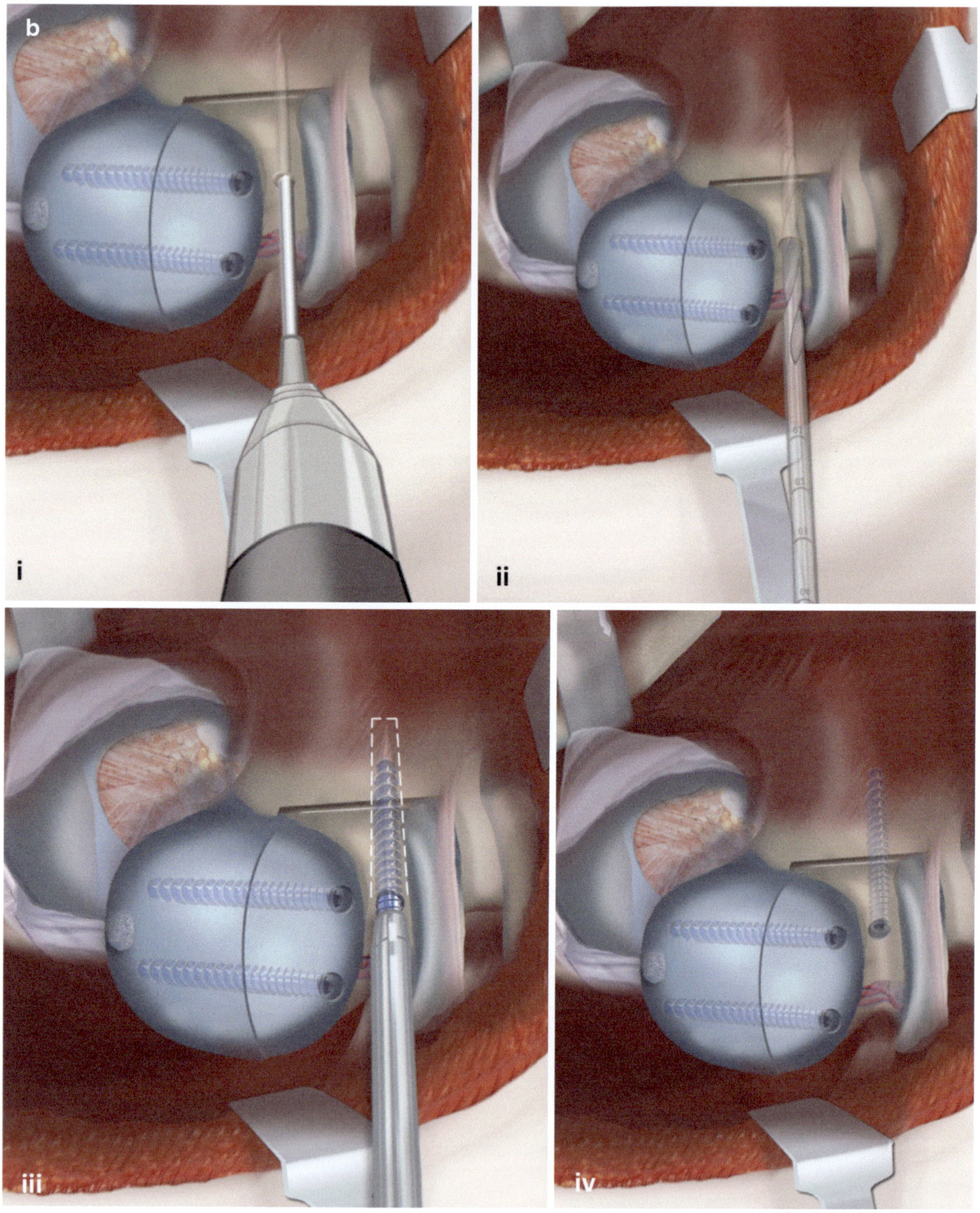

Fig. 38.17 (continued)

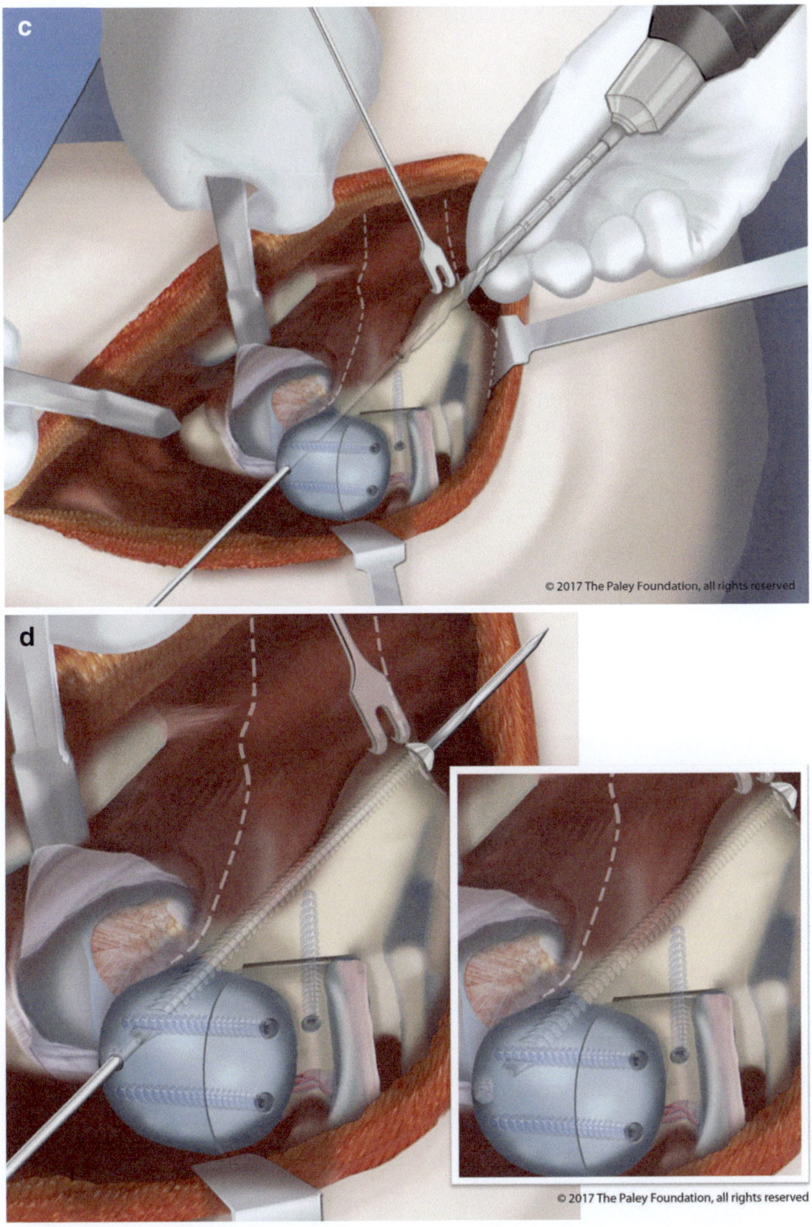

Fig. 38.17 (continued)

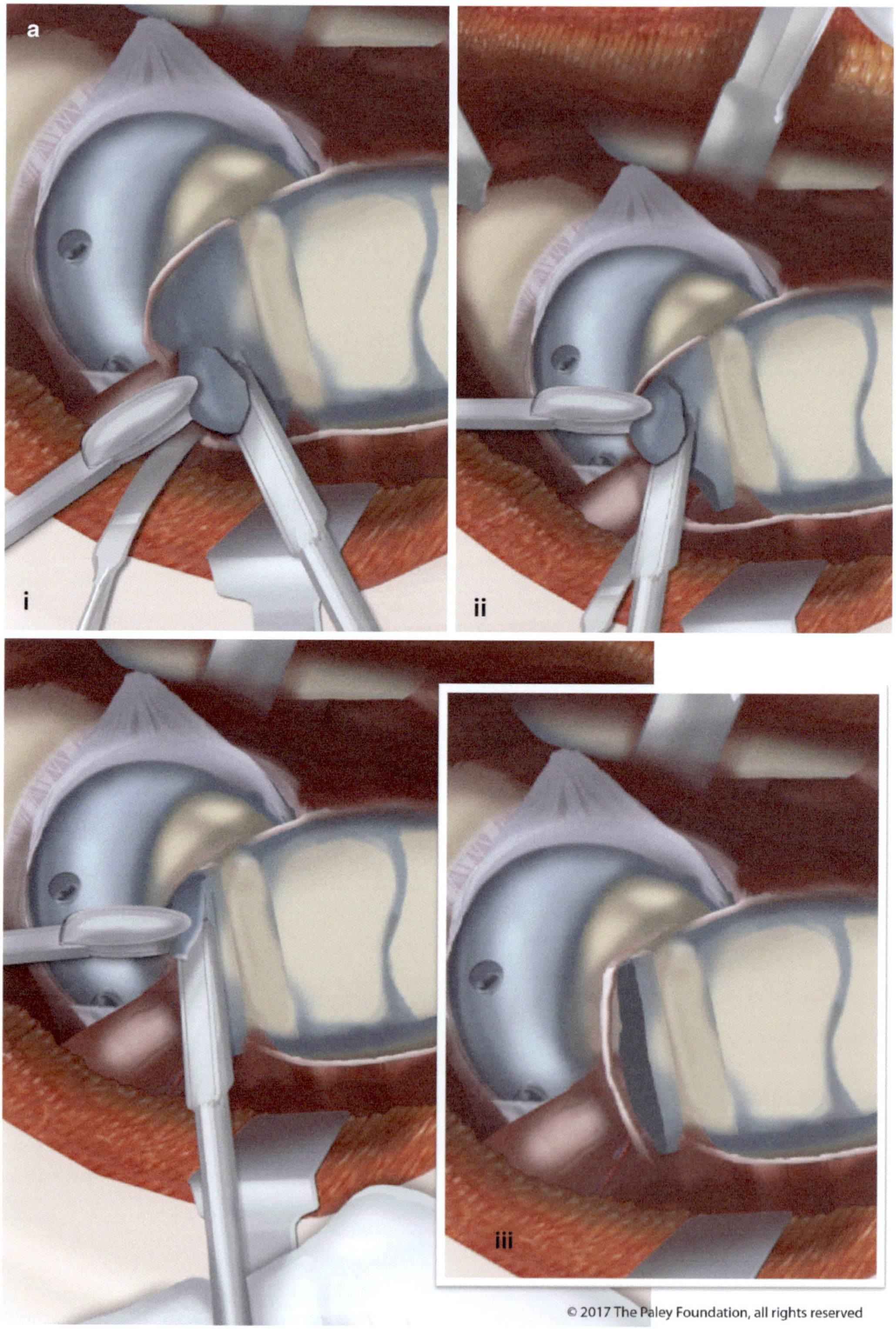

Fig. 38.18 (**a**) The femoral head is reduced into joint. The stable trochanter is excised carefully so as not to injure the retinacular vessels. (**b**) A superior view shows the femoral head mostly covered by the acetabulum after the femoral head reduction osteotomy (© 2017 The Paley Foundation, with permission. All rights reserved)

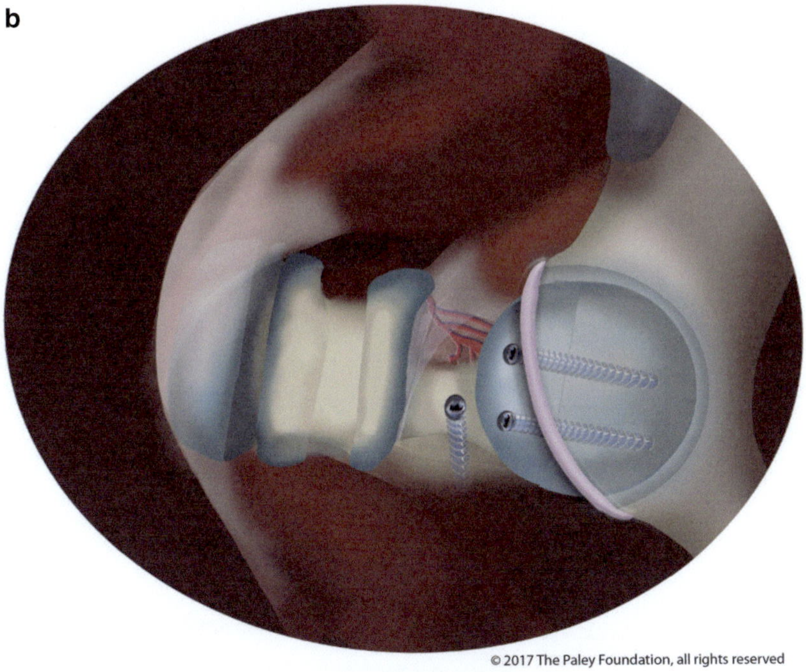

Fig. 38.18 (continued)

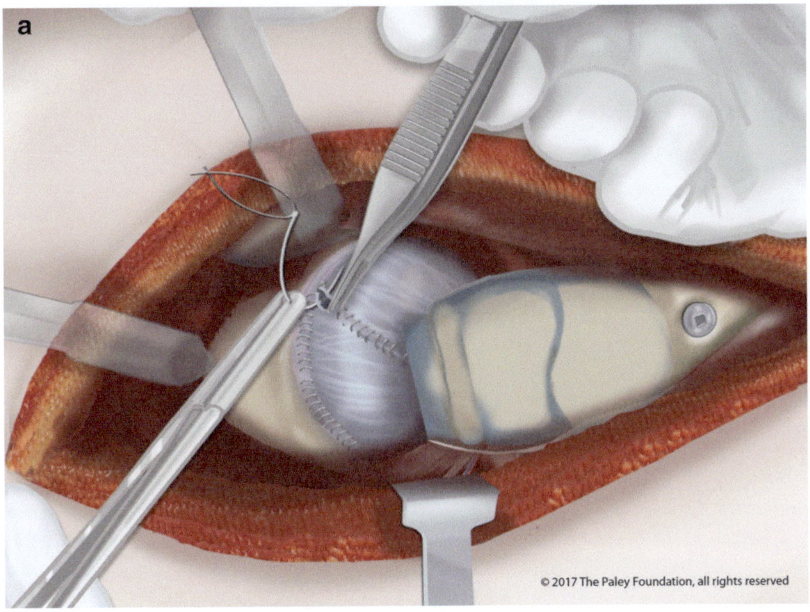

Fig. 38.19 (**a**) The capsule is closed and any redundant capsule is advanced to maintain joint stability. (**b**) The greater trochanter (GT) is advanced laterally and distally and then fixed with two 3.2 mm drill bits. The tip of the GT should be at the level of the center of the femoral head. (**c**) The drill bits are replaced with two 4.5 mm screws with washers which fix and compress the GT in place (© 2017 The Paley Foundation, with permission. All rights reserved)

b

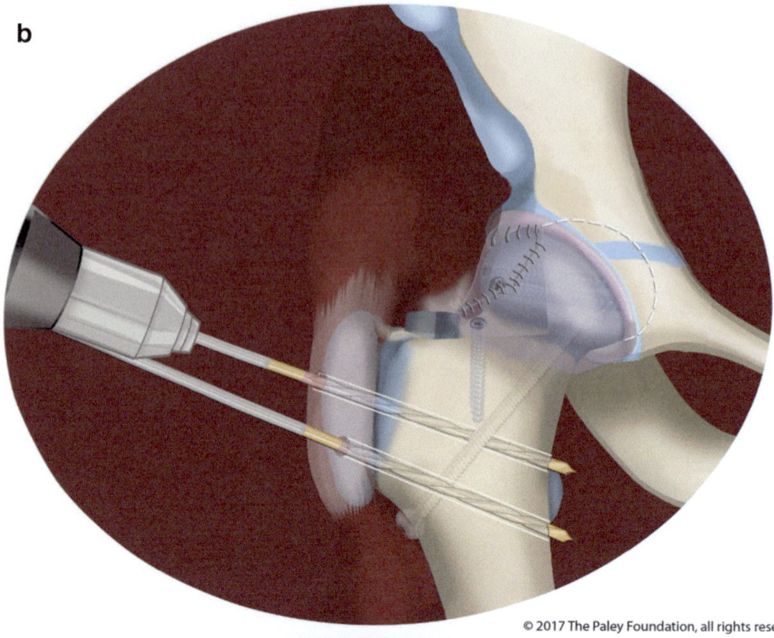

c

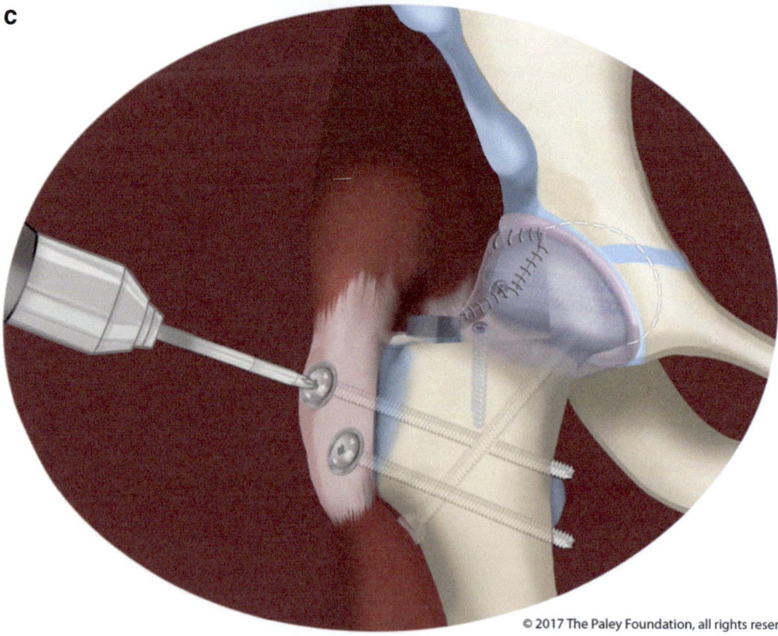

Fig. 38.19 (continued)

Step 28: Resect the Stable Trochanter Reduce the femoral head into joint. In this position resect the stable trochanter with great care not to damage the retinacular flap (Fig. 38.18).

Step 29: Capsular Repair Repair the Z capsulotomy taking up some of the redundancy to prevent subluxation (Fig. 38.19a).

Step 30: Transfer the Mobile Trochanter Fix the mobile trochanter into place more distal and lateral than before. Aim to lower the tip of the GT to the level of the center of the femoral head. Insert two 3.2 mm drill bits and fix the trochanter at the desired level (Fig. 38.19b). Use another same length drill bit, to measure the length of each screw and then replace each drill bit with a 4.5 mm screw with washer (Fig. 38.19c).

Postoperative Care

Place the operative leg on a continuous passive motion (CPM) machine in the recovery room. The patient stays on CPM for 20 h a day for about a week. After that they use CPM half the day on and half the day off and all night long for five more weeks. When ambulating the patient uses a unilateral hip 5° hip abduction brace. Physical therapy is instituted allowing only passive hip abduction and flexion. No external rotation or adduction past the midline is permitted for 6 weeks. The patient is allowed touch down weight bearing for 12 weeks. Active range of motion is permitted between 6 and 12 weeks. Muscle strengthening and full weight bearing without crutches begin after 12 weeks.

Postoperative Considerations

After healing of the FHRO, the hip should be assessed for the need for a periacetabular osteotomy (PAO). The need for a PAO may be obvious or subtle after the FHRO. It is not recommended to do the PAO at the time of the FHRO unless there is gross instability. In most cases the PAO is performed six or more months after the FHRO.

Limb length discrepancy can be treated by contralateral femoral epiphysiodesis in skeletally immature patients. Lengthening using an implantable lengthening rod is another option preferably after skeletal maturity.

Postoperative Imaging

Patient 1 This patient is now 2 years after FHRO (see Fig. 38.3c). Intraoperative measurements confirmed this was a Type A and two parallel cuts were made (see Fig. 38.3f–r). An osteochondroplasty was required of the anterolateral femoral head (see Fig. 38.3q–r). The femoral head was insufficiently covered due to previous acetabular remodeling. A PAO was performed 8 months after the FHRO (see Fig. 38.3c). One year after the FHRO, the patient underwent a 3 cm femoral lengthening with an internal lengthening rod to treat her limb length discrepancy (see Fig. 38.3e). The patient currently has no limp or pain, and has equal and symmetric full hip range of motion compared to the opposite side. Final radiographs confirm good reduction, coverage and joint space maintenance of the hip (see Fig. 38.3e).

Patient 2 This patient is now 10 years after FHRO (see Fig. 38.4c, d). Intraoperative measurements confirmed this was a Type B femoral head requiring non-parallel wedge type resection of the central segment (see Fig. 38.4e–i). Four years after his FHRO he underwent lengthening with an implantable limb lengthening device to equalize his limb lengths. Ten years after the FHRO he has no pain in his right hip. He walks with no limp. He has equal and full range of motion to his opposite hip (see Fig. 38.4j). His hip abduction and external rotation movements increased significantly after surgery. His hip no longer has obligatory external rotation with flexion. He participates in sports. His hip remains round and well contained clinically and radiographically (Fig. 38.4k, l). He has equal leg lengths and excellent lower limb alignment (see Fig. 38.4m).

Pearls and Pitfalls

- Prognosis improves with better preserved femoral and acetabular cartilage. Degenerative changes in the non-resected areas theoretically worsen the prognosis.
- The younger the patient (age 10–16 years) often the better the outcome.
- Preoperative planning of the size of the wedge or rectangle to be taken is essential in aiding operative execution.
- The retinacular flap is a key component to the operation and should be performed in stages as described in the operative discussion.
- The femoral neck screw protect against fracture of the femoral neck.
- The capsule at the end of the reduction is capacious and should be advanced to prevent lateral subluxation.
- Be certain the trochanter is well fixed. In older/larger patients three screws are preferred.
- The presence of an open physis is not a contraindication due to risk of avascular necrosis as once thought. It is important to close the physis to avoid a bifid femoral head from developing.
- The Ganz type of FHRO should be used when the femoral head elongation is perpendicular to the femoral head. When it is used for cases where the femoral head is elongated not parallel to the femoral neck, it runs a greater risk of narrowing and fracturing the neck [1–4, 6] due to the inclined orientation of the cut. The Paley type of FHRO presented here is a more horizontal cut and more appropriate geometrically for the majority of cases where the femoral head is elongated not parallel to the femoral neck. This should reduce the risk of fracture and injury to blood supply in these cases.

Indications and Contraindications (Table 38.1)

Table 38.1 Femoral head reduction osteotomy: surgical indications and contraindications

Parameter	Good indication	Relative contraindication
Femoral head shape	Elliptical, saddle, medial head round in sagittal plane	Medial part not round in sagittal plane
Coxa magna	Lateral or anterior	Posterior and medial enlargement
Acetabulum	Round ± dysplastic	Incongruous, cystic, degenerative
Pain	Impingement	Arthritic outside of central region
Range of motion	Good flexion-extension	Poor flexion-extension
Physis	Closed	Open

Acknowledgements The authors wish to thank Pamela Boullier Ross, who created all of the illustrations used in this chapter. The authors would also like to thank the Paley Foundation for funding the cost of the illustrations and for giving permission for their use in this chapter.

References

1. Leunig M, Ganz R. Relative neck lengthening and intracapital osteotomy for severe Perthes and Perthes-like deformities. Bull NYU Hosp Jt Dis. 2011;69(Suppl 1):S62–7.
2. Paley D. Intra-articular osteotomies of the hip, knee, and ankle. Oper Tech Orthop. 2011;21:184–96.
3. Paley D. The treatment of femoral head deformity and coxa magna by the Ganz femoral head reduction osteotomy. Orthop Clin North Am. 2011;42(3):389–99. viii.
4. Ganz R, Huff TW, Leunig M. Extended retinacular soft tissue flap for intra-articular hip surgery: surgical technique, indications and results of application. Instr Course Lect. 2009;58:241–55.
5. Burian M, Dungl P, Chomiak J, Ostadal M, Kubes R, Schwarz O. Operative treatment for saddle-shaped femoral heads. Acta Chir Orthop Traumatol Cechoslov. 2016;83(4):247–53. [in Czech].
6. Siebenrock KA, Anwander H, Zurmuhle CA, Tannast M, Slongo T, Steppacher SD. Head reduction osteotomy with additional containment surgery improves sphericity and containment and reduces pain in Legg-Calves-Perthes disease. Clin Orthop Relat Res. 2015;473(4):1274–83.

39 Articulated Hip Joint Distraction

Dan S. Epstein and Reggie C. Hamdy

Introduction

Articulated hip distraction, or arthrodiastasis, is not a new concept. It was first described in Verona in 1979 [1] and since then has been used in the management of sequelae of Perthes disease, epiphysiolysis, developmental dysplasia of the hip, fracture of the femoral neck, osteoarthrosis and chondrolysis, multiple epiphyseal dysplasia, sickle cell disease, and lupus erythematosus [1–3].

It is considered a salvage procedure in adolescents with a severely deformed or collapsed femoral head, as a consequence of the conditions mentioned above, and is an alternative to hip fusion or hip arthroplasty when reconstruction with osteotomies is likely to fail.

General goals of treatment are to improve pain, to increase the range of motion (ROM), to allow the patient to return to normal activity, and—equally important—to postpone conversion to a definitive surgical procedure such as total hip replacement or hip arthrodesis [4, 5].

The beneficial effects of articulated hip distraction are due to a combination of two factors: distraction and ROM. The distraction offloads the hip joint, eliminates the joint reaction forces, prevents friction between the destroyed articular cartilage of the collapsed femoral head and the articular cartilage of the acetabulum, stretches the ligaments and muscles, and allows all weight bearing to occur through the external fixator.

Joint distraction has shown to decrease proinflammatory mediators in canine models and is suggested to promote cartilaginous repair [6, 7].

ROM in flexion and extension is made possible through the hinge in the monolateral fixator that is centered on the center of rotation of the femoral head. It has been shown that passive ROM allows for a decrease of inflammation, and also allows for reossification to occur [8–10]. Several preclinical and clinical studies have demonstrated the beneficial effect of passive ROM on the articular cartilage and synovial membrane in several other joints, including the knee, elbow, and ankle [11, 12]. We believe the active ROM does not have deleterious effects since the joint is offloaded.

D. S. Epstein
McGill University, Montreal, QC, Canada

Shriners Hospital for Children – Canada, Montreal, QC, Canada

R. C. Hamdy (✉)
McGill University, Montreal, QC, Canada

Shriners Hospital for Children – Canada, Montreal, QC, Canada

Division of Orthopaedic Surgery, McGill University Health Centre, Montreal, QC, Canada

The Montreal Children's Hospital, Montreal, QC, Canada
e-mail: rhamdy@shriners.mcgill.ca

R. C. Hamdy, N. Saran (eds.), *Pediatric Pelvic and Proximal Femoral Osteotomies*,
https://doi.org/10.1007/978-3-319-78033-7_39

Brief Clinical History

A 10-year-old male patient, otherwise healthy, presented with increasing left hip pain for the preceding 6 months. He had an unremarkable medical history. Examination revealed an antalgic gait and severely restricted hip ROM with 90° of flexion, no abduction or adduction, and internal and external hip rotation of 10° each. The physical examination for the right hip, knees, and ankles was normal. Radiographs revealed severe Perthes disease of the left femoral head with complete collapse and destruction of the lateral pillar (Herring type C) (Figs. 39.1 and 39.2). He was immediately started on physiotherapy in an attempt to regain as much ROM as possible. The problems and various options were discussed with the patient and his family, and it was decided to proceed with articulated hip distraction.

Following adductor release of adductor longus and gracilis, a monolateral hinged external fixator was applied to the left hip. An acute distraction of 1.0 cm was performed intra-operatively followed by gradual distraction until the Shenton line was restored. The patient had intensive physiotherapy and was allowed partial weight bearing. The hip joint was kept in extension during the night by locking the hinge. The fixator was removed after 4 months, and full weight bearing and night bracing was continued for 3 months postremoval of the fixator. Approximately 6 months after removal of the external fixator the patient had flexion of 130°, abduction of 30°, internal rotation of 30°, and external fixation of 20°. At 2 year follow-up, despite some loss in abduction of 10° and a mild Trendelenburg gait, he remained pain-free and fully active.

Preoperative Imaging

Anteroposterior (AP) and abduction internal rotation view (AIR) (see Fig. 39.1).

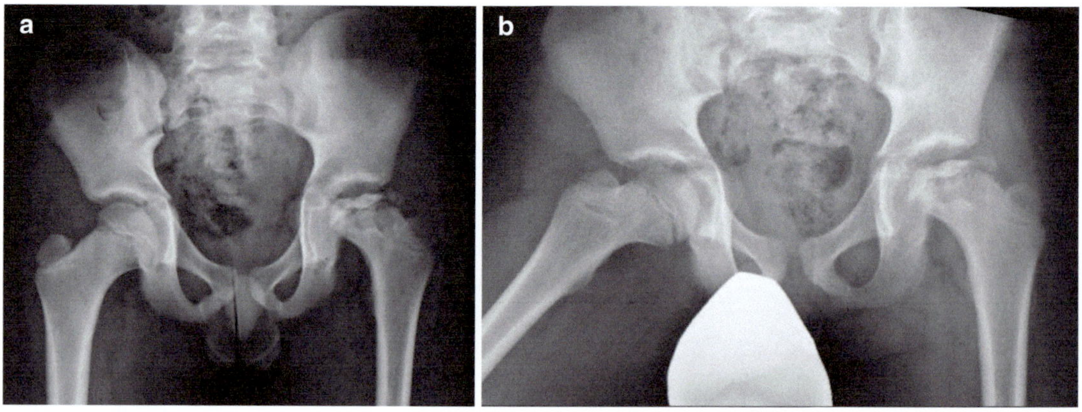

Fig. 39.1 (**a**) Anteroposterior pelvis X-ray showing Perthes disease of the left femoral head with loss of the lateral pillar and hip subluxation. (**b**) Abduction internal rotation view. Note the lack of abduction on the left hip

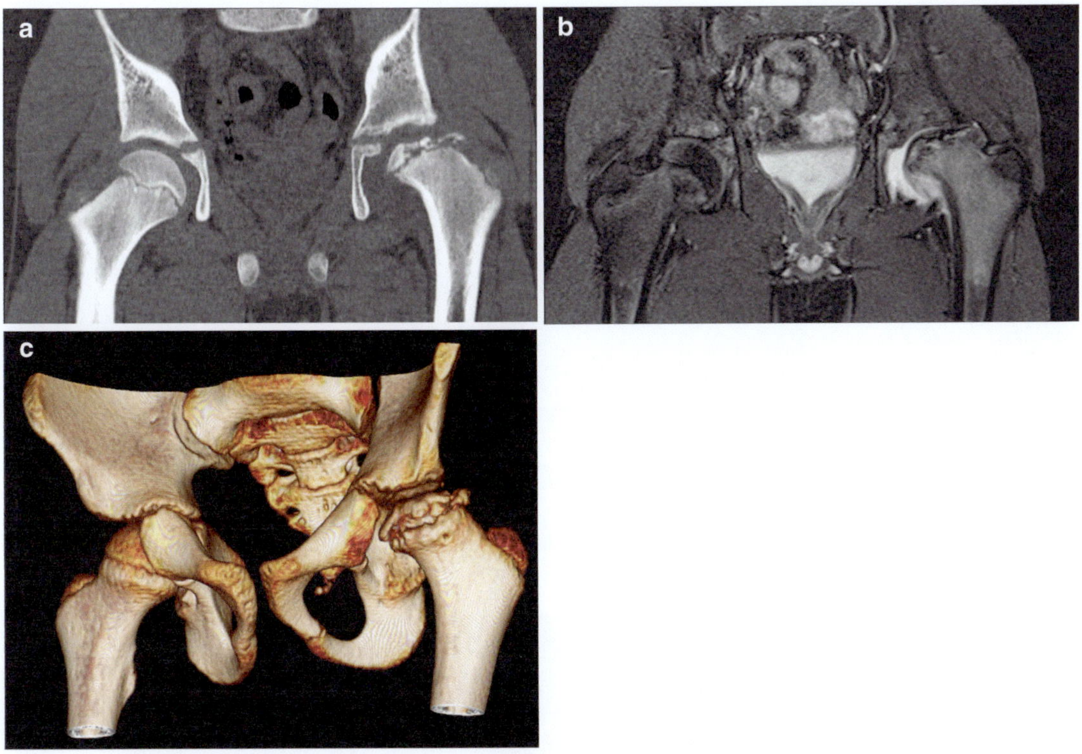

Fig. 39.2 (**a**) On a coronal view of a computed tomography scan, the left femoral head is deformed with collapse of the lateral pillar and extrusion of the femoral head. (**b**) On a coronal view of a magnetic resonance image, the left femoral head is flattened, irregular, partially sclerotic. There is bone marrow edema and hip effusion. (**c**) A three-dimensional reconstruction image of the left hip demonstrates the deformity and extrusion of the femoral head

Goals of Treatment

1. To prevent further deformity to the femoral head by offloading the hip joint
2. To regain ROM of the hip joint
3. To relieve pain
4. To keep the femoral head contained—as much as possible—and to prevent hinged abduction
5. To delay the possible need for a more definitive procedures such as hip fusion or joint arthroplasty

Treatment Strategy

The problems to be addressed in this particular case were increasing hip pain; stiffness; loss of function; and a progressively deformed, collapsed, and extruded femoral head with subluxation of the hip joint. At that stage, only a few options are available, and all of them are salvage procedures [11]. Hip fusion is an excellent procedure, especially for isolated unilateral disease of the hip joint in an otherwise healthy adolescent, but is not without side effects. Joint arthroplasty at that very young age should be avoided and delayed as much as possible. An alternative to hip fusion and joint arthroplasty is articulated hip distraction that has been previously shown—in many severely affected cases—to relieve pain, increase ROM, and, most importantly, to return the patient to almost normal function. It is still considered a salvage procedure; however, we believe it is the best available alternative that may delay definitive treatment with either hip fusion or joint arthroplasty.

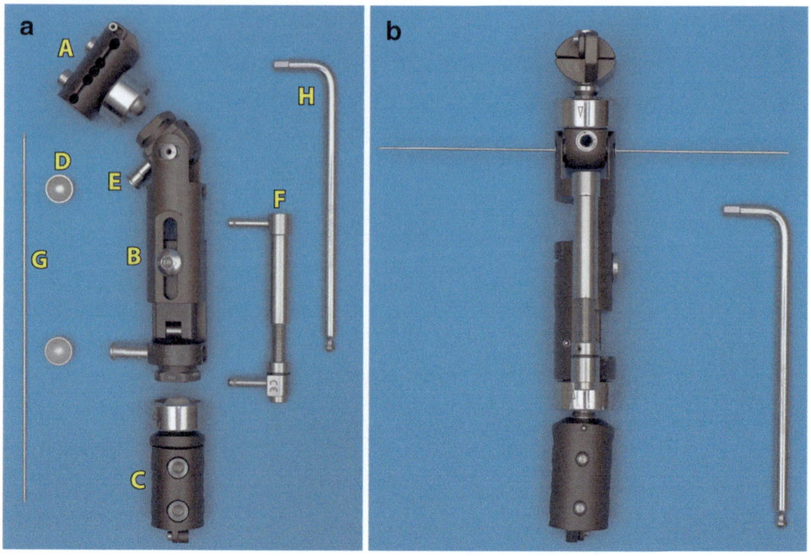

Fig. 39.3 Pre-assembled and assembled articulated monolateral hinged external fixation. Template (**a**): *A* Procallus T-clamp. *B* Procallus fixator (90.000 series) central body. *C* Straight clamp. *D* Bush. *E* Cam. *F* Compression distraction unit. *G* 2 mm Kirschner wire (KW). *H* 6 mm Allen wrench. Template (**b**): The external fixator assembled and with the KW inside the hinge connecting the T-clamp to the central body

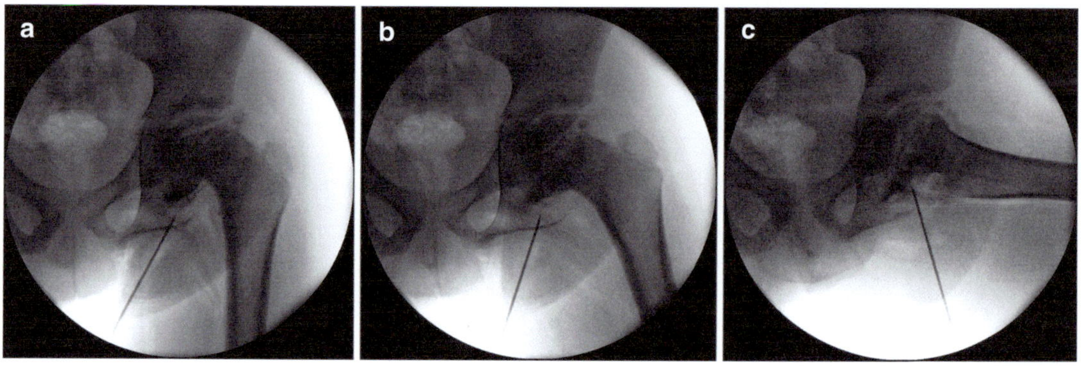

Fig. 39.4 Intra-operative arthrography of the left hip joint after adductor release. (**a**) Anterior-posterior (AP) view. (**b**) Abduction. (**c**) Frog view

Surgical Details

- Under general anesthesia and antibiotic prophylaxis, the patient is positioned supine on a radiolucent table top with the entire affected hemipelvis draped free to allow abduction of the hip joint during surgery.
- Preoperative fixator assembly. In our case, we used a ProCallus Fixator (Orthofix, Lewisville TX, USA) (Fig. 39.3), which was composed of a T-clamp, a central body, and a straight clamp.
- A hip arthrogram (Fig. 39.4) through a subadductor approach is performed to assess the femoral head's shape and hinge abduction.
- An adductor longus and gracilis tenotomy is performed through a medial approach.
- Under fluoroscopy, a 2 mm Kirschner (K) wire is inserted just distal to the estimated center of the femoral head while keeping an abduction of about 15–20° (Fig. 39.5). The K-wire should be inserted parallel to the coronal plane and perpendicular to the femoral shaft.
- The articulated body is mounted over the K-wire (Fig. 39.6).
- Three guide wires are inserted into the supra-acetabular region at the widest part of the bone which on an oblique view resembles a triangle. AP and 45° external oblique ("triangular view") fluoroscopy views verify that there is no penetration of the hip joint. The K-wires are inserted through the T-clamp which is used as a guiding device. Each K-wire is inserted in

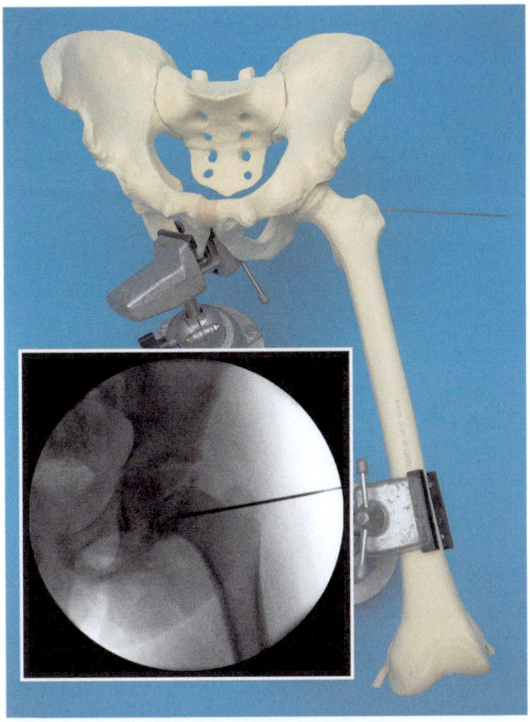

Fig. 39.5 *Insert*. Under fluoroscopy, a 2 mm Kirschner (K) wire is inserted into the center of rotation of the femoral head, which because of the collapse of the femoral head is situated slightly distal to the center of the femoral head (about 0.5 cm). *Large image*. On a bone model the K wire is inserted in the same way while keeping hip joint abduction of about 15–20°

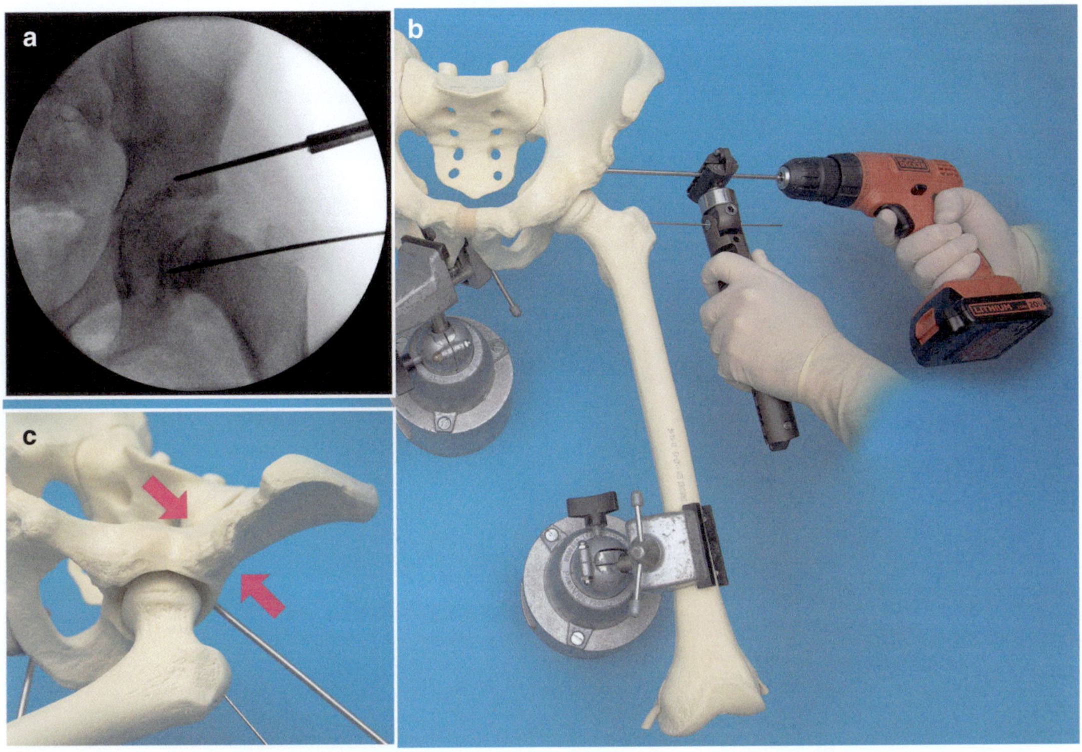

Fig. 39.6 Insertion of half pins to the supra-acetabular region. (**a**) Under fluoroscopy, we begin with inserting 2 mm K-wires through the T clamp. A tissue protector is inserted, and then drilling and insertion of the half pins. (**b**) The monolateral external fixator hinge is mounted on the 2 mm Kirschner wire. The pelvic wires and pins are inserted using the T-clamp as a guiding device. (**c**) Insertion of the half pin is done at the widest part of the supra-acetabular region just above the acetabulum

the coronal plane. The angle of penetration to the ilium can be variable.

- Bending of the K-wires should be avoided.
- A small skin incision is made with a scalpel at the entry points of the guide wires; blunt dissection is performed to make a track in the soft tissue.
- A trochar and a 4.8 mm drill bit are inserted, and drilling of the ilium bone is performed.
- A 6 mm pelvic half pin (hydroxyapatite-coated) is inserted with a T-wrench (Fig. 39.7). Three half pins are needed to secure the proximal clamp.
- The half pins are inserted at the widest part of the supra-acetabular bone. The device is mounted on the K-wire (in the center of the femoral head), and cannot be moved proximally or distally. Further adjustments of the angle of half pin insertion, if needed, can be done via the ball and socket joint of the device (Fig. 39.8).
- Three 5–6 mm femoral half pin are inserted distally (Fig. 39.9) perpendicular to the femoral shaft.
- After tightening the proximal and distal clamps to the half pins, the movement of the hip joint should be coupled with the movement of the hinged external fixator (Fig. 39.10) and should offer no resistance.
- Acute distraction of about 1.0–2.0 cm is applied. If more distraction is needed to restore the Shenton line, this is performed gradually in the postoperative period (Fig. 39.11).
- The ball and socket joint is cemented.

Postoperative Care and Imaging

- Follow up with an AP pelvis every 4 weeks.
- Continue distraction at 0.5 mm a day until the Shenton line is restored.
- Maintain intensive supervised physiotherapy for exercising flexion and extension of the hip joint.
- Partial weight bearing is allowed.
- The frame is locked in extension during the night using a distraction unit.
- The frame is kept for about 4–5 months until ossification of the lateral pillar is seen on AP X-ray (Fig. 39.12).
- After removal of the external fixation, the patient continues with exercises for the hip joint with weight bearing as tolerated.
- Follow-up meetings with AP X-rays every 3–6 months until healing (Figs. 39.13, 39.14).

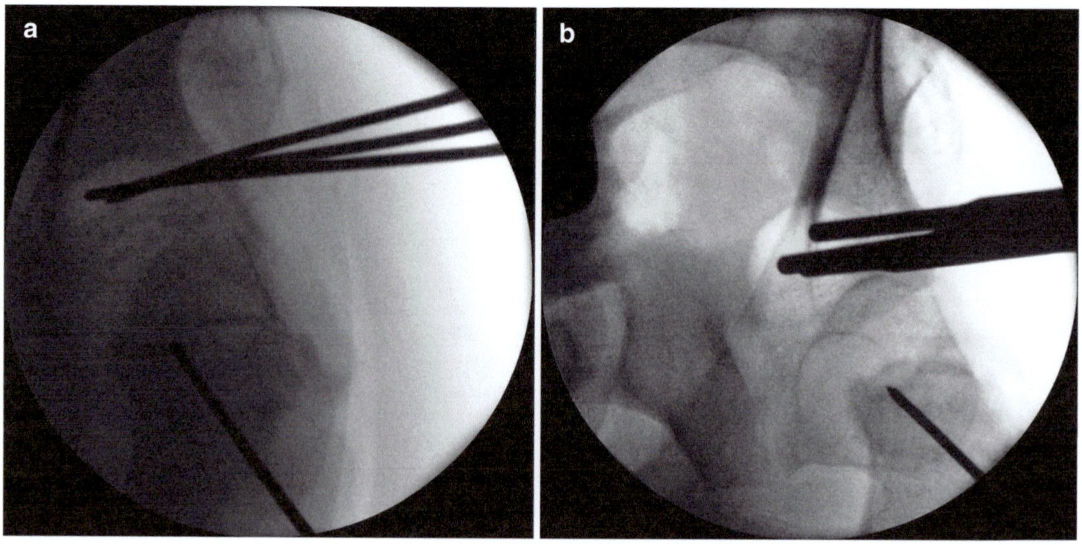

Fig. 39.7 Fluoroscopy images of the wires (**a**) and pins (**b**) in the supra-acetabular region. Forty five degree external oblique ("triangular views") of the supra-acetabular region are taken by angulating the intra-operative fluoroscopy machine

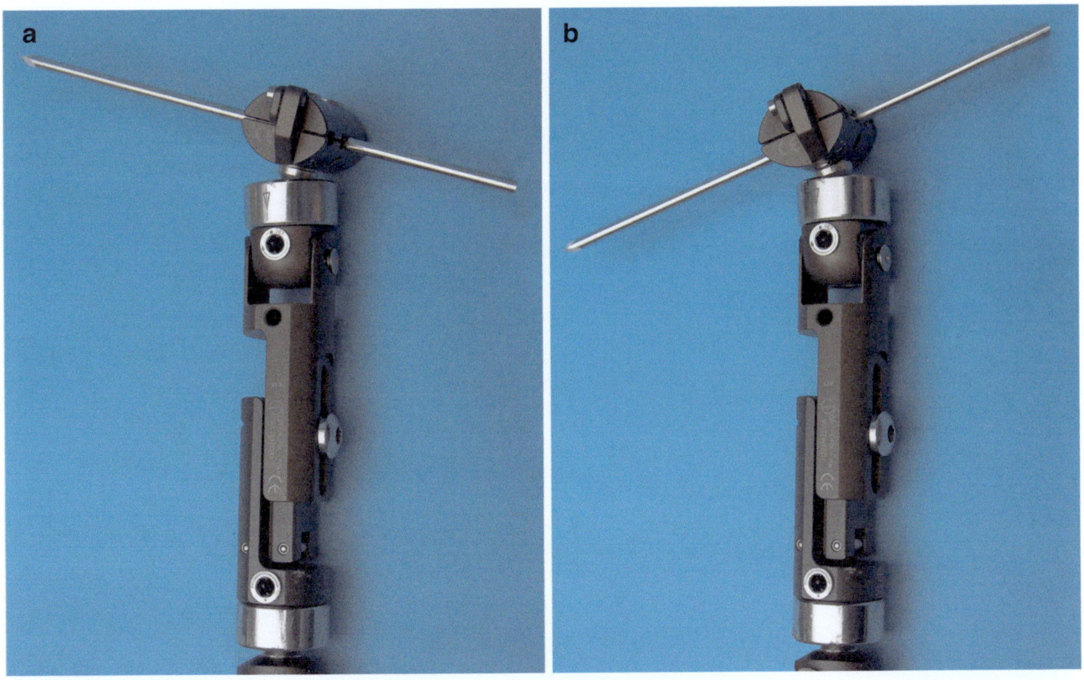

Fig. 39.8 Controlling the angle of insertion, of the K-wires, and then later with half pins to the pelvis is achieved by adjusting the ball and socket joint of the T-clamp in different directions as shown in (**a**, **b**)

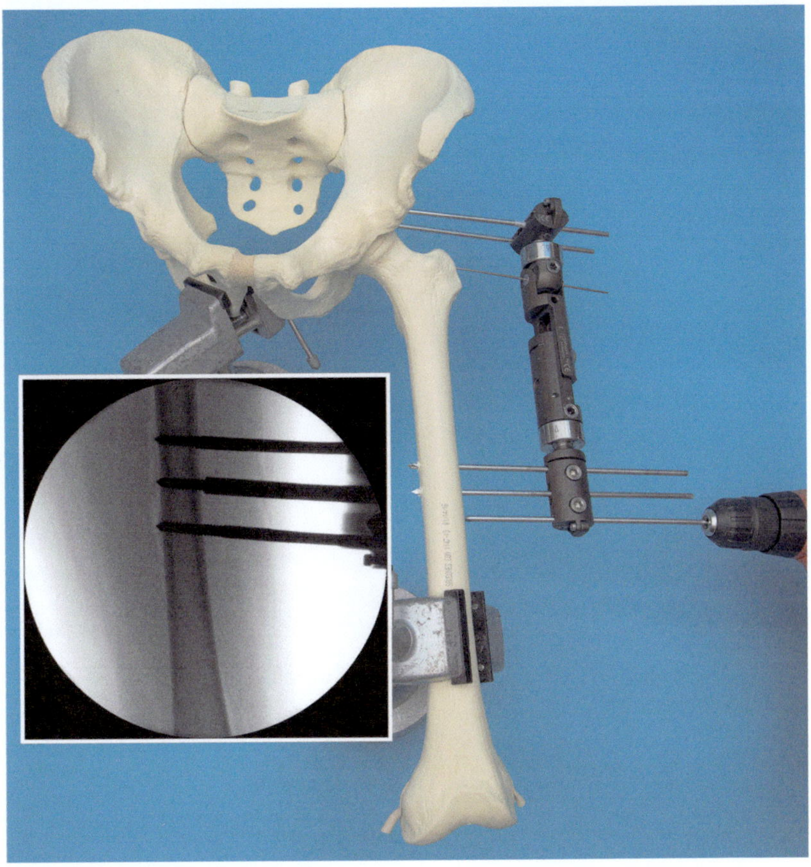

Fig. 39.9 Insertion of the three half pins. *Large image*. Through the straight clamp three half pins are inserted. *Insert*. Under fluoroscopy

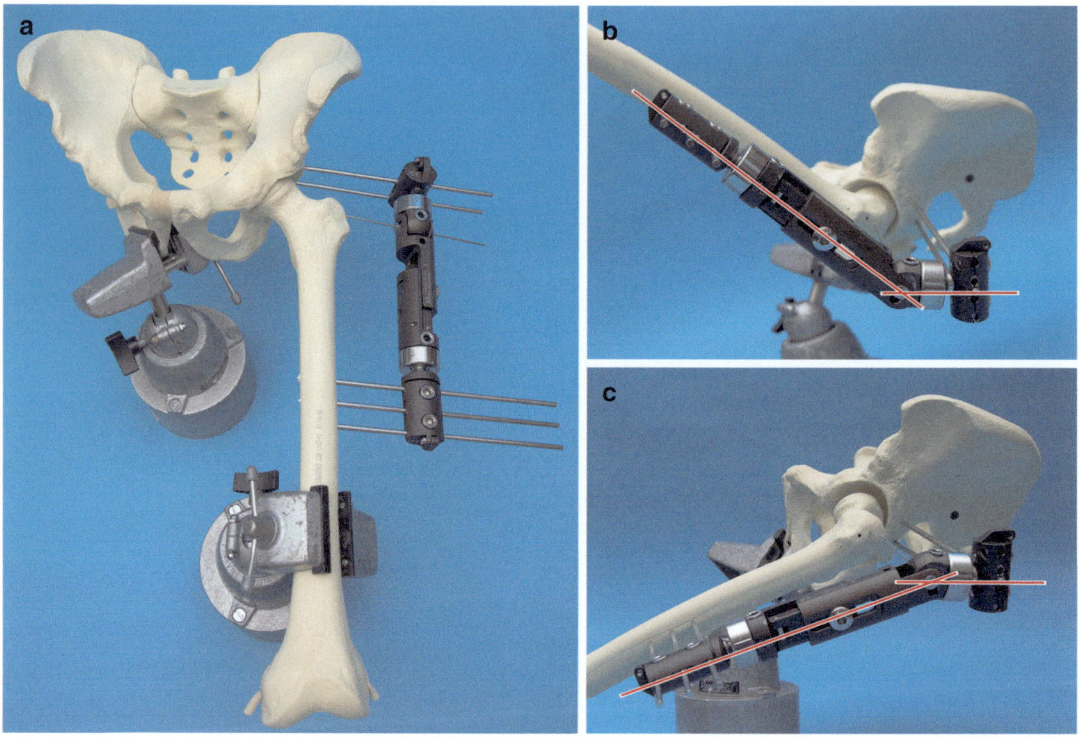

Fig. 39.10 Final view of the fixation of the pelvis and femur with the monolateral hinged external fixator. (**a**) View in the coronal plane. (**b**) Lateral view of the hip joint in flexion. (**c**) Hip joint in extension

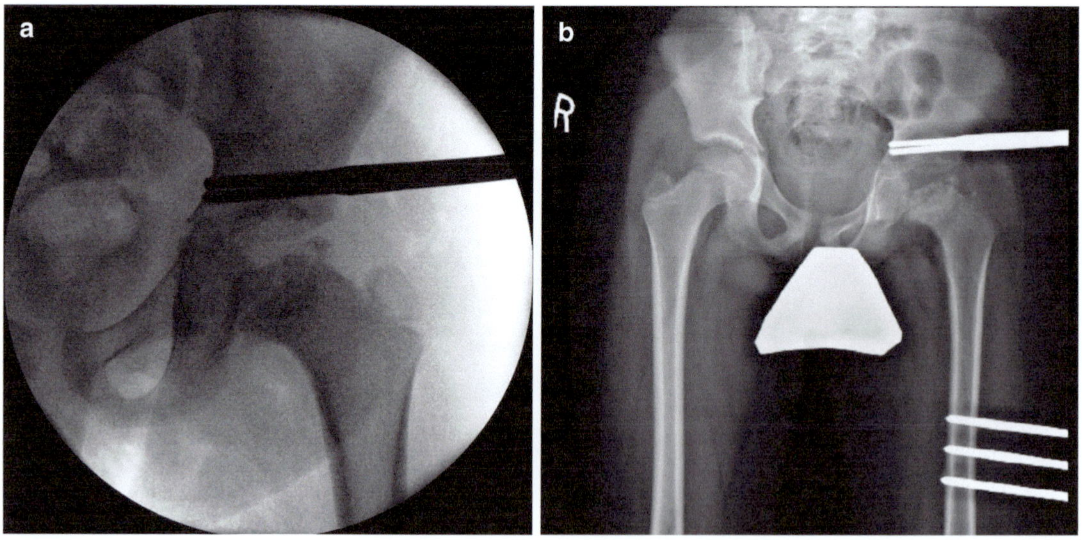

Fig. 39.11 (**a**) Intra-operative acute distraction of the hip joint under fluoroscopy. (**b**) Anteroposterior pelvis X-ray with restoration of the Shenton line

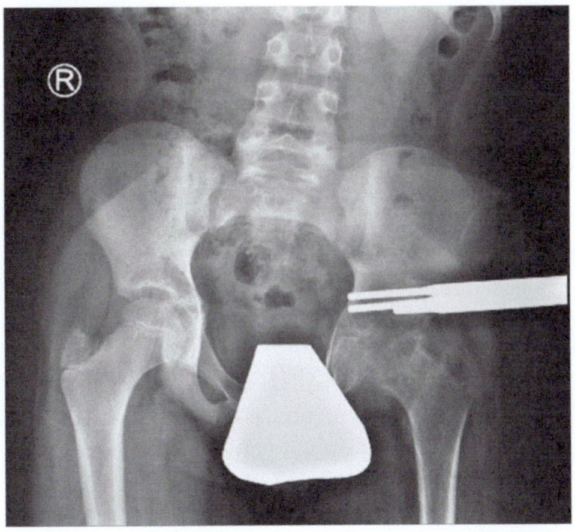

Fig. 39.12 Anteroposterior view demonstrating reossification of the lateral pillar

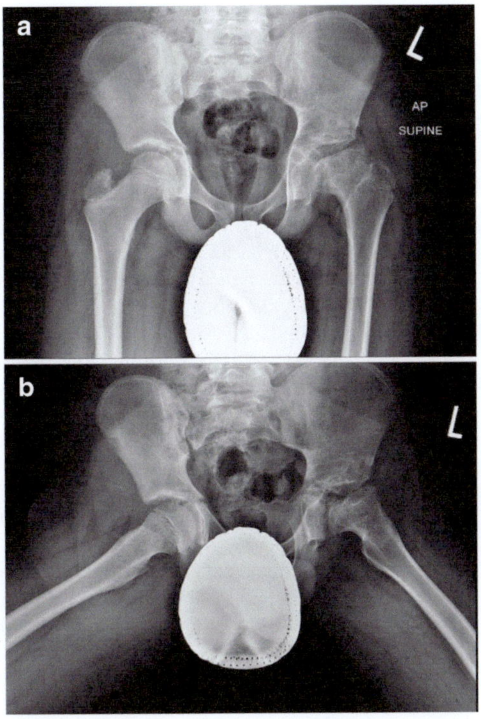

Fig. 39.13 Eighteen months post op. (**a**) Anteroposterior and (**b**) frog views

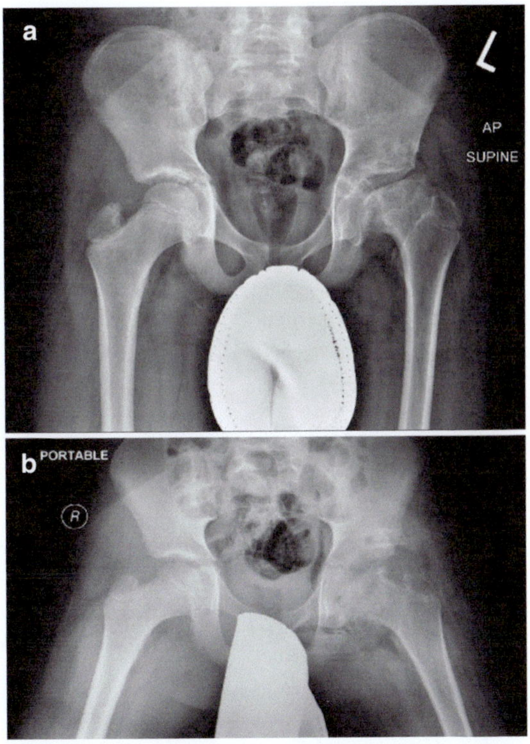

Fig. 39.14 At two-year follow-up. The left femoral head is deformed with coxa irregularis, coxa magna, coxa breva. (**a**) Anteroposterior view. (**b**) Abduction internal rotation view

Pearls and Pitfalls

1. Assembling the external fixator before surgery and deciding what is the correct size to use for the patient may save operative time.
2. Placement of the hinge is crucial; otherwise flexion and extension postoperatively will not be possible. The K-wire has to be inserted just below (0.5 cm) the center of the femoral head and the position checked in both the coronal and sagittal planes. The K-wire should be perpendicular to the femoral shaft while keeping the femur abducted.

3. Whenever distraction of the hip is performed, either acutely during the surgical procedure or gradually postoperatively, an anterior block has to be used in order to prevent the hip from going into flexion during the distraction. This is done by locking the device with a distraction unit.
4. Proper insertion of the guide wires and half pins in the supra-acetabular region is critical in order to prevent undue penetration of the half pins in the pelvis. Forty five degree external oblique, triangular views of the supra-acetabular regions must be obtained intra-operatively, and the K-wire technique must be used while inserting the guide wire.
5. In order to prevent dislodgment of the ball and socket joints, cement is used to keep these segments "locked."
6. Compliance with the physiotherapy program is extremely important.

Indications and Contraindications (Table 39.1)

Table 39.1 Articulated hip joint distraction: Surgical indications and contraindications

Indications
As an alternative for hip fusion and joint arthroplasty in adolescents and young patients with pain stiffness and severely deformed femoral head
Contraindications
Noncompliant patient/caregivers
Bone pathology precluding pin fixation
Active infection
Relative contraindication
Obesity

References

1. Aldegheri R. Artrodiatasi d'anca. Orthopedia e Traumatoligia Oggi. 1981;1:103.
2. Cañadell J, Gonzales F, Barrios RH, Amillo S. Arthrodiastasis for stiff hips in young patients. Int Orthop. 1993;17(4):254–8.
3. Thacker MM, Feldman DS, Madan SS, Straight JJ, Scher DM. Hinged distraction of the adolescent arthritic hip. J Pediatr Orthop. 2005;25(2):178–82.
4. Gomez JA, Matsumoto H, Roye DP Jr, Vitale MG, Hyman JE, van Bosse HJ, et al. Articulated hip distraction: a treatment option for femoral head avascular necrosis in adolescence. J Pediatr Orthop. 2009;29(2):163–9.
5. Segev E, Ezra E, Wientroub S, Yaniv M. Treatment of severe late onset Perthes' disease with soft tissue release and articulated hip distraction: early results. J Pediatr Orthop. 2004;13(3):158–65.
6. van Valvurg AA, van Roy JLAM, Lafever FPJG, Bijlsma JWJ. Beneficial effect of intermittent fluid pressure, of a low but physiological magnitude, on cartilage and inflammation in osteoarthritis. J Rheumatol. 1998;25:515–21.
7. van Valburg AA, van Roermund PM, Marijnissen AC, Wenting MJ, Verbout AJ, Lafeber FP, Bijlsma JW. Joint distraction in treatment of osteoarthritis (II): effects on cartilage in a canine model. Osteoarthr Cartil. 2000;8(1):1–8.
8. Salter RB. The biologic concept of continuous passive motion of synovial joints. The first 18 years of basic research and its clinical application. Clin Orthop Relat Res. 1989;242:12–25.
9. Salter RB, Simmonds DF, Malcolm BW, Rumble EJ, MacMichael D, Clements ND. The biological effect of continuous passive motion on the healing of full-thickness defects in articular cartilage. An experimental investigation in the rabbit. J Bone Joint Surg Am. 1980;62(8):1232–51.
10. Salter RB. Continuous passive motion: from origination to research to clinical applications. J Rheumatol. 2004;31(11):2104–5.
11. Judet R, Judet T. The use of a hinge distraction apparatus after arthrolysis and arthroplasty. (author's transl). Rev Chir Orthop Reparatrice Apparat Mot. 1978;64(5):353–65.
12. Morrey BF. Distraction arthroplasty. Clinical applications. Clin Orthop Relat Res. 1993;293:46–54.

Index

R. C. Hamdy, N. Saran (eds.), *Pediatric Pelvic and Proximal Femoral Osteotomies*,
https://doi.org/10.1007/978-3-319-78033-7

G

H

MIX
Papier aus verantwortungsvollen Quellen
Paper from responsible sources
FSC® C105338

If you have any concerns about our products,
you can contact us on
ProductSafety@springernature.com

In case Publisher is established outside the EU,
the EU authorized representative is:
Springer Nature Customer Service Center GmbH
Europaplatz 3, 69115 Heidelberg, Germany

Printed by Libri Plureos GmbH
in Hamburg, Germany